# Gerontology and Geriatrics

# Gerontology and Geriatrics

Editor: Oliver Fincher

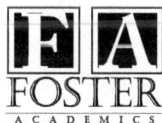

**FA**
**FOSTER**
A C A D E M I C S

www.fosteracademics.com

www.fosteracademics.com

**FA**
FOSTER
ACADEMICS

Cataloging-in-Publication Data

Gerontology and geriatrics / edited by Oliver Fincher.
        p. cm.
Includes bibliographical references and index.
ISBN 978-1-63242-595-9
1. Gerontology. 2. Aging. 3. Geriatrics. 4. Older people--Diseases.
5. Older people--Health and hygiene. I. Fincher, Oliver.
RC952 .G47 2019
618.97--dc23

Foster Academics,
118-35 Queens Blvd., Suite 400,
Forest Hills, NY 11375, USA

ISBN 978-1-63242-595-9 (Hardback)

# Contents

# Preface

This book has been a concerted effort by a group of academicians, researchers and scientists, who have contributed their research works for the realization of the book. This book has materialized in the wake of emerging advancements and innovations in this field. Therefore, the need of the hour was to compile all the required researches and disseminate the knowledge to a broad spectrum of people comprising of students, researchers and specialists of the field.

Gerontology refers to the study of the biological, psychological, cognitive and sociocultural aspects of aging. An important sub-field of gerontology is biogerontology, which is concerned with the biological process of aging, its evolutionary origin and the possible potential interventions in the process. It investigates the causes, effects and mechanisms of aging. Geriatrics is a field of medicine, which is focused on the health care for the elderly. As an individual ages, there is a gradual decline in the physiological reserve in organs. This results in the development of diseases and complications. Instability, immobility, impaired intellect and memory, and incontinence are the major impairments that occur in the elderly. Many of these problems can be addressed with medications and adequate care. This book is a valuable compilation of topics, ranging from the basic to the most complex advancements in the fields of gerontology and geriatrics. From theories to research, case studies related to all medical aspects of relevance to these fields have been included herein. It will prove to be immensely beneficial to students and researchers in this field.

At the end of the preface, I would like to thank the authors for their brilliant chapters and the publisher for guiding us all-through the making of the book till its final stage. Also, I would like to thank my family for providing the support and encouragement throughout my academic career and research projects.

Editor

# Continuity and utilization of health and community care in elderly patients with heart failure before and after hospitalization

Emma Säfström[1,2,3]* iD, Tiny Jaarsma[4] and Anna Strömberg[2,5]

## Abstract

**Background:** The period after hospitalization due to deteriorated heart failure (HF) is characterized as a time of high generalized risk. The transition from hospital to home is often problematic due to insufficient coordination of care, leading to a fragmentation of care rather than a seamless continuum of care. The aim was to describe health and community care utilization prior to and 30 days after hospitalization, and the continuity of care in patients hospitalized due to de novo or deteriorated HF from the patients' perspective and from a medical chart review.

**Methods:** This was a cross-sectional study with consecutive inclusion of patients hospitalized at a county hospital in Sweden due to deteriorated HF during 2014. Data were collected by structured telephone interviews and medical chart review and analyzed with the Spearman's rank correlation coefficient and Chi square. A P value of 0. 05 was considered significant.

**Results:** A total of 121 patients were included in the study, mean age 82.5 (±6.8) and 49% were women. Half of the patients had not visited any health care facility during the month prior to the index hospital admission, and 79% of the patients visited the emergency room (ER) without a referral. Among these elderly patients, a total of 40% received assistance at home prior to hospitalization and 52% after discharge. A total of 86% received written discharge information, one third felt insecure after hospitalization and lacked knowledge of which health care provider to consult with and contact in the event of deterioration or complications. Health care utilization increased significantly after hospitalization.

**Conclusion:** Most patients had not visited any health care facility within 30 days before hospitalization. Health care utilization increased significantly after hospitalization. Flaws in the continuity of care were found; even though most patients received written information at discharge, one third of the patients lacked knowledge about which health care provider to contact in the event of deterioration and felt insecure at home after discharge.

**Keywords:** Heart failure, Health care utilization, Hospitalization, Continuity of care, Discharge, Elderly patients

* Correspondence: emma.safstrom@liu.se
[1]Sörmland County Council, Nyköping Hospital, Nyköping, Sweden
[2]Department of Medical and Health Sciences, Division of Nursing Science, Linköping University, Linköping, Sweden
Full list of author information is available at the end of the article

## Background

Heart failure (HF) it is the end stage of several cardiac diseases, and an increasing number of people are diagnosed with HF worldwide [1]. In developed countries the prevalence of HF is estimated to be 1–2% [2] and increases with age. The mean age of patients diagnosed with HF is 77 years, and in the population over the age of 80 years the prevalence is 20% [3]. Patients with HF often suffer from multiple illnesses leading to polypharmacy and frailty [4]. Heart failure is characterized by alternating periods of clinical stability and instability. Periods of deterioration have serious consequences in terms of increased mortality and morbidity as well as great suffering for the individuals, and may result in patients needing hospitalization [5]. The patients' situation after hospitalization is complex and it is difficult for them to get the overall picture without comprehensive context-oriented discharge planning [6]. The period post-discharge after hospitalization is characterized as a time of high generalized risk and instability [7]. Readmission rates are high after hospitalization due to HF deterioration, with about one quarter of patients being readmitted within one month [5]. The HF patients often receive care from multiple providers and facilities; thus, there is a potential danger of fragmentation of care [4]. Patients with HF have been found to visit the emergency room (ER), outpatient clinic and/or primary care multiple times every year [8–10] and 25% of the HF patients receive home care after hospitalization [11]. To reduce fragmentation, patients with HF need a seamless chain of care across hospital and primary care. This can only be achieved through close collaboration between the healthcare providers so that the follow-up and management of every patient is optimal and integrated [7, 12]. A seamless continuity of care is most at risk during the patients' transition from an institutional care setting to the home [13].

A few previous studies have reported health care utilization [8–10] for patients with HF, and community care utilization is occasionally described [11, 14] but no studies have been found that describe both health and community care in HF patients in the period associated with hospitalization. Community care includes assistance with housekeeping, personal hygiene and/or dressing. Home health care includes health care provided by registered nurses. Furthermore, the American Heart Association (AHA) recognizes the lack of evidence for best practice of transition from hospital to home in HF patients, advocating further research to optimize the discharge process and the transition from one setting to another [4]. To reduce the fragmentation and make the HF care follow a better continuum between different caregivers, we need more insights into the HF patient's own perspective on the journey through the community and health care system. The objectives were to describe, from the patients' perspective and from a medical chart review, health and community care utilization prior to and 30 days after hospitalization, and the continuity of care in patients hospitalized due to de novo or deteriorated HF.

## Method

### Design and study setting

In this cross-sectional study, data were collected by structured standardized telephone interviews with patients and from their medical charts. The study was conducted at a district county hospital in central Sweden with approximately 120 hospital beds. The hospital had no specialized cardiology ward, so patients with HF were cared for in a general medicine ward. According to the hospital routine all patients had to receive written discharge information when discharged from the medical ward. The discharge information should include: information on diagnosis, medical treatment and exams performed during the hospitalization, changes in medication, and a plan for follow-up. A total of seven different primary care centers were located within the hospital catchment area. Most of them had a specially trained HF nurse during the study period. Elderly, fragile patients within the hospital catchment area may also be assisted in their home by community care and/or home health care. Community care included assistance with housekeeping, personal hygiene and/or dressing. Home health care included health care provided by registered nurses. During the time of the study, HF care could also be carried out by the mobile home care team where registered nurses and nurse assistants worked during the daytime, seven days a week. The mobile home care team was hospital-based and had resources to monitor patients in their homes and provide diuretics intravenously when needed.

### Study participants

This study enrolled patients hospitalized due to an episode of de novo HF or with deteriorating HF (ICD: I50.0, I50.1, I50.9, I42.0) as the primary cause of admission, or patients who developed significant HF symptoms during hospitalization for another primary diagnosis. Exclusion criteria were dementia, non-Swedish speaking, short anticipated survival, not answering the telephone, or discharge to nursing home.

### Procedure

Consecutive inclusion was carried out from January to June 2014 and from August to December 2014. A list of patients discharged from the medical wards was reviewed four times a week. Eligible patients were contacted by telephone by the first author within one week after discharge. If the patient did not answer the telephone after three calls, no further attempts were made. The patients were given verbal information about the study, and if they gave verbal consent, the phone call continued with the structured standardized interview. After the interview, additional data were collected from the medical chart. A review of health care utilization was conducted 30 days after discharge.

### Instruments

A questionnaire with 20 items addressing the time after discharge from hospital was used in the study [15]. The questionnaire was developed by The Swedish Association of Local Authorities and Regions (SALAR). The nine questions reported in this article are presented in Fig. 1. A second questionnaire was also used with items on symptoms before admission, reasons for admission and time of patient delay (Additional file 1). This questionnaire was developed by a research group in cardiovascular nursing research in collaboration with a patient representative and tested for face validity with a group of HF nurses and cardiologists [16]. Furthermore, the charts were reviewed by the first author for sociodemographic and clinical variables including multimorbidity as well as pharmacological treatment at admission and discharge. Multimorbidity was defined as co-occurrence of medical conditions and included diseases classified as etiology [17]. Renal failure was defined as ICD-10 code N17-N19. Assistance at home prior to and after hospitalization was listed as community care or home health care or assistance by the mobile home care team. Patient delay, which was defined as 'the time between first symptoms and hospital admission' was categorized in four different groups: one day, <one week, 1–2 weeks, > two weeks.

### Ethical issues

The study was designed and conducted in accordance with the principles of the World Medical Association Declaration of Helsinki [18]. Permission was granted by the Regional Ethical Review Board. All included patients were given verbal information regarding the study and gave verbal informed consent. It was underlined that participation was voluntary, could be terminated at any time without justification, and that not participating would in no way affect the patients' future care. The patients were guaranteed confidentiality.

### Data analysis

Statistical analyses were performed using SPSS version 22.0. The characteristics of enrolled patients are presented as frequency and percentages for categorical variables and by mean and standard derivations for continuous variables. Spearman's rank correlation coefficient was used for analysis of correlations between patient delay and symptoms on admission. A chi square test was used to compare health care utilization before and after the index hospitalization. A $P$ value of 0.05 was considered significant.

### Results

#### Demographic characteristics

A total of 370 patients (49% women, mean age $79 \pm 10.7$) were hospitalized due to HF during the inclusion period. A total of 249 patients were not eligible for inclusion. The main reasons for exclusion were not answering the telephone or being discharged to a nursing home. In total, 121 patients were included in the study, mean age 82.5 ($\pm$6.8) and 49% women. The ejection fraction (EF) was assessed by echocardiography in 59% of the patients. Within this group of patients, 25% had preserved EF and 75% had reduced EF (mean EF $36 \pm 11$). The demographical and clinical variables of the enrolled patients are presented in Table 1. The mean number of co-morbidities, besides HF was 2.9 ($\pm$ 1.3), with cardiac co-morbidities such as hypertension (63%) and previous

- How has your situation at home been after discharge?
- What has worked well after discharge?
- What has worked poorly after discharge?
- When you were admitted to hospital did you receive treatment and help with the problem(s) you were seeking care for?
- Where you involved in the discharge planning?
- Did you receive written information about your planned follow-up care when being discharged to home?
- Do you know whom to contact if you have questions?
- Did you receive a medication list at discharge?
- Are you satisfied with the conversation with the physician at discharge?

**Fig. 1** Questions from SALAR reported in the article. The questions are translated by the authors and are available in Swedish via the website http://www.webbkollen.com/ [15]

**Table 1** Sociodemographic and clinical characteristic of hospitalized heart failure patients ($n = 121$)

| Characteristics | |
|---|---|
| Age in years, mean (SD) | 82.5 (± 6.8) |
| Woman, n (%) | 59 (49%) |
| Cohabiting with family or others, n (%) | 62 (51%) |
| Co-morbidities | n (%) |
| Hypertension | 76 (63%) |
| MI / ischemic heart disease | 62 (51%) |
| Atrial fibrillation | 59 (49%) |
| Diabetes without complications | 26 (22%) |
| Stroke | 24 (20%) |
| COPD | 20 (17%) |
| Renal failure | 18 (15%) |
| Malignancy | 16 (13%) |
| Other | 14 (12%) |
| Period of time since diagnosed | n (%) |
| < 1 year | 44 (36%) |
| 1–5 years | 33 (27%) |
| > 5 years | 38 (31%) |
| Pharmacological treatment at discharge | n (%) |
| ACEI/ARB | 91 (75%) |
| MRA | 34 (28%) |
| Beta-blocker | 100 (83%) |
| Total number of medication at discharge mean (SD) | 11.58 (± 4.37) |

*MI* myocardial infarction, *COPD* chronic obstructive pulmonary disease, *ACEI*; Angiotensin converting enzyme inhibitor, *ARB* Angiotensin receptor blocker, *MRA* Mineralocorticoid receptor antagonist

myocardial infarction (MI) and/or ischemic heart disease (51%) being the most common. The most frequent symptoms at admission were breathlessness (64%) and fatigue (36%) (Table 2). The median length of stay was four days and the median number of hospitalizations within six months prior to the index hospitalization was one, ranging from one to eight.

## Health care and community care utilization prior to the index hospital admission

Most of the patients had not visited any health care facility the month prior to the index hospital admission (Table 3) and some patients had visited several different health care facilities. A total of 7% of the patients had visited the ER without being admitted. A total of 40% of the patients had assistance at home from community care or home health care prior to index hospital admission. At the visit to the ER that ended with the index hospital admission, only 21% of the patients had a note of referral.

A total of 33% of the patients were admitted on the same day of symptom onset, 33% within one week, 9%

**Table 2** Symptoms at admission in hospitalized heart failure patients (n = 121)

| Symptoms | n (%) |
|---|---|
| Breathlessness | 77 (64%) |
| Fatigue | 44 (36%) |
| Chest pain | 38 (31%) |
| Leg edema | 35 (29%) |
| Orthopnea | 30 (25%) |
| Cough | 20 (17%) |
| Weight gain | 13 (11%) |
| Dizziness | 12 (10%) |
| Nausea | 10 (8%) |
| Palpation | 7 (6%) |
| Pulmonary edema | 7 (6%) |
| Abdominal edema | 2 (2%) |

within two weeks and 24% delayed for more than two weeks from symptom onset. There were significant correlations between being admitted within the first week of symptom onset and prior MI and four typical symptoms of HF (Table 4). According to correlation analyses, patient delay was shorter when the patient experienced acute symptoms and signs such as chest pain and pulmonary edema, and longer when having symptoms of

**Table 3** Assistance at home and health care utilization 30 days prior and 30 days after the index hospitalization for patients with heart failure (n = 121)

| | |
|---|---|
| Assistance at home prior index hospitalization | n (%) |
| Community care prior hospitalization | 43 (35%) |
| Home health care prior hospitalization | 22 (18%) |
| Mobile home care team prior hospitalization | 5 (4%) |
| Assistance at home after index hospitalization | n (%) |
| Community care after hospitalization | 56 (46%) |
| Home health after hospitalization | 29 (24%) |
| Mobile home care team after hospitalization | 22 (18%) |
| Health care facility visits 30 days prior to index hospitalization | n (%) |
| No prior visits to health care facility | 62 (52%) |
| Primary care | 34 (29%) |
| Hospitalized | 16 (13%) |
| ER (without being admitted) | 8 (7%) |
| Internal medicine outpatient clinic | 3 (3%) |
| Health care facility visits 30 days after index hospitalization | n (%) |
| Primary care | 27 (22%) |
| Rehospitalized | 28 (23%) |
| ER (without being admitted) | 19 (16%) |
| Internal medicine outpatient clinic | 18 (15%) |

*ER* Emergency room

Continuity and utilization of health and community care in elderly patients with heart failure before...

5

**Table 4** Factors significantly correlated with being admitted within the first week of symptom onset in patients hospitalized due to heart failure (n = 121)

| | | |
|---|---|---|
| Prior MI, rho (p) | 0.275 | (0.003) |
| Chest pain, rho (p) | 0.214 | (0.020) |
| Pulmonary edema, rho (p) | 0.206 | (0.025) |
| Total number of symptoms, rho (p) | - 0.199 | (0.031) |
| Fatigue, rho (p) | - 0.203 | (0.027) |
| Leg edema, rho (p) | −0.204 | (0.026) |

leg edema and fatigue. No statistically significant correlation was found between patient delay and age or sex.

### Continuity of care

The total number of patients who received assistance at home from community care or home health care increased from 40% at admission to 52% after hospitalization. Prior to hospitalization, 35% of the patients received assistance from community care, increasing to 46% after discharge. Patients receiving assistance from home health care increased from 18% at admission to 24% after discharge. The number of patients receiving assistance from the mobile home care team increased from 4% prior to hospitalization to 18% after discharge (Table 3).

During the telephone interview within one week after discharge, half of the patients described their situation at home after discharge as functioning well, 29% reported their situation as both good and bad, and 20% said that their situation at home was functioning poorly. In total 50% of the patients experienced difficulties after discharge, most often due to burdensome symptoms of HF such as fatigue and dyspnea (Table 5). Difficulties were also due to medications, e.g. not having received necessary prescriptions or not being able to understand the list of medications. Two thirds of the patients stated they

**Table 5** Concerns and symptoms in patients with heart failure after discharge (n = 121)

| Symptoms | n (%) |
|---|---|
| Fatigue | 38 (31%) |
| Shortness of breath | 15 (12%) |
| Dizzy | 7 (6%) |
| Lack of appetite | 5 (4%) |
| Concerns | n (%) |
| Concerns regarding the medications | 13 (11%) |
| Not enough community care after discharge | 5 (4%) |
| The need of assistive equipment not met | 4 (3%) |
| Not enough home health care after discharge | 1 (1%) |
| Overburdened relative | 1 (1%) |

had participated in the planning of their discharge and 57% were satisfied with the discharge conversation. A total of 86% reported having received written discharge information and 89% had received a list of their medications. Two-thirds of the patients reported that they had knowledge of which health care provider to consult in case of deterioration or complications. Two thirds reported feeling safe and secure with their current health care and community care contacts.

Health care utilization prior to and post-discharge is presented in fig. 2. At discharge, 10% of the patients had no documented plan for follow-up, 48% were referred to the primary care (57% women, mean age $83.8 \pm 6.7$) and 36% to the outpatient medical clinic (47% women, mean age $80.7 \pm 6.7$). Seven percent had non-categorized types of follow-up; by telephone calls or at other outpatient clinics. Five patients were referred for follow-up to both the primary care and an outpatient clinic.

### Readmissions and health care utilization after discharge

A review of health care utilization 30 days post-discharge revealed a significant increase of health care utilization after hospitalization. Only 35% of the patients had visited a health care facility within one month prior to index hospitalization, and 55% of the patients had visited a health care facility within 30 days after hospitalization (p 0.002). Within 30 days after the index hospitalization, 22% of the patients had visited the primary care, 16% had visited the ER without being admitted, and 15% had visited the internal medicine outpatient clinic. A total of 18% had been visited by the mobile home care team. In total, 23% of the patients were readmitted within 30 days (Table 3). Most patients were readmitted due to HF or other cardiovascular problems as their primary or secondary diagnosis; only three patients were readmitted due to a condition not related to HF. Two patients came to the ER with a note of referral and the rest sought care on their own initiative. The mean time to readmission was 13 ($\pm$9) days. The most common symptoms at readmission were fatigue (40%), breathlessness (39%) and weight gain (17%). Among patients with planned follow-up in primary care, one in four (26%) had visited the primary care within 30 days after discharge. In patients with planned follow-up in outpatient internal medicine clinic, 36% had visited the outpatient medicine clinic within 30 days after discharge.

### Discussion and conclusion
#### Discussion

This cross-sectional study, combining the perspective of elderly patients as well as data from the medical charts on health and community care, revealed novel aspects of the continuity of care in patients hospitalized due to HF. The aspects included patients' care seeking, health and community care utilization, as well as patients' experiences of

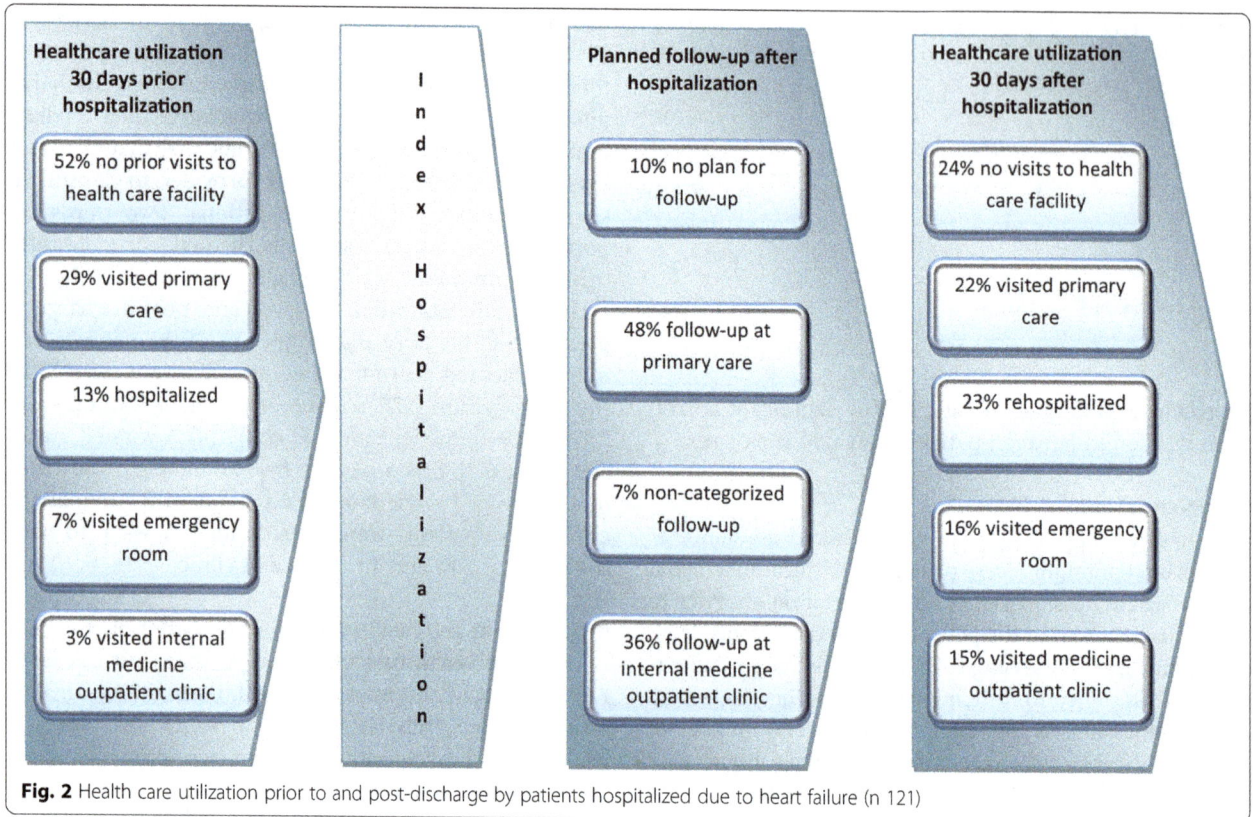

**Fig. 2** Health care utilization prior to and post-discharge by patients hospitalized due to heart failure (n 121)

Healthcare utilization 30 days prior hospitalization

- 52% no prior visits to health care facility
- 29% visited primary care
- 13% hospitalized
- 7% visited emergency room
- 3% visited internal medicine outpatient clinic

Index Hospitalization

Planned follow-up after hospitalization

- 10% no plan for follow-up
- 48% follow-up at primary care
- 7% non-categorized follow-up
- 36% follow-up at internal medicine outpatient clinic

Healthcare utilization 30 days after hospitalization

- 24% no visits to health care facility
- 22% visited primary care
- 23% rehospitalized
- 16% visited emergency room
- 15% visited medicine outpatient clinic

continuity of care. All these aspects need to be further addressed in order to improve the HF care.

A majority of studies on HF patients have exclusion criteria based on comorbidity, and 25% apply an upper age limit [19], leading to underrepresentation of the HF population [20]. The high mean age in our study highlights the situation for elderly patients burdened with multimorbidity.

It was striking to see that most patients turned to the ER in the first instance when their condition deteriorated and not to the primary care center or outpatient HF clinic in which they were enlisted. The number of patients who came to the ER without referral have increased from 62% in 1999 [21] to 79% in this present study. The ER should not be the first health care facility to contact when symptoms of deteriorated HF occur. This results in meeting a substantial number of different physicians and nurses over time, which may contribute to flaws in the continuity of care so that patients experience the care as fragmented [22]. Horowitz et al. found that patients preferred to contact the ER instead of their primary care, when treatment was immediately available at the ER and the accessibility of primary care was perceived to be low [23]. Low accessibility of primary care is confirmed in our study, when only 26% of the patients with a planned follow at primary care had actually visited the primary care within 30 days after discharge.

Among the patients enrolled in this study, 86% of them recalled receiving written information at discharge, but only two-thirds knew which health care provider to consult when deterioration or complications occurred. Similar flaws in the continuity of care were found in a study from 2008 where 30% of the patients reported no knowledge of this key information [24]. This either implies that the discharge information lacked this important information, or that the patients were unable to assimilate the information. Prior trials reveal coherent communication behavior as an essential factor in the discharge process [13, 25], and lack of proper discharge information has been found to be a contributing factor to readmissions [25]. Since the HF patients are often old and fragile it is even more important to ensure that information given is correctly understood [26]. It has previously been found that patients sometimes do not read the information they receive [27] which further emphasizes the importance of the use of techniques such as teach-back during discharge conversation [28]. Both the European Society of Cardiology (ESC) and AHA state that discharge planning is crucial to secure the continuity of care. As a part of comprehensive discharge planning, the patient should be provided with information on sufficient self-care behavior and a detailed plan for follow-up, which should include facilitated access to care [2, 4]. The ESC even suggests that HF patients are not medically fit for discharge if they have not been provided with tailored education [2].

For old and cognitively impaired patients it is important not only to provide information adjusted to their preferences and cognitive ability, but also provide to teach skills in how to manage self-care and assess the need of support from caregivers and community services [29, 30].

Prior studies suggest that the patient delay may be due to difficulties in recognizing symptoms of decompensated HF, and that the patients use a "wait and see" mentality [31, 32]. However, insights from this study also reveal that one third of the patients did not know which health care provider to contact if they had questions or deterioration occurred, and this uncertainty may be a contributing factor to patient delay.

### Follow-up in primary care

The proportion of patients referred for follow-up in primary care and at the internal medicine outpatient clinic respectively has been about the same for the last 20 years. In 1995, 57% of the patients were referred to the primary care [21], and 48% of the patients enrolled in this study were referred to the primary care. The patient preference seems to be follow-up at internal medicine outpatient clinics. Two recent studies on follow-up found that patients declined study participation due to the risk of being assigned follow-up at primary care [12, 33]. However, these days, when the competence of primary care has been enhanced with HF nurses and the quality of the care can be ensured [34, 35], it would be advantageous and cost-effective to refer stable HF patients who are on optimal dosing of medicines to the primary care, which complies with the guidelines from ESC [2]. Furthermore, guideline adherence and patient adherence to medication have been found to be maintained when follow-up is managed within primary care [12, 36]. The availability of primary care is too low [37], and only one fourth of the patients with planned follow-up at primary care actually had a follow-up visit at primary care within 30 days post-discharge. The exact reason for this is unclear, but prior studies have found flaws in discharge communication and information transfer from hospital to primary care and lack of resources [38, 39], which could prolong the time from discharge to follow-up. Early follow-up, and follow-up with home visiting programs and multidisciplinary interventions have been found to reduce readmission and mortality [40].

### Problems after discharge

Many of the patients still experienced troublesome symptoms after discharge. Fatigue and shortness of breath was frequently reported, and these were also the most common symptoms in patients readmitted within 30 days after the index hospitalization. Distressing symptoms have been described as a common reason for rehospitalization [41]. To still experience the same symptoms suffered on admission

when discharged, might increase the feeling of uncertainty at home. Besides symptoms, concern regarding medication was a factor that made the situation at home bothersome for many of the patients (Table 5). This is in line with a recent review that found that medication-related difficulties after discharge are common in HF patients [42]. Since the goals of pharmacological treatment are relief of symptoms, to improve survival and decrease the need for hospital admission [2] it is elementary that patients are given the best preconditions to handle the pharmacological regime after discharge. Before discharge it should be ensured that the patients have all they need to manage the medical treatment [43]. Symptoms of deterioration, as well as medication-related problems are factors contributing to hospital readmission [25, 44]. The period after hospitalization is characterized as a time of high generalized risk [7], and health care utilization seemed to increase 30 days after hospitalization, when 55% of the patients had visited a health care facility. Some increase in health care utilization such as planned follow-up visits and home health care is a positive reflection of intensified attention to patient monitoring and follow-up after discharge and may improve outcomes. However, it must be considered as a flaw in HF care and a flaw in the continuity of care that a total of 35% of the patients were rehospitalized or visited the ER within the first month after discharge. Furthermore, it is deplorable that so few of the patients had their planned follow up visit at primary care or an outpatient clinic within the first month after discharge.

### Study limitations

There are potential limitations to the present findings. The number of patients was relatively small, and they were all treated at the same hospital. The health care facility system varies between counties, making generalization limited. Another weakness of this study is the fact that we did not retrieve data regarding whether the patients had contacted any health care facility or "Swedish Healthcare Direct 1177" by telephone. Only data on physical visits were collected and it is possible that the number of patients who had contacted health care facilities was higher. Another limitation is the fact that there was poor documentation in the medical records of the New York Heart Association (NYHA) functional classification in the medical charts. According to HF guidelines, NYHA classification should be used to describe the severity of symptoms and exercise intolerance and there is an association among NYHA class and hospitalization and death [2]. The NYHA classification would have been a useful variable in correlation analysis and it is possible that it might have influenced the results. Furthermore, the NYHA classification might be a variable that affects the patient's experience of their situation at home after hospitalization.

*Recommendations to overcome flaws in the continuity of care:*

- Ensure that patient has understood the discharge information correctly.
- Discharge information should include contact information of an appropriate health care provider
- Ensure that discharge information or referral is available in primary care immediately after discharge
- Continuity of care should be a prioritized area of improvement work

## Conclusion

The findings of this study, describing the care utilization and continuity of care in the real-world elderly hospitalized HF patients, showed that most patients had not visited any health care facility during the month prior to the index hospital admission, and that health care utilization increased significantly after hospitalization. The number of patients who received assistance at home increased after hospitalization and patients were most often referred for follow-up in primary care. We also found that, although most patients received written information at discharge, many of them felt insecure after discharge and lacked knowledge about which health care provider to consult in the case of deterioration or complications.

### Abbreviations
AHA: American Heart Association; EF: Ejection Fraction; ER: Emergency room; ESC: The European Society of Cardiology; HF: Heart failure; ICD: International Statistical Classification of Diseases and Related Health Problems; MI: Myocardial infarction; NYHA: New York Heart Association

### Funding
This work was funded by Linköping University and Sörmland County Council. The funders had no role in the design of the study, data collection, analysis or interpretation of the data.

### Authors' contributions
ES and AS planned, designed and received funding for the study, and ES collected and analyzed the data with supervision from TJ and AS. ES, drafted the manuscript and TJ and AS revised it critically for important intellectual content. All authors have read and approved the final version of the manuscript.

### Competing interests
The authors declare that they have no competing interests.

### Author details
[1]Sörmland County Council, Nyköping Hospital, Nyköping, Sweden. [2]Department of Medical and Health Sciences, Division of Nursing Science, Linköping University, Linköping, Sweden. [3]Centre for Clinical Research Sörmland, Uppsala University, Eskilstuna, Sweden. [4]Department of Social and Welfare Studies, Linköping University, Linköping, Sweden. [5]Department of Cardiology, Linköping University, Linköping, Sweden.

### References
1. Bui AL, Horwich TB, Fonarow GC. Epidemiology and risk profile of heart failure. Nat Rev Cardiol. 2011;8(1):30–41.
2. Ponikowski PVA, Anker SD, Bueno H, Cleland JG, Coats AJ, Falk V, González-Juanatey JR, Harjola VP, Jankowska EA, Jessup M, Linde C, Nihoyannopoulos P, Parissis JT, Pieske B, Riley JP, Rosano GM, Ruilope LM, Ruschitzka F, Rutten FH, van der Meer P. 2016 ESC guidelines for the diagnosis and treatment of acute and chronic heart failure: The Task Force for the diagnosis and treatment of acute and chronic heart failure of the European Society of Cardiology (ESC) Developed with the special contribution of the Heart Failure Association (HFA) of the ESC. European J heart failure. 2016;
3. Zarrinkoub R, Wettermark B, Wandell P, Mejhert M, Szulkin R, Ljunggren G, Kahan T. The epidemiology of heart failure, based on data for 2.1 million inhabitants in Sweden. Eur J Heart Fail. 2013;15(9):995–1002.
4. Yancy CW, Jessup M, Bozkurt B, Butler J, Casey DE Jr, Drazner MH, Fonarow GC, Geraci SA, Horwich T, Januzzi JL, et al. 2013 ACCF/AHA guideline for the management of heart failure: a report of the American College of Cardiology Foundation/American Heart Association task force on practice guidelines. J Am Coll Cardiol. 2013;62(16):e147–239.
5. Ponikowski P, Anker SD, AlHabib KF, Cowie MR, Force TL, Hu S, Jaarsma T, Krum H, Rastogi V, Rohde LE, et al. Heart failure: preventing disease and death worldwide. ESC Heart Failure. 2014;1(1):4–25.
6. Hekmatpou D, Mohammadi E, Ahmadi F, Arefi SH. Lack of sensitivity to readmission: a grounded theory study for explaining the process of readmitting patients suffering from congestive heart failure. Eur J Cardiovasc Nurs. 2009;8(5):355–63.
7. Dharmarajan K, Krumholz HM. Strategies to reduce 30-day readmissions in older patients hospitalized with heart failure and acute myocardial infarction. Current geriatrics reports. 2014;3(4):306–15.
8. Agvall B, Borgquist L, Foldevi M, Dahlstrom U. Cost of heart failure in Swedish primary healthcare. Scand J Prim Health Care. 2005;23(4):227–32.
9. Mejhert M, Persson H, Edner M, Kahan T. Epidemiology of heart failure in Sweden--a national survey. Eur J Heart Fail. 2001;3(1):97–103.
10. Bogner HR, Miller SD, De Vries HF, Chhatre S, Jayadevappa R. Assessment of cost and health resource utilization for elderly patients with heart failure and diabetes mellitus. J Card Fail. 2010;16(6):454–60.
11. Eastwood CA, Howlett JG, King-Shier KM, McAlister FA, Ezekowitz JA, Quan H. Determinants of early readmission after hospitalization for heart failure. The Canadian journal of cardiology. 2014;30(6):612–8.
12. Luttik ML, Jaarsma T, van Geel PP, Brons M, Hillege HL, Hoes AW, de Jong R, Linssen G, Lok DJ, Berge M et al: Long-term follow-up in optimally treated and stable heart failure patients: primary care vs. heart failure clinic. Results of the COACH-2 study. Eur J Heart Fail 2014, 16(11):1241–1248.
13. Spehar AM, Campbell RR, Cherrie C, Palacios P, Scott D, Baker JL, Bjornstad B, Wolfson J: Advances in Patient Safety - Seamless Care: Safe Patient Transitions from Hospital to Home. In: Advances in Patient Safety: From Research to Implementation (Volume 1: Research Findings). Edited by Henriksen K, Battles JB, Marks ES, Lewin DI. Rockville (MD): Agency for Healthcare Research and Quality (US); 2005.
14. Li H, Morrow-Howell N, Proctor EK. Post-acute home care and hospital readmission of elderly patients with congestive heart failure. Health & social work. 2004;29(4):275–85.
15. Webbkollen. Intervjufrågor - Sjukhus - Ring upp.
16. Strömberg A MJ, Fridlund B, Dahlström U: Cause of deterioration and treatment seeking behaviour in patients hospitalised due to heart failure. In: Congress of the European Society of Cardiology: September Wien 2007.
17. Stewart S, Riegel B, Boyd C, Ahamed Y, Thompson DR, Burrell LM, Carrington MJ, Coats A, Granger BB, Hides J et al: Establishing a pragmatic framework to optimise health outcomes in heart failure and multimorbidity (ARISE-HF): a multidisciplinary position statement. Int J Cardiol 2016, 212:1–10.
18. Association. WM: World Medical Association. Declaration of Helsinki - ethical principles for medical research involving human subjects, 2013. 2013.https://www.wma.net/policies-post/wma-declaration-of-helsinki-ethical-principles-for-medical-research-involving-human-subjects/.
19. Cherubini A, Oristrell J, Pla X, Ruggiero C, Ferretti R, Diestre G, Clarfield AM, Crome P, Hertogh C, Lesauskaite V, et al. The persistent exclusion of older patients from ongoing clinical trials regarding heart failure. Arch Intern Med. 2011;171(6):550–6.
20. Heiat A, Gross CP, Krumholz HM. Representation of the elderly, women, and minorities in heart failure clinical trials. Arch Intern Med. 2002;162(15):1682–8.

21. Mejhert M, Holmgren J, Wandell P, Persson H, Edner M. Diagnostic tests, treatment and follow-up in heart failure patients--is there a gender bias in the coherence to guidelines? Eur J Heart Fail. 1999;1(4):407–10.

22. McDonagh TA, Blue L, Clark AL, Dahlstrom U, Ekman I, Lainscak M, McDonald K, Ryder M, Stromberg A, Jaarsma T, et al. European Society of Cardiology Heart Failure Association Standards for delivering heart failure care. Eur J Heart Fail. 2011;13(3):235–41.

23. Horowitz CR, Rein SB, Leventhal H. A story of maladies, misconceptions and mishaps: effective management of heart failure. Social science & medicine (1982). 2004;58(3):631–43.

24. Hadjistavropoulos HD, Biem HJ, Kowalyk KM. Measurement of continuity of care in cardiac patients: reliability and validity of an in-person questionnaire. The Canadian journal of cardiology. 2004;20

25. Gheorghiade M, Vaduganathan M, Fonarow GC, Bonow RO. Rehospitalization for heart failure: problems and perspectives. J Am Coll Cardiol. 2013;61(4):391–403.

26. Vidan MT, Sanchez E, Fernandez-Aviles F, Serra-Rexach JA, Ortiz J, Bueno H. FRAIL-HF, a study to evaluate the clinical complexity of heart failure in nondependent older patients: rationale, methods and baseline characteristics. Clin Cardiol. 2014;37(12):725–32.

27. Hekmatpou D, Mohammadi E, Ahmadi F, Arefi SH. Termination of professional responsibility: exploring the process of discharging patients with heart failure from hospitals. Int J Nurs Pract. 2010;16(4):389–96.

28. White M, Garbez R, Carroll M, Brinker E, Howie-Esquivel J. Is "teach-back" associated with knowledge retention and hospital readmission in hospitalized heart failure patients? The Journal of cardiovascular nursing. 2013;28(2):137–46.

29. Lainscak M, Blue L, Clark AL, Dahlstrom U, Dickstein K, Ekman I, McDonagh T, McMurray JJ, Ryder M, Stewart S, et al. Self-care management of heart failure: practical recommendations from the patient Care Committee of the Heart Failure Association of the European Society of Cardiology. Eur J Heart Fail. 2011;13(2):115–26.

30. Dickson VV, Riegel B. Are we teaching what patients need to know? Building skills in heart failure self-care. Heart Lung. 2009;38(3):253–61.

31. Nieuwenhuis MM, Jaarsma T, van Veldhuisen DJ, van der Wal MH. Factors associated with patient delay in seeking care after worsening symptoms in heart failure patients. J Card Fail. 2011;17(8):657–63.

32. Sethares KA, Sosa ME, Fisher P, Riegel B. Factors associated with delay in seeking care for acute decompensated heart failure. The Journal of cardiovascular nursing. 2014;29(5):429–38.

33. Stewart S, Carrington MJ, Marwick TH, Davidson PM, Macdonald P, Horowitz JD, Krum H, Newton PJ, Reid C, Chan YK, et al. Impact of home versus clinic-based management of chronic heart failure: the WHICH? (Which heart failure intervention is most Cost-Effective & Consumer Friendly in reducing hospital care) multicenter, randomized trial. J Am Coll Cardiol. 2012;60(14):1239–48.

34. Stromberg A, Martensson J, Fridlund B, Levin LA, Karlsson JE, Dahlstrom U. Nurse-led heart failure clinics improve survival and self-care behaviour in patients with heart failure: results from a prospective, randomised trial. Eur Heart J. 2003;24(11):1014–23.

35. Mariani M, Vella G, Bianchi C, Verde S, De Maria R, Pirelli S. Implementation of beta-blockade in elderly heart failure patients: role of the nurse specialist. Eur J Cardiovasc Nurs. 2008;7(3):196–203.

36. Gjesing A, Schou M, Torp-Pedersen C, Kober L, Gustafsson F, Hildebrandt P, Videbaek L, Wiggers H, Demant M, Charlot M, et al. Patient adherence to evidence-based pharmacotherapy in systolic heart failure and the transition of follow-up from specialized heart failure outpatient clinics to primary care. Eur J Heart Fail. 2013;15(6):671–8.

37. Siciliani L, Borowitz M, Moran V. Waiting time policies in the health sector: what works: OECD; 2013.

38. Bell CM, Schnipper JL, Auerbach AD, Kaboli PJ, Wetterneck TB, Gonzales DV, Arora VM, Zhang JX, Meltzer DO. Association of communication between hospital-based physicians and primary care providers with patient outcomes. J Gen Intern Med. 2009;24(3):381–6.

39. Kripalani S, LeFevre F, Phillips CO, Williams MV, Basaviah P, Baker DW. Deficits in communication and information transfer between hospital-based and primary care physicians: implications for patient safety and continuity of care. Jama. 2007;297(8):831–41.

40. Feltner C, Jones CD, Cené CW, Zheng Z-J, Sueta CA, Coker-Schwimmer EJL, Arvanitis M, Lohr KN, Middleton JC, Jonas DE. Transitional care interventions to prevent readmissions for persons with heart FailureA systematic review and meta-analysisTransitional Care for Persons with Heart Failure. Ann Intern Med. 2014;160(11):774–84.

41. Retrum JH, Boggs J, Hersh A, Wright L, Main DS, Magid DJ, Allen LA. Patient-identified factors related to heart failure readmissions. Circ Cardiovasc Qual Outcomes. 2013;6(2):171–7.

42. Albert NM. A systematic review of transitional-care strategies to reduce rehospitalization in patients with heart failure. Heart & Lung: The Journal of Acute and Critical Care. 2016;45(2):100–13.

43. Mebazaa A, Yilmaz MB, Levy P, Ponikowski P, Peacock WF, Laribi S, Ristic AD, Lambrinou E, Masip J, Riley JP, et al. Recommendations on pre-hospital & early hospital management of acute heart failure: a consensus paper from the Heart Failure Association of the European Society of Cardiology, the European Society of Emergency Medicine and the Society of Academic Emergency Medicine. European journal of heart failure. 2015;17(6):544–58.

44. Robinson S, Howie-Esquivel J, Vlahov D. Readmission risk factors after hospital discharge among the elderly. Population health management. 2012;15(6):338–51.

# 2

# Retrospective assessment of patient characteristics and healthcare costs prior to a diagnosis of Alzheimer's disease in an administrative claims database

Radhika Nair[1], Virginia S. Haynes[2,4*], Mir Siadaty[1], Nick C. Patel[1], Adam S. Fleisher[2], Derek Van Amerongen[3], Michael M. Witte[2], AnnCatherine M. Downing[2], Leslie Ann Hazel Fernandez[1], Vishal Saundankar[1] and Daniel E. Ball[2]

**Abstract**

**Background:** The objective of this study was to examine patient characteristics and health care resource utilization (HCRU) in the 36 months prior to a confirmatory diagnosis of Alzheimer's disease (AD) compared to a matched cohort without dementia during the same time interval.

**Methods:** Patients newly diagnosed with AD (with ≥2 claims) were identified between January 1, 2013 to September 31, 2015, and the date of the second claim for AD was defined as the index date. Patients were enrolled for at least 36 months prior to index date. The AD cohort was matched to a cohort with no AD or dementia codes (1:3) on age, gender, race/ethnicity, and enrollment duration prior to the index date. Descriptive analyses were used to summarize patient characteristics, HCRU, and healthcare costs prior to the confirmatory AD diagnosis. The classification and regression tree analysis and logistic regression were used to identify factors associated with the AD diagnosis.

**Results:** The AD cohort ($N = 16{,}494$) had significantly higher comorbidity indices and greater odds of comorbid mental and behavioral diagnoses, including mild cognitive impairment, mood and anxiety disorders, behavioral disturbances, and cerebrovascular disease, heart disease, urinary tract infections, and pneumonia than the matched non-AD or dementia cohort ($N = 49{,}482$). During the six-month period before the confirmatory AD diagnosis, AD medication use and diagnosis of mild cognitive impairment, Parkinson's disease, or mood disorder were the strongest predictors of a subsequent confirmatory diagnosis of AD. Greater HCRU and healthcare costs were observed for the AD cohort primarily during the six-month period before the confirmatory AD diagnosis.

**Conclusion:** The results of this study demonstrated a higher comorbidity burden and higher costs for patients prior to a diagnosis of AD in comparison to the matched cohort. Several comorbidities were associated with a subsequent diagnosis of AD.

**Keywords:** Alzheimer's disease, Comorbidities, Costs

* Correspondence: ginger.haynes@lilly.com
[2]Eli Lilly and Company, Indianapolis, USA
[4]Lilly Corporate Center, Drop Code 1730, Indianapolis, IN 46285, USA
Full list of author information is available at the end of the article

# Background

Development of Alzheimer's disease (AD) occurs more frequently in the elderly. With an increasing elderly population in the U.S., the prevalence and associated healthcare costs of AD are expected to rise significantly in the absence of any intervention or medication to slow or stop cognitive and functional decline in these patients [1]. Many of the compounds in development to address this issue aim to target the underlying AD pathophysiology, such as modulation of amyloid and tau protein deposition, and therefore may have the potential to slow the progression of disease. In anticipation of this potential shift away from the treatment paradigm of the currently available AD-indicated medications, which are mainly used for symptom management, the ability to accurately identify individuals earlier in the course of disease, prior to irreversible neuronal dysfunction, becomes critical [2, 3]. Therefore, clinical tools are needed to help identify patients earlier in the spectrum of illness and facilitate the ongoing development of disease modifying agents with the ability to alter AD progression.

For research studies that utilize administrative claims data, current diagnostic codes make it challenging to identify patients with AD until the later stages of the illness and require unique approaches to study trends before diagnosis occurs. Prior studies have used various methods to delineate how patients with AD are identified. These include, prospective observational cohorts, [4] using samples derived from electronic medical records of family practitioners, [5] Medicare databases, [6] Medicaid databases, [7] and commercial managed healthcare databases [8–10].

Among the studies utilizing administrative data, Gilden et al. [6] identified four major pathways that led to an AD diagnosis among Medicare Fee For Service (FFS) beneficiaries: AD as the initial diagnosis or cognitive disturbance followed by AD; dementia with suspected etiologies, followed by AD; dementia without known cause, followed by AD; and a triple pathway which included cognitive disturbance followed by dementia of unknown cause, followed by AD. Jaakkimainen et al. [5] described an algorithm of "one hospitalization code or three physician claims codes at least 30 days apart in a two year period OR a prescription filled for an Alzheimer's disease and related dementias (AD-RD) specific medication" with high sensitivity, specificity, and positive predictive value to identify AD-RD. These studies highlight the challenge of identifying patients with AD from administrative claims data.

Along with the identification of patients with AD, several studies have aimed to characterize the management of these patients prior to diagnosis. In the 12–18 month period prior to the initial diagnosis of AD, patients tend to have increases in healthcare resource utilization (HCRU) and healthcare costs [6, 9, 11]. A study by Gilden et al. (2015) [6] demonstrated a rapid increase in total monthly Medicare expenditures shortly before AD diagnosis, followed by a rapid decline in expenditures. In both Medicare and Medicaid populations, individuals with AD or AD-RD incurred higher expenditures than matched controls in the 12 months prior to diagnosis [7, 9, 11]. A majority of these increases have been attributed to outpatient services, inpatient, and acute care services [7, 11].

The objective of the current study was to understand the pre-diagnostic journey of a cohort of patients who were newly diagnosed with AD. The characterization of this pre-diagnostic journey of patients with AD builds on previous research through the examination of clinical characteristics, socioeconomic attributes, and behavioral characteristics. In addition, this study captures HCRU and costs during the 36 months prior to a confirmatory AD diagnosis in comparison to a matched cohort without AD or dementia. With a longer window of examination prior to a confirmed diagnosis of AD, the current study also aimed to identify potential indicators available in administrative claims data that may help to predict patients who will be subsequently diagnosed with AD.

# Methods

This was a retrospective, observational study using a linked database comprised of information from two databases, retrospective claims and the AmeriLINK data provided by Knowledge Base Management (KBM). The claims data includes billing for inpatient and outpatient office visits and outpatient prescription medication filled for millions of participants. The data includes claims for patients enrolled in commercial or Medicare plans. For the purposes of this study, we included individuals enrolled in commercial or Medicare Advantage and Prescription Drug plans (MAPD) with both medical and pharmacy coverage. Medicare Advantage plans are insurance plans offered to consumers through private companies that cover medical and hospital services that are included under Medicare parts A and B and include additional coverage not available in Medicare, typically including a prescription drug plan. The US federal government reimburses private companies approved to sell Medicare Advantage plans for those services covered in Medicare parts A and B. The consumer's premium covers additional services and benefits that are unique to the Medicare Advantage Plan [12].

All medical and pharmacy claims included in the study are fully adjudicated and paid. The enrollment, medical, and pharmacy claims data of individuals enrolled in the MAPD were linked using a unique identifier to three variables from AmeriLINK data from KBM. AmeriLINK data consists of consumer, census, and computed behavioral data using publicly available information (i.e., public records), retail transaction data (i.e., credit card purchases), and computed variables derived from census-type information and/or the combination of data to generate new variables. For this study we included three variables from AmeriLINK namely, estimated household income, percent 2010 white collar and blue collar employed (the percentage of the population in the census-area employed in a white collar or blue collar industry). The study protocol that included a description of the research database and methods was reviewed and approved by an external institutional review board.

Patients 55–89 years of age with two or more claims for AD [International Statistical Classification of Diseases, Ninth Revision, Clinical Modification (ICD-9-CM) 331.0×] on different dates within 18 months of each other between January 1, 2013 and September 30, 2015, were identified (Fig. 1). The date of the second claim for AD was set as the index date. Patients were required to have continuous enrollment for at least 36 months prior to the index date, and had no medical claims with diagnosis codes for AD during the pre-index period (with the exception of the first medical claim for AD).

This AD cohort was matched at the individual patient level with a cohort during the same time interval with no AD or dementia codes (matched cohort) on age (same age in years), gender, race/ethnicity, and enrollment duration prior to the index date (± 3 months). Each individual patient in the AD cohort was matched based on demographics with three individual patients from the control group of patients without any AD or dementia codes. The cohorts were matched only on demographics to allow for a clearer evaluation of the patient's clinical characteristics prior to the diagnosis of AD, while minimizing any demographic differences.

AD is a form of dementia; therefore, it is likely that patients with a diagnosis of dementia, might actually have AD. To ensure our matched cohort did not have undiagnosed AD dementia, we required that they have no diagnosis codes for dementia. Conversely, for the AD cohort, it is possible that physicians would document dementia without confidence in classifying as AD, so we did not want to

exclude patients with two diagnoses of AD dementia due to the presence of a less specific dementia code.

This matched non-AD or dementia cohort were required to have a medical claim within 30 days of the index date of the matched patient from the AD cohort and no medical claims with diagnosis codes for AD, mild cognitive impairment (MCI; ICD-9-CM: 331.83), or AD-related or unrelated dementia codes for the entire length of enrollment. The index date for the matched patient was the date of their medical claim which was within 30 days of their matched AD cohort member's second diagnosis.

### Variables

Medical and pharmacy claims data, along with AmeriLINK data, were examined prior to the confirmatory AD diagnosis in order to understand demographic, clinical, and socioeconomic/behavioral characteristics of these patients. Prior to the confirmatory diagnosis of AD, baseline demographics including age, gender, race/ethnicity (MAPD only), region of residence, insurance type (MAPD or commercial), and low income subsidy status were evaluated. Low income subsidy status refers to patients with limited resources and an income below 150% of the U.S. federal poverty threshold who were eligible for additional premium and cost-share assistance for prescription drugs. Patients eligible for both Medicare and Medicaid (dual eligible) were also identified.

Comorbidities were evaluated using the Deyo Charlson Comorbidity Index (DCCI) score [13–15] and the RxRisk-V Score [16]. The DCCI score is based on 17 categories of comorbidities, which are used to calculate a score that reflects the cumulative increased likelihood of one-year mortality [13]. The evolution of the Deyo-Charlson methodology has permitted researchers to use the score as an assessment of overall patient health risk. The RxRisk-V Score [16] is a pharmacy-based comorbidity index that involves the identification of 45 distinct medical condition categories via their associated medication treatments. Of the 45 conditions, three that are defined based on claims for durable medical equipment (neurogenic bladder, ostomy, and urinary incontinence) were not included in this study given these claims are not captured in pharmacy claims data.

The prevalence of pre-specified chronic comorbidities and the proportions of patients with annual wellness visits and cognitive assessments prior to the diagnosis of AD were compared between the AD cohort and the matched cohort. The proportion of patients who filled prescriptions for AD medications [cholinesterase inhibitors (donepezil, galantamine, rivastigmine) or N-methyl-D-aspartate (NMDA) antagonist (memantine)] during the pre-index period was also compared across both cohorts.

To evaluate trends in utilization, HCRU and healthcare costs were measured at 6-month intervals prior to

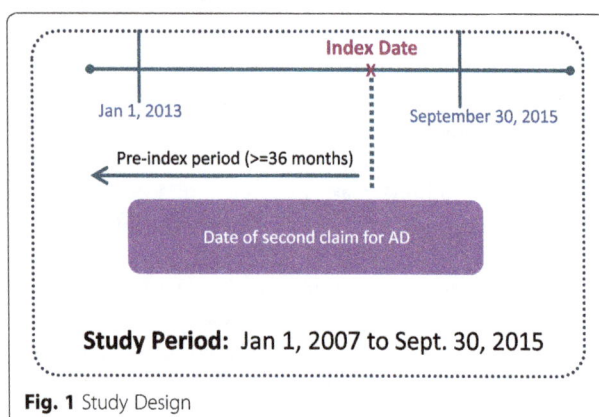

**Fig. 1** Study Design

the confirmatory diagnosis of AD. Medical HCRU included the number of outpatient, inpatient, and emergency department (ED) visits. Pharmacy HCRU included the calculated number of unique medication classes filled by a patient. The total costs (paid by plan and patient) included medical (outpatient, inpatient, and ED), pharmacy, and total healthcare costs (medical plus pharmacy); these costs were adjusted to 2015.

Socioeconomic and behavioral characteristics play an important role in patient behavior related to the consumption of health care. As such, we used variables identified from the AmeriLINK data including household income, occupation in the census area where the patient resided (blue collar vs. white collar), and education. Furthermore, we used behavior segmentation developed by Humana that provides insights on how individuals naturally group themselves based on their general propensity to engage in their health/healthcare system and with the health plan. The behavior segmentation includes multiple distinct behavioral groups, and are further classified into whether individuals have chronic health issues (chronic) or not (healthy). At the time of this study, the behavior segmentation was applied only to the MAPD population; however, the number of patients in this study enrolled in a commercial plan was low (1.0%). The behavior segmentation was included in the analyses to control for individual variations, but the results for the segments themselves are not provided due to their proprietary nature.

## Analyses

Descriptive analyses were used to compare the pre-index demographic, clinical, and socioeconomic/behavioral characteristics of the AD and matched cohorts. HCRU and healthcare costs for the 0–36 months prior to the index date were analyzed for both cohorts. Mean and median cost components were computed, and mean cost components were compared across groups using t-test.

The associations between patient characteristics and AD diagnosis were tested using multivariate logistic regression models. Given the large number of variables and uncertainty as to their potential interactions, a classification and regression tree (CART) [17, 18] method was used to refine the selection of variables for inclusion in the logistic regression model. The CART analysis is a decision tree method that uses recursive partitioning of data into strata, enabling a study population to be categorized into meaningful subsets. The advantages of using CART are that it is a non-parametric technique not dependent on assumptions regarding distribution of the variables in a dataset, and it can be used to assess both dichotomous and continuous outcome variables [18].

In addition to the selection of variables for inclusion, the CART analysis further aided in identifying the most important explanatory variables in the dataset, which were most predictive of a diagnosis of AD. The top 15 explanatory variables from the CART analysis, along with their two-way interactions, were included in the logistic regression models.

For the final logistic regression model, the forward selection method was used with entry criteria of $P \leq 0.05$ and retention criteria of $P \leq 0.2$. In the results for the regression analysis, the ratios of odds ratios (RORs) are reported for interactions. The RORs is an estimate derived from dividing one odds ratio (OR) by another (i.e., OR X/OR Y) when calculating the interaction of one factor with another. In the logistic regression models, the ROR is the exponent of the beta of the two-way interaction term. For example, variable X has OR of 50 and variable Y has OR of 100; both ORs are larger than the neutral value of 1. The ratio of OR X/OR Y is 50/100, or 0.5; this ROR is smaller than 1; however, having an ROR less than 1 does not mean the interaction of variables X and Y has led to a decrease in the odds of having the outcome.

## Results

A total of 16,558 patients newly diagnosed with AD were identified, and of these, 16,494 patients were matched with 49,482 patients in the matched cohort (with no AD or dementia-related diagnoses). Patients in both cohorts were 79.9 [standard deviation (SD) 6.1] years old, with a higher proportion of women (59.4%), and of white race (84.1%, Table 1). The majority of patients were enrolled in MAPD (~ 99%), and the average length of pre-index enrollment was 68.9 (SD 19.4) months.

Sociodemographically (Table 1), the AD cohort was from communities with fewer white-collar, employed professionals. Based on behavior segmentation, a larger proportion of the AD cohort was classified as having chronic disease (53.3% vs. 37.1%), compared with the matched cohort, and the patterns of behavior regarding their healthcare varied within the classifications of Healthy and Chronic. An index diagnosis for AD was made by the primary care physician in 35.1% of the patients and 77.5% of patients had multiple visits to the index physician prior to index date. The average time between the two claims for AD was 92 [SD 125] days.

A significantly higher proportion of the matched cohort had a claim for an annual wellness visit compared to the AD cohort (35.0% vs. 29.5%, $P < 0.001$, Table 2), but a greater proportion of the AD cohort had cognitive assessments (2.6% vs. 0.2%, $P < 0.001$, Table 2). The majority of patients in the AD cohort (64.0%) had filled a prescription for at least one AD medication during the pre-index period.

The AD cohort had significantly higher DCCI scores (3.8 vs. 3.0, $P < 0.001$) and RxRisk-V Scores (9.8 vs. 8.3, $P < 0.001$) than the matched cohort (Table 2), indicating a higher comorbidity burden. Among the pre-specified

**Table 1** Demographic, socioeconomic and behavioral characteristics of Alzheimer's disease and matched cohorts

| Characteristic | AD | Matched Cohort (no AD or dementia) | P value* |
|---|---|---|---|
| N | 16,494 | 49,482 | – |
| Age in years, mean [SD] | 79.9 [6.1] | 79.9 [6.1] | 0.830 |
| Gender, n (%) | | | |
| Female | 9800 (59.4) | 29,400 (59.4) | 1.000 |
| Male | 6694 (40.6) | 20,082 (40.6) | |
| Race/ Ethnicity, n (%) | | | |
| White | 13,879 (84.1) | 41,637 (84.1) | 1.000 |
| Black | 1970 (11.9) | 5910 (11.9) | |
| Hispanic | 317 (1.9) | 951 (1.9) | |
| Other | 328 (1.9) | 984 (1.9) | |
| Geographic Region, n (%) | | | |
| Northeast | 328 (1.9) | 1081 (2.2) | < 0.001 |
| Midwest | 4080 (24.7) | 13,227 (26.7) | |
| South | 10,859 (65.8) | 30,862 (62.4) | |
| West | 1227 (7.4) | 4312 (8.7) | |
| Plan Type, n (%) | | | |
| MAPD | 16,391 (99.4) | 48,923 (98.9) | < 0.001 |
| Commercial | 103 (0.6) | 559 (1.1) | |
| Plan Characteristics (MAPD), n (%) | | | |
| Low Income Subsidy Status Only | 2566 (15.5) | 4531 (9.1) | < 0.001 |
| Dual Eligibility (Medicare and Medicaid) Only | 32 (0.2) | 61 (0.1) | 0.030 |
| Length of Pre-index Enrollment – mean [SD] | 68.9 [19.4] | 68.9 [19.4] | 0.980 |
| Estimated Household Income, n (%) | | | |
| < $15,000 | 3465 (21.0) | 10,748 (21.7) | 0.003 |
| $15,000–$29,999 | 2589 (15.7) | 7948 (16.0) | |
| $30,000–$49,999 | 3433 (20.8) | 10,467 (21.1) | |
| $50,000–$99,999 | 3749 (22.7) | 12,250 (24.7) | |
| > =$100,000* | 1084 (6.6) | 3757 (7.6) | |
| Unknown | 2174 (13.2) | 4312 (8.7) | |
| Census 2010 Percent Blue Collar Employed, n (%) | | | |
| 0–14% | 2940 (17.8) | 10,086 (20.3) | < 0.001 |
| 15–20% | 2802 (16.9) | 9361 (18.9) | |
| 21–26% | 3077 (18.6) | 9765 (19.7) | |
| 27–33% | 3030 (18.4) | 8846 (17.8) | |
| 34–99% | 2471 (14.9) | 7112 (14.3) | |
| Unknown | 2174 (13.2) | 4312 (8.7) | |
| Census 2010 Percent White Collar Employed, n (%) | | | < 0.001 |
| 0–48% | 3149 (19.1) | 9305 (18.8) | |
| 49–56% | 3167 (19.2) | 9505 (19.2) | |
| 57–64% | 2981 (18.1) | 9620 (19.4) | |
| 65–74% | 2875 (17.4) | 9406 (19.0) | |
| 75–99% | 2148 (13.0) | 7334 (14.8) | |
| Unknown | 2174 (13.2) | 4312 (8.7) | |

Retrospective assessment of patient characteristics and healthcare costs prior to a diagnosis...

15

**Table 1** Demographic, socioeconomic and behavioral characteristics of Alzheimer's disease and matched cohorts *(Continued)*

| Characteristic | AD | Matched Cohort (no AD or dementia) | P value* |
|---|---|---|---|
| Index AD diagnosing Provider, n (%) (*N* = 16,558) | | | |
|   Primary Care | 5800 (35.1) | | |
|   Geriatrics | 526 (3.2) | | |
|   Neurology | 2225 (13.5) | | |
|   Psychiatry | 813 (4.9) | | |
|   Psychology | 240 (1.5) | | |
|   Other | 6906 (41.8) | | |
| Multiple Visits to Index AD-diagnosing provider | 12,838 (77.5) | | |
| Only one Visit to Index AD-diagnosing provider | 3720 (22.5) | | |
| Time between first and second claim with AD diagnosis | Average: 92 days SD: 125 Median: 34 days | | |

Abbreviations: *AD* Alzheimer's disease, *MAPD* Medicare Advantage Prescription Drug, *SD* Standard deviation
Cohorts were matched on age, gender, race and length of pre-index enrollment
¥ Categories were merged; *Chi square test used for categorical variables; Wilcoxon rank sum test used for continuous variables; Significance level set at *P* < 0.05
Please note that for identifying most commonly seen provider were identified prior to matching (*N* = 16,558) and we have identified only outpatient visits. The index diagnoses for 35 patients were not at an outpatient facility. The specialties of 15.7% of the index AD-diagnosing providers were unknown because the specialty data were missing from the claims database

comorbidities evaluated, hypertension, dyslipidemia, and other forms of heart disease were the most prevalent in both cohorts (Table 3). Other pre-specified comorbidities with notable differences each occurring more frequently in the AD cohort included mood disorders (+ 22.3% difference), cerebrovascular disease (+ 20.5% difference), urinary tract infection (+ 14.8% difference), anxiety disorder (+ 11.4% difference), and MCI (+ 10.5% difference).

When comparing the average pre-index HCRU (Fig. 2) the number of outpatient visits, hospitalizations, and ED visits at 6-month intervals were similar between the cohorts until six months prior to the index date. For the AD cohort, the number of these visits increased during the six months prior to the index date. A similar trend was observed for healthcare costs, with an increase in mean and median medical costs for the AD cohort occurring during the – 6-month interval prior to the index

date (Fig. 3). During this time period, the average total healthcare cost per person was significantly higher for the AD cohort than for the matched cohort ($10,054 vs. $4833, *P* < 0.0001).

Using the CART analysis, up to 67 potential predictors of an AD diagnosis were evaluated, and the top 15 variables by importance were identified for inclusion in the logistic regression model (Fig. 4). From the tree, we see that use of AD medication is the most important predictor of an AD diagnosis and that an MCI or behavioral disturbance diagnosis, presence of an emergency department visit, and patient age provided additional information to classify patients as likely to receive an AD diagnosis. Due to its size, only the first part of the full tree is illustrated. The model showed excellent specificity (97%) and acceptable sensitivity (77%), and the overall area under the curve was 0.917. The 15 top performing variables and their

**Table 2** Clinical characteristics of Alzheimer's disease and matched cohorts

| | AD (*n* = 16,494) | | Matched Cohort (No AD or Dementia) (*n* = 49,482) | | P value* |
|---|---|---|---|---|---|
| | Mean [SD] | Median | Mean [SD] | Median | |
| Deyo Charlson Comorbidity Index | 3.8 [3.0] | 3.0 | 3.0 [2.9] | 2.0 | < 0.001 |
| RxRisk-V Score | 9.8 [4.0] | 10.0 | 8.3 [3.7] | 8.0 | < 0.001 |
| Number of Unique Medications Used (Drug Classes) | 22.0 [14.0] | 20.0 | 18.2[10.7] | 17.0 | |
| Wellness Visit and Assessments, n (%) | | | | | |
|   Annual Medicare Wellness Visit | 4832 (29.5) | | 17,132 (35.0) | | < 0.001 |
|   Cognitive Assessment | 435 (2.6) | | 114 (0.2) | | < 0.001 |
| AD medication use at baseline | 10,559 (64.0) | | 884 (1.8) | | |

Abbreviations: *AD* Alzheimer's disease, *MCI* Mild Cognitive Impairment, *SD* Standard deviation
RxRisk-V Score was calculated for those with at least one prescription
*Chi square test used for categorical variables; Wilcoxon rank sum test used for continuous variables; Significance level set at *P* < 0.05

**Table 3** Prevalence of pre-specified comorbidities for Alzheimer's disease and matched cohorts

| Comorbidity, n (%) | AD (n = 16,494) | Matched Cohort (No AD or Dementia) (n = 49,482) | P value* |
|---|---|---|---|
| Hypertension | 14,816 (89.8) | 43,198 (87.4) | < 0.001 |
| Dyslipidemia | 13,951 (84.6) | 41,824 (84.6) | 0.986 |
| Other forms of heart disease | 9434 (57.2) | 23,597 (47.7) | < 0.001 |
| Osteoarthritis | 8372 (50.8) | 23,389 (47.3) | < 0.001 |
| Urinary tract infection | 8146 (49.4) | 17,096 (34.6) | < 0.001 |
| Cerebrovascular disease | 7207 (43.7) | 11,479 (23.2) | < 0.001 |
| Ischemic heart disease | 6963 (42.2) | 17,841 (36.1) | < 0.001 |
| Diabetes | 6866 (41.6) | 18,698 (37.8) | < 0.001 |
| Mood disorder | 6483 (39.3) | 8391 (17.0) | < 0.001 |
| Osteoporosis | 5788 (35.1) | 16,325 (33.0) | < 0.001 |
| Any chronic obstructive pulmonary disease | 5728 (34.7) | 15,405 (31.2) | < 0.001 |
| Acute respiratory infection | 5137 (31.1) | 16,576 (33.5) | < 0.001 |
| Cancer | 4390 (26.6) | 14,271 (28.9) | < 0.001 |
| Anxiety disorder | 4356 (26.4) | 7428 (15.0) | < 0.001 |
| Heart failure | 3957 (24.0) | 8907 (18.0) | < 0.001 |
| Peripheral vascular disease | 3547 (21.5) | 8155 (16.5) | < 0.001 |
| Atherosclerosis | 3435 (20.8) | 8615 (17.4) | < 0.001 |
| Pneumonia | 2931 (17.8) | 5506 (11.1) | < 0.001 |
| Insomnia | 2132 (12.9) | 4704 (9.5) | < 0.001 |
| Mild Cognitive Impairment | 1727 (10.5) | 0 (0.0) | < 0.001 |
| Diseases of pulmonary circulation | 1689 (10.2) | 4248 (8.6) | < 0.001 |
| Chronic ulcer of skin | 1505 (9.1) | 2486 (5.0) | < 0.001 |
| Behavioral disturbance | 1369 (8.3) | 0 (0.0) | < 0.001 |
| Venous Thromboembolism | 969 (5.9) | 1999 (4.0) | < 0.001 |
| Parkinson's disease | 872 (5.3) | 568 (1.1) | < 0.001 |
| Gastric, duodenal, peptic, or gastrojejunal ulcer | 854 (5.2) | 1710 (3.5) | < 0.001 |
| Epilepsy | 845 (5.1) | 688 (1.4) | < 0.001 |
| Rheumatoid arthritis | 771 (4.7) | 2155 (4.4) | 0.087 |
| Lung cancer | 233 (1.4) | 720 (1.5) | 0.686 |

Abbreviations: *AD* Alzheimer's disease, *MCI* Mild Cognitive Impairment
*Chi square test used; Significance level set at P < 0.05

interactions were used to run a logistic regression model (Fig. 5, Additional file 1: Table S1).

The results of the logistic regression analysis (Additional file 1: Table S1) showed AD medication use had the greatest association with increased likelihood of AD diagnosis (OR = 161.157, P < 0.001) followed by the presence of comorbidities such as MCI (OR = 111.626, P < 0.001), Parkinson's disease (OR = 10.081, P < 0.001), mood disorder (OR = 3.083, P < 0.001), cerebrovascular disease (OR = 1.856, P = 0.007), and/or a urinary tract infection (UTI, OR = 1.246, P < 0.001) and ED visits (OR = 1.131, P < 0.001).

Although there were significant two-way interactions involving AD medication use, ED visit, and mood disorder, estimates at the mean values and distinct categories of interacting variables with these terms were

consistently significant and greater than one. Similarly, odds ratios for Parkinson's disease were consistently greater than one and 5 of the 8 were statistically significant. Thus, the direction of main effects related to AD medication use, ED visit, mood disorder, and Parkinson's disease can be interpreted. There were no significant two-way interactions with MCI or UTI, facilitating the interpretation of these effects.

The main effect of cerebrovascular disease is not interpretable due to significant two-way interactions and odds ratios that varied in direction. Specifically, the presence of a cerebrovascular disease diagnosis indicated lower likelihood of an AD diagnosis in patients with a cognitive assessment as part of the annual wellness visit (3 of 4 odds ratios significant). Conversely, among

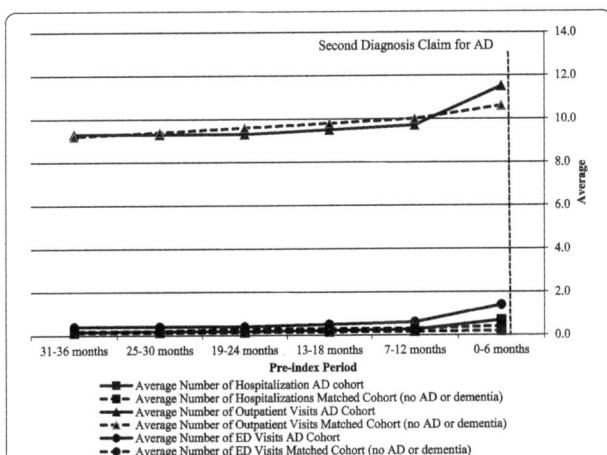

**Fig. 2** Trends in healthcare resource use per person at six-month intervals for AD and matched cohorts. Abbreviations: AD-Alzheimer's disease, ED-Emergency department

patients who did not have a cognitive assessment as part of the annual wellness visit, the cerebrovascular diagnosis indicated a greater likelihood of AD diagnosis (3 of 4 odds ratios significant).

Increasing age (OR = 0.937, $P < 0.001$) decreased the odds of being diagnosed with AD, but this finding should

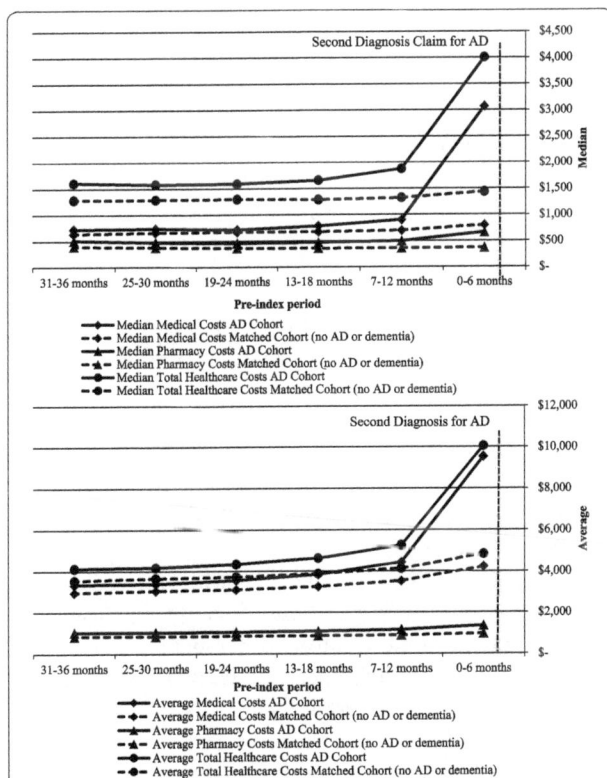

**Fig. 3** Title: Trends in healthcare cost per person at six-month intervals for AD and matched (No AD or Dementia) cohorts (Adjusted to 2015 dollars). Abbreviations: AD – Alzheimer's disease

be interpreted with caution as the AD and matched cohorts were matched on age. Additionally, there were significant two way interactions between age and Parkinson's disease, and between age and cerebrovascular disease. When examining the 96 odds ratios involving age and combinations of values for each of AD Medication use, mood disorder, cerebrovascular disorder, Parkinson's disease, and income, the majority are significant, 71 were less than one, indicating increased age was associated with lower likelihood of AD and 6 were less than 1. The patient subgroups in which increased age was associated with greater likelihood of AD were those who had not received AD medications and did not have a diagnosis of mood disorder, cerebrovascular disease or Parkinson's disease and this OR was significant in four of the 6 income categories. The other subgroups in which increased age was associated with greater likelihood of AD were those in the upper two income categories who had not received AD medications, did not have a diagnosis of mood disorder or Parkinson's disease but did have a cerebrovascular diagnosis.

## Discussion

With our study's longer duration of time to observe patients' engagement with the healthcare system, we were able to add to the existing understanding of a patients' journey prior to confirmatory AD diagnosis. Our study results significantly add to existing literature as the sample of 16,494 patients with a confirmatory diagnosis of AD is notable in terms of its longevity; the median duration of the pre-index period for the AD and matched cohorts was 72 months. In contrast, similar studies by Lin et al. (2016) [11] observed patients 24 months before and after their AD diagnosis, and Gilden et al. (2015) [6] required 12 months of data prior to and following AD diagnosis.

Over a third of the sample received their confirmatory AD diagnosis in the primary care setting, in comparison to less than one fourth receiving this diagnosis from a geriatric or mental health specialist. Also, we found that almost two-thirds of the AD patients received AD-related medications prior to their confirmatory diagnosis, and only 10% of patients in the AD group received an MCI diagnosis prior to their confirmatory diagnosis, all of which may suggest a reluctance to diagnose memory related issues [19]. Some factors that may contribute to the reluctance to make a diagnosis of AD include physician's decision not to create or increase the emotional stress of a patient. Alternatively, reluctance to make a diagnosis of AD may be reflective of insufficient training or time to confidently make a diagnosis through appropriate assessments resulting in a delayed diagnosis, especially given the ongoing challenge to diagnose based on exclusions [19, 20]. Without a biomarker or pathognomonic test, the diagnosis is always going to be somewhat questionable.

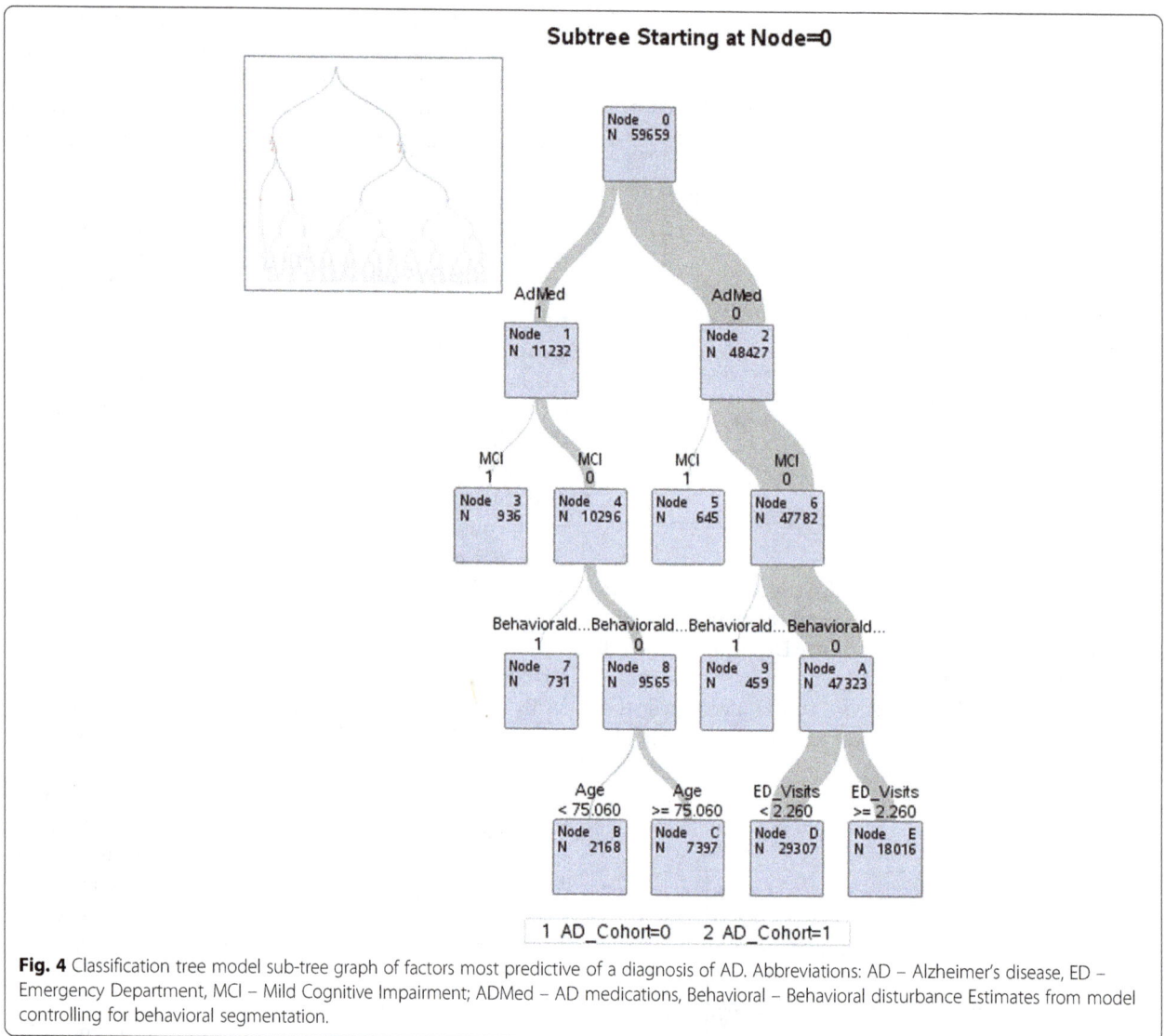

**Fig. 4** Classification tree model sub-tree graph of factors most predictive of a diagnosis of AD. Abbreviations: AD – Alzheimer's disease, ED – Emergency Department, MCI – Mild Cognitive Impairment; ADMed – AD medications, Behavioral – Behavioral disturbance Estimates from model controlling for behavioral segmentation.

The AD cohort was generally in poorer health than the matched cohort, which was reflected in the significantly higher comorbidity indices and greater odds of comorbid mental and behavioral diagnoses, cerebrovascular disease, and other diseases such as heart disease, UTIs, and pneumonia. This is a similar clinical profile to that observed in the post-index follow-up period by Suehs et al. (2013) [9], with exception of MCI and behavioral disturbance, which were not examined. The presence of various comorbidities in patients with AD highlights the importance that treatment plans for such patients should not be only focused on the expected cognitive decline, but should warrant a multidisciplinary approach to routinely assess for comorbid conditions.

Consistent with other administrative claims studies examining HCRU and cost in the year prior to the first AD diagnosis, [8, 9] this study showed that HCRU for patients with AD was significantly higher than that for the matched cohort. Similarly, Lin and others demonstrated that for patients with AD-RD, from the 5% Medicare sample, HCRU was greater than the control population during the 24 months prior to their first diagnosis, particularly during the most proximal 12 months [11]. This was driven by inpatient, home health, and post-acute care, with virtually no difference in outpatient or physician office visits. In contrast, a prospective study by Zhu et al (2015), [21] that included Medicare beneficiaries who received clinical evaluations for AD every 18 months, found significant differences only in home health and durable medical equipment use. Observed differences in HCRU in these studies could be due to case ascertainment (AD-RD, AD by clinical evaluation, or AD determined based on the presence of two ICD-9 codes), specific study population evaluated (MAPD, a multi-ethnic cohort from northern Manhattan, FFS Medicare), or changes in the approach to medical care of elderly patients over time.

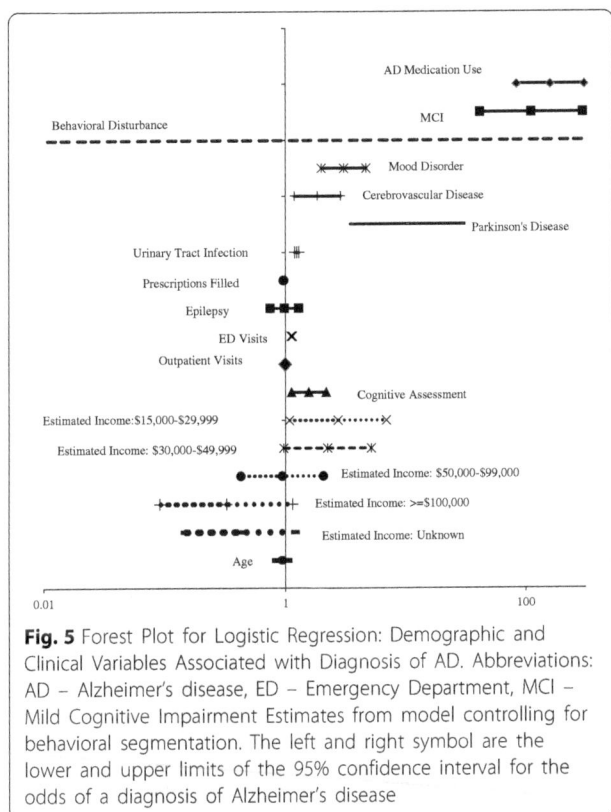

**Fig. 5** Forest Plot for Logistic Regression: Demographic and Clinical Variables Associated with Diagnosis of AD. Abbreviations: AD – Alzheimer's disease, ED – Emergency Department, MCI – Mild Cognitive Impairment Estimates from model controlling for behavioral segmentation. The left and right symbol are the lower and upper limits of the 95% confidence interval for the odds of a diagnosis of Alzheimer's disease

three physician claims separated by 30 days or more in the same 24-month period. The sensitivity and positive predictive value of the algorithm was improved by inclusion of a prescription for a cholinesterase inhibitor. In the CART model, which had good sensitivity and higher specificity, AD medication use, diagnosis of MCI, Parkinson's disease, and a mood disorder were the strongest predictors of an AD diagnosis.

In extending the interpretation of AD medication use by exploring their interactions with other predictors, we found that the magnitude of association of AD medication use with an AD diagnosis varied, depending on whether patients also had cerebrovascular disease, Parkinson's disease, mood disorder, or UTI. The odds of AD diagnosis associated with AD medication use was uniformly lower in the subgroups of patients with Parkinson's disease, UTI, mood disorder or cerebrovascular disease in comparison to patients who were similar on all variables but that particular diagnosis. The predictor of AD medication use may reflect physician and/or patient preference to treat with symptomatic medication prior to receiving a definitive diagnosis, [6] while the most important psychiatric and neurological diagnoses likely reflect disease progression.

The current study's findings should be interpreted in the light of the following limitations. Characteristic of retrospective, claims-based research, the results may have been influenced by missing data, potential errors in coding, and unmeasured factors, such as psychosocial variables and other clinical variables. In addition, there is an established, multi-factorial gap in diagnosis and observance of AD symptoms. Furthermore, the commonality of the identified comorbidities in the non-AD population may limit the ability to use these as screening measures for potential AD. This study focused on patients with a confirmatory diagnosis for AD and did not include undiagnosed patients or those with only one claim for AD diagnosis. The index date for this study was the confirmatory diagnosis of AD, which meant the costs would include the assessment and other AD-related costs from the first diagnosis of AD. Despite this, our findings are consistent with that of Lin et al., who evaluated costs prior to diagnosis of AD [11]. Additionally, data in this study were obtained from a single health insurance company, and although Humana is a large national health plan with members from various geographic regions, the results may not be generalizable to the overall U.S. population, or to subpopulations within certain geographic regions of the U.S. Moreover, the results may not be generalizable to all Medicare populations due to differences in benefit structure of MAPD and non-MAPD health plans. The matching criteria used in the current study, as well as the method for selecting the

In our study, the total average cost for patients at six months prior to AD diagnosis was greater ($5221 in 2015 dollars) than for the matched cohort. One plausible explanation for this difference may be related to the comorbidity burden. Matching between the AD cohort and the non-AD or dementia cohort was not based on comorbidity, which allowed for a better understanding of the relative comorbidity differences across the cohorts. Additionally, costs associated with the subsequent AD diagnosis are also contributory to the difference. In comparison, the study by Lin et al. identified individuals on the basis of their first recorded AD-RD diagnosis code and found the difference in average pre-diagnosis costs in the six months prior to index was $3571 (in 2014 dollars) [11]. The comparison of AD-RD to control subjects in the 5% Medicare sample included comorbidity in the identification of the matched cohort, supporting the premise that additional costs are incurred as a result of a subsequent AD diagnosis [11].

Our analysis of examining potential predictors of AD is similar to the findings of the study by Jaakkimainen et al. (2016), [5] which showed that the best performing algorithm in Canadian administrative claims data from primary care practices was either a hospitalization or

AD cohort, may be considered as additional study limitations. We matched the population only on demographic characteristics and not clinical characteristics such as comorbidities. This was so that we can understand the differences in comorbidities between patients, however, these comorbidities may have contributed to increases in healthcare resource use and costs. Additionally, we used second date of claim for AD as index date as opposed to the first. Healthcare resource and costs since the first visit with a claim of AD may have contributed to the increases observed during the six months prior to the second claim with AD. However, in some sensitivity analyses conducted (not shown), the results did not change when first claim for AD was set as index date.

As an administrative claims study, we are only able to associate healthcare resource use with different cohorts defined by diagnostic codes. In the current study, our intent was to understand the total healthcare resource use, so we did not limit to claims specifically related to AD. Other types of observational research that include reason for cost are needed to understand if these increased costs are due to AD.

## Conclusion

Given the growing elderly population and the concomitant increases in prevalence of AD and associated cost of care, it is important to understand the patients' journey to diagnosis of this disease.

This study demonstrated that prior to the diagnosis of AD, patients had a higher number of comorbidities and incurred higher costs in comparison to a demographically matched cohort. Certain comorbidities that occurred at a higher rate in the AD cohort, namely psychiatric and neurological in nature, may serve as flags to help identify patients most likely to develop AD using administrative claims data. We observed a trend of increasing healthcare costs during the 6-month period prior to the confirmatory diagnosis of AD, offering yet another potential signal that can be gleaned from administrative claims data.

Without a biomarker or a test to detect AD, diagnosis is challenging, since it is essentially a diagnosis of exclusion. This suggests that AD is underdiagnosed, and the true impact of this disease may be greater than what the current study reports. With the pipeline of AD drug development aimed at disease modification, additional research is needed to further understand other clinical presentations that might potentially predict diagnosis of AD more robustly or even earlier than the 36-month-year period used in this study. Furthermore, with early recognition of AD, a better understanding of the stage of illness at which patients are diagnosed with AD, along with these early predictors, can help guide the treatment pathway.

## Abbreviations

AD: Alzheimer's Disease; AD-RD: Alzheimer's Disease and Related Dementias; CART: Classification and Regression Tree; DCCI: Deyo Charlson Comorbidity Index; ED: Emergency Department; FFS: Medicare Fee for Service; HCRU: Healthcare Resource Utilization; ICD-9-CM: International Statistical Classification of Diseases, Ninth Revision, Clinical Modification; KBM: Knowledge Base Management; MAPD: Medicare Advantage with Prescription Drug Coverage; MCI: Mild Cognitive Impairment; NMDA: N-methyl-D-aspartate; RORs: Ratios of Odds Ratios; SD: Standard Deviation; UTI: Urinary Tract Infection

## Acknowledgements

The authors would like to acknowledge Mary Costantino, PhD for her editorial support.

## Funding

This study was funded by Eli Lilly and Company. Employees of Eli Lilly and Company who coauthored this manuscript collaborated in the design of the study, in the interpretation of data, and in writing the manuscript.

## Authors' contributions

Authors RN, VH, MS, NP, AF, DVA, MW, AD, LHF, VS, and DB were involved in the study design and interpretation. VS extracted data and MS analyzed the data. RN and VH were major contributors in writing the manuscript. Authors RN, VH, MS, NP, AF, DVA, MW, AD, LHF, VS, and DB reviewed, provided significant contributions and approved the final manuscript.

## Competing interests

○ Virginia S. Haynes, Adam S. Fleisher, Michael Witte, AnnCatherine Downing, are full-time employees and stockholders of Eli Lilly and Company.
○ Daniel E. Ball is a stockholder of Eli Lilly and Company.
○ Radhika Nair and Nick Patel are employees of Comprehensive Health Insights, Humana Inc., which received funding and Sponsorship from Eli Lilly and Humana to conduct this study.
○ Vishal Saundankar, Mir Siadaty, and Leslie Hazel-Fernandez, were employees of Comprehensive Health Insights, Humana Inc. at the time of the study.
○ Daniel E. Ball was an employee of Eli Lilly and Company at the time of the study.

## Author details

¹Comprehensive Health Insights, Louisville, USA. ²Eli Lilly and Company, Indianapolis, USA. ³Humana Inc., Louisville, USA. ⁴Lilly Corporate Center, Drop Code 1730, Indianapolis, IN 46285, USA.

## References

1. 2016 Alzheimer's disease facts and figures. Alzheimer's & dementia : the journal of the Alzheimer's Association 2016, 12(4):459–509.
2. Dubois B, Feldman HH, Jacova C, Cummings JL, Dekosky ST, Barberger-Gateau P, Delacourte A, Frisoni G, Fox NC, Galasko D, et al. Revising the definition of Alzheimer's disease: a new lexicon. The Lancet Neurology. 2010;9(11):1118–27.
3. Sperling RA, Aisen PS, Beckett LA, Bennett DA, Craft S, Fagan AM, Iwatsubo T, Jack CR Jr, Kaye J, Montine TJ, et al. Toward defining the preclinical stages of Alzheimer's disease: recommendations from the National Institute on Aging-Alzheimer's Association workgroups on diagnostic guidelines for Alzheimer's disease. Alzheimer's & dementia : the journal of the Alzheimer's Association. 2011;7(3):280–92.
4. Roberts RO, Geda YE, Knopman DS, Cha RH, Pankratz VS, Boeve BF, Tangalos EG, Ivnik RJ, Rocca WA, Petersen RC. The incidence of MCI differs by subtype and is higher in men: the Mayo Clinic study of aging. Neurology. 2012;78(5):342–51.
5. Jaakkimainen RL, Bronskill SE, Tierney MC, Herrmann N, Green D, Young J, Ivers N, Butt D, Widdifield J, Tu K. Identification of physician-diagnosed Alzheimer's disease and related dementias in population-based

Retrospective assessment of patient characteristics and healthcare costs prior to a diagnosis...

21

administrative data: a validation study using family physicians' electronic medical records. Journal of Alzheimer's disease: JAD. 2016;54(1):337–49.

6. Gilden DM, Kubisiak JM, Sarsour K, Hunter CA. Diagnostic pathways to Alzheimer disease: costs incurred in a Medicare population. Alzheimer Dis Assoc Disord. 2015;29(4):330–7.

7. Geldmacher DS, Kirson NY, Birnbaum HG, Eapen S, Kantor E, Cummings AK, Joish VN. Pre-diagnosis excess acute care costs in Alzheimer's patients among a US Medicaid population. Applied health economics and health policy. 2013;11(4):407–13.

8. Frytak JR, Henk HJ, Zhao Y, Bowman L, Flynn JA, Nelson M. Health service utilization among Alzheimer's disease patients: evidence from managed care. Alzheimer's & dementia : the journal of the Alzheimer's Association. 2008;4(5):361–7.

9. Suehs BT, Davis CD, Alvir J, van Amerongen D, Patel NC, Joshi AV, Faison WE, Shah SN. The clinical and economic burden of newly diagnosed Alzheimer's disease in a medicare advantage population. American journal of Alzheimer's disease and other dementias. 2013;28(4):384–92.

10. Suehs BT, Shah SN, Davis CD, Alvir J, Faison WE, Patel NC, van Amerongen D, Bobula J. Household members of persons with Alzheimer's disease: health conditions, healthcare resource use, and healthcare costs. J Am Geriatr Soc. 2014;62(3):435–41.

11. Lin PJ, Zhong Y, Fillit HM, Chen E, Neumann PJ. Medicare expenditures of individuals with Alzheimer's disease and related dementias or mild cognitive impairment before and after diagnosis. J Am Geriatr Soc. 2016; 64(8):1549–57.

12. What is Medicare Advantage. [https://www.medicare.gov/Pubs/pdf/11474.pdf].

13. Deyo RA, Cherkin DC, Ciol MA. Adapting a clinical comorbidity index for use with ICD-9-CM administrative databases. J Clin Epidemiol. 1992;45(6):613–9.

14. Klabunde CN, Potosky AL, Legler JM, Warren JL. Development of a comorbidity index using physician claims data. J Clin Epidemiol. 2000;53(12): 1258–67.

15. Quan H, Parsons GA, Ghali WA. Validity of information on comorbidity derived from ICD-9-CCM administrative data. Med Care. 2002;40(8):675–85.

16. Sloan KL, Sales AE, Liu CF, Fishman P, Nichol P, Suzuki NT, Sharp ND. Construction and characteristics of the RxRisk-V: a VA-adapted pharmacy-based case-mix instrument. Med Care. 2003;41(6):761–74.

17. Faries DE, Chen Y, Lipkovich I, Zagar A, Liu X, Obenchain RL. Local control for identifying subgroups of interest in observational research: persistence of treatment for major depressive disorder. Int J Methods Psychiatr Res. 2013;22(3):185–94.

18. Morgan J. Classification and regression tree analysis (technical report 1). In.: Boston University School of Public Health. Department of Health Policy & Management.

19. Lang L, Clifford A, Wei L, Zhang D, Leung D, Augustine G, Danat IM, Zhou W, Copeland JR, Anstey KJ, et al. Prevalence and determinants of undetected dementia in the community: a systematic literature review and a meta-analysis. BMJ Open. 2017;7(2):e011146.

20. Dubois B, Padovani A, Scheltens P, Rossi A, Dell'Agnello G. Timely diagnosis for Alzheimer's disease: a literature review on benefits and challenges. Journal of Alzheimer's disease : JAD. 2016;49(3):617–31.

21. Zhu CW, Cosentino S, Ornstein K, Gu Y, Scarmeas N, Andrews H, Stern Y. Medicare utilization and expenditures around incident dementia in a multiethnic cohort. J Gerontol A Biol Sci Med Sci. 2015;70(11):1448–53.

# 3

# Relationship of muscle function to circulating myostatin, follistatin and GDF11 in older women and men

Elizaveta Fife[1][*] ⓘ, Joanna Kostka[1,2], Łukasz Kroc[1], Agnieszka Guligowska[1], Małgorzata Pigłowska[1], Bartłomiej Sołtysik[1], Agnieszka Kaufman-Szymczyk[3], Krystyna Fabianowska-Majewska[3] and Tomasz Kostka[1]

## Abstract

**Background:** Myostatin, its inhibitor follistatin, and growth/differentiation factor 11 (GDF11) have been proposed as factors that could potentially modify biological aging. The study aimed to test whether there is a relationship between these plasma circulating proteins and muscle strength, power and optimal shortening velocity ($\upsilon_{opt}$) of older adults.

**Methods:** The cross-sectional study included 56 women and 45 men aged 60 years and older. Every participant underwent examination which included anthropometric and bioimpedance analysis measurements, functional and cognitive performance tests, muscle strength of upper and lower extremities, muscle power testing with two different methods and blood analyses.

**Results:** Women had higher plasma levels of myostatin and GDF11 than men. Men had higher plasma level of follistatin than women. In women, plasma level of myostatin was negatively correlated with left handgrip strength and $\upsilon_{opt}$. Follistatin was negatively correlated with maximum power output ($P_{max}$), power relative to kg of body mass ($P_{max} \cdot kg^{-1}$) (friction-loaded cycle ergometer) and power at 70% of the 1-repetition maximum (1RM) strength value (P70%) of leg press (Keiser pneumatic resistance training equipment), and positively correlated with the Timed Up & Go (TUG) test. GDF11 was negatively correlated with body mass, body mass index, waist circumference, fat mass and the percentage of body fat. In men, there were no significant correlations observed between circulating plasma proteins and muscle function measures.

**Conclusions:** The circulating plasma myostatin and follistatin are negatively associated with muscle function in older women. There is stronger relationship between these proteins and muscle power than muscle strength. GDF11 has a higher association with the body mass and composition than muscle function in older women.

**Keywords:** Functional performance, Sarcopenia, Quadriceps muscle power, Optimal shortening velocity, Aging

## Background

Population aging is transforming the world significantly. It is undeniable that the patient's age is a primary risk factor for sarcopenia, frailty and disability. In recent years, there are various attempts by different research groups to figure out the nature of that link. Those efforts included the search for the circulating blood factors that could be identified as biomarkers of aging [1]. Myostatin, its inhibitor follistatin, and growth/differentiation factor 11 (GDF11) have been proposed as such factors that could potentially modify biological age [2, 3].

Myostatin is a strong negative regulator of skeletal muscle development and size [4]. It is a member of the transforming growth factor-β (TGFβ) family, acting through the activin type II A and B receptors. It is highly expressed in skeletal muscle, but also present in adipose tissue and cardiac muscle [5]. Follistatin is a glycosylated plasma protein, a member of the TGFβ family [6]. It is abundant in different tissues such as placenta, ovary, testis and skeletal muscles. It inhibits myostatin from

---
* Correspondence: elizaveta.fife@umed.lodz.pl; elizavetafife@gmail.com
[1]Department of Geriatrics, Healthy Ageing Research Centre, Medical University of Lodz, ul. Pieniny 30, 91-647 Łódź, Poland
Full list of author information is available at the end of the article

binding to the activin type II B; therefore, neutralizing it in circulation [7]. GDF11 is strongly related to myostatin, also a member of the TGFβ family [8]. It is expressed in the pancreas, intestine, kidney, skeletal muscle, and nervous system [9]. In recent years, GDF11 has been described as a circulating age-associated factor with different proposed roles [1].

The changes in the body composition that occur with aging can negatively affect daily functioning and health status of older people. Loss of strength and skeletal muscle mass have been identified as prime risk factors for falls and impaired mobility in older people [10]. Falls are frequent reason for the emergency department visits of older adults [11]. Skeletal muscle strength is identified as the maximum capacity to develop force [12]. It is associated with activities of daily living and mobility [13]. Muscle power is defined as the ability to exert force as fast as possible [14]. Muscle power and contraction velocity are strong independent predictors of functional performance such as gait speed, chair-rise time, and stair-climb time in older adults [15–17]. Muscle power is also associated with dynamic balance and postural sway. It is thought to be a better predictor of fall risk than muscle strength [18].

In available literature, there are no records of studies that would consider all three mentioned above proteins and their relationship to those measures of muscle function. Therefore, the main aim of the study was to test whether there is a relationship between circulating myostatin, follistatin and GDF11, with muscle strength, power and optimal shortening velocity ($v_{opt}$) of older adults.

## Methods

### Participants

One-hundred and six subjects were consecutively recruited between October 2015 and May 2016 for the study through the local newspapers' advertisements. To be eligible, subjects needed to be 60 years and older, community dwelling, able to understand and execute commands, and willing to participate and give blood samples. Exclusion criteria included: acute illness, unstable cardiovascular or metabolic disease, myocardial infarction in the past 6 months, upper or lower limb amputation, neuromuscular and musculoskeletal disorders disrupting the voluntary movements, and cognitive impairment. Out of those 106, 5 subjects were excluded due to the contraindications to muscle power testing. Therefore, 101 participants, all of them Caucasian, were finally included to the study. The average number of chronic illnesses was $2.9 \pm 1.9$. Fifteen participants (14.9%) were diagnosed with coronary heart disease, 13 (12.9%) had chronic heart failure, seven (6.9%) suffered from stroke, 10 (9.9%) had chronic pulmonary disease,

19 (18.8%) had gastrointestinal disease, and 8 (7.9%) had history of cancer. Fifty-three participants (52%) were treated for hypertension, 55 (54%) for hypercholesterolemia, and 19 (18.8%) for diabetes mellitus type 2. Osteoarthritis was diagnosed in 36 subjects (35.6%) and 19 (18.8%) had osteoporosis. Each participant signed written informed consent, which was an obligatory requirement for the study participation. The Medical University of Lodz Ethics Committee approved this study.

### Protocol

The examination lasted approximately 4 h per patient. It was performed in the Geriatric Outpatient Clinic, Central Veterans' Hospital in Lodz (Poland). The participants reported to the Clinic after 8 h of overnight fasting for blood sampling. Then the interview on socioeconomic status, current and previous illnesses and current medications was conducted. The contradictions for bioimpedance testing (implanted cardiac device, high fever) were identified for each participant. All participants underwent medical examination, which included blood pressure measurement to identify possible contraindications to the muscle power testing. Thereafter, participants could eat breakfast (all subjects were instructed to bring sandwiches, beverages, and comfortable sportswear to the appointment). The anthropometric, skinfolds and muscle strength measurements were intermitted by functional and cognitive performance tests. The same researcher/research assistant was always responsible for conducting the measurements to avoid interobserver/-analyzer variability. Before the muscle power assessment, all the subjects underwent a 5-min warm-up on the friction-loaded cycle ergometer.

### Anthropometric measurements

The anthropometric measurements including height and body mass were obtained. Each patient was weighed on calibrated SECA chair scales without shoes and outdoor clothes to the nearest 0.1 kg. Height was measured with the stadiometer to the nearest 0.5 cm. Body mass index (BMI) was calculated as body mass in kilograms divided by the height in meters squared. Calf circumference (CC) was measured on the widest part of the left leg to the nearest centimeter without compressing the subcutaneous tissue with flexible plastic tape. Waist circumference (WC) was measured midway between the lower rib cage and the iliac crest to the nearest centimeter with flexible plastic tape. Hips circumference (HC) was measured on the widest part of the buttocks. Skinfolds measurements were obtained using Baseline Skinfold Caliper at four sites: triceps, biceps, subscapular and supraileum. The percentage of body fat was estimated from the skinfolds measurements, according to the Durnin and Womersley method [19].

## Body composition

The body composition of 93 study participants due to preexisting contradictions was also analyzed by validated electrical bioimpedance device (Maltron Bioscan 920, Maltron International Ltd., Rayleigh, Essex UK). Two injector electrodes were placed on the dorsal surface of the foot and wrist. Two detector electrodes were placed between the styloid process of radius and ulna, and between the medial and lateral malleolus. During the measurement, each subject remained in the supine position with feet apart and hands at their sides.

## Functional performance

Functional performance for each subject was assessed by several tests and scales: Activities of Daily Living (ADL) scale [20], Instrumental Activities of Daily Living (IADL) scale [21], Timed Up & Go (TUG) test [22], and Tinetti test [23]. ADL consists of 6 questions concerning basic daily activities: self-feeding, dressing, bathing, toileting, continence, and transferring. It is graded from 0 to 6 points. A poor score reflects the necessity of supervision by caregiver in performing basic daily activities by a patient. IADL scale includes 8 areas of instrumental activities of daily living: ability to use telephone, shopping, food preparation, housekeeping, mode of transportation, responsibility for own medication, ability to handle finances and laundry. It is graded from 0 (low function, dependent) to 8 (high function, independent) points. The TUG test assesses mobility: standing up from a chair, walking a 3-m distance, returning, and sitting down as quickly as possible. The test was timed using stopwatch to the nearest 0.1 s. The Tinetti test includes the assessments of balance and gait with the maximum of 28 points.

## Cognitive assessment

Global cognitive function was assessed by the Folstein Mini-Mental State Examination (MMSE) with scores ranging from 0 to 30 points [24]. The Geriatric Depression Scale (GDS) Short Form is a questionnaire consisting of 15 yes/no questions, which assesses depression in the previous week. A score greater than 5 indicates the increasing likelihood and severity of depression in the examined patient [25].

## Muscle strength

Muscle strength was measured with two different methods. Muscle strength of upper extremities was assessed by a handgrip test (evaluating flexors of the hand and forearm) using Jamar Hydraulic Hand Dynamometer (Lafayette Instrument, Lafayette, IN, USA). The handgrip

test was performed in duplicate for both hands with best result recorded. The participant was in the standing position with arms along the side not touching the body. Participants were asked to squeeze the dynamometer with as much force as possible with a 20–30s pause between trials to avoid muscle fatigue. All subjects were given verbal encouragement during the trials to ensure full activation and generation of maximal muscle strength. The results of each trial were recorded to the nearest kilogram.

Muscle strength of lower extremities was quantitatively determined by the one repetition maximum (1RM) measure of bilateral leg extension (evaluating quadriceps) and leg press (evaluating quadriceps, hamstrings, gluteals) using Keiser pneumatic resistance training equipment fitted with A300 electronics (Keiser Sports Health Equipment, Fresno, CA). The 1RM is described as the maximum load than can be lifted once throughout the full range of motion while sustaining the correct technique [26]. For the leg extension, the subjects were asked to sit in the upright position and on the cue to extend right knee as fast and forceful as possible. The subjects were asked to cross their upper extremities on the chest, and to not lift the gluteals off the seat while performing the movement. The same procedure was repeated with the left leg. For the leg press, the starting position of the seat was adjusted to where the knee joint is as a 90°-degree angle between thigh and shin. The subjects were instructed to cross their upper extremities on the chest, and to extend fully both legs simultaneously but without locking the knee joints. The examiner progressively increased the resistance between 5 to 10 kg for each repetition until the subject could no longer move the lever arm for leg extension or pedals for leg press through the full range of motion. Each trial was separated by the 30-s rest period.

## Muscle power

Muscle power was measured with two different methods: using Keiser pneumatic resistance training equipment fitted with A300 electronics (Keiser Sports Health Equipment, Fresno, CA) and friction-loaded cycle ergometer. First method included measurements of leg extension and leg press at 40 and 70% of the 1RM. These two percentages of the 1RM were chosen to represent muscle power production of low force/high velocity (40%) and high force/low velocity (70%) [13]. Muscle power at 40 and 70% is related to functional performance such as stair-climb time, chair-rise time, and habitual gait speed. Muscle power at 40% 1RM is suggested to be a better predictor of walking performance [26]. Those assessments were performed with five repetitions using the same Keiser pneumatic resistance training equipment. The subjects were instructed to complete the movement of each repetition as fast as possible, then to slowly lower the weight. All the attempts were verbally cued. All subjects were highly motivated during the exercise testing to enhance their performance. Each trial was separated by the 30-s rest period. For the leg extension, the maximum values for each side were recorded for further analyses. For the leg press, the highest measured simultaneously for both legs values were recorded for further analyses.

The second method included measurement of muscle power using the friction-loaded cycle ergometer (Monark type 818E Stockholm, Sweden) [17, 27]. The ergometer was instrumented with a strain gauge (KMM20 type, 200 N, WObit, Poznań, Poland) and an incremental encoder (Rotapuls 141-H-200ZCU46L2 type, 200pts/turn, Lika Electronic, Carre, Italy) for measurement of the friction force applied by the tension of the belt that surrounded the flywheel and the flywheel displacement, respectively. Instantaneous pedaling velocity ($v$), force (F), and the power output (P) were calculated each 5 ms and then averaged over each downstroke period. The saddle height of ergometer was adjusted to the maximum comfort of each subject. The subjects were familiarized with the ergometer by the 5-min of submaximal cycling and sprints of 3–4 s against different friction loads. Following the warm-up and 5-min rest, the subjects were instructed to perform 8 s sprints from a standardized starting position, each separated by at least 5-min break. Friction loads were 0.25 $N \cdot kg^{-1}$ and 0.35 $N \cdot kg^{-1}$ of body mass. The $v$-P combinations obtained during two sprints were fitted by a least square mathematical procedure to establish the $v$-P relationship. The highest value of P (maximum power output - $P_{max}$) and optimal shortening velocity (velocity at which the power reaches a maximum value - $v_{opt}$) were calculated from a third-order polynomial function. $P_{max}$ was also expressed as relative to the body mass: $P_{max} \cdot kg^{-1} (W \cdot kg^{-1})$. $v_{opt}$ was given in the number of rotations per minute (rpm) [17].

## Laboratory analysis
### Plasma samples
The venous 5 ml blood samples were drawn after overnight fasting into tubes containing EDTA. Samples were centrifuged at 3500 rpm for 20 min at 4 °C in the Eppendorf 5430R centrifuge (Eppendorf AG, Hamburg, Germany) and divided into aliquots. The isolated plasma was stored at – 80 °C until analyzed.

### Plasma analysis
Plasma was analyzed using immunoassays, which utilize the quantitative sandwich enzyme immunoassay technique. A monoclonal antibody specific to the protein was pre-coated onto a microplate. The samples and standards were pipetted into the wells and any of the proteins of interest present could bind by the immobilized antibody. After washing away any unbound substances, an enzyme-linked monoclonal antibody specific to the proteins of interest is added to the wells. Following the consequent wash to remove the unbound antibody-protein complexes, the substrate solution was added to the wells and developed color was proportioned to the amount of proteins bound. The intensity of color was measured using absorption photometry technique.

Plasma myostatin levels were measured using 4-h immunoassay kits (Immundiagnostik AG, Bensheim, Germany) according to the included protocol by manufacturer. Samples were diluted 1:10 prior to assay. Samples were analyzed in duplicate. An eight-point calibration curve was prepared using three-fold dilutions, starting with a prepared standard sample and two controls with known concentration ranges 0.7–6.9 ng/ml and 7.0–17.0 ng/ml, respectively. The assay sensitivity was 0.37 ng/ml with the intra- and inter-assay precision variations less than 11% and 15%, respectively. The absorption was read using GloMax®-Multi Detection System microplate reader (Promega Corporation, Madison, WI, USA) at 450 nm against 620 nm as a reference.

Plasma follistatin levels were measured by 6-h solid-phase Quantikine ELISA (R&D Systems, Minneapolis, MN, USA) according to the protocol. Samples were analyzed in duplicate. An eight-point calibration curve was prepared using three-fold dilutions, starting with a prepared standard sample of 16.000 pg/ml. The detectable dose ranged from 10 to 83 pg/ml with a mean of 29 pg/ml, and the intra- and inter-assay variations were less than 3% and 10%, respectively. The absorption was read using GloMax®-Multi Detection System microplate reader (Promega Corporation, Madison, WI, USA) at 450 nm against 560 nm as a reference.

Plasma GDF-11 levels were measured by 5-h Human Growth/differentiation factor 11 ELISA kit (Wuhan EIAab Science Co., Ltd., Wuhan, China) according to the protocol. Samples were analyzed in duplicate. An eight-point calibration curve was prepared using three-fold dilutions, starting with a prepared standard sample of 1000 pg/ml. The detectable dose ranged from 15.6–1000 pg/ml with the sensitivity less than 10 pg/ml. The intra- and inter-assay variations were ≤ 4.7% and ≤ 6.9%, respectively. The absorption was read using GloMax®-Multi Detection System microplate reader (Promega Corporation, Madison, WI, USA) at 450 nm.

## Statistical analysis
Statistical analysis was carried out using Statistica 12 software. The data was verified for normality of distribution and equality of variances. Variables that did not meet the assumption of normality were analyzed with

nonparametric statistics. The one-way analysis of variance (ANOVA) and Kruskall-Wallis test were used to compare groups. Spearman correlations were used to measure the strength and direction of the relationship between two variables. The limit of significance was set at $p = 0.05$ for all analyses.

## Results

Baseline characteristics of the participants is presented in Table 1. Subjects ranged in age from 61 to 89 years with the mean age of 69 years, who were mostly women (56 females, 45 males). Men were characterized by higher body mass and height than women, however BMI was virtually the same. Women had higher percentage of body fat measured by both methods used in the study than men. Men had wider WC, higher fat free mass and muscle mass than women. Males were also characterized by higher muscle strength and power of upper and lower extremities than women. Men were slightly faster in TUG performance. Women performed better in MMSE, had higher (i.e. worse) GDS scores and experienced higher number of falls per year than men. Women had higher plasma levels of myostatin and GDF11 than men. Men had higher plasma level of follistatin than women.

Spearman correlation coefficients for females are presented in Table 2. The plasma level of myostatin was negatively correlated with left handgrip strength and $v_{opt}$. The plasma level of follistatin was negatively correlated with $P_{max}$, $P_{max} \cdot kg^{-1}$ and P70% leg press, and positively correlated with the TUG test. The plasma level of GDF11 was negatively correlated with body mass, BMI, WC, fat mass and the percentage of body fat measured by both methods. Interestingly, GDF11 correlated positively with the percentage of fat free mass. All the correlations observed for women were at weak or moderate level of strength.

Spearman correlations coefficients for males are presented in Table 3. There were no correlations observed between plasma levels of myostatin, follistatin, GDF11 and measured parameters. The similar trends as in females were observed in men, but the correlations were too weak to reach the statistically significant level.

## Discussion

This is the first study which investigates whether the circulating plasma proteins: myostatin, follistatin and GDF11 are related to muscle strength, power and $v_{opt}$ in older adults. We demonstrated the inverse relationship between myostatin and muscle strength of the upper extremities and between myostatin and quadriceps $v_{opt}$ in women but not in men. We found the negative correlation between follistatin and muscle power in older women. We also demonstrated a distinctive link

between GDF11 and body composition in women but not in men.

Myostatin is known as a key negative regulator of muscle mass. Loss of function of myostatin induces skeletal muscle hyperplasia and hypertrophy [5]. Since

**Table 1** Baseline characteristics of the participants ($n = 101$)

|  | Women $n = 56$ | Men $n = 45$ |
|---|---|---|
| Age (y) | 68.2 ± 4.4 | 70.9 ± 6.8 |
| Body mass (kg) | 71.1 ± 12.8 | 83.7 ± 14*** |
| Body Mass Index (kg/m²) | 28.3 ± 4.7 | 28.5 ± 4.0 |
| Waist circumference (cm) | 89.5 ± 10.8 | 101 ± 10.6*** |
| Waist-to-hip ratio | 0.86 ± 0.08 | 0.99 ± 0.06*** |
| Body fat % | 43.1 ± 8.1 | 24.75 ± 4.6*** |
| Fat free mass (kg) | 42.6 ± 3.9 ($n = 52$) | 60.3 ± 8.9 ($n = 41$)*** |
| Fat free mass (%) | 61.1 ± 6.8 ($n = 52$) | 73.1 ± 4.7 ($n = 41$)*** |
| Fat mass (kg) | 28.3 ± 9.9 ($n = 52$) | 22.7 ± 7.3 ($n = 41$)** |
| Fat mass (%) | 38.9 ± 6.8 ($n = 52$) | 26.9 ± 4.7 ($n = 41$)*** |
| Muscle mass (kg) | 18.1 ± 1.8 ($n = 52$) | 29.4 ± 4.1 ($n = 41$)*** |
| ADL (pts) | 5.8 ± 0.4 | 5.9 ± 0.23 |
| IADL (pts) | 7.9 ± 0.2 | 7.93 ± 0.27 |
| Timed Up & Go test (s) | 6.2 ± 0.97 | 6.53 ± 1.99 |
| Tinetti test (pts) | 27.6 ± 1.1 | 27.58 ± 1.7 |
| MMSE (pts) | 29.9 ± 0.1 | 29.4 ± 1.2*** |
| GDS (pts) | 2.8 ± 2.6 | 2.33 ± 2.53 |
| Falls (n/year) | 0.6 ± 0.7 | 0.24 ± 0.5* |
| Handgrip strength L (kG) | 29.5 ± 6.7 | 45.6 ± 9.97*** |
| Handgrip strength R (kG) | 30.5 ± 7.3 | 47.4 ± 10.8*** |
| Leg Extension 1RM R (kG) | 32.3 ± 9.4 | 55.5 ± 13.4*** |
| Leg Extension 1RM L (kG) | 31.2 ± 8.8 | 54.1 ± 13.5*** |
| Leg Press 1RM (kG) | 134.1 ± 30.9 | 215.8 ± 56.3*** |
| P40% LE R (W) | 138.6 ± 41.5 | 260.7 ± 76.9*** |
| P70% LE R (W) | 154.5 ± 47.9 | 302.1 ± 87.7*** |
| P40% LE L (W) | 133.9 ± 40.2 | 242.8 ± 72.7*** |
| P70% LE L (W) | 144.5 ± 44.1 | 272.1 ± 83.6*** |
| P40% LP (W) | 612.4 ± 175.9 | 1165.8 ± 321.8*** |
| P70% LP (W) | 695.7 ± 202 | 1259.3 ± 338.1*** |
| $P_{max}$ (W) | 271.4 ± 88.4 | 446.2 ± 159.5*** |
| $P_{max} \cdot kg^{-1}$ (W·kg⁻¹) | 3.9 ± 1.2 | 5.4 ± 1.9*** |
| $v_{opt}$ (rpm) | 71.5 ± 12.6 | 83.7 ± 18.2*** |
| Myostatin (ng/ml) | 42.9 ± 25.6 | 39.8 ± 17.4 |
| Follistatin (pg/ml) | 1429.6 ± 436.9 | 1695.5 ± 659.6* |
| GDF11 (pg/ml) | 52.5 ± 24.2 | 40.2 ± 19.4* |

Data presented as mean + SD
*Note.* ADL Activities of daily living, *GDF11* growth/differentiation factor 11, *GDS* Geriatric Depression Scale, *IADL* Instrumental Activities of daily living, *MMSE* Mini-Mental State Examination
\*$p < 0.05$, \*\*$p < 0.01$, \*\*\*$p < 0.001$

**Table 2** Spearman correlation coefficients for women (n = 56)

| | Myostatin (ng/ml) | Follistatin (pg/ml) | GDF11 (pg/ml) |
|---|---|---|---|
| Age (y) | − 0.039 | 0.185 | − 0.089 |
| Body mass (kg) | 0.002 | − 0.070 | − 0.301* |
| Body Mass Index (kg/m²) | 0.022 | − 0.013 | − 0.354** |
| Waist circumference (cm) | − 0.043 | 0.083 | − 0.372** |
| Waist-to-hip ratio | −0.103 | 0.260 | −0.202 |
| Body fat % | −0.084 | 0.035 | −0.458*** |
| Fat free mass (kg) (n = 52) | −0.075 | −0.173 | − 0.128 |
| Fat free mass (%) (n = 52) | 0.073 | −0.083 | 0.359** |
| Fat mass (kg) (n = 52) | −0.071 | 0.006 | −0.331** |
| Fat mass (%) (n = 52) | −0.073 | 0.083 | −0.359** |
| Muscle mass (kg) (n = 52) | −0.025 | −0.123 | − 0.199 |
| ADL (pts) | −0.024 | 0.161 | 0.016 |
| IADL (pts) | −0.132 | 0.114 | 0.081 |
| Timed Up&Go test (s) | −0.071 | 0.366** | −0.163 |
| Tinetti test (pts) | 0.163 | −0.199 | −0.127 |
| MMSE (pts) | 0.038 | −0.138 | 0.038 |
| GDS (pts) | 0.040 | 0.034 | 0.049 |
| Falls (n/year) | −0.239 | 0.066 | −0.133 |
| Handgrip strength L (kG) | −0.296* | −0.063 | − 0.080 |
| Handgrip strength R (kG) | −0.203 | 0.036 | 0.030 |
| Leg Extension 1RM R (kG) | −0.049 | −0.075 | − 0.143 |
| Leg Extension 1RM L (kG) | −0.051 | − 0.204 | −0.170 |
| Leg Press 1RM (kG) | 0.031 | −0.216 | −0.135 |
| P40% LE R (W) | −0.056 | −0.179 | − 0.124 |
| P70% LE R (W) | −0.169 | − 0.135 | −0.206 |
| P40% LE L (W) | −0.058 | −0.151 | − 0.242 |
| P70% LE L (W) | −0.046 | − 0.147 | −0.151 |
| P40% LP (kG) | −0.091 | −0.216 | − 0.177 |
| P70% LP (kG) | −0.117 | − 0.279* | −0.250 |
| $P_{max}$ (W) | −0.141 | − 0.387** | − 0.186 |
| $P_{max} \cdot kg^{-1}$ (W·kg⁻¹) | −0.156 | − 0.405** | −0.049 |
| $v_{opt}$ (rpm) | −0.329* | −0.183 | − 0.220 |
| Myostatin (ng/ml) | – | −0.061 | 0.080 |
| Follistatin (pg/ml) | −0.061 | – | 0.032 |
| GDF11 (pg/ml) | 0.080 | 0.032 | – |

*Note. ADL* Activities of daily living, *GDF11* growth/differentiation factor 11, *GDS* Geriatric Depression Scale, *IADL* Instrumental Activities of daily living, *MMSE* Mini-Mental State Examination
*p < 0.05, **p < 0.01, ***p < 0.001

**Table 3** Spearman correlation coefficients for men (n = 45)

| | Myostatin (ng/ml) | Follistatin (pg/ml) | GDF11 (pg/ml) |
|---|---|---|---|
| Age (y) | 0.007 | −0.021 | −0.159 |
| Body mass (kg) | −0.009 | −0.058 | − 0.104 |
| Body Mass Index (kg/m²) | −0.050 | − 0.075 | −0.164 |
| Waist circumference (cm) | 0.029 | 0.009 | −0.131 |
| Waist-to-hip ratio | −0.028 | 0.143 | −0.000 |
| Body fat % | −0.074 | −0.119 | − 0.036 |
| Fat free mass (kg) (n = 41) | −0.174 | 0.041 | 0.028 |
| Fat free mass (%) (n = 41) | −0.162 | −0.023 | 0.078 |
| Fat mass (kg) (n = 41) | 0.052 | 0.020 | −0.020 |
| Fat mass (%) (n = 41) | 0.162 | 0.023 | −0.078 |
| Muscle mass (kg) (n = 41) | −0.119 | 0.037 | 0.029 |
| ADL (pts) | 0.216 | 0.040 | 0.057 |
| IADL (pts) | −0.181 | −0.227 | −0.233 |
| Timed Up&Go test (s) | −0.101 | 0.139 | −0.031 |
| Tinetti test (pts) | −0.046 | 0.092 | −0.254 |
| MMSE (pts) | −0.017 | 0.114 | 0.293 |
| GDS (pts) | 0.209 | 0.154 | 0.117 |
| Falls (n/year) | 0.091 | 0.171 | 0.131 |
| Handgrip strength L (kG) | 0.153 | −0.202 | 0.044 |
| Handgrip strength R (kG) | 0.113 | −0.110 | −0.015 |
| Leg Extension 1RM R (kG) | −0.062 | −0.264 | − 0.045 |
| Leg Extension 1RM L (kG) | −0.187 | − 0.193 | −0.135 |
| Leg Press 1RM (kG) | 0.034 | −0.052 | −0.051 |
| P40% LE R (W) | −0.016 | −0.251 | 0.055 |
| P70% LE R (W) | 0.008 | −0.230 | 0.101 |
| P40% LE L (W) | −0.196 | −0.232 | − 0.132 |
| P70% LE L (W) | −0.189 | − 0.253 | −0.128 |
| P40% LP (kG) | −0.022 | −0.178 | 0.163 |
| P70% LP (kG) | −0.008 | −0.085 | − 0.04 |
| $P_{max}$ (W) | −0.101 | − 0.127 | −0.013 |
| $P_{max} \cdot kg^{-1}$ (W·kg⁻¹) | − 0.156 | −0.115 | − 0.017 |
| $v_{opt}$ (rpm) | −0.094 | 0.016 | −0.127 |
| Myostatin (ng/ml) | – | 0.008 | 0.183 |
| Follistatin (pg/ml) | 0.008 | – | 0.171 |
| GDF11 (pg/ml) | 0.183 | 0.171 | – |

*Note. ADL* Activities of daily living, *GDF11* growth/differentiation factor 11, *GDS* Geriatric Depression Scale, *IADL* Instrumental Activities of daily living, *MMSE* Mini-Mental State Examination
*p < 0.05, **p < 0.01, ***p < 0.001

its discovery, it became a unique and desirable therapeutic target. It can be interfered by neutralizing its activity antibodies [5]. Becker et al. [28] reported the increase of lean body mass and improvement of some performance measures in older individuals after the treatment by the humanized monoclonal myostatin antibody LY2495655. In future, it may be potentially indicated for treatment of hip arthroplasty, cancer cachexia, and elderly fallers [29]. Serum myostatin has been reported to increase, decrease or remain unchanged with age [1, 30–33]. Bowser et al. [34] showed in mice that there is age-associated increase in myostatin levels and the myostatin:follistatin ratio in slow-twitch soleus muscle and reversed pattern in the fast-twitch extensor digitorum longus muscle. Conflicting results have also been provided considering association of myostatin to body composition, muscle mass and strength as well as physical performance [2, 30, 31, 35]. Binns et al. showed that neither serum myostatin nor protein intake influenced the total body lean mass among older men and women [36]. Bergen et al. [33] obtained a significant positive correlation with grip strength and knee extensor strength in young men but not in older men or women. However, Han et al. [32] reported the negative correlation between handgrip strength and serum myostatin level in hemodialysis patients. The accelerator-brake (or yin and yang) hypothesis has been put forward to explain on one hand, the restrictive myostatin activity to excessive muscle growth (role of chalone) and on the other hand, lower myostatin expression in response to unfavorable metabolic environment, e.g. metabolic syndrome, inflammatory cytokines or uremia [32, 35, 37–39]. Undoubtedly, the potential modulating role of androgens and estrogens on myostatin and other proteins that maintain muscle function is of interest. Testosterone is one of the well-known anabolic hormones, which can increase muscle protein muscle synthesis and muscle mass [40]. Lakshman et al. [41] showed significant correlation between free testosterone and myostatin levels in younger men. On the contrary, Smith et al. [40] found neither testosterone nor estradiol have any effect on myostatin mRNA expression in postmenopausal women. According to the other study, the increased level of estradiol correlates with decreased level of myostatin mRNA expression in younger females [42]. Further studies are necessary to interpret those conflicting reports on the role of androgens and estrogens in the activity of myostatin and other muscle-related proteins.

Another factor should be mentioned, such as activin A, which is thought to replicate a biological activity of myostatin on skeletal muscle. Gilson et al. [43] demonstrated that follistatin-induced muscle hypertrophy resulted in activin A inhibition in wild-type mice. In addition, it was shown that human anti-ActRII antibody bimagrumab (BYM338) inhibits myostatin- and activin A- muscle atrophy and significantly increases skeletal muscle mass in mice [44]. Activin A and myostatin bind to type II activin receptors with greater affinity of activin A to the type IIA. Activin A circulates in the bloodstream and its concentration increases in acute conditions such as inflammation, respiratory and renal failure, and some types of cancer [34, 45]. Baccarelli et al. [46] showed that increased serum concentration of activin A is associated with age in both men and postmenopausal women. Activin A was not a subject of this study; however, it might be useful to consider examining it in future analyses.

Follistatin was demonstrated to prevent myostatin binding to the activin type II B receptor, which as a result neutralizes its activity in circulation. It was observed that follistatin overexpression in mice promotes increase in muscle mass [7]. Similarly to myostatin, in the majority of recent studies, follistatin was not found to be age-dependent [2, 31], though this data is also conflicting [33]. In several studies follistatin was not found to reflect dynapenia in older women or men [2, 31]. Interestingly, Miyamoto et al. reported negative association between plasma follistatin and muscle strength in patients with chronic kidney disease, which is not consistent with observed effects of follistatin in inducing muscle hypertrophy [38]. Likewise, Liaw et al. [35] found a negative correlation between follistatin and gait speed among older adults. On the other hand, follistatin increased after resistance training in older women and performance gains have been attributed to the blocked degradation pathways via follistatin [47]. All these discrepancies may be explained by the fact that increased follistatin may accompany elevated myostatin levels [38]. Increased follistatin levels occur also in inflammatory diseases and have been suggested to counteract catabolism in chronic kidney disease [35, 38].

GDF11 and myostatin are closely related TGF-β superfamily proteins [48]. Their homology is very impressive, differing by 11 residues within the amino acid sequence. Nevertheless, myostatin is expressed primarily in skeletal muscle and acts to limit muscle growth. GDF11 is expressed more widely and plays multiple roles [49], including suggested aging regulation of multiple mammalian tissues [48]. Unlike myostatin, GDF11 declines in aging mice [50]. In contrast, Schafer et al. [1] showed that GDF11 levels do not decline throughout aging and there was no difference between sexes in healthy adults.

GDF11 has been proposed to be both a rejuvenating factor and a biomarker of advanced biological aging [1, 3]. Using parabiosis (exposure of the aged mouse to a young circulation), Sinha et al. [50] demonstrated that circulating GDF11 is a rejuvenating factor for skeletal muscle. Parabiosis (increased GDF11 levels in aged mice) reversed functional impairments and restored genomic integrity in aged muscle stem cells and increased strength and endurance exercise capacity [50]. The 4-week exposure to the blood circulation of young mice resulted in the cardiac hypertrophy regression in old mice. GDF11 was identified as a responsible circulating factor. Restoration of GDF11 in old mice to youthful levels repeated the effects of parabiosis and reversed age-related hypertrophy [51].

Nevertheless, there are considerable new data showing that GDF11 can aggravate rather than regenerate skeletal muscle injury in old animals [3]. It was shown to inhibit muscle regeneration in a dose-dependent manner [52]. There are also doubts whether GDF11 therapy can reverse cardiac pathologies while elevated blood levels of GDF11 may generate a cachectic effect in skeletal and cardiac muscles in both young and old animals [3]. In one clinical study, Schafer et al. [1] demonstrated that older adults with slow gait, weak grip strength and higher prevalence of cardiac conditions had higher GDF11 levels. In the same study individuals with higher body weight were characterized by a trend towards lower GDF11 plasma levels. These authors suggested that GDF11 circulating levels may be associated with deficits in multiple physiological functions [1].

Age-related gradual decline of muscle loss associates more with fast twitch (type II) fibers than with type I ones. Fast twitch fibers mainly determine velocity of contraction and muscle power [27]. Therefore, these two measures have been proposed to be more crucial factors determining functional performance than muscle strength [16, 17]. To the best of our knowledge our study is the first one to report on the relationship of directly measured muscle power and optimal shortening velocity to circulating myostatin, follistatin and GDF11. In one study with young non-athletic men, the polymorphism in the myostatin gene was associated with the ability to produce peak power assessed with vertical jumps [53]. In a large clinical trial, Becker et al. [28] reported the improvement of power-demanding performance measures (stair climbing, five-chair rise, fast gait speed) in the older individuals after the treatment with the humanized monoclonal antibody LY2495655. For less power-intensive performance-based measures (6-min walking distance, usual gait speed) and muscle strength no important treatment effects were observed [28].

Our data show a consistently negative trend for the association of all the three proteins to muscle function measures, with significant relationship of myostatin to $v_{opt}$ and of follistatin to $P_{max}$, $P_{max} \cdot kg^{-1}$ and P70% leg press in women. For muscle strength, only one significant relationship was found for the myostatin-left handgrip strength association in women, with no significant relationship of circulating proteins to lower extremity isometric strength measures. Therefore, power and shortening velocity might be more affected by circulating myostatin and follistatin than isometric strength. This association being also more visible in older women than in men.

In our study GDF11 was inversely related to body mass, BMI and the percentage of body fat in women. Positive relationship to the percentage of fat free mass may be related to the strong negative association between the percentage of fat free mass and body mass in women ($r = -0.86$; $p < 0.0001$). Therefore, lower body mass was related to higher relative percentage of fat free mass. The association between GDF11, absolute values of fat free mass and muscle mass tended to be negative. This supports the data of some previous animal and clinical studies [1, 3] and suggests that GDF11 circulating levels may be associated with increased catabolism in older adults. Only a minor relationship to functional tests (the only significant relationship being between follistatin and TUG test in women) may be related to the fact that our subjects were highly functioning elders with no apparent functional limitations.

Sex-related differences observed in this study are in accord with some previous reports. Schirwis et al. [54] reported that the effects of myostatin deficiency on maximal force and power are greater in young (as compared to old) and female (as compared to male) mice. Bergen et al. [33] showed that older females compared to younger have higher myostatin levels and older men have lower myostatin levels compared to younger ones. Nevertheless, one should note that our data show a consistently negative trend for the association of all the three proteins to muscle function measures both in women and men. Future epidemiological studies with larger samples of participants should solve this problem and elucidate whether these associations are valid in both sexes.

The main strength of this study was the fact that it considered simultaneously the relationship between plasma circulating proteins myostatin, follistatin, and GDF11 and muscle strength and power in older adults. Several limitations of our study should be considered. One limitation was the relatively small number of the participants. Another one is the cross-sectional nature of analysis performed in this study and modest correlations presented as uncorrected for multiple comparisons. Participants were volunteers, usually more healthy and willing to participate than general population of older subjects. Possible coexisting factors such as inflammation should also be considered in the design of future prospective studies. Finally, we used commercially available GDF11 reagent and ongoing discussion concerning the validity of different reagents should be acknowledged.

## Conclusions

The circulating myostatin and follistatin are negatively associated with muscle function in older women. The relationship between circulating plasma proteins is more visible for muscle power than muscle strength. GDF11 appeared to have a higher association with the body mass and composition than muscle function in older women. Future studies should explore whether these changes are the adaptation to age-related increased catabolism and whether they are potentially reversible.

## Abbreviations

1RM: one repetition maximum; ADL: Activities of Daily Living; BMI: body mass index; CC: calf circumference; F: force; GDF11: growth/differentiation factor 11; GDS: Geriatric Depression Scale; HC: hips circumference; IADL: Instrumental Activities of Daily Living; MMSE: Mini-Mental State Examination; P: power; $P_{max}$: maximum power; rpm: rotations per minute; TGFβ: transforming growth factor-β; TUG: Timed Up & Go; WC: waist circumference; υ: velocity; $υ_{opt}$: optimal shortening velocity

## Acknowledgements

None declared.

## Funding

This work was supported by Medical University of Lodz, Łódź, Poland, grants 502–03/6–077-01/502–64-099, 503/6–077-01/503–61-002. The funding had no role in any of the following: design of the study; collection, analysis, and interpretation of the data; and preparation, review of the manuscript.

## Authors' contributions

All authors have contributed to the conception and design of this study. EF performed statistical analysis and wrote the first draft of the manuscript. TK revised the manuscript and provided the meritorical support. EF, JK, ŁK, AG, MP, BS participated in recruitment and examinations of patients. EF, AK-S, KF-M performed laboratory analysis. All authors interpreted data. All authors approved the final version of the manuscript.

## Competing interests

The authors declare that they have no competing interests.

## Author details

[1]Department of Geriatrics, Healthy Ageing Research Centre, Medical University of Lodz, ul. Pieniny 30, 91-647 Łódź, Poland. [2]Department of Physical Medicine, Medical University of Lodz, Hallera 1, Łódź, Poland. [3]Department of Biomedical Chemistry, Medical University of Lodz, Mazowiecka 6/8, Łódź, Poland.

## References

1. Schafer MJ, Atkinson EJ, Vanderboom PM, Kotajarvi B, White TA, et al. Quantification of GDF11 and Myostatin in human aging and cardiovascular disease. Cell Metab. 2016;23(6):1207–15.
2. Hofmann M, Halper B, Oesen S, Franzke B, Stuparits P, et al. Serum concentrations of insulin-like growth factor-1, members of the TGF-beta superfamily and follistatin do not reflect different stages of dynapenia and sarcopenia in elderly women. Exp Gerontol. 2015;64:35–45.
3. Harper SC, Brack A, MacDonnell S, Franti M, Olwin BB, et al. Is growth differentiation factor 11 a realistic therapeutic for aging-dependent muscle defects? Circulat Res. 2016;118(7):1143–50.
4. Hittel DS, Axelson M, Sarna N, Shearer J, Huffman KM, et al. Myostatin decreases with aerobic exercise and associates with insulin resistance. Med Sci Sports Exerc. 2010;42(11):2023–9.
5. White TA, LeBrasseur NK. Myostatin and sarcopenia: opportunities and challenges - a mini-review. Gerontology. 2014;60(4):289–93.
6. Hansen J, Rinnov A, Krogh-Madsen R, Fischer CP, Andreasen AS, et al. Plasma follistatin is elevated in patients with type 2 diabetes: relationship to hyperglycemia, hyperinsulinemia, and systemic low-grade inflammation. Diabetes Metab Res Rev. 2013;29(6):463–72.
7. Hansen J, Brandt C, Nielsen AR, Hojman P, Whitham M, et al. Exercise induces a marked increase in plasma follistatin: evidence that follistatin is a contraction-induced hepatokine. Endocrinology. 2011;152(1):164–71.
8. Egerman MA, Cadena SM, Gilbert JA, Meyer A, Nelson HN, et al. GDF11 increases with age and inhibits skeletal muscle regeneration. Cell Metab. 2015;22(1):164–74.
9. McPherron AC. Metabolic functions of Myostatin and Gdf11. Immunol Endocr Metab Agents Med Chem. 2010;10(4):217–31.
10. Ivey FM, Roth SM, Ferrell RE, Tracy BL, Lemmer JT, et al. Effects of age, gender, and myostatin genotype on the hypertrophic response to heavy resistance strength training. J Gerontol A Biol Sci Med Sci. 2000;55(11): M641–8.
11. Pua YH, Ong PH, Clark RA, Matcher DB, Lim EC. Falls efficacy, postural balance, and risk for falls in older adults with falls-related emergency department visits: prospective cohort study. BMC Geriatr. 2017;17(1):291.
12. Fielding RA, LeBrasseur NK, Cuoco A, Bean J, Mizer K, et al. High-velocity resistance training increases skeletal muscle peak power in older women. J Am Geriatr Soc. 2002;50(4):655–62.
13. Herman S, Kiely DK, Leveille S, O'Neill E, Cyberey S, et al. Upper and lower limb muscle power relationships in mobility-limited older adults. J Gerontol A Biol Sci Med Sci. 2005;60(4):476–80.
14. Bean JF, Kiely DK, Herman S, Leveille SG, Mizer K, et al. The relationship between leg power and physical performance in mobility-limited older people. J Am Geriatr Soc. 2002;50(3):461–7.
15. Reid KF, Fielding RA. Skeletal muscle power: a critical determinant of physical functioning in older adults. Exerc Sport Sci Rev. 2012;40(1):4–12.
16. Clémençon M, Hautier CA, Rahmani A, Cornu C, Bonnefoy M. Potential role of optimal velocity as a qualitative factor of physical functional performance in women aged 72 to 96 years. Arch Phys Med Rehabil. 2008;89:1594–9.
17. Kostka JS, Czernicki JW, Kostka TJ. Association of muscle strength, power, and optimal shortening velocity with functional abilities of women with chronic osteoarthritis participating in a multi-modal exercise program. J Aging Phys Act. 2014;22(4):564–70.
18. de Vos NJ, Singh NA, Ross DA, Stavrinos TM, Orr R, et al. Optimal load for increasing muscle power during explosive resistance training in older adults. J Gerontol A Biol Sci Med Sci. 2005;60(5):638–47.
19. Durnin J, Womersley J. Body fat assessed from total body density and its estimation from skinfold thickness: measurements on 481 men and women aged from 16 to 72 years. Brit J Nutr. 1974;32(01):77–97.
20. Katz S, Ford AB, Moskowitz RW, Jackson BA, Jaffe MW. Studies of illness in the aged. The index of Adl: a standardized measure of biological and psychosocial function. JAMA. 1963;185:914–9.
21. Lawton MP, Brody EM. Assessment of older people: self-maintaining and instrumental activities of daily living. Gerontologist. 1969;9(3):179–86.
22. Podsiadlo D, Richardson S. The timed "up & go": a test of basic functional mobility for frail elderly persons. J Am Geriatr Soc. 1991;39(2):142–8.
23. Tinetti ME. Performance-oriented assessment of mobility problems in elderly patients. J Am Geriatr Soc. 1986;34(2):119–26.
24. Folstein MF, Robins LN, Helzer JE. The mini-mental state examination. Arch Gen Psychiatry. 1983;40(7):812.
25. Yesavage JA, Brink TL, Rose TL, Lum O, Huang V, et al. Development and validation of a geriatric depression screening scale: a preliminary report. J Psychiatr Res. 1982;17(1):37–49.
26. Cuoco A, Callahan DM, Sayers S, Frontera WR, Bean J, et al. Impact of muscle power and force on gait speed in disabled older men and women. J Gerontol A Biol Sci Med Sci. 2004;59(11):1200–6.
27. Hautier CA, Linossier MT, Belli A, Lacour JR, Arsac LM. Optimal velocity for maximal power production in non-isokinetic cycling is related to muscle fibre type composition. Eur J Appl Physiol Occup Physiol. 1996;74:114–8.
28. Becker C, Lord SR, Studenski SA, Warden SJ, Fielding RA, et al. Myostatin antibody (LY2495655) in older weak fallers: a proof-of-concept, randomised. phase 2 trial Lancet Diabetes Endocrinol. 2015;3(12):948–57.
29. Beaudart C, McCloskey E, Bruyere O, Cesari M, Rolland Y, et al. Sarcopenia in daily practice: assessment and management. BMC Geriatr. 2016;16(1):170.
30. Yarasheski KE, Bhasin S, Sinha-Hikim I, Pak-Loduca J, Gonzalez-Cadavid NF. Serum myostatin-immunoreactive protein is increased in 60-92 year old women and men with muscle wasting. J Nutr Health Aging. 2002;6(5):343–8.
31. Ratkevicius A, Joyson A, Selmer I, Dhanani T, Grierson C, et al. Serum concentrations of myostatin and myostatin-interacting proteins do not differ between young and sarcopenic elderly men. J Gerontol A Biol Sci Med Sci. 2011;66(6):620–6.
32. Han DS, Chen YM, Lin SY, Chang HH, Huang TM, et al. Serum myostatin levels and grip strength in normal subjects and patients on maintenance haemodialysis. Clin Endocrinol. 2011s;75(6):857–63.

33. Bergen HRIII, Farr JN, Vanderboom PM, Atkinson EJ, White TA, et al. Myostatin as a mediator of sarcopenia versus homeostatic regulator of muscle mass: insights using a new mass spectrometry-based assay. Skelet Muscle. 2015;5:21.

34. Bowser M, Herberg S, Arounleut P, Shi X, Fulzele S, et al. Effects of the activin A-myostatin-follistatin system on aging bone and muscle progenitor cells. Exp Gerontol. 2013;48(2):290-7.

35. Liaw FY, Kao TW, Fang WH, Han DS, Chi YC, et al. Increased follistatin associated with decreased gait speed among old adults. Eur J Clin Investig. 2016;46(4):321-7.

36. Binns A, Gray M, Henson AC, Fort IL. Changes in lean mass and serum myostatin with habitual protein intake and high-velocity resistance training. J Nutr Health Aging. 2017;21(10):1111-7.

37. Han DS, Chu-Su Y, Chiang CK, Tseng FY, Tseng PH, et al. Serum Myostatin is reduced in individuals with metabolic syndrome. PLoS One. 2014;9(9): e108230.

38. Miyamoto T, Carrero JJ, Qureshi AR, Anderstam B, Heimburger O, et al. Circulating follistatin in patients with chronic kidney disease: implications for muscle strength, bone mineral density, inflammation and survival. Clin J Am Soc Nephrol. 2011;6(5):1001-8.

39. Mak RH, Rotwein P. Myostatin and insulin-like growth factors in uremic sarcopenia: the yin and yang in muscle mass regulation. Kidney Int. 2006;70(3):410-2.

40. Smith GI, Yoshino J, Reeds DN, Bradley D, Burrows RE, et al. Testosterone and progesterone, but not estradiol, stimulate muscle protein synthesis in postmenopausal women. J Clin Endocrinol Metab. 2014;99(1):256-65.

41. Lakshman KM, Bhasin S, Corcoran C, Collins-Racie LA, Tchistiakova L, et al. Measurement of myostatin concentrations in human serum: circulating concentrations in young and older men and effects of testosterone administration. Mol Cell Endocrinol. 2009;302(1):26-32.

42. Willoughby DS, Wilborn CD. Estradiol in females may negate skeletal muscle myostatin mRNA expression and serum myostatin propeptide levels after eccentric muscle contractions. J Sports Sci Med. 2006;5(4):672-81.

43. Gilson H, Schakman O, Kalista S, Lause P, Tsuchida K, et al. Follistatin induces muscle hypertrophy through satellite cell proliferation and inhibition of both myostatin and activin. Am J Physiol Endocrinol Metab. 2009;297(1):E157-64.

44. Lach-Trifilieff E, Minetti GC, Sheppard K, Ibebunjo C, Feige JN, et al. An antibody blocking activin type II receptors induces strong skeletal muscle hypertrophy and protects from atrophy. Mol Cell Biol. 2014;34(4):606-18.

45. Loumaye A, de Barsy M, Nachit M, Lause P, Frateur L, et al. Role of Activin a and myostatin in human cancer cachexia. J Clin Endocrinol Metab. 2015;100(5):2030-8.

46. Baccarelli A, Morpurgo PS, Corsi A, Vaghi I, Fanelli M, et al. Activin a serum levels and aging of the pituitary-gonadal axis: a cross-sectional study in middle-aged and elderly healthy subjects. Exp Gerontol. 2001;36(8):1403-12.

47. Hofmann M, Schober-Halper B, Oesen S, Franzke B, Tschan H, et al. Effects of elastic band resistance training and nutritional supplementation on muscle quality and circulating muscle growth and degradation factors of institutionalized elderly women: the Vienna active ageing study (VAAS). Eur J Appl Physiol. 2016;116(5):885-97.

48. Walker RG, Poggioli T, Katsimpardi L, Buchanan SM, Oh J, et al. Biochemistry and biology of GDF11 and Myostatin: similarities, differences and questions for future investigation. Circulat Res. 2016;118(7):1125-42.

49. Lee YS, Lee SJ. Regulation of GDF-11 and myostatin activity by GASP-1 and GASP-2. Proc Natl Acad Sci U S A. 2013;110(39):E3713-22.

50. Sinha M, Jang YC, Oh J, Khong D, Wu EY, et al. Restoring systemic GDF11 levels reverses age-related dysfunction in mouse skeletal muscle. Science. 2014;344(6184):649-52.

51. Loffredo FS, Steinhauser ML, Jay SM, Gannon J, Pancoast JR, et al. Growth differentiation factor 11 is a circulating factor that reverses age-related cardiac hypertrophy. Cell. 2013;153(4):828-39.

52. Glass DJ. Elevated GDF11 Is a Risk Factor for Age-Related Frailty and Disease in Humans. Cell Metab. 2016;24(1):7-8.

53. Santiago C, Ruiz JR, Rodriguez-Romo G, Fiuza-Luces C, Yvert T, et al. The K153R polymorphism in the myostatin gene and muscle power phenotypes in young, non-athletic men. PLoS One. 2011;6(1):e16323.

54. Schirwis E, Agbulut O, Vadrot N, Mouisel E, Hourdé C, et al. The beneficial effect of myostatin deficiency on maximal muscle force and power is attenuated with age. Exp Gerontol. 2013;48(2):183-90.

# 4

# The OptimaMed intervention to reduce inappropriate medications in nursing home residents with severe dementia: results from a quasi-experimental feasibility pilot study

Machelle Wilchesky[1,2], Gerhard Mueller[3], Michèle Morin[4,5], Martine Marcotte[4], Philippe Voyer[4,5], Michèle Aubin[4], Pierre-Hugues Carmichael[4], Nathalie Champoux[6], Johanne Monette[7], Anik Giguère[4,5], Pierre Durand[4,5], René Verreault[4,5], Marcel Arcand[8] and Edeltraut Kröger[4,5*] [iD]

## Abstract

**Background:** Medication regimens in nursing home (NH) residents with severe dementia should be frequently reviewed to avoid inappropriate medication, overtreatment and adverse drug events, within a comfort care approach. This study aimed at testing the feasibility of an interdisciplinary knowledge exchange (KE) intervention using a medication review guidance tool categorizing medications as either "generally", "sometimes" or "exceptionally" appropriate for NH residents with severe dementia.

**Methods:** A quasi-experimental feasibility pilot study with 44 participating residents aged 65 years or over with severe dementia was carried out in three NH in Quebec City, Canada. The intervention comprised an information leaflet for residents' families, a 90-min KE session for NH general practitioners (GP), pharmacists and nurses focusing on the medication review guidance tool, a medication review by the pharmacists for participating residents with ensuing team discussion on medication changes, and a post-intervention KE session to obtain feedback from team staff. Medication regimens and levels of pain and of agitation of the participants were evaluated at baseline and at 4 months post-intervention. A questionnaire for team staff explored perceived barriers and facilitators. Statistical differences in measures comparing pre and post-intervention were assessed using paired t-tests and Cochran's-Q tests.

(Continued on next page)

\* Correspondence: edeltraut.kroger.ciussscn@ssss.gouv.qc.ca
[4]Centre d'excellence sur le vieillissement de Québec, Centre intégré universitaire de santé et de services sociaux de la Capitale-Nationale, 1050, Chemin Ste-Foy, room L2-30, Quebec City, Quebec G1S 4L8, Canada
[5]Laval University, 1050, avenue de la Médecine, Quebec City, Quebec G1V 0A6, Canada
Full list of author information is available at the end of the article

(Continued from previous page)

**Results:** The KE sessions reached 34 NH team staff (5 GP, 4 pharmacists, 6 heads of care unit and 19 staff nurses). Forty-four residents participated in the study and were followed for a mean of 104 days. The total number of regular medications was 372 pre and 327 post-intervention. The mean number of regular medications per resident was 7.86 pre and 6.81 post-intervention. The odds ratios estimating the risks of using any regular medication or a "sometimes appropriate" medication post-intervention were 0.81 (95% CI: 0.71–0.92) and 0.83 (95% CI: 0.74–0.94), respectively.

**Conclusion:** A simple KE intervention using a medication review guidance tool categorizing medications as being either "generally", "sometimes" or "exceptionally" appropriate in severe dementia was well received and accompanied by an overall reduction in medication use by NH residents with severe dementia. Levels of agitation were unaffected and there was no clinically significant changes in levels of pain. Staff feedback provided opportunities to improve the intervention.

**Keywords:** Intervention, Inappropriate medication use, Long-term care, Dementia

## Background

Medication use is considered optimal when the prescribed medications are well tolerated and have a clear indication based on scientific evidence. Age-related physiological changes, however, may result in altered pharmacokinetic and pharmacodynamic responses to medications, thereby reducing their tolerability in older patients [1]. Moreover, some commonly prescribed medications offer limited benefit in the face of shortened life expectancy [2–4]. Medications presenting unfavorable adverse event risk to benefit ratios are associated with negative health outcomes [5–8]. Prevalence of potentially inappropriate medication prescriptions to seniors (aged 65 and over) is estimated as being high [9–11]. Furthermore, seniors with dementia, who may be incapable of verbalizing symptoms associated with adverse drug effects [12] are at even greater risk of inappropriate prescribing [3, 13–16].

Optimal medication use in seniors with severe dementia residing in nursing homes (NHs) presents an ongoing challenge. Health professionals, who may not always acknowledge severe dementia as being a terminal disease, may expose patients to unnecessarily aggressive treatments [17, 18]. Medication regimens in these patients should be frequently reconsidered to take into account changes in patients' condition, avoid overtreatment and adverse drug events, and improve symptom control and comfort [15]. A body of research has produced guidance for medication appropriateness in seniors, most notably the Beers criteria [19] and the STOPP/START consensus [20]. While these lists indicate medications that are inappropriate for seniors, they do not, however, specifically address the issue of medication appropriateness for seniors with severe dementia who are even more vulnerable and have shortened life expectancy, like those living in NHs.

Building upon prior research that did address this issue in patients with severe dementia [21, 22], our previous study engaged a panel of experts to categorize medications that are of questionable benefit for Quebec NH seniors with severe dementia [23]. Briefly, the 15-member multidisciplinary Delphi panel agreed on the categorization of 63 medications or medication classes as being either "generally", "sometimes," or "exceptionally" appropriate for these patients as shown in Additional file 1. The aim of the present pilot study was to test the feasibility of an interdisciplinary knowledge exchange (KE) intervention using this list, and to measure its impact on medication use, and on pain and agitation levels in this population.

## Methods

### Study design

A quasi-experimental (pre-post) study was conducted within three Quebec City NHs between January and December 2014.

### Setting

In Canada, public NHs are financed at the provincial level, leading to differences in their organization and management of care across the country. In the province of Quebec, general practitioners (GPs) and clinical pharmacists work on a part-time basis in public NHs that provide 24-h nursing care for people with complex needs. The present study was proposed to the local Health and Social Services Board (HSSB), which suggested the name of three NHs that agreed to participate. The study was approved by the HSSB and the *CHU de Québec* research centre ethics review boards (Ethics Certificate # C13-12-1886 / 2013–2014-25).

### Participant eligibility and recruitment procedures

To be eligible, residents within the three participating NHs had to be 65 years of age or older, have a diagnosis of severe dementia (of any etiology) recorded within their medical chart, and have resided in this NH for at least 2 months. The level of dementia severity is not usually available in the NH medical chart therefore, the Functional Autonomy Measurement System (*Système de Mesure de l'Autonomie Fonctionnelle*, SMAF) was used as a proxy measure [24]. SMAF is a broadly validated tool that predicts the needs of seniors and disabled persons on the basis of the WHO's classification of impairments, disabilities and handicaps. It measures performance on 29 functions of 1) activities of daily living, 2) mobility, 3) communication, 4) mental functions, and 5) instrumental activities of daily living. This leads to a numeric Iso-SMAF profile, which is used since 2005 to assess admission eligibility to Quebec NHs. Residents with Iso-SMAF profiles 13 and 14 (corresponding to stage 7 on the Reisberg FAST scale [25]) were included for study. There was no Iso-SMAF profile on record for three potentially eligible residents admitted before 2005, these residents Iso-SMAF profile was therefore evaluated by the NH nurses directly involved with their care.

Letters of invitation to participate in the study, along with a two-page informational leaflet about medication use in seniors with severe dementia, were sent to the families or legal guardians of eligible residents. A flow chart depicting study recruitment procedures is presented in Fig. 1.

### Medication review guidance

A medication review guidance (MRG) tool was developed from the medication appropriateness list agreed upon by the Delphi panel [23], for use in the province of Quebec NHs. In addition to being in French, the tool uses the American Hospital Formulary Service (AHFS) medication classes, and examples of drugs used in Quebec NHs as well as summary explanations (available at: http://www.ciusss-capitalenationale.gouv.qc.ca/sites/default/files/medication_demence_severe_oct2015.pdf).

### Knowledge exchange intervention

An interdisciplinary 90-min continuous education and Knowledge Exchange (KE) session, held by a geriatrician with extensive experience in continuous education (MMorin) and a pharmacist (EK), was conducted at each participating institution and included the institution's physicians, nurses and pharmacists. First, the context of the study as well as issues pertaining to the complexity of prescribing for seniors with severe dementia (e.g. frailty, multimorbidity, polypharmacy, metabolic changes) were presented. Second, the MRG tool (summarized in Additional file 1) and its intended use were explained. Finally, a clinical vignette representing a typical NH resident was used to illustrate how the MRG tool could facilitate medication reviews and the ensuing discussions.

Participating NH pharmacists were then asked to perform a medication review, using the MRG tool provided,

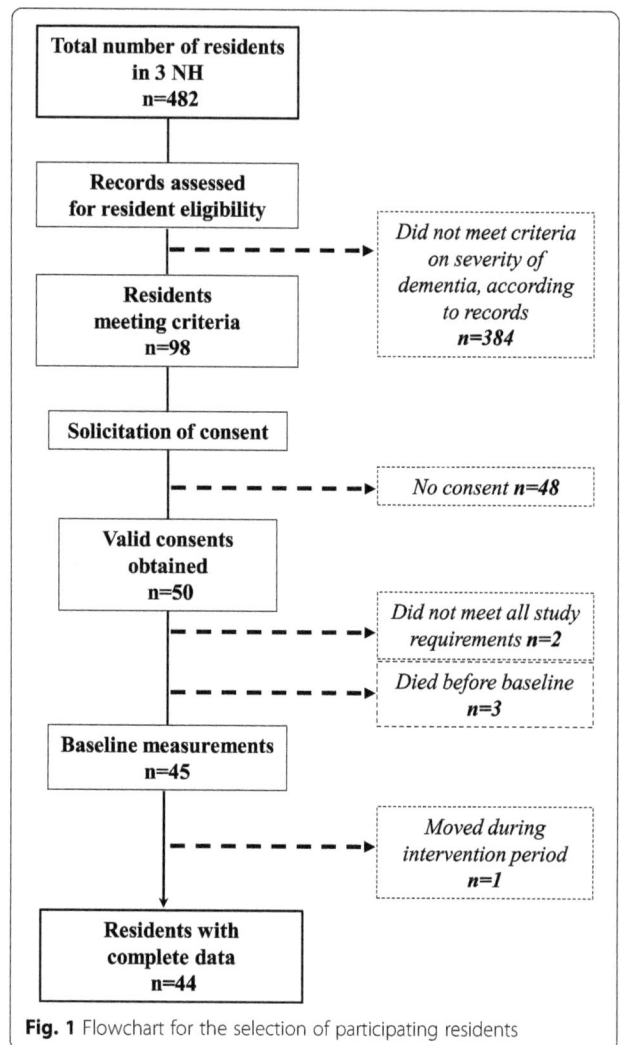

**Fig. 1** Flowchart for the selection of participating residents

for all study residents. The ensuing recommendations would be discussed with families and during NH multidisciplinary meetings involving the treating physician and, whenever possible, the treating nurse. The final decision regarding changes in medication regimen would be taken by each resident's physician, applying clinical judgment and considering all relevant information on the resident's clinical, psychological and social circumstances, level of care, and family considerations. The clinical decision and deprescribing processes were left to the care team discretion.

Finally, a second KE session was held at the end of the follow-up period where all participating health professionals were asked to complete a questionnaire and to provide feedback for the purposes of intervention improvement.

### Measurements

Data pertaining to age, sex and medical comorbidities [26] were collected from medical records of participating residents at baseline. The Observation Grid for

Medication-Taking [27] was used by the study nurse to assess problems with medication taking in participating residents.

Baseline and post follow-up medication use were derived from the NH pharmacy database, and each current ("active") prescription per participating resident was categorized according to the appropriateness list presented in Additional file 1 [23].

In order to evaluate whether deprescribing as a result of our intervention had resulted in adverse effects, levels of pain and of agitation were measured in participating residents during both the pre and post-intervention periods. Levels of pain and agitation were assessed during a total of four fifteen-minute observation periods, both at rest and during mobilization, and on two different days. The 60 items from the French version of the Pain Assessment Checklist for Seniors with Limited Ability to Communicate (PACSLAC-F) were used to evaluate the level of pain [28, 29]. PACSLAC-F, already used in many NHs, is based on the observation of residents' facial expression, activity or body movement, social behaviour, personality or mood, physiological changes or changes in eating, sleeping or vocal behaviour. No cut-off has been defined for this tool. Levels of agitation were measured by the total number of times any Cohen-Mansfield Agitation Inventory (CMAI) item was observed during the observation periods and scores over 45 should reflect severe agitation [30, 31]. Whenever possible, multidisciplinary meetings were attended by the study nurse to document discussions surrounding the pharmacist recommendations.

Finally, intervention relevance and feasibility were evaluated by NH GPs, pharmacists and nurses attending the post-intervention KE session via completion of a semi-structured questionnaire that included the opportunity to respond to open-ended questions.

## Data analyses

Descriptive statistics were computed for all variables collected at baseline (Table 1) and for all resident outcomes for both the pre and post-intervention periods (Table 2). Statistical differences in measures comparing pre and post-intervention were assessed using paired t-tests and Cochran's-Q tests for continuous and categorical outcomes, respectively. Odds ratios modeled using generalized linear mixed models (GLMM) were used to estimate the odds of having a prescription within each of the 3 medication appropriateness categories comparing the pre vs. post-intervention period. The GLMM model allowed for intra-prescription correlation, but assumed that prescriptions for a given individual were independent. Given the small sample size, no further adjustment could be performed. For similar reasons, the model included only effects for the appropriateness category,

**Table 1** Baseline characteristics, $n = 44$ participating residents

|  | Mean or % | SD |
|---|---|---|
| Age (years, mean) | 86.9 | 6.9 |
| Female (%) | 70.5 | n/a |
| Follow-up (days, mean) | 104 | 13.5 |
| Medication administration problems (scale of 0 to 13, mean)[a] | 0.23 | 0.86 |
| Charlson Comorbidity Score (mean) | 7.45 | 2.46 |
| Residents with severe agitation (> 45[b], %) | 13.6 | 12.8 |
| Discomfort/pain (scale of 0 to 60, mean)[c] | 8.1 | 2.3 |

SD, standard deviation
[a]Total number of problematic behaviors observed during medication administration [27]
[b]Sum of the number of times the Cohen-Mansfield Agitation Inventory items [31] were observed during the four 15-min observation periods
[c]Sum of observations of PACSLAC-F items [29] during the four 15-min observation periods

time, a category by time interaction, and no adjustment for confounding variables. All analyses were conducted using SAS 9.4.

## Results

Thirty-four NH health professionals participated in the first KE session: 5 GPs, 4 clinical pharmacists, 6 heads of NH care units (registered nurses or administrators), and 19 staff nurses (registered or auxiliary nurses). A total of 98 residents met the initial eligibility criteria as determined by medical records, and consent for study participation was obtained, from those who were entitled to take care decisions for these residents, for 50 eligible residents. Five potential participants were lost during the pre-intervention period: for two residents meeting the required Iso-SMAF profile, the level of dementia severity turned out to be below stage 7 on the FAST scale; three residents died before the intervention start date. In addition, one patient moved during the intervention period. For all remaining 44 residents, at least one medication review took place during the study period, and medication data both at baseline and at follow-up were available. Five participants died during the follow-up period before their level of pain and of agitation could be assessed. Baseline characteristics of the 44 participating residents are presented in Table 1. The participants have resided in the NH between 2 months and 16 years (mean 4.13 years; SD 3.13).

Mean follow-up for all 44 residents was 104 days (SD 13.5). The study nurse reported that pharmacists revised the medication regimens of all 44 participating residents using the provided medication review guidance tool. Pharmacist recommendations were discussed during scheduled meetings with the responsible GP; however, nurses did not generally attend these meetings but they were consulted as needed. The observation grid for medication-taking [27] did not provide much additional

**Table 2** Intervention outcomes among 44 participating residents

| Medication use | Pre-intervention | Post follow-up | p-value[***] |
|---|---|---|---|
| Total number of regular medications (n) | 372 | 327 | 0.0003 |
| Total number of "generally appropriate" medications (n) | 99 | 112 | 0.0741 |
| Total number of "sometimes appropriate" medications (n) | 194 | 167 | 0.0003 |
| Total number of "exceptionally appropriate" medications (n) | 12 | 10 | 0.4795 |
| Number of medications per participant (mean ± SD) | 7.86 ± 3.78 | 6.82 ± 3.75 | 0.0007 |
| Proportion of participants using "generally appropriate" medications (%) | 90.9 | 93.2 | 0.3173 |
| Proportion of participants using "sometimes appropriate" medications (%) | 97.7 | 97.7 | 1.000 |
| Proportion of participants using "exceptionally appropriate" medications (%) | 20.5 | 18.2 | 0.5637 |
| Level of agitation (mean ± SD)[*] | 21.1 ± 19.5 | 21.3 ± 15.9 | 0.7139 |
| Level of pain (scale 0 to 60, mean ± SD)[**] | 8.1 ± 2.3 | 9.7 ± 2.5 | < 0.0001 |

SD, standard deviation
[*]Sum of the number of times the Cohen-Mansfield Agitation Inventory items [31] were observed during the four 15-min observation periods
[**]Sum of observations of PACSLAC-F items [29] during the four 15-min observation periods
[***]p-values were estimated using Cochran's Q test for categorical variables and paired T-test for continuous variables

information since administration of crushed tablets mixed with yogurt or fruit purees was already used for residents with dysphagia.

Medication regimens of participating residents included 240 different medications, of which 22 (9%) were considered "generally", 109 (45%) "sometimes", and 29 (12%) "exceptionally" appropriate according to the medication appropriateness list (Additional file 1). Seventeen (7%) of the prescribed medications corresponded to those for which the Delphi panel had not been able to reach a consensus, including cholinesterase inhibitors, vitamin and mineral supplements. The remaining 63 medications (26%) were either products used for pressure ulcer or other dermatological indications not included in the appropriateness list (17), or other medications (47) for which appropriateness had been considered neither by the Delphi panel nor by previous research [22, 23]. For statistical analyses, these 80 medications were grouped together and categorized as "other medications".

Table 2 shows that, in this cohort, the proportion of residents exposed to the three categories of "generally", "sometimes", or "exceptionally" appropriate medications did not change much. There was a significant decrease in the total number of "sometimes" appropriate medications (from 194 pre to 167 post-intervention) and for "other" medications (from 31 to 21, not shown). There was, however, a significant reduction in the overall medication burden. The total number of regular medications decreased by 12.1%, from 372 at baseline to 327 at the end of follow-up (OR: 0.81; 95% CI: 0.70–0.92). The mean number of regular medications per participant decreased from 7.86 to 6.81 ($p = 0.007$)).

Mean levels of agitation did not change, six of the 44 participants showed severe agitation (score > 45) at baseline as compared to five residents with severe agitation

among the 39 observed at follow-up. There was a slight yet statistically significant increase in the level of pain post-intervention (Table 2).

Odds ratios and corresponding 95% confidence intervals estimating the risk associated with having at least one prescription at the end the follow-up as compared to baseline were 0.82 (0.52–1.30), 0.83 (0.74–0.94), 1.16 (1.00–1.36) and 0.53 (0.42–0.67) for "exceptionally appropriate", "sometimes-appropriate", "generally appropriate", and "other medications", respectively (Table 3).

Reduction in the use of antipsychotic agents however was minimal: detailed analyses showed that three antipsychotic agents were stopped, two were increased and for one the dosage was reduced. There were very few active prescriptions for cholinesterase inhibitors or memantine with only five prescriptions at baseline and four at the end of follow-up (Additional file 2).

The post-intervention KE session was attended by 22 health professionals, overall the intervention was positively evaluated (Table 4) In response to the open-ended questions, two thirds of the respondents mentioned inter-professional relations (e.g. team meetings, nurse involvement) as being very important, and one third indicated that information exchange had been clear and rigorous. Perceived barriers associated with medication review and adjustment included workload, difficulties in communication between shifts, staff turnover, and the fact that GPs and pharmacists are often off-site. Discontinuation of antipsychotic agents was identified as being difficult (Table 4).

## Discussion

Medication revision where consideration is given to reducing less appropriate medications for NH residents suffering from severe dementia, which underlies the

**Table 3** Odds ratio for the risk of having a prescription pre versus post-intervention

| Medication use among 44 participants | Odds ratio | 95% CI |
|---|---|---|
| All medications | 0.81 | (0.71–0.92) |
| By appropriateness category[a]: | | |
| "Generally appropriate" medication | 1.16 | (1.00–1.36) |
| "Sometimes appropriate" medication | 0.83 | (0.74–0.94) |
| "Exceptionally appropriate" medication | 0.82 | (0.52–1.30) |
| "Other" medication[b] | 0.53 | (0.42–0.67) |

[a]According to the medication appropriateness list [23]
[b]"Other" medications comprised those for which the Delphi panel had not reached a consensus as well as the medications not considered in the appropriateness list [23]

present research, stems from the desire to provide comfort care in the presence of severe dementia [3, 21, 22, 32–34]. This approach is not based on an estimate of remaining life expectancy, but on the consideration that residents with severe dementia benefit more from increased comfort than from increased life expectancy [22]. Medication appropriateness categories, as presented in the medication review guidance tool, should and do not replace clinical judgement by the resident's physician and care team, who would take all clinical, psychological and social characteristics of the resident into account. This idea is reflected by the terms used:

the Delphi panel members expressed the necessity to always make individualized therapeutic decisions and were unable to retain a "never" nor an "always" category [23]. The idea of considering certain medications, beyond criteria on potentially inappropriate medications for seniors such as those by Beers [19], as only "sometimes" or "exceptionally" appropriate for seniors suffering from severe dementia, is based on the conviction that these seniors should benefit from a comfort care approach [22, 32]. The clinical presentation of severe dementia, as indicated by the Reisberg scale [35], should trigger a change towards this care approach. When the risk to benefit ratio is in doubt (e.g. maintaining warfarin in the presence of atrial fibrillation for secondary stroke prevention with the need for frequent monitoring of blood level posing a heavy burden), it is the physician's clinical judgement determining whether to continue or deprescribe. These decisions are difficult and must include the family, if available, the care team, and all information regarding the senior's well-being.

The aim of this study was to establish the feasibility and acceptability of an interdisciplinary knowledge-exchange intervention to reduce medication load for NH senior residents with severe dementia. Our results indicate that the intervention was feasible and well accepted by health care professionals. The overall reduction in the number of medications per resident (12%) is encouraging as it may

**Table 4** Evaluation of the intervention by health professionals attending the post-intervention KE session

| # | Questions with multiple choice answers | Summary of responses |
|---|---|---|
| 1 | What do you think about the objective of optimizing medication for NH residents with severe dementia? | **All respondents** found that the study objective was a good idea. |
| 2 | Did you attend the first KE session? | **The majority of respondents** had participated in the first education session. |
| 3 | What about the relevance of the first KE session? | **All respondents** found the first education session either relevant or very relevant. |
| 4 | Had the first KE session influenced your attitude regarding the medication of residents with severe dementia? | The first education session influenced the attitude of **all but one respondent** who was already convinced of the merits of medication optimization. |
| 5 | Have you studied the provided MRG tool? | **Over half of the respondents** reported having read the provided MRG tool. |
| 6 | Has the MRG tool been useful in your practice? | **All respondents** found the provided MRG tool either useful or very useful. |
| 7 | How often did you use the MRG tool during the intervention period? | The degree of use of the MRG tool was **highly variable**, possibly depending on the respondents' responsibilities and experience. |
| 8 | Did the study nurse interfere with your work? | **All respondents** agreed on the noninterference of the study nurse. |
| 9 | Was your workload increased by the intervention? | **More than half of respondents** did not notice an increase in their workload; only one mentioned a greatly increased workload. |
| 10 | Was the residents' behavior changed by the intervention? | **More than half of respondents** did not observe changes in the residents' behavior. One respondent mentioned positive changes for some patients but negative for others, another found it difficult to evaluate. |
| 11 | Was the quality of life of the residents changed by the intervention? | **None of the respondents** mentioned a deterioration of the quality of life of residents. |
| 12 | Do you feel that NH staff should be sensitized to the complexity of medication for the residents with severe dementia? | **There was unanimity** on the need to educate NH staff regarding this issue. |
| 13 | Do you feel that NH staff should receive more information regarding the medication of residents with severe dementia? | **The majority of respondents** agreed, only two respondents were not sure. |

translate to less discomfort related to medication taking and monitoring and to time savings for care staff.

As shown in Additional file 2, these reductions concerned most significantly the category of "sometimes" appropriate medications, notably antidiabetic (from 12 to 7 prescriptions, 42%), antihypertensive (from 28 to 21, 25%), antidepressant (from 19 to 16, 16%) and laxative medications (from 46 to 42, 9%). Multivitamins, a medication class for which no Delphi consensus was achieved, were reduced from 21 to 7 prescriptions (67%). As for psychotropic drugs, a very small decrease in the number of regular prescriptions for antidepressants and antipsychotics was observed. There was no modification in the number of regular prescriptions for anxiolytic agents, which were considered "generally" appropriate [22, 23]. Thus, the OptimaMed intervention did not have a meaningful impact on the use of psychotropic drugs, but the study took place in settings already sensitive to the considerable risk of serious adverse effects associated with these medications [36–39]. It is interesting to note that the baseline average of 8 regular prescriptions per participating resident was lower than the 2012 Canadian NH average of 10 or more different medications in this population [11]. Despite low baseline medication use, a further reduction in medication load and in the use of only "sometimes appropriate" medications was observed.

Some NH antipsychotic deprescribing studies have generated encouraging results [40, 41] although one study did report an increase in neuropsychiatric symptoms in the intervention group [42]. Further interventions emphasize deprescribing of antipsychotics for neuropsychiatric symptoms of dementia. In Canada, this is facilitated by the recently published guidelines for the deprescribing of antipsychotics in dementia [43]. Given that at the time of this study, in 2014, these or other guidelines specific to the Canadian context had not yet been published, we were unable to include them in our pilot intervention. Study physicians had to follow prior available clinical guidance to progressively deprescribe certain medications, such as antipsychotics, for which a slight reduction was observed.

Previous deprescribing interventions have concluded that it is relatively safe to deprescribe antihypertensives (including diuretics), statins, and benzodiazepines in seniors [16, 44, 45]. In the present study, we observed no changes in the level of agitation, but a statistically significant increase in the measured level of pain. This increase of 1.6 point (the PACSLAC-F scale ranging from 0 to 60 points), over 4 months is not clinically worrisome, however, particularly in the context of the evolution of severe dementia.

Our intervention built upon the promising work by Garfinkel and colleagues, who incorporated evidence for medication indication, effectiveness, and adverse effects as well as patient circumstances and continuation preferences in an algorithm to improve drug therapy in frail seniors [46, 47]. In a Dutch cluster randomized trial to discontinue inappropriate medications, physicians in collaboration with pharmacists performed one multidisciplinary, multistep medication review for NH residents [48]. After a mean follow-up of 144 days, at least one inappropriate medication (according to the STOPP criteria [49]) was discontinued for 39% of participants, as compared to 29.5% in the control group, for an adjusted relative risk of 1.23 (95% CI 1.02–1.75), while there was no deterioration of clinical outcomes. In a randomised controlled trial on deprescribing, the intervention group had a mean reduction of 1.9 (SD 4.1) medications compared to an increase of 0.1 (SD 3.5) in the control group, for an estimated difference of 2.0 (95% CI 0.08–3.8) without significant differences for other outcomes [50]. However, none of these studies specifically addressed the particularly vulnerable subgroup of NH residents with severe dementia who may necessitate more specific criteria of medication appropriateness [22].

To our knowledge, our study is the first intervention based on a medication review guidance tool developped in Canada for NH seniors with advanced dementia. There are several limitations, however, that apply to the results of this study which must be interpreted cautiously. First, using a quasi-experimental design. it was not possible to determine whether the observed increase in the mean level of pain was a consequence of the intervention or of the evolution of the disease. Second, the sample size was too small to allow for adjustments for potential confounders. Third, the short follow-up duration did not permit to evaluate how sustainable the observed effects would be in the long run. On the other hand, the life expectancy of NH senior residents with severe dementia is limited, indeed 11% of our participants died during the 104-day period. Fourth, due to the NH GPs and pharmacists limited availability, the interval between the medication review and the measurement of outcomes varied between participants. Fifth, we were able to evaluate the levels of pain and of agitation at baseline and at the end of follow-up only. The same well-trained nurse performed pre and post measurements with the help of validated tools, but those were snapshots of behaviours likely to fluctuate from day to day. Finally, with the aim of testing the feasibility of implementing the OptimaMed intervention in Quebec NHs, we did not document the clinical decision-making process itself nor the specific reasons why medications were continued or deprescribed.

Several barriers and facilitators, identified by the NH care teams, may be addressed to improve the intervention. Adding specific information regarding the challenges of neuropsychiatric symptoms to KE sessions may prove useful. In addition to providing families with medication use information, it was also suggested that it would be important to consider further involvement of families in discussions regarding medication use. Research on challenges regarding KE with families and the ethical aspects of adjusting medication is ongoing, [51–53] and may help improve shared decision making in NHs. The quality of information exchange within the care team was identified as being a critical barrier, but workload, staff turnover and the limited availability of GPs and pharmacists were also mentioned as organisational/structural barriers. Improvements in those matters would, however, require changes in governmental policies.

## Conclusions

This quasi-experimental study tested the feasibility of an interdisciplinary intervention comprising KE and a tool to facilitate medication review for NH senior residents with severe dementia. Its results are encouraging with regard to reduction of overall medication burden, feasibility and NH staff interaction. The OptimaMed intervention may have the potential to improve medication use among this particularly vulnerable population of seniors. Ongoing regulatory changes regarding the roles and autonomy of pharmacists and nurses in North America, including the province of Quebec, may further this intervention. The conduct of clinical examinations by nurses and the adjustment of medication dosage by pharmacists may palliate the limited availability of GPs in NHs, and provide for a more harmonious work flow between all health care professionals.

## Abbreviations

AHFS: American Hospital Formulary Service; CIUSSSCN: *Centre intégré universitaire de santé et de services sociaux de la Capitale-Nationale*; CI: Confidence Intervals; CMAI: Cohen-Mansfield Agitation Inventory; FAST: Functional Assessment Staging Test; GLMM: Generalized Linear Mixed Models; GP: General Practitioner; HSSB: Health and Social Services Board; KE: Knowledge Exchange; MRG: Medication Review Guidance; NH: Nursing Home; OR: Odds Ratio; *p*: Probability; PACSLAC-F: Pain Assessment Checklist for Seniors with Limited Ability to Communicate-French; SD: Standard Deviation; SMAF: *Système de Mesure de l'Autonomie Fonctionnelle*; STOPP/START: Screening Tool Of Older People's Prescription/Screening Tool To Alert To Right Treatment

## Acknowledgements

The authors would like to thank the local Health and Social Services Board and all the staff at the three participating nursing homes who made this research possible. Special thanks to Mrs. Lise Grenier Gosselin, clinical pharmacist at the HSSB, for her contribution to the development of the medication review guidance tool and the extraction of medication data from the NH pharmacy database, and to Mrs. Denise Milliard, the study nurse, who collected all the other data.

## Funding

This study received financial and logistic support from the Alzheimer Society of Canada (EK; 2016 to 2018), the Quebec City Centre for Excellence in Aging of the *Centre intégré universitaire de santé et de services sociaux de la Capitale-Nationale (CIUSSSCN)* (EK), from the *Réseau québécois de recherche sur le vieillissement du Fonds de recherche québecois – santé* (EK and study team), from the *Fondation des hôpitaux St-Sacrement et Enfant-Jésus* (EK), the Donald Berman Foundation (MW), the *Fondation Laure Gaudreault* (EK) and the Canadian Consortium on Neurodegeneration and Aging (EK). None of the financial contributors participated in collection, analysis or interpretation of data or in writing the manuscript. The authors declare that they have no conflict of interest.
Some of the results in this manuscript have been presented at the annual meetings of the Canadian Geriatrics Society (2015) and the Canadian Academy of Geriatric Psychiatry (best poster award, October 2016).

## Authors' contributions

All authors participated in the development of the study, which was originally an idea of RV, MA and EK. EK, MMarcotte and MMorin participated in the actual intervention and PHC did the main analyses. MW and EK wrote the manuscript and all authors participated in data interpretation and commented the manuscript. All authors read and approved the final manuscript.

## Competing interests

The authors declare that they have no competing interests. None of the financing or supporting institutions had any influence on the study's objective, design, results or conclusion.

## Author details

[1]Department of Family Medicine and Division of Geriatric Medicine, McGill University, 5858, Chemin de la Côte-des-Neiges, Montreal, Quebec H3S 1Z1, Canada. [2]Donald Berman Maimonides Centre for Research in Aging, 5795 Caldwell Avenue, Montreal, Quebec H4W 1W3, Canada. [3]Department of Nursing Science and Gerontology, UMIT-The Health & Life Sciences University, Eduard-Wallnoefer-Zentrum 1, A-6060 Hall in Tyrol, Tyrol, Austria. [4]Centre d'excellence sur le vieillissement de Québec, Centre intégré universitaire de santé et de services sociaux de la Capitale-Nationale, 1050, Chemin Ste-Foy, room L2-30, Quebec City, Quebec G1S 4L8, Canada. [5]Laval University, 1050, avenue de la Médecine, Quebec City, Quebec G1V 0A6, Canada. [6]Faculté de médecine, Université de Montréal, 2900 Boulevard Edouard-Montpetit, Montreal, Quebec H3T 1J4, Canada. [7]Division of Geriatric Medicine, McGill University, Jewish General Hospital, 3755 Côte-Ste-Catherine, Montreal, Quebec H3T 1E2, Canada. [8]Centre de recherche sur le vieillissement, affilié à l'Université de Sherbrooke, 1036, rue Belvédère Sud, Sherbrooke, Quebec J1H 4C4, Canada.

## References

1. Mangoni AA, Jackson SH. Age-related changes in pharmacokinetics and pharmacodynamics: basic principles and practical applications. Br J Clin Pharmacol. 2004;57(1):6–14.
2. Lee SP, Bain KT, Maio V. Appropriate discontinuation of medications at the end of life: a need to establish consensus criteria. Am J Med Qual. 2007; 22(6):393–4.
3. Holmes HM. Rational prescribing for patients with a reduced life expectancy. Clin Pharmacol Ther. 2009;85(1):103–7.
4. Maddison AR, Fisher J, Johnston G. Preventive medication use among persons with limited life expectancy. Prog Palliat Care. 2011;19(1):15–21.
5. Gurwitz JH, Field TS, Harrold LR, Rothschild J, Debellis K, Seger AC, et al. Incidence and preventability of adverse drug events among older persons in the ambulatory setting. JAMA. 2003;289(9):1107–16.
6. Passarelli MC, Jacob-Filho W, Figueras A. Adverse drug reactions in an elderly hospitalised population: inappropriate prescription is a leading cause. Drugs Aging. 2005;22(9):767–77.
7. Hanlon JT, Pieper CF, Hajjar ER, Sloane RJ, Lindblad CI, Ruby CM, et al. Incidence and predictors of all and preventable adverse drug reactions in

frail elderly persons after hospital stay. J Gerontol A Biol Sci Med Sci. 2006; 61(5):511–5.

8.  Olivier P, Bertrand L, Tubery M, Lauque D, Montastruc JL, Lapeyre-Mestre M. Hospitalizations because of adverse drug reactions in elderly patients admitted through the emergency department: a prospective survey. Drugs Aging. 2009;26(6):475–82.

9.  Fahlman C, Lynn J, Finch M, Doberman D, Gabel J. Potentially inappropriate medication use by Medicaid+choice beneficiaries in the last year of life. J Palliat Med. 2007;10(3):686–95.

10. Gallagher P, Barry P, O'Mahony D. Inappropriate prescribing in the elderly. J Clin Pharm Ther. 2007;32(2):113–21.

11. Canadian Institute for Health Information. Drug Use Among Seniors on Public Drug Programs in Canada, 2012. Ottawa: CIHI; 2014.

12. Knight EL, Avorn J. Quality indicators for appropriate medication use in vulnerable elders. Ann Intern Med. 2001;135(8 Pt 2):703–10.

13. Brauner DJ, Muir JC, Sachs GA. Treating nondementia illnesses in patients with dementia. JAMA. 2000;283(24):3230–5.

14. Lau DT, Mercaldo ND, Harris AT, Trittschuh E, Shega J, Weintraub S. Polypharmacy and potentially inappropriate medication use among community-dwelling elders with dementia. Alzheimer Dis Assoc Disord. 2010;24(1):56–63.

15. Toscani F, Di Giulio P, Villani D, Giunco F, Brunelli C, Gentile S, et al. Treatments and prescriptions in advanced dementia patients residing in long-term care institutions and at home. J Palliat Med. 2013;16(1):31–7.

16. Tjia J, Cutrona SL, Peterson D, Reed G, Andrade SE, Mitchell SL. Statin discontinuation in nursing home residents with advanced dementia. J Am Geriatr Soc. 2014;62(11):2095–101.

17. Fialova D, Topinkova E, Gambassi G, Finne-Soveri H, Jonsson PV, Carpenter I, et al. Potentially inappropriate medication use among elderly home care patients in Europe. JAMA. 2005;293(11):1348–58.

18. Blass DM, Black BS, Phillips H, Finucane T, Baker A, Loreck D, et al. Medication use in nursing home residents with advanced dementia. Int J Geriatr Psychiatry. 2008;23(5):490–6.

19. American Geriatrics Society 2015 Updated Beers Criteria for Potentially Inappropriate Medication Use in Older Adults. J Am Geriatr Soc. 2015;63(11): 2227–46.

20. O'Mahony D, O'Sullivan D, Byrne S, O'Connor MN, Ryan C, Gallagher P. STOPP/START criteria for potentially inappropriate prescribing in older people: version 2. Age Ageing. 2015;44(2):213–8.

21. Arcand M, Roy-Petit J, Voyer G, Allard J, Ethier S. Doit-on prescrire des médicaments à visée préventive dans un contexte de démence modérée ou grave? La revue de gériatrie. 2007;32(3 Mars):189–200.

22. Holmes HM, Sachs GA, Shega JW, Hougham GW, Cox Hayley D, Dale W. Integrating palliative medicine into the care of persons with advanced dementia: identifying appropriate medication use. J Am Geriatr Soc. 2008;56(7):1306–11.

23. Kroger E, Wilchesky M, Marcotte M, Voyer P, Morin M, Champoux N, et al. Medication use among nursing home residents with severe dementia: identifying categories of appropriateness and elements of a successful intervention. J Am Med Dir Assoc. 2015;16(7):629 e1–17.

24. Dubuc N, Hebert R, Desrosiers J, Buteau M, Trottier L. Disability-based classification system for older people in integrated long-term care services: the Iso-SMAF profiles. Arch Gerontol Geriatr. 2006;42(2):191–206.

25. Reisberg B. Functional assessment staging (FAST). Psychopharmacol Bull. 1988;24(4):653–9.

26. Charlson ME, Pompei P, Ales KL, MacKenzie CR. A new method of classifying prognostic comorbidity in longitudinal studies: development and validation. J Chronic Dis. 1987;40(5):373–83.

27. Arcand M, Grégoire A, Béliveau MJ, Marcotte M, Kröger E. Problèmes liés à la prise de médicaments chez les résidents d'établissements de soins de longue durée. Quebec City: Centre d'excellence sur le vieillissement de Québec du Centre intégré universitaire de santé et de services sociaux de la Capitale-Nationale (CIUSSSCN); 2013 [Observational grid for nurses in long term care]. Available from: https://www.ciusss-capitalenationale.gouv.qc.ca/sites/default/files/docs/CEVQ/observation_prise_medicaments.pdf.

28. Fuchs-Lacelle S, Hadjistavropoulos T, Lix L. Pain assessment as intervention: a study of older adults with severe dementia. Clin J Pain. 2008;24(8):697–707.

29. Aubin M, Verreault R, Savoie M, LeMay S, Hadjistavropoulos T, Fillion L, et al. [Validity 'and Utilities' clinic of a grid observation (PACSLAC-F) to evaluate the pain in seniors with dementia's living in the Long-Term Care ]. Can J Aging. 2008 Spring;27(1):45–55.

30. Cohen-Mansfield J, Marx MS, Rosenthal AS. A description of agitation in a nursing home. J Gerontol. 1989;44(3):M77–84.

31. Deslauriers S, Landreville P, Dicaire L, Verreault R. Validité et fidélité de l'Inventaire d'agitation de Cohen-Mansfield. Can J Aging. 2001;20(3):374–84.

32. Arcand M, Monette J, Monette M, Sourial N, Fournier L, Gore B, et al. Educating nursing home staff about the progression of dementia and the comfort care option: impact on family satisfaction with end-of-life care. J Am Med Dir Assoc. 2009;10(1):50–5.

33. Arcand M, Verreault R. Améliorer les soins de fin de vie en démence avancée. Ger Psychol Neuropsychiatr Vieil. 2014;12(suppl 1):37.

34. van der Steen JT, Radbruch L, Hertogh CM, de Boer ME, Hughes JC, Larkin P, et al. White paper defining optimal palliative care in older people with dementia: a Delphi study and recommendations from the European Association for Palliative Care. Palliat Med. 2014;28(3):197–209.

35. Reisberg B, Ferris SH, de Leon MJ, Crook T. The global deterioration scale for assessment of primary degenerative dementia. Am J Psychiatry. 1982;139(9): 1136–39.

36. Kales HC, Gitlin LN, Lyketsos CG. Assessment and management of behavioral and psychological symptoms of dementia. BMJ. 2015;350:h369.

37. Ballard CG, Gauthier S, Cummings JL, Brodaty H, Grossberg GT, Robert P, et al. Management of agitation and aggression associated with Alzheimer disease. Nat Rev Neurol. 2009;5(5):245–55.

38. Gill SS, Bronskill SE, Normand SL, Anderson GM, Sykora K, Lam K, et al. Antipsychotic drug use and mortality in older adults with dementia. Ann Intern Med. 2007;146(11):775–86.

39. Rochon PA, Normand SL, Gomes T, Gill SS, Anderson GM, Melo M, et al. Antipsychotic therapy and short-term serious events in older adults with dementia. Arch Intern Med. 2008;168(10):1090–6.

40. Monette J, Monette M, Sourial N, Vandal AC, Wolfson C, Champoux N, et al. Effect of an interdisciplinary educational program on antipsychotic prescribing among residents with dementia in two long-term care centers. J Appl Gerontol. 2013;32(7):833–54.

41. Ballard C, Lana MM, Theodoulou M, Douglas S, McShane R, Jacoby R, et al. A randomised, blinded, placebo-controlled trial in dementia patients continuing or stopping neuroleptics (the DART-AD trial). PLoS Med. 2008;5(4):587–99.

42. Pan YJ, Wu CS, Gau SS, Chan HY, Banerjee S. Antipsychotic discontinuation in patients with dementia: a systematic review and meta-analysis of published randomized controlled studies. Dement Geriatr Cogn Disord. 2014;37(3–4):125–40.

43. Bjerre LM, Farrell B, Hogel M, Graham L, Lemay G, McCarthy L, et al. Deprescribing antipsychotics for behavioural and psychological symptoms of dementia and insomnia: evidence-based clinical practice guideline. Can Fam Physician. 2018;64(1):17–27.

44. Tannenbaum C, Martin P, Tamblyn R, Benedetti A, Ahmed S. Reduction of inappropriate benzodiazepine prescriptions among older adults through direct patient education: the EMPOWER cluster randomized trial. JAMA Intern Med. 2014;174(6):890–8.

45. Iyer S, Naganathan V, McLachlan AJ, Le Couteur DG. Medication withdrawal trials in people aged 65 years and older: a systematic review. Drugs Aging. 2008;25(12):1021–31.

46. Garfinkel D. Poly-de-prescribing to treat polypharmacy: efficacy and safety. Ther Adv Durg Saf. 2017:1–19.

47. Garfinkel D, Ilhan B, Bahat G. Routine deprescribing of chronic medications to combat polypharmacy. Ther Adv Drug Saf. 2015;6(6):212–33.

48. Wouters H, Scheper J, Koning H, Brouwer C, Twisk JW, van der Meer H, et al. Discontinuing inappropriate medication use in nursing home residents. A cluster randomized controlled trial. Ann Intern Med. 2017;167(9):609–17.

49. Gallagher P, O'Mahony D. STOPP (screening tool of older Persons' potentially inappropriate prescriptions): application to acutely ill elderly patients and comparison with Beers' criteria. Age Ageing. 2008;37(6):673–9.

50. Gallagher PF, O'Connor MN, O'Mahony D. Prevention of potentially inappropriate prescribing for elderly patients: a randomized controlled trial using STOPP/START criteria. Clin Pharmacol Ther. 2011;89(6):845–54.

51. Reeve E, Low LF, Hilmer SN. Beliefs and attitudes of older adults and carers about deprescribing of medications: a qualitative focus group study. Br J Gen Pract. 2016;66(649):e552–60.

52. Turner JP, Edwards S, Stanners M, Shakib S, Bell JS. What factors are important for deprescribing in Australian long-term care facilities? Perspectives of residents and health professionals. BMJ Open. 2016;6(3): e009781.

53. Simard M, Marcotte M, Pluye P, Sirois C, Champoux N, Arcand M, et al. Chapitre 13 : Attitudes et comportements des aînés et de leurs proches face à la polypharmacie ou à la déprescription: une revue mixte de la littérature. In: Bujold M, QN Hong, V Ridde, CJ Bourque, MJ Dogba, I Vedel et P Pluye, editors. Oser les défis des méthodes mixtes en sciences sociales et sciences de la santé. Cahiers scientifiques de l'ACFAS. Montréal, Canada: ACFAS; 2018. p. 223–43.

# 5

# Variation in the health outcomes associated with frailty among home care clients: relevance of caregiver distress and client sex

Colleen J. Maxwell[1,2]* ⓘ, Michael A. Campitelli[2], Christina Diong[2], Luke Mondor[2,3], David B. Hogan[4], Joseph E. Amuah[5], Sarah Leslie[6], Dallas Seitz[7], Sudeep Gill[8], Kednapa Thavorn[9], Walter P. Wodchis[10], Andrea Gruneir[11], Gary Teare[12] and Susan E. Bronskill[2]

## Abstract

**Background:** The identification of contextual factors that modify associations between client frailty and their health and service use outcomes is essential for informed home health care and policy planning. Our objective was to examine variation in the associations between frailty and select 1-year health outcomes by caregiver distress and client sex among community-residing older care recipients.

**Methods:** We conducted a retrospective cohort study using linked population-based clinical and health administrative databases for all long-stay home care clients ($n = 234,552$) aged 66+ years assessed during April 2010–2013 in Ontario, Canada. Frailty was assessed using a previously validated 72-item frailty index (FI). Presence of caregiver distress was derived from clinical assessment items administered by trained home care assessors. Multivariable log-binomial regression models were used to examine variations in the associations between frailty and outcomes of interest (mortality, nursing home [NH] placement, all-cause and prolonged hospitalization) by caregiver distress, with further model stratification by client sex.

**Results:** Frailty prevalence varied little by sex (19.3% women, 19.9% men) despite significant sex-differences in clients' sociodemographic and health characteristics. In both sexes, frailty was significantly associated with all outcomes, particularly NH placement (RR = 3.84, 95%CI 3.75–3.93) and death (RR = 2.32, 95%CI 2.27–2.37), though risk ratios were greater for women. Caregiver distress was more common with increasing frailty and for male clients, and a significant independent predictor of NH placement and prolonged hospitalization in both sexes. The association between frailty and NH placement (but not other outcomes) varied by caregiver distress for both men and women ($p < 0.001$ interaction terms), showing a greater magnitude of association among clients without (vs. with) a distressed caregiver.

**Conclusions:** As caregiver distress varies by client sex, represents a key driver of NH placement (even among relatively robust clients), and modifies the impact of other risk factors such as frailty, it should be routinely assessed. Further, sex-differences should be considered when developing and evaluating community-based services for older adults and their caregivers.

**Keywords:** Home care, Frailty, Caregiver distress, Sex, Gender, Nursing home, Hospitalization, Mortality, Retrospective cohort

* Correspondence: colleen.maxwell@uwaterloo.ca
[1]Schools of Pharmacy and Public Health & Health Systems, University of Waterloo, 200 University Ave. W, Waterloo, ON N2L 3G1, Canada
[2]Institute for Clinical Evaluative Sciences, 2075 Bayview Ave, Toronto, ON M4N 3M5, Canada
Full list of author information is available at the end of the article

## Background

In Canada and the United States, the provision of in-home professional and supportive services for older adults is an important and growing part of the healthcare system [1, 2]. Proposals for healthcare reforms in both countries have called for a significant expansion of publicly funded home care, including the provision of additional support for family caregivers [3–5]. Underlying these reforms is the hope that enhanced community-based care may reduce both acute and nursing home facility admissions among vulnerable older adults [6–9]. As government payers face competing demands for their (limited) health budgets, identifying individuals at heightened risk for admission to facility-based care and thus, most likely to benefit from community-based services, has become a key priority [7, 10].

The identification of frailty offers a promising approach to risk stratification in this care setting [11, 12]. Frailty refers to a state of increased vulnerability to stressors arising from multi-system dysfunction leading to declines in homeostatic reserve and resiliency [12]. In previous work, we demonstrated both the feasibility and predictive validity of a frailty index measure derived from assessment data routinely collected on older home care recipients [10, 13]. In addition to predicting mortality and transitions to higher levels of care, this frailty measure was positively associated with the likelihood of caregiver distress. Intriguing questions emerging from this earlier work include the extent to which caregiver-related factors modify the associations between client frailty and relevant health outcomes such as hospitalization and NH placement and whether associations further vary by client sex. Given sex-related differences in health and the nature and availability of informal support [14–16], it is plausible that the impact of caregiver distress on frailty-related outcomes may differ by client sex.

Family and friends play a significant role in providing supportive care to vulnerable older adults in the community [4, 5, 17]. This role is viewed positively by many informal (or unpaid) caregivers who derive a sense of fulfillment from providing needed care or services [18–20]. At the same time, the increasingly complex nature of care recipient needs coupled with demanding caregiving roles and expectations can precipitate stress and poor outcomes for both care providers and recipients [21–24]. Consequently, the presence and extent of caregiver distress or burden requires consideration when assessing the larger impact of community-based care reforms for older adults. Caregiver distress has been shown to be an independent predictor of health outcomes and costs among community-dwelling older adults, particularly for those with dementia [25–28]. However, few large scale studies have examined its importance among the general population of older home care clients, and data

are especially scarce on its role as an effect modifier of associations between frailty and health outcomes in this care setting [11].

Among the few studies that have examined moderators of frailty-related outcomes, the focus has largely been on the relevance of psychosocial resources (including perceived social support and wellbeing) and findings were inconclusive [29, 30]. There is also some preliminary data to suggest that more positive responses on a summary protection index (combining a diverse number of items reflecting an older adult's socioeconomic status, lifestyle behaviours and environmental factors) may mitigate frailty-related mortality and health decline for robust or pre-frail older persons [31]. The relevance of such findings to more vulnerable older adults receiving home care is unknown. Further exploration of the impact of informal care characteristics on frailty-related outcomes among female and male home care recipients could inform policy development and resource allocation for this population [10, 32]. Additionally, illustrating effect modification by these contextual factors might enhance support for targeted and tailored community-based services for older adults [33].

Our primary objective was to examine the degree to which caregiver distress modifies the associations between frailty and select 1-year health outcomes among a population-based cohort of older home care clients. A secondary objective was to investigate variation in the role of this modifying factor between female and male clients.

## Methods

### Study design, setting and population

We conducted a retrospective cohort study of long-stay home care clients in Ontario, Canada using linked health administrative and clinical databases (see Additional file 1: Table S1). These databases were linked using encoded identifiers and analyzed at the Institute for Clinical Evaluative Sciences (ICES).

In Ontario, semi-annual assessments with the Resident Assessment Instrument for Home Care (RAI-HC) are provincially mandated for all clients receiving long-stay services (i.e., ≥ 60 days in a single episode). The RAI-HC is administered by trained staff and provides standardized validated data on clients' sociodemographic characteristics, health conditions, physical and cognitive status, behaviors, and service use [34]. RAI-HC assessment data are included in the ICES repository. A summary of the organization and funding of Ontario home care at the time of this study is provided in Additional file 1: Table S1.

We identified all clients assessed between April 1, 2010 and March 31, 2013 ($n = 296,964$) and captured data from their earliest RAI-HC (index date). Given our focus on clients receiving services in the community and age requirements for data availability, we excluded those aged < 66 ($n = 55,343$; 18.6%) or > 105 ($n = 24$; 0.01%) years, receiving case management only ($n = 4444$; 1.5%), in a nursing home facility during the prior year ($n = 2351$; 0.8%), with data quality issues ($n = 183$; 0.06%), or a non-Ontario postal code ($n = 67$; 0.02%). The resulting sample included 234,552 clients.

This study was approved by the Research Ethics Board at Sunnybrook Health Sciences Centre and the University of Waterloo, Office of Research Ethics (ORE File #19950). Informed consent by participants was not required as this project was conducted under section 45 of Ontario's Personal Health Information Protection Act and approved by ICES' Privacy and Compliance Office.

## Frailty

Frailty was assessed with a validated 72-item frailty index (FI) based on items derived from the index RAI-HC assessment [10]. The FI was calculated as the proportion of accumulated to potential health deficits. Deficits included physical, cognitive, behavioural and psychosocial characteristics. As in previous work [10, 13], robust, pre-frail and frail clients were defined based on FI scores of < 0.2, 0.2–0.3, and > 0.3, respectively.

## Covariates

Clients' age, sex, and date of death were determined from administrative data (Additional file 1: Table S1). Comorbidity was assessed with the Aggregated Diagnosis Groups (ADGs) derived using the Johns Hopkins Adjusted Clinical Group algorithms [35] and based on health service use in the two years prior to clients' index date (The Johns Hopkins ACG® System, v10). Data regarding clients' marital status, health conditions and caregiver characteristics were obtained from their index RAI-HC.

## Caregiver measures

Caregiver characteristics included the presence of a primary caregiver (and their relationship to, and living arrangement with, the client) and average hours of care per day for instrumental and basic activities of daily living (ADL) provided in the past week by family, friends and neighbours. Unfortunately, we did not have information on caregivers' age or sex, though some assumptions could be made about both based on the information that was available to us from the RAI-HC (as described above). Caregiver distress was determined by a positive response to at least one the following two RAI-HC items: a caregiver reports or is perceived by the home care assessor to be unable to continue in caring activities (due to various reasons, e.g., a decline in health of caregiver, a lack of desire to continue, geographical

inaccessibility, other competing family or work requirements or personal health issues) and/or caregiver reported feelings of distress, anger or depression. This is a standard and widely accepted measure of caregiver distress (burden) when using RAI-HC data and has been employed in numerous national and provincial health system quality reports [3, 4, 36, 37] and previous studies on home care in Canada [14, 38, 39].

## Outcomes

Outcomes assessed over the 1-year included death, nursing home (NH) placement, any (inpatient) hospitalization and prolonged hospital stay as derived from the administrative databases. In Ontario, the NH setting primarily encompasses long-stay residents requiring 24-h nursing and personal care and/or supervision. A prolonged hospitalization is defined for a patient who no longer requires the intensity of services provided in acute care but is unable to be discharged because adequate care is not available elsewhere (often because a NH bed is unavailable) [40].

## Analysis

Descriptive analyses examined the distribution of baseline characteristics and 1-year outcomes among the total sample and by frailty level. Associations between frailty and each of the binary outcomes were examined using log-binomial regression models to estimate risk ratios. Models were adjusted for age, sex and comorbidity to be consistent with previous work [10]. Associations between caregiver distress and the four outcomes were examined in separate models that were initially adjusted for age, sex and comorbidity and then also for frailty level.

To examine effect modification by caregiver distress, we derived a set of mutually exclusive variables to cross-classify clients by frailty and presence/absence of caregiver distress. For example, clients were classified into one of 6 categories defined by frailty level (robust, pre-frail, frail) and caregiver distress (yes, no) and four separate regression models (one for each outcome) were examined including this categorical variable while also adjusting for age, sex and comorbidity. This allows for direct estimation of the effect of frailty on outcomes at each level of the covariate and comparison of risk ratios within and between levels of the covariate. For this categorical variable, the reference group was selected to represent those expected to have the lowest risk (e.g., robust and caregiver not distressed). These analyses were then stratified by client sex.

We employed alternative modeling strategies (i.e., including an interaction term between frailty and caregiver distress) to derive tests of statistical significance for this interaction term. We were cautious when interpreting findings from these tests as even small differences would be expected to be highly significant given our sample size.

All analyses were conducted using SAS version 9.4 (SAS Institute Inc., Cary, NC).

## Results

The mean age of clients was 82 (±7.4) years, 65% were women and almost half were widowed (Additional file 1: Table S2). Most reported having a primary caregiver (98%) and for half of these clients, this caregiver lived in the same residence. The primary caregiver was most commonly a child or child-in-law (55.3%) followed by a spouse (31.2%), other relative (7.9%) and friend or neighbor (5.7%) [data not shown]. Clients received an average of 2.4 h of care from family or friends per day, and almost one quarter had a distressed caregiver. High levels of client morbidity were evident. Frailty was positively associated with client age, comorbidity level, informal care hours, and likelihood for the primary caregiver to live with the client and to be distressed.

Female clients were more likely to be older, widowed, and to not reside with their primary caregiver (Table 1). For women, relative to men, this caregiver was more likely to be a child or child-in-law (65.9% vs. 35.7%) as

**Table 1** Baseline characteristics of long-stay home care clients in Ontario (2010–2013), by sex and frailty status (n = 234,552)

| Characteristic | Women (n = 151,427) | | | Men (n = 83,125) | | |
|---|---|---|---|---|---|---|
| | FI Frailty Status (n, column %) | | | FI Frailty Status (n, column %) | | |
| | Robust (n = 69,709; 46.0%) | Pre-Frail (n = 52,549; 34.7%) | Frail (n = 29,169; 19.3%) | Robust (n = 38,967; 46.9%) | Pre-Frail (n = 27,606; 33.2%) | Frail (n = 16,552; 19.9%) |
| Age group | | | | | | |
| 66–74 | 12,154 (17.4) | 8163 (15.5) | 3800 (13.0) | 9250 (23.7) | 5354 (19.4) | 2920 (17.6) |
| 75–84 | 28,943 (41.5) | 21,722 (41.3) | 11,067 (37.9) | 17,084 (43.8) | 12,526 (45.4) | 7350 (44.4) |
| 85+ | 28,612 (41.0) | 22,664 (43.1) | 14,302 (49.0) | 12,633 (32.4) | 9726 (35.2) | 6282 (38.0) |
| Mean age ± SD | 82.1 ± 7.4 | 82.6 ± 7.3 | 83.6 ± 7.4 | 80.5 ± 7.5 | 81.3 ± 7.2 | 81.7 ± 7.2 |
| Marital status | | | | | | |
| Married | 18,930 (27.2) | 13,867 (26.4) | 7647 (26.2) | 23,450 (60.2) | 17,254 (62.5) | 10,916 (65.9) |
| Never married/other | 3739 (5.4) | 2256 (4.3) | 1134 (3.9) | 2601 (6.7) | 1402 (5.1) | 756 (4.6) |
| Widowed | 42,506 (61.0) | 32,987 (62.8) | 18,817 (64.5) | 9893 (25.4) | 7038 (25.5) | 3935 (23.8) |
| Separated/Divorced | 4534 (6.5) | 3439 (6.5) | 1571 (5.4) | 3023 (7.8) | 1912 (6.9) | 945 (5.7) |
| Primary Caregiver | | | | | | |
| No primary caregiver | 1857 (2.7) | 926 (1.8) | 372 (1.3) | 1276 (3.3) | 515 (1.9) | 235 (1.4) |
| Yes, does not live with | 40,437 (58.0) | 28,388 (54.0) | 14,430 (49.5) | 13,799 (35.4) | 8868 (32.1) | 4962 (30.0) |
| Yes, lives with | 27,415 (39.3) | 23,235 (44.2) | 14,367 (49.3) | 23,892 (61.3) | 18,223 (66.0) | 11,355 (68.6) |
| Average hours of informal care per day,[a] | | | | | | |
| mean ± SD | 1.60 ± 1.80 | 2.39 ± 2.59 | 3.25 ± 3.83 | 2.01 ± 2.07 | 3.09 ± 2.96 | 3.82 ± 4.09 |
| Caregiver is distressed | | | | | | |
| No | 62,992 (90.4) | 40,566 (77.2) | 17,557 (60.2) | 32,833 (84.3) | 17,999 (65.2) | 7985 (48.2) |
| Yes | 6717 (9.6) | 11,983 (22.8) | 11,612 (39.8) | 6134 (15.7) | 9607 (34.8) | 8567 (51.8) |
| # ADG comorbidity categories | | | | | | |
| 0–5 | 11,766 (16.9) | 7554 (14.4) | 3743 (12.8) | 5089 (13.1) | 3082 (11.2) | 1485 (9.0) |
| 6–9 | 23,646 (33.9) | 16,163 (30.8) | 8142 (27.9) | 11,862 (30.4) | 7742 (28.0) | 4023 (24.3) |
| 10+ | 34,297 (49.2) | 28,832 (54.9) | 17,284 (59.3) | 22,016 (56.5) | 16,782 (60.8) | 11,044 (66.7) |
| Most prevalent diagnoses | | | | | | |
| Hypertension | 41,260 (59.2) | 35,755 (68.0) | 20,623 (70.7) | 20,160 (51.7) | 16,614 (60.2) | 10,660 (64.4) |
| Arthritis | 37,575 (53.9) | 32,496 (61.8) | 18,075 (62.0) | 13,382 (34.3) | 11,834 (42.9) | 7418 (44.8) |
| Diabetes | 13,281 (19.1) | 14,177 (27.0) | 8876 (30.4) | 10,229 (26.3) | 9120 (33.0) | 6142 (37.1) |
| Coronary artery disease | 11,900 (17.1) | 14,032 (26.7) | 8859 (30.4) | 9357 (24.0) | 9346 (33.9) | 6486 (39.2) |
| Osteoporosis | 19,175 (27.5) | 17,665 (33.6) | 10,829 (37.1) | 2355 (6.0) | 2379 (8.6) | 1663 (10.0) |

Abbreviations: *FI* = frailty index, *SD* = standard deviation, *ADG* = Aggregated Diagnosis Groups
[a]Hours of care for instrumental and basic activities of daily living in past week by family, friends and neighbours
Note: for all comparisons across frailty level, *p* < 0.001

opposed to a spouse (19.5% vs. 52.6%) [data not shown]. Average hours of informal care received per day were higher for men than women as was the likelihood for a distressed caregiver (e.g., 51.8% of frail men and 39.8% of frail women had a distressed caregiver). Higher levels of comorbidity were observed among men although some conditions were more prevalent among women (e.g., hypertension, arthritis, and osteoporosis). Although statistically significant, there was little difference in frailty prevalence between women (19.3%) and men (19.9%).

## Associations between frailty, caregiver distress and outcomes

During the 1-year follow-up, 18% of clients died, 17% were admitted to a NH, 42% experienced at least 1 hospitalization and 14% had a prolonged hospital stay. The proportion of clients experiencing each outcome increased significantly with frailty level (Additional file 1: Table S3). The distribution of outcomes by sex, caregiver distress, and frailty are presented in Additional file 1: Tables S4 and S5. With the exception of NH placement, all outcomes were more common among men.

Following adjustment for age, sex and comorbidity, higher frailty levels were significantly associated with all outcomes, most notably NH placement and death (Table 2, base models). Further stratification by sex showed similar findings although for all outcomes except prolonged hospitalization, risk ratios associated with frailty were higher among women than men. Overall and for both sexes, including frailty and caregiver distress in the same model (Table 2, full models) had little effect on frailty-related risk estimates for most outcomes with the exception of NH placement where risk estimates were somewhat attenuated.

In similarly adjusted base models, caregiver distress was significantly associated with client risk for all outcomes, with stronger associations observed for NH placement and weaker associations noted for other outcomes, especially any hospitalization (Table 2, base models). Similar findings were observed for models further stratified by sex. Following further adjustment for client frailty (Table 2, full models), caregiver distress remained significantly associated with NH placement and prolonged hospitalization only.

## Modification of frailty-outcome associations by caregiver distress

The associations between frailty and death, hospitalization and prolonged hospitalization were not modified by caregiver distress (Table 3). For example, the risk of prolonged hospitalization for frail vs. robust clients was 1.42 among those without a distressed caregiver and 1.49 (1.68/1.13) among those with a distressed caregiver. For some outcomes, interaction terms were

statistically significant (i.e., for any hospitalization, $p = 0.002$ for frail*caregiver distress; for prolonged hospitalization, $p = 0.002$ for pre-frail*caregiver distress) largely reflecting the sample size rather than meaningful variation.

The association between frailty and NH placement was modified by caregiver distress, both overall and when stratified by client sex (Table 3; Fig. 1). Specifically, while increasing frailty was associated with increased risk of placement among those with and without a distressed caregiver, the magnitude of the association was greater among clients *without* than with a distressed caregiver ($p < 0.001$, all interaction terms). For example, the risk of placement for frail vs. robust clients was 4 fold among those *without* a distressed caregiver, and 2.3 fold (4.79/2.10) among those with a distressed caregiver. Relative to the reference group (client robust and caregiver not distressed), the combination of frailty and a distressed caregiver was associated with a 5 fold increased risk of placement for women and a 4 fold increased risk for men.

## Discussion

Building on our earlier work [10], higher frailty levels were significantly and independently associated with all health outcomes examined among both women and men. Risk estimates were strongest for NH placement and death and higher for women than men for most outcomes. Interestingly, despite significant sex-related differences in clients' sociodemographic and health characteristics, frailty prevalence did not vary by client sex with approximately 1 in 5 women and men classified as frail. However, caregiver distress, which increased significantly with increasing frailty and hours of informal care, was considerably more common among male than female clients.

After adjusting for covariates (including frailty), clients with a distressed caregiver were 40% more likely to be placed in a NH and 10% more likely to experience a prolonged hospitalization and these findings were comparable for female and male clients. The presence of caregiver distress did not appear to modify the associations between frailty and death or hospitalization events. There was, however, evidence of important effect modification by caregiver distress for the association between frailty and NH placement. Overall, and for women and men separately, the impact of frailty on placement was of a greater magnitude among those without (vs. with) a distressed caregiver.

There is general agreement that caregiver burden is an important predictor of institutionalization, particularly among older adults with dementia [25–27]. Our findings demonstrate that this association extends to the wider population of older home care clients not selected for

**Table 2** Associations between client frailty status, caregiver distress and risk of health outcomes during 1 year follow-up, overall and by client sex

| | Outcomes at 1 year | | | | | | | |
| | Death | | NH Placement | | Any Hospitalization | | Prolonged Hospitalization[a] | |
| | Base Models[b] Risk Ratio (95% CI) | Full Models[c] Risk Ratio (95% CI) | Base Models[b] Risk Ratio (95% CI) | Full Models[c] Risk Ratio (95% CI) | Base Models[b] Risk Ratio (95% CI) | Full Models[c] Risk Ratio (95% CI) | Base Models[b] Risk Ratio (95% CI) | Full Models[c] Risk Ratio (95% CI) |
|---|---|---|---|---|---|---|---|---|
| **OVERALL** | | | | | | | | |
| Client Frailty (FI) | | | | | | | | |
| Robust (ref) | | | | | | | | |
| Pre-frail | 1.45 (1.42–1.48) | 1.46 (1.43–1.49) | 2.20 (2.15–2.26) | 2.08 (2.03–2.13) | 1.17 (1.16–1.19) | 1.17 (1.16–1.19) | 1.42 (1.39–1.45) | 1.40 (1.37–1.43) |
| Frail | 2.32 (2.27–2.37) | 2.34 (2.29–2.40) | 3.84 (3.75–3.93) | 3.39 (3.31–3.48) | 1.22 (1.20–1.23) | 1.22 (1.20–1.23) | 1.51 (1.47–1.55) | 1.47 (1.43–1.51) |
| Caregiver Distress | | | | | | | | |
| No (ref) | | | | | | | | |
| Yes | 1.21 (1.19–1.24) | 0.97 (0.95–0.98) | 1.95 (1.92–1.99) | 1.40 (1.37–1.42) | 1.06 (1.05–1.07) | 1.00 (0.99–1.01) | 1.23 (1.20–1.25) | 1.10 (1.08–1.13) |
| **WOMEN** | | | | | | | | |
| Client Frailty (FI) | | | | | | | | |
| Robust (ref) | | | | | | | | |
| Pre-frail | 1.51 (1.47–1.56) | 1.52 (1.47–1.56) | 2.25 (2.18–2.32) | 2.13 (2.07–2.20) | 1.20 (1.19–1.22) | 1.20 (1.18–1.22) | 1.43 (1.39–1.48) | 1.41 (1.37–1.45) |
| Frail | 2.61 (2.53–2.69) | 2.62 (2.54–2.70) | 4.06 (3.94–4.17) | 3.58 (3.47–3.69) | 1.26 (1.24–1.28) | 1.25 (1.23–1.27) | 1.52 (1.47–1.57) | 1.47 (1.42–1.52) |
| Caregiver Distress | | | | | | | | |
| No (ref) | | | | | | | | |
| Yes | 1.29 (1.25–1.32) | 0.99 (0.96–1.02) | 2.02 (1.97–2.06) | 1.41 (1.38–1.45) | 1.08 (1.07–1.10) | 1.02 (1.00–1.03) | 1.25 (1.21–1.28) | 1.12 (1.08–1.15) |
| **MEN** | | | | | | | | |
| Client Frailty (FI) | | | | | | | | |
| Robust (ref) | | | | | | | | |
| Pre-frail | 1.40 (1.35–1.44) | 1.41 (1.37–1.45) | 2.14 (2.05–2.22) | 2.00 (1.92–2.08) | 1.14 (1.12–1.16) | 1.14 (1.12–1.16) | 1.40 (1.35–1.45) | 1.38 (1.33–1.43) |
| Frail | 2.07 (2.03–2.13) | 2.10 (2.04–2.17) | 3.48 (3.35–3.62) | 3.07 (2.95–3.20) | 1.17 (1.15–1.19) | 1.18 (1.15–1.20) | 1.50 (1.44–1.56) | 1.46 (1.40–1.52) |
| Caregiver Distress | | | | | | | | |
| No (ref) | | | | | | | | |
| Yes | 1.16 (1.13–1.19) | 0.95 (0.93–0.98) | 1.85 (1.80–1.91) | 1.37 (1.32–1.41) | 1.04 (1.02–1.05) | 0.99 (0.97–1.00) | 1.21 (1.17–1.24) | 1.08 (1.05–1.12) |

Abbreviations: FI = frailty index, NH = nursing home, ADG = Aggregated Diagnosis Groups

[a]Excludes clients hospitalized *without a prolonged bed stay* (overall sample, n = 66,764)

[b]Risk estimates also adjusted for age, sex (overall models only) and ADG comorbidity, p < 0.001 for all estimates

[c]Risk estimates from models including age, sex (overall models only), ADG comorbidity, FI frailty status and caregiver distress, p < 0.001 for all estimates except:
- caregiver distress relationship to any hospitalization for overall model (p = 0.8096); among women (p = 0.0415); among men (p = 0.1765)
- caregiver distress relationship to death among women (p = 0.4072)

**Table 3** Associations between client frailty status - caregiver distress categorical variable and risk of health outcomes during 1 year follow-up, overall and by client sex

| | Outcomes at 1 year, risk ratio (95% CI) | | | |
| --- | --- | --- | --- | --- |
| | Death | NH Placement | Any Hospitalization | Prolonged Hospitalization[a] |
| Client Frailty (FI) and Caregiver Distress, Overall[b] | | | | |
| CG not distressed & Robust | 1 | 1 | 1 | 1 |
| CG not distressed & Pre-Frail | 1.47 (1.43, 1.50) | 2.20 (2.14, 2.27) | 1.18 (1.16, 1.19) | 1.43 (1.40, 1.47) |
| CG not distressed & Frail | 2.36 (2.30, 2.42) | 4.00 (3.88, 4.11) | 1.20 (1.18, 1.21) | 1.42 (1.38, 1.47) |
| CG distressed & Robust | 0.99 (0.95, 1.04) | 2.10 (2.01, 2.20) | 0.99 (0.96, 1.01) | 1.13 (1.08, 1.19) |
| CG distressed & Pre-Frail | 1.41 (1.37, 1.46) | 3.26 (3.16, 3.37) | 1.16 (1.14, 1.18) | 1.48 (1.43, 1.53) |
| CG distressed & Frail | 2.26 (2.20, 2.32) | 4.79 (4.65, 4.93) | 1.24 (1.22, 1.26) | 1.68 (1.62, 1.73) |
| Ratio [Fr v Robust] CG not distressed | 2.36 | 4.00 | 1.20 | 1.42 |
| Ratio (Fr v Robust) CG distressed | 2.28 | 2.28 | 1.25 | 1.49 |
| Client Frailty (FI) and Caregiver Distress, Women[b] | | | | |
| CG not distressed & Robust | 1 | 1 | 1 | 1 |
| CG not distressed & Pre-Frail | 1.52 (1.47, 1.58) | 2.22 (2.15, 2.30) | 1.20 (1.18, 1.22) | 1.43 (1.39, 1.48) |
| CG not distressed & Frail | 2.64 (2.55, 2.73) | 4.15 (4.01, 4.29) | 1.23 (1.20, 1.25) | 1.43 (1.37, 1.49) |
| CG distressed & Robust | 1.03 (0.95, 1.11) | 2.16 (2.04, 2.30) | 0.98 (0.95, 1.02) | 1.13 (1.06, 1.21) |
| CG distressed & Pre-Frail | 1.50 (1.42, 1.57) | 3.42 (3.29, 3.57) | 1.20 (1.17, 1.23) | 1.51 (1.44, 1.58) |
| CG distressed & Frail | 2.59 (2.49, 2.69) | 5.05 (4.88, 5.24) | 1.30 (1.27, 1.33) | 1.71 (1.64, 1.79) |
| Ratio [Fr v Robust] CG not distressed | 2.64 | 4.15 | 1.23 | 1.43 |
| Ratio (Fr v Robust) CG distressed | 2.51 | 2.34 | 1.33 | 1.51 |
| Client Frailty (FI) and Caregiver Distress, Men[b] | | | | |
| CG not distressed & Robust | 1 | 1 | 1 | 1 |
| CG not distressed & Pre-Frail | 1.41 (1.36, 1.46) | 2.18 (2.08, 2.29) | 1.15 (1.13, 1.17) | 1.43 (1.37, 1.49) |
| CG not distressed & Frail | 2.09 (2.01, 2.17) | 3.69 (3.51, 3.88) | 1.15 (1.13, 1.18) | 1.41 (1.34, 1.49) |
| CG distressed & Robust | 0.95 (0.89, 1.01) | 1.98 (1.85, 2.12) | 0.98 (0.95, 1.01) | 1.13 (1.06, 1.21) |
| CG distressed & Pre-Frail | 1.33 (1.27, 1.39) | 3.00 (2.85, 3.16) | 1.12 (1.09, 1.14) | 1.44 (1.37, 1.52) |
| CG distressed & Frail | 2.01 (1.94, 2.09) | 4.34 (4.14, 4.56) | 1.18 (1.15, 1.21) | 1.64 (1.56, 1.72) |
| Ratio [Fr v Robust] CG not distressed | 2.09 | 3.69 | 1.15 | 1.41 |
| Ratio (Fr v Robust) CG distressed | 2.12 | 2.19 | 1.20 | 1.45 |

Abbreviations: *FI* = frailty index, *NH* = nursing home, *CG* = caregiver;
[a]Excludes clients hospitalized *without* a prolonged bed stay (overall sample, n = 66,764)
[b]Models adjusted for age, sex (overall models only) and ADG comorbidity; all estimates $p < 0.001$ except:
- caregiver distressed - robust for death: overall ($p = 0.8345$); women ($p = 0.4499$); men ($p = 0.0871$)
- caregiver distressed - robust for any hospitalization: overall ($p = 0.3063$); women ($p = 0.4029$); men ($p = 0.1932$)

cognitive impairment. Although we lacked specific information on caregiver sex, previous literature [27, 41–44] and our descriptive findings suggest that much of this informal care (and associated distress) falls disproportionately on female caregivers. For example, among older male clients, the primary caregiver was more commonly a spouse whereas among older female clients, the primary caregiver was more likely to be a child or child-in-law. As a prolonged hospitalization often precedes a transition to NH, it is not surprising that caregiver distress was also associated with this outcome [45]. Importantly clients with a distressed caregiver and who were also frail showed the highest risks for both NH placement and prolonged hospitalization, relative to the lowest risk group.

At first glance, the observation that the association between frailty and NH placement was greater among clients *without* than *with* a distressed caregiver seems counterintuitive. However, this largely reflects the significant contribution of caregiver distress to placement among less frail clients. For example, robust clients with (vs. without) a distressed caregiver were twice as likely to be admitted to a NH.

We observed higher risk estimates for death, NH placement and hospitalization associated with frailty among women relative to men. For death and hospitalization, this

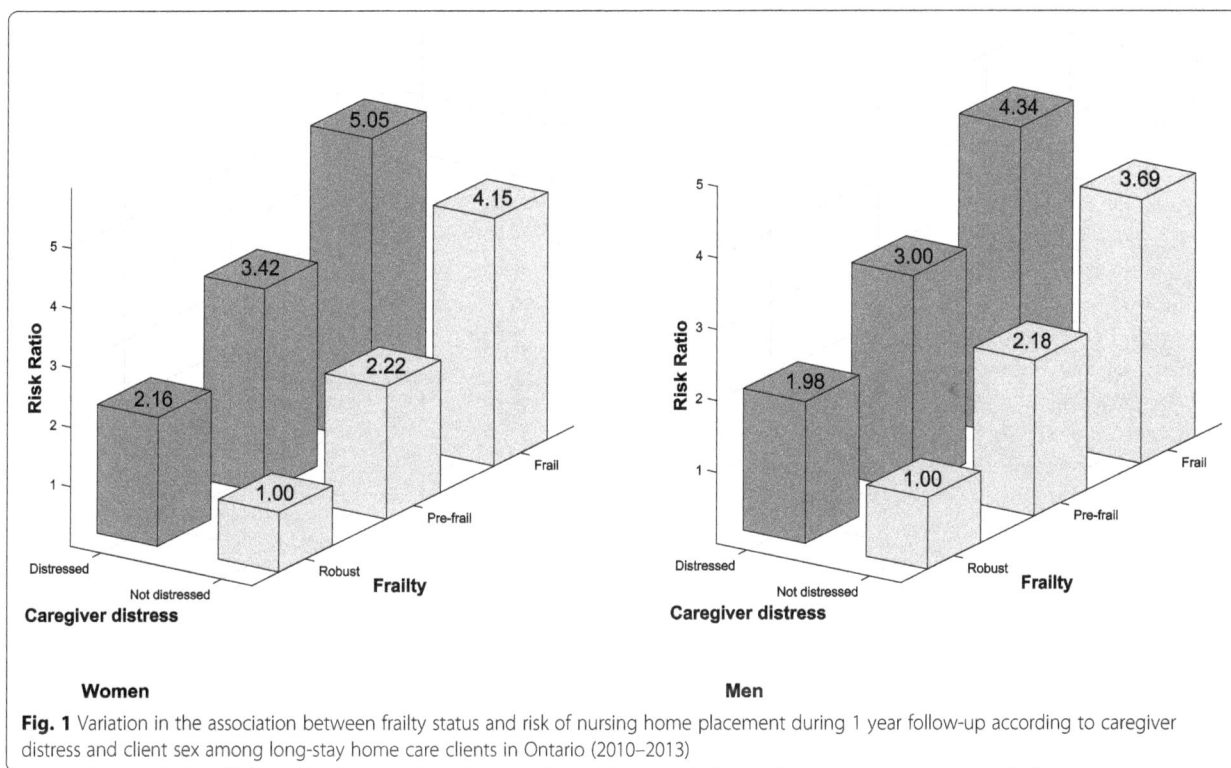

**Fig. 1** Variation in the association between frailty status and risk of nursing home placement during 1 year follow-up according to caregiver distress and client sex among long-stay home care clients in Ontario (2010–2013)

may reflect higher baseline risks for these outcomes among men. This would not explain the greater impact of frailty on placement among women as baseline risk was similar for men and women. The increased risk among women may be related to their increased likelihood to be widowed and to differences in their caregiver characteristics relative to male clients. There is some literature suggesting that female caregivers [25] and those who live with the care recipient [16], a scenario more likely for male clients in our study, may be less likely to pursue NH placement. This pattern may persist even with increasing client frailty level, leading to higher levels of distress for (female) caregivers as they strive to keep their loved one at home [42–44].

Strengths of our study include the population-based sample of older home care clients and availability of comprehensive clinical, functional, and psychosocial measures derived from the linked databases. Our analyses employed a frailty measure previously validated for this population [10]. Our focus on community-dwelling care recipients adds to the existing literature on the relevance of caregiver distress to health outcomes among older adults.

Limitations include the absence of detailed data on the informal caregivers, including their sex and the nature of, and amount of time spent on, caregiving activities. Similarly, for both informal and formal care providers, we did not have access to qualitative aspects of their relationships with clients which may be important to caregiver distress and client outcomes [18, 19, 44]. This

would include both positive and negative aspects of caregiving, which may show different patterns for female and male caregivers and between spouses and children [20, 41]. Despite these noted concerns, it is important to investigate the modifying effect of caregiver distress (as assessed with the RAI-HC) on client outcomes given its availability for population-based analyses. With the widespread implementation of the RAI-HC instrument in Canada and beyond, demonstrating the utility of these caregiver items for informing community-based practice and policy decisions is an important research priority. It should also be noted that our data do not allow us to comment on the relevance of caregiver support (or burden) to vulnerable older adults in the community not receiving formal care [43]. Additional research is required to more fully understand what underlies these observed associations and the potential impact of interventions designed to either minimize caregiver distress or delay frailty progression.

## Conclusions

Our findings highlight the extensive involvement of unpaid caregivers in providing assistance to home care clients and the impact of this care on their health and on care recipient outcomes. On average, caregivers provided almost 2.5 h of care per day, which increased to 3.5 h for clients who were frail. Among frail clients, almost half had distressed caregivers, an estimate double that noted for the total sample. With continued shifts from institutional to community-based care and increased levels of clinical complexity and frailty among older home care recipients, the prevalence of caregiver distress is likely to increase [46]. Our findings that caregiver distress is a significant driver of NH placement, even among relatively robust clients, and modifies the impact of other risk factors such as client frailty, demonstrate the importance of implementing routine assessments of caregiver burden and family-centered interventions as core elements of optimal community-based care [33, 46–48]. Despite ongoing calls for increased publicly-funded services and support for family caregivers, our findings and those of others [1–4, 36] point to lingering concerns of significant unmet needs among both care recipients and their caregivers.

As we also observed important sex-differences in caregiver relationships and likelihood for distress and in the magnitude of associations between frailty and NH placement, it is essential that both caregiver and care recipient sex be considered in research and planning of services for vulnerable home care populations [49, 50]. More extensive and innovative changes in relevant home and social care policies and funding arrangements will be needed to permit greater flexibility in how support services are packaged and targeted to meet the unique needs of care recipient and caregiver dyads.

### Abbreviations
ADGs: Aggregated Diagnosis Groups; CG: Caregiver; FI: Frailty index; NH: Nursing home; RAI-HC: Resident assessment instrument for home care; SD: Standard deviation

### Acknowledgments
The authors wish to acknowledge Matthew Kumar (Institute for Clinical Evaluative Sciences, Toronto) for his assistance with data presentation.

### Funding
This work was supported by a Canadian Institutes of Health Research (CIHR) grant [MOP-136854]. This study was conducted at the Institute for Clinical Evaluative Sciences (ICES), which is funded by an annual grant from the Ontario Ministry of Health and Long-Term Care (MOHLTC). The opinions, results and conclusions reported in this paper are those of the authors and are independent from the funding sources. No endorsement by ICES or the Ontario MOHLTC is intended or should be inferred. Parts of this material are based on data and information compiled and provided by the Canadian Institute for Health Information (CIHI). However, the analyses, conclusions, opinions and statements expressed herein are those of the authors, and not necessarily those of CIHI. The sponsors played no role in the study design; in the collection, analysis and interpretation of data; in the writing of the report; or in the decision to submit the report for publication.

### Authors' contributions
CJM, SEB, MAC, DBH, and LM conceived and designed the study; CD, with assistance from MAC and LM, carried out the statistical analyses; DBH, JEA, SL, DS, SG, KT, WPW, AG, and GT made substantial contributions to the interpretation of data; CJM wrote the initial version of the manuscript and MAC, CD, LM, DBH, JEA, SL, DS, SG, KT, WPW, AG, GT and SEB were involved in revising the manuscript for important intellectual content; CJM, MAC, CD, LM, DBH, JEA, SL, DS, SG, KT, WPW, AG, GT and SEB have read and approved the final version of the manuscript to be published and have agreed to be accountable for all aspects of the work.

### Competing interests
The authors declare that they have no competing interests.

### Author details
[1]Schools of Pharmacy and Public Health & Health Systems, University of Waterloo, 200 University Ave. W, Waterloo, ON N2L 3G1, Canada. [2]Institute for Clinical Evaluative Sciences, 2075 Bayview Ave, Toronto, ON M4N 3M5, Canada. [3]Health System Performance Research Network, Toronto, ON, Canada. [4]Division of Geriatric Medicine, Department of Medicine, University of Calgary, HSC-3330 Hospital Drive NW, Calgary, AB T2N 4N1, Canada. [5]School of Epidemiology, Public Health & Preventive Medicine, University of Ottawa, 451 Smyth Road, Ottawa, ON K1H 8M5, Canada. [6]School of Public Health & Health Systems, University of Waterloo, 200 University Ave. W, Waterloo, ON N2L 3G1, Canada. [7]Division of Geriatric Psychiatry, Queen's University & Providence Care Hospital, 752 King Street W, Kingston, ON K7L 4X3, Canada. [8]Department of Medicine, Queen's University & Providence Care Hospital, 752 King Street W, Kingston, ON K7L 4X3, Canada. [9]Ottawa Hospital Research Institute, 501 Smyth Road, PO Box201B, Ottawa, ON K1H 8L6, Canada. [10]Institute of Health Policy Management & Evaluation, University of Toronto, 155 College Street, Toronto, ON M5T 3M6, Canada. [11]Department of Family Medicine, University of Alberta, 8440 112 St. NW, Edmonton, AB T6G 2R7, Canada. [12]Department of Community Health & Epidemiology, College of Medicine, University of Saskatchewan, Health Science Building, 107 Wiggins Rd, Saskatoon, SK S7N 5E5, Canada.

### References
1. Expert Group on Home & Community Care. Bringing Care Home. In: Report of the expert group on Home & Community Care; 2015. http://health.gov.on.ca/en/public/programs/ccac/docs/hcc_report.pdf. Accessed 7 Oct 2017.
2. Institute of Medicine (IOM) and National Research Council (NRC). The future of home health care: workshop summary. Washington, DC: The National Academies Press; 2015. http://nationalacademies.org/hmd/reports/2015/future-home-health-care.aspx. Accessed 7 Oct 2017
3. Canadian Institute for Health Information (CIHI). (2017). Seniors in transition: exploring pathways across the care continuum. Ottawa, ON. Available at: https://www.cihi.ca/sites/default/files/document/seniors-in-transition-report-2017-en.pdf. Accessed 7 Oct 2017.
4. Canadian Institute for Health Information (CIHI). (2010). Analysis in Brief: Supporting informal caregivers – the heart of home care. Available at: https://secure.cihi.ca/free_products/Caregiver_Distress_AIB_2010_EN.pdf. Accessed 7 Oct 2017.
5. National Academies of Sciences, Engineering, and Medicine. 2016. Families caring for an aging America. Washington, DC: The National Academies Press. Available at: http://nationalacademies.org/hmd/reports/2016/families-caring-for-an-aging-america.aspx Accessed 7 Oct 2017.
6. Accreditation Canada and the Canadian Home Care Association. Advancing Quality Improvement and Integrated Care. In: Home Care in Canada; 2015. http://www.cdnhomecare.ca/media.php?mid=4328. Accessed 7 Oct 2017.
7. Greiner MA, Qualls LG, Iwata I, et al. Predicting nursing home placement among home- and community-based services program participants. Am J Manag Care. 2014;20:e535–46.
8. Lohman MC, Scherer EA, Whiteman KL, et al. Factors associated with accelerated hospitalization and re-hospitalization among medicare home health patients. J Gerontol A Biol Sci Med Sci. 2018;73(9):1280-86. https://doi.org/10.1093/gerona/glw335. [Epub ahead of print]
9. Seow H, Barbera L, Howell D, et al. Using more end-of-life homecare services is associated with using fewer acute care services: a population-based cohort study. Med Care. 2010;48:118–24.
10. Campitelli MA, Bronskill SE, Hogan DB, et al. The prevalence and health consequences of frailty in a population-based older home care cohort: a comparison of different measures. BMC Geriatr. 2016;16:133.
11. Hogan DB, Maxwell CJ, Afilalo J, et al. A scoping review of frailty and acute care in middle-aged and older individuals with recommendations for further research. Can Geriatr J. 2017;20:22–37.
12. Bergman H, Ferrucci L, Guralnik J, et al. Frailty: an emerging research and clinical paradigm--issues and controversies. J Gerontol A Biol Sci Med Sci. 2007;62:731–7.
13. Hogan DB, Freiheit EA, Strain LA, et al. Comparing frailty measures in their ability to predict adverse outcome among older residents of assisted living. BMC Geriatr. 2012;12:56.

14. Gruneir A, Forrester J, Camacho X, et al. Gender differences in home care clients and admission to long-term care in Ontario. Canada: a population-based retrospective cohort study BMC Geriatrics. 2013;13:48.

15. Noël-Miller C. Spousal loss, children, and the risk of nursing home admission. J Gerontol B Psychol Sci Soc Sci. 2010;65B:370–80.

16. Allen SM, Lima JC, Goldscheider FK, et al. Primary caregiver characteristics and transitions in community-based care. J Gerontol B Psychol Sci Soc Sci. 2012;67:362–71.

17. Ankuda CK, Levine DA. Trends in caregiving assistance for home-dwelling, functionally impaired older adults in the United States, 1998-2012. JAMA. 2016;316:218–20.

18. Monin JK, Poulin MJ, Brown SL, Langa KM. Spouses' daily feelings of appreciation and self-reported well-being. Health Psychol. 2017;36:1135–9.

19. Monin JK, Schulz R, Feeney BC. Compassionate love in individuals with Alzheimer's disease and their spousal caregivers: associations with caregivers' psychological health. Gerontologist. 2015;55:981–9.

20. Lin IF, Fee HR, Wu H-S. Negative and positive caregiving experiences: a closer look at the intersection of gender and relationships. Fam Relat. 2012; 61:343–58.

21. Monin JK, Levy B, Doyle M, Schulz R, Kershaw T. The impact of both spousal caregivers' and care recipients' health on relationship satisfaction in the Caregiver Health Effects Study. J Health Psychol 2017 Mar 1; [Epub ahead of print]:1–12. https://doi.org/10.1177/1359105317699682

22. Beach SR, Schulz R. Family caregiver factors associated with unmet needs for care of older adults. J Am Geriatr Soc. 2017;65:560–6.

23. Monin J, Doyle M, Levy B, et al. Spousal associations between frailty and depressive symptoms: longitudinal findings from the cardiovascular health study. J Am Geriatr Soc. 2016;64:824–30.

24. Wolff JL, Spillman BC, Freedman VA, Kasper JD. A national profile of family and unpaid caregivers who assist older adults with health care activities. JAMA Intern Med. 2016;176:372–9.

25. Cepoiu-Martin M, Tam-Tham H, Patten S, et al. Predictors of long-term care placement in persons with dementia: a systematic review and meta-analysis. Int J Geriatr Psychiatry. 2016;31:1151–71.

26. Gaugler JE, Yu F, Krichbaum K, et al. Predictors of nursing home admission for persons with dementia. Med Care. 2009;47:191–8.

27. Yaffe K, Fox P, Newcomer R, et al. Patient and caregiver characteristics and nursing home placement in patients with dementia. JAMA. 2002;287:2090–7.

28. Ankuda CK, Maust DT, Kabeto MU, et al. Association between spousal caregiver well-being and care recipient healthcare expenditures. J Am Geriatr Soc. 2017;65:2220–6.

29. Dent E, Hoogendijk EO. Psychosocial factors modify the association of frailty with adverse outcomes: a prospective study of hospitalized older people. BMC Geriatr. 2014;14:108.

30. Hoogendijk EO, van Hout HPJ, van der Horst HE, et al. Do psychosocial resources modify the effects of frailty on functional decline and mortality? J Psychosom Res. 2014;77:547–51.

31. Wang C, Song X, Mitnitski A, et al. Effect of health protective factors on health deficit accumulation and mortality risk in older adults in the Beijing longitudinal study of aging. J Am Geriatr Soc. 2014;62:821–8.

32. Dent E, Hoogendijk EO. Psychosocial resources: moderators or mediators of frailty outcomes? J Am Med Dir Assoc. 2015;16:258–9.

33. Schulz R, Czaja SJ. Family caregiving: A vision for the future. Am J Geriatr Psychiatry. 2018;26(3):358-63. [Epub ahead of print]: 1–6.

34. Canadian Institute for Health Information (CIHI). Data quality documentation, home care reporting system, 2012–2013. Ottawa, ON; 2013. https://secure.cihi.ca/free_products/HCRS-External-Data-Quality-Report_2012_EN_web.pdf. Accessed 7 Oct 2017.

35. Austin PC, van Walraven C, Wodchis WP, et al. Using the Johns Hopkins aggregated diagnosis groups (ADGs) to predict mortality in a general adult population cohort in Ontario, Canada. Med Care. 2011;49:932–9.

36. Health Quality Ontario. The Reality of Caring: Distress among the caregivers of home care patients. Toronto: Queen's Printer for Ontario; 2016. http://www.hqontario.ca/Portals/0/documents/system-performance/reality-caring-report-en.pdf. Accessed 28 July 2018

37. Health Council of Canada. What are the home care priorities for seniors in Canada? In: Seniors in need, caregivers in distress. Toronto: Health Council of Canada; 2012. http://www.bcforum.ca/Resources/HCC_HomeCare_FA2012.pdf. Accessed 28 July 2018.

38. Vu M, Hogan DB, Patten SB, et al. A comprehensive profile of the sociodemographic, psychosocial and health characteristics of Ontario home care clients with dementia. Chronic Dis Inj Can. 2014;34(2–3):132–44.

39. Mitchell LA, Hirdes J, Poss JW, et al. Informal caregivers of clients with neurological conditions: profiles, patterns and risk factors for distress from a home care prevalence study. BMC Health Serv Res. 2015;15:350.

40. Walker JD, Morris K, Frood J. Alternative level of care in Canada: A summary. Healthcare Quarterly. 2009;12(2):21-23.

41. Chappell NL, Dujela C, Smith A. Caregiver well-being: intersections of relationship and gender. Res Aging. 2015;37:623–45.

42. Penning MJ, Wu Z. Caregiver stress and mental health: impact of caregiving relationship and gender. Gerontologist. 2016;56:1102–13.

43. Sutcliffe C, Giebel C, Bleijlevens M, et al. Caring for a person with dementia on the margins of long-term care: a perspective on burden from 8 European countries. J Am Med Dir Assoc. 2017; https://doi.org/10.1016/j.jamda.2017.06.004. [Epub ahead of print]

44. Adelman RD, Tmanova LL, Delgado D, Dion S, Lachs MS. Caregiver burden: a clinical review. JAMA. 2014;311:1052–60.

45. McCloskey R, Jarrett P, Stewart C, et al. Alternate level of care patients in hospitals: what does dementia have to do with this? Can Geriatr J. 2014;17: 88–94.

46. Health Quality Ontario. (2016). Measuring up 2016: a yearly report on how Ontario's health system is performing. Toronto, ON: Queen's Printer for Ontario. Available at: http://www.hqontario.ca/System-Performance/Yearly-Reports/Measuring-Up-2016. Accessed 7 Oct 2017.

47. Mason DJ. Long-term care: investing in models that work. JAMA. 2017;318: 1529–30.

48. Wolff JL, Feder J, Schulz R. Supporting family caregivers of older Americans. N Engl J Med. 2016;375:2513–5.

49. Ringer TJ, Hazzan AA, Kennedy CC, et al. Care recipients' physical frailty is independently associated with subjective burden in informal caregivers in the community setting: a cross-sectional study. BMC Geriatr. 2016;16:186.

50. Hoover M, Rotermann M. Seniors' use of and unmet needs for home care, 2009. Health Rep. 2012;23:3–8.

# 6

# Hand dexterity, not handgrip strength, is associated with executive function in Japanese community-dwelling older adults: a cross-sectional study

Kimi Estela Kobayashi-Cuya[1,2] (iD), Ryota Sakurai[1*], Naoko Sakuma[1], Hiroyuki Suzuki[1], Masashi Yasunaga[1], Susumu Ogawa[1], Toru Takebayashi[2] and Yoshinori Fujiwara[1]

## Abstract

**Background:** An association between handgrip strength, hand dexterity and global cognition is suggested; however, it is unclear whether both hand motor functions are associated with executive function, which is important for performing daily activities. Understanding this association will help identify motor risk factors for impairment of executive function in late adulthood. We aim to investigate the relationship of handgrip strength and hand dexterity with executive function in physically and mentally healthy community-dwelling older adults.

**Methods:** Three hundred and twenty-six older adults (287 women, mean age ± SD, 70.1 ± 5.6) underwent handgrip strength and hand dexterity tests using a hand dynamometer and the Purdue Pegboard Test (PPT), respectively. Executive function was evaluated with the Trail Making Test (TMT)-A, TMT-B and Digit symbol; global cognition was assessed with the Mini-Mental State Examination (MMSE).

**Results:** Age-group differences showed that the younger groups (60–64, 65–69 and 70–74) had a significant better PPT and executive function performance than the oldest group (75 and older), whereas no significant age differences were observed for handgrip strength. Multiple regression analysis adjusted for potential covariates, including MMSE scores, showed that TMT-A, TMT-B, and Digit symbol were significantly associated with PPT scores; however, no significant association was observed between executive function variables and handgrip strength.

**Conclusions:** Hand dexterity is vulnerable to the effects of aging and, contrary to handgrip strength, it strongly associates with executive function, independent of global cognition. Our results suggest that assessing hand dexterity may help identify individuals at higher risk of impairment of executive function among high-functioning older adults.

**Keywords:** Cognitive function, Community-dwelling older adults, Executive function, Hand dexterity, Handgrip strength

* Correspondence: r_sakurai@hotmail.co.jp
[1]Research Team for Social Participation and Community Health, Tokyo Metropolitan Institute of Gerontology, 35-2 Sakae-cho, Itabashi-ku, Tokyo 173-0015, Japan
Full list of author information is available at the end of the article

## Background

Cognitive decline is a major clinical and public health concern that threatens the quality of life of older adults and their families and poses significant challenges to aging societies [1]. Several behavioral studies have been conducted to understand the risk factors for cognitive decline and the incidence of dementia and found that impairment of motor function is closely related to these changes [2–4]. A better understanding of the association between motor and cognitive performance in older adults without cognitive impairment could help accurately detect at early-stage which individuals have motor risk factors associated with cognitive decline.

Cross-sectional studies have indicated that either handgrip strength [5, 6] or hand dexterity [7] is associated with global cognitive performance. Also, clinical studies have reported significant differences in motor impairment (loss in muscle control or movement) between cognitively normal older adults and those with mild cognitive impairment (MCI) [3, 8]. These findings are reasonable because handgrip strength and coordination are needed to successfully perform daily activities that require cognitive engagement such as writing, cooking, gardening, making craft-works, and playing instruments. The nature of these hand movements requires visual search [9], motor speed skills [10], attention allocation and motor planning [11]. Therefore, executive function, which consists of cognitive processes of attention, working memory, planning, judgment, task flexibility, and inhibition [12], seems to be strongly influenced by the level of hand motor function.

Although there is a growing body of epidemiological evidence for the association between hand motor function and cognitive function [13], it is still unclear which hand motor variable including handgrip strength and hand dexterity is strongly associated with executive function. Executive function is a cognitive domain that is important for maintaining a safe and independent living in older adults [12]; however, reduced executive function seems to be prevalent even among healthy, community-dwelling older adults without overt cognitive impairment [4]. For this reason, it is crucial to evaluate the association between hand motor function and cognitive performance in cognitively intact subjects in order to provide more evidence of the motor risk factors associated with cognitive decline in late adulthood.

Therefore, our aim is to understand which hand motor variable (focusing on handgrip strength and hand dexterity of the dominant hand) is strongly associated with executive function in healthy community-dwelling older adults aged 60 years and over with intact global cognition. We also examined whether significant variability exists in hand motor and executive function variables across age groups in our sample. As mentioned earlier, executive function is a significant predictor of functional status and independent living determined by ADLs (activities of daily living) and IADLs (instrumental ADLs) [14]; thus, understanding its association with hand motor function would contribute to identify older adults at higher risk of impairment of executive function.

## Methods

### Study design and population

The sample consisted of 326 physically and mentally healthy Japanese community-dwelling older adults recruited from our volunteer database available from a longitudinal and randomized controlled trial of the REsearch of PRoductivity by INTergenerational Sympathy (REPRINTS) program at Tokyo Metropolitan Institute of Gerontology (TMIG) between 2004 and 2017. Participants were recruited from three types of areas—urban (Bunkyo, Chuo, Itabashi and Toshima Wards, Tokyo), suburban (Kawasaki city, Kanagawa), and rural (Nagahama city, Shiga)—through community newsletters and meetings. The REPRINTS program is a longitudinal study, with no significant effects on hand motor function, which evaluates the effects of an intergenerational book-reading program on cognitive function in community-dwelling older adults aged 65 years and older [15]. A randomized, short-term study of this program includes middle-aged adults and over. In the present study, the analyzed data was combined from the two databases, so the number of cases for one variable (Digit symbol, see below) was 207.

The exclusion criteria included history of cerebrovascular disorder, history of hospitalization due to an acute medical condition (e.g., stroke and heart disease) within 3 months before the study; motor/neuromuscular problems (e.g., hand tremors); significant hearing loss and visual deficits; and mental disorders and cognitive impairment indicated with a Mini-Mental State Examination (MMSE) score of 25 or lower [16]. Handedness was determined according to the Edinburgh Handedness Inventory [17]. In this regard, to examine the motor function of the dominant hand, participants with ambidexterity were excluded. However, only the data of the dominant right hand is reported due to the lack of left-handed participants (see Results). Written informed consent was obtained from all participants before examination. The study was conducted in accordance with the Declaration of Helsinki (1983). The Ethics Committee of the Tokyo Metropolitan Institute of Gerontology approved the research protocol.

### Hand motor tests

#### The Purdue Pegboard Test (PPT)

The PPT (Lafayette Instrument Company, Model 32,020) is a hand and finger dexterity test [18]. It consists of a

19.7 × 44.9 cm board with 25 slotted holes in a 5 × 5 array. The participants were instructed to insert one pin at a time starting from the top hole in either the right or left row, depending on the starting hand, as fast as possible for 30 s without option to pick up any dropped pins. The order of the starting hand was counterbalanced across participants. There was one practice session for each hand in which participants could practice until they were able to insert five pins in a row. The number of pins correctly inserted in 30 s was recorded for each trial, and the average of two trials was used for analysis.

### Handgrip strength

Handgrip strength was measured on the dominant hand using the Smedley dynamometer (ES-100, Evernew Co., Ltd., Koto., Tokyo, Japan) to the nearest 0.5 kg of force. Subjects were instructed to deeply inhale and fully exhale while squeezing the dynamometer with as much force as possible on their dominant hand. The average of two trials was used for analysis.

## Neuropsychological tests for measuring executive function

### The Trail Making Test (TMT)

The TMT has been widely used for assessing executive function and involves cognitive skills including visual search, perceptual/motor skills, processing speed, attention, switching, and working memory [19, 20]. It consists of two parts: The TMT-A, which requires the subject to draw a line connecting consecutive encircled numbers (1 to 25) randomly distributed in a sheet form, and the TMT-B, which requires the subject to alternate between numbers (1 to 13) and letters of Hiragana, a Japanese syllabary, (i.e., 1-A) as quickly and as accurate as possible. The TMT-A has been associated with cognitive skills involved in executive function such as visual search, processing speed, sustained attention and working memory [19–22], while the TMT-B requires additional executive function skills such as task switching, cognitive flexibility and greater working memory [23]. The time (in seconds) required for the participant to complete each task was used for analysis.

### Digit symbol - Wechsler Adult Intelligence Test-Revised (WAIS-R)

The Digit symbol subtest of the WAIS-R consists of a row of squares containing symbols paired with digits from 1 to 9 and another row of blank squares randomly assigned with digits from 1 to 9. After a practice session, the participant fills in the blank squares with the symbol that corresponds to each digit. The Digit symbol test has been used to evaluate executive function [24], where sustained attention, visuomotor coordination, and response speed contribute to the performance of the test

[25]. The total score was the number of squares correctly matched in 90 s.

## Covariates

All participants were interviewed by a physician to assess heath related characteristics that could be associated with hand dexterity and executive function including demographics such as age, sex and years of education. Functional health status was evaluated using the Tokyo Metropolitan Institute of Gerontology Index of Competence (TMIG-IC), in which scores ranging from 0 to 13 indicate functional capacity in IADLs (i.e., being able to shop, prepare meals), intellectual activities (i.e., reading newspapers, books) and social roles (i.e., visiting friends) [26]. Comorbidities consisted of the presence or absence of self-reported diseases including heart disease, diabetes, hypertension, and stroke. Depressive mood was assessed using a 15-item short version of the Geriatric Depression Scale (GDS-15), a measurement of depressive feelings during the past week. Higher GDS scores indicate greater depression. Scores of five and above are indicative of depressive symptoms [27, 28]. Global cognition was evaluated using the MMSE, a cognitive screening test both for the evaluation of general or global cognitive performance and for detecting dementia [29]. The test consists of 30 items of various domains including orientation, attention, immediate recall, delayed recall, language, and visuospatial ability. It has been shown that the total scores of the MMSE and the Montreal Cognitive Assessment (MoCA), a brief cognitive screening test with higher sensitivity to detect MCI than the MMSE [30], are significantly correlated even among participants who score > 24 [29]. We have therefore included MMSE as a covariate to adjust for global cognitive function despite their restricted range of score in the present study.

## Statistical analysis

All data were analyzed using the Statistical Package for the Social Sciences (SPSS) 23.0 (SPSS Inc., Chicago, Ill., USA). Simple correlations were conducted among hand motor function and cognitive variables. To examine the differences in hand motor and cognitive variables among four age-groups, a one-way ANOVA was performed. A Bonferroni correction for $p < 0.008$ was applied in post-hoc comparisons (0.05/6) to avoid type 1 error, where the denominator 6 represents the six pairwise comparisons resulting after comparing the four age-groups. Multiple regression analyses controlling for age, sex, years of education, TMIG-index of competence, depression, comorbidities, and MMSE tested the associations between executive function (i.e., TMT-A, TMT-B and Digit Symbol as dependent variables) and hand motor function (i.e., handgrip strength and hand dexterity as independent variables). Regression analyses were performed separately for each independent and dependent variable (Model 1). In total, six regressions were run in Model 1. Also, to eliminate the confounding variable between hand motor variables, regression models including both handgrip strength and hand dexterity as independent variables together were then performed separately for each dependent variable (Model 2). Thus, three regressions were run in Model 2. Statistical significance was set at $p < 0.05$.

## Results

Five participants who showed significant cognitive decline impairment (MMSE < 26) and 12 participants who were ambidextrous were excluded from the analyses. Thus, a total of 326 right-handed older adults were included in the analyses. Table 1 shows age-group differences in hand motor variables, cognitive variables and covariates. After dividing the sample into four age-groups, performance in PPT, TMT-A, and Digit symbol were significantly higher in the younger groups (ages 60–64, 65–69, and 70–74) than the oldest group (≥75), whereas no significant age-group differences were observed in handgrip strength. TMT-B scores were also significantly different between age-groups 60–64, 65–69 and the older groups, whereas MMSE scores were significantly different between 60 and 64 and ≥ 75. Years of education was significantly different between the youngest group (60–64) and the older groups

(70–74 and ≥ 75). The proportion of participants with heart disease and hypertension tended to be higher in older groups.

Figure 1 shows the scatter plots of the associations between executive function variables (TMT-A, TMT-B, Digit symbol) and hand motor variables (handgrip strength and PPT performance) in older adults. Correlation analyses showed that PPT performance, which was assessed by the number of inserted pegs, was significantly correlated with TMT-A, TMT-B and Digit symbol. Contrarily, handgrip strength was not significantly correlated with TMT-B and Digit symbol; only TMT-A showed a significant but low correlation coefficient with handgrip strength. On the other hand, Fig. 2 shows no significant association between handgrip strength and PPT performance.

Table 2 shows the results of the multiple regression analyses evaluating the association between executive function (i.e., TMT-A, TMT-B and Digit symbol) and hand motor function (i.e., handgrip strength and hand dexterity). Lower PPT performance was associated with longer both TMT-A and TMT-B times and lower Digit symbol score. These associations remained significant after adjusting for potential covariates and additional adjustment for handgrip strength. On the other hand, no association was observed between executive function variables and handgrip strength, even after additional adjustment for PPT scores. Covariates including age ($p < 0.001$), sex ($p = 0.016$), GDS

**Table 1** Comparison of covariates, hand and cognitive variables among age categories ($N = 326$)

| Variables | Age categories | | | | p-value |
|---|---|---|---|---|---|
| | 60–64 (n = 54) | 65–69 (n = 104) | 70–74 (n = 101) | ≥ 75 (n = 67) | |
| Years of education | 14.4 ± 2.5 | 13.4 ± 2.2 | 13.3 ± 2.5 | 12.8 ± 2.7* | 0.004 |
| TMIG-IC | 12.2 ± 0.8 | 12.3 ± 0.9 | 12.4 ± 0.9 | 12.2 ± 1.3 | 0.645 |
| GDS | 2.3 ± 2.1 | 3.1 ± 2.5 | 2.5 ± 2.3 | 3.0 ± 2.3 | 0.09 |
| Heart disease, n (%) | 2 (3.7) | 1 (1.0) | 11 (10.9) | 7 (10.4) | 0.012[a] |
| Diabetes, n (%) | 2 (3.7) | 9 (8.7) | 6 (5.9) | 5 (7.5) | 0.670[a] |
| Hypertension, n (%) | 11 (20.4) | 23 (22.1) | 27 (26.7) | 28 (41.8) | 0.020[a] |
| Stroke, n (%) | 3 (5.6) | 6 (5.8) | 5 (5.0) | 3 (4.5) | 0.983[a] |
| Hand motor variables, mean ± SD | | | | | |
| Handgrip strength (Kg) | 23.4 ± 4.7 | 22.6 ± 5.3 | 22.9 ± 7.0 | 20.9 ± 6.3 | 0.104 |
| PPT (Number of pegs) | 14.5 ± 1.5 | 13.7 ± 2.1 | 13.1 ± 1.9* | 11.9 ± 1.9*,†,‡ | < 0.001 |
| Cognitive variables, mean ± SD | | | | | |
| MMSE | 29.2 ± 0.9 | 28.8 ± 1.3 | 28.9 ± 1.0 | 20.6 ± 1.38* | 0.023 |
| TMT-A | 30.2 ± 7.7 | 35.3 ± 13.2 | 37.9 ± 11.1* | 43.2 ± 12.4*,†,‡ | < 0.001 |
| TMT-B | 74.5 ± 18.6 | 91.9 ± 37.6* | 107.4 ± 39.9*,† | 121.6 ± 40.8*,† | < 0.001 |
| Digit symbol[b] | 67.7 ± 9.3 | 60.2 ± 13.8 | 55.3 ± 10.9* | 45.6 ± 8.4*,†,‡ | < 0.001 |

Values are expressed as mean ± SD

*TMIG-IC* Tokyo Metropolitan Institute of Gerontology - Index of Competence, *GDS* Geriatric Depression Scale, *MMSE* Mini-Mental State Examination, *TMT* Trail Making Test

Bonferroni correction for post-hoc tests: *$p < 0.008$ vs. 60–64; †$p < 0.008$ vs. 65–69; ‡$p < 0.008$ vs. 70–74

[a]The Chi-square test was performed

[b]The total number of subjects analyzed was 207

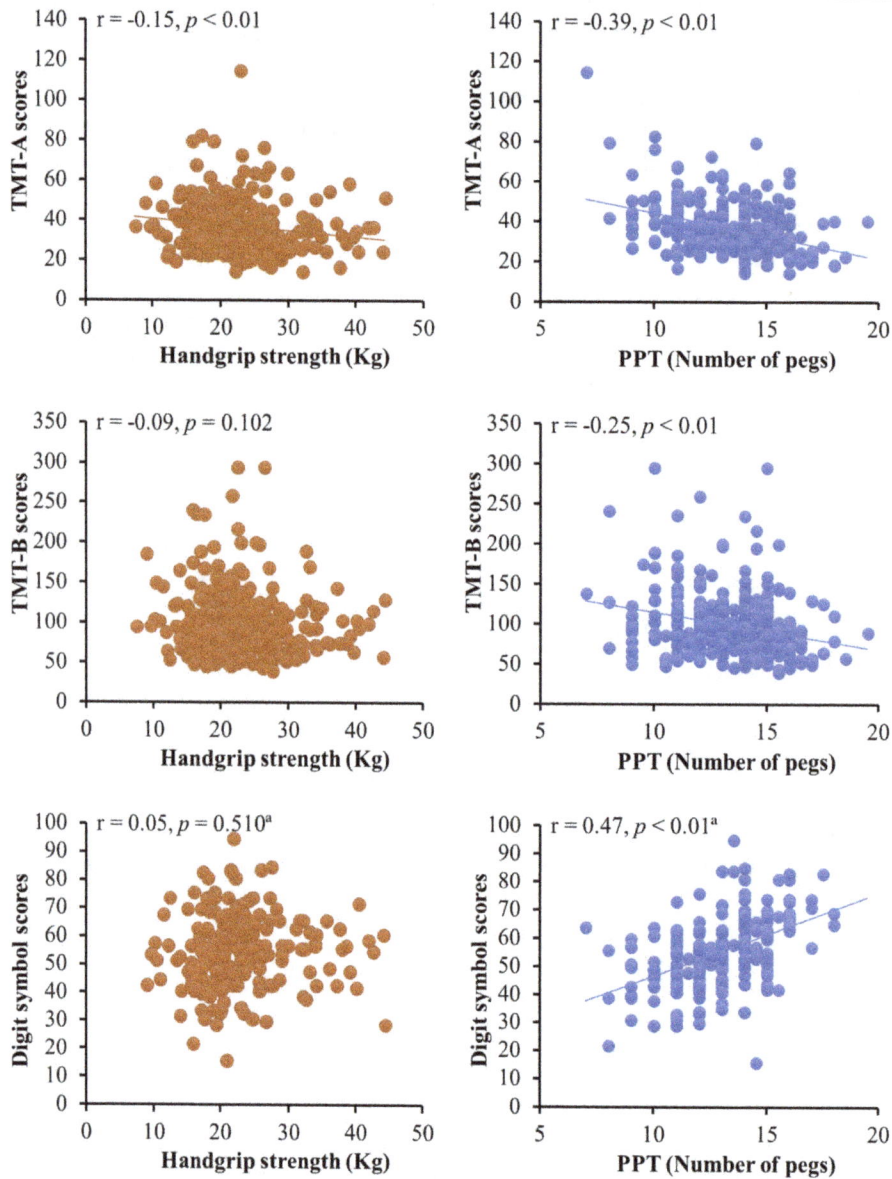

**Fig. 1** Scatter diagrams of the relationships between hand motor variables (handgrip strength, PPT performance) and executive function variables (TMT-A, TMT-B, Digit symbol). Each plot shows the best-fit simple regression line, the correlation coefficient (*r*) and the statistical significance (*p*). [a]The total number of subjects analyzed was 207

($p = 0.025$), stroke ($p = 0.039$) and MMSE scores ($p = 0.005$) significantly contributed to the association between TMTA and PPT performance, whereas only age ($p < 0.001$) and MMSE scores ($p = 0.13$) contributed to the association between TMTB and PPT performance. Age ($p < 0.001$), stroke ($p < 0.001$) and diabetes ($p = 0.013$) significantly contributed to the association between digit symbol and PPT performance.

## Discussion

The objective of this study was to evaluate which hand motor variable (handgrip strength or hand dexterity) has

a stronger association with executive function performance in community-dwelling older adults. Our results revealed that hand dexterity assessed by PPT performance, and not handgrip strength, was significantly associated with executive function among high-functioning older adults. Regression analysis confirmed this association after further adjustment for covariates including handgrip strength. These findings suggest that hand dexterity may be considered a measurable motor risk factor for the early detection of executive function impairment among older adults with intact global cognitive performance. To our knowledge, the present study provides the

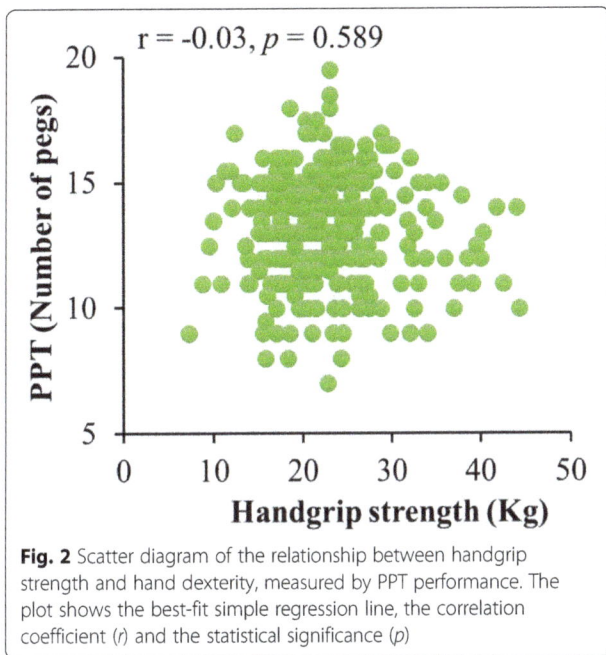

**Fig. 2** Scatter diagram of the relationship between handgrip strength and hand dexterity, measured by PPT performance. The plot shows the best-fit simple regression line, the correlation coefficient (r) and the statistical significance (p)

first evidence that hand dexterity is more strongly associated with executive function performance than handgrip strength among physically and mentally healthy community-dwelling older adults.

The rationale of this association resides in that hand dexterity requires not only the sensorimotor coordination of hands and fingers with the eyes [31], but it also requires complex cognitive processes observed in executive function such as attention, working memory, planning, judgment, task flexibility, and inhibition [12]. These cognitive processes seem to play a significant role in the successful performance of fine motor movements rather than that of muscle strength. This finding may also be attributed to the commonality of the association between the prefrontal cortex of the brain with executive function [32] and hand dexterity [33], as well as the association between nerve myelination with executive function [34] and hand dexterity [35]. All these shared

complex mechanisms make hand dexterity more closely related to executive function impairment than handgrip strength.

The association between the hand motor variables (handgrip strength and hand dexterity) was also evaluated since they are essential hand components for performing manual activities. In this regard, a previous study reported an association between handgrip strength and hand dexterity in a sample with a wide age range (ages 18 to 93) [36]; however, in the present study with community-dwelling older adults, handgrip strength was not significantly associated with hand dexterity. A possible explanation is that our participants were high-functioning individuals with no significant differences in handgrip strength. Although reduction in muscle mass is associated with reduced handgrip strength, possibly influencing hand dexterity performance in older adults, the significant association between hand dexterity and executive function found in the present study suggests that the integration of complex cognitive and sensory mechanisms constitutes a crucial component of hand motor function. This may be further supported by the age-group differences in executive function and hand dexterity performance observed in the present study, suggesting hand dexterity as a useful motor variable to evaluate executive function in different age subgroups of older adults.

Executive function has been strongly associated with independent living [14], and it is considered a stronger predictor of functional impairment than MMSE in healthy subjects and in patients with MCI and Alzheimer's disease [12, 37]. Therefore, the association observed in the present study between executive function and hand dexterity also suggests the role of hand dexterity in maintaining executive function in high-functioning older adults.

The strength of this study includes the analysis of hand motor and cognitive variables in a large sample of active and cognitive intact community-dwelling older adults. This study also provides an understanding of the

**Table 2** Multiple Linear Regression Model Summary for TMT-A, TMT-B and Digit symbol

| Dependent variables | Independent variables | | | | | | | |
|---|---|---|---|---|---|---|---|---|
| | Model 1 | | | | Model 2 | | | |
| | HG | | PPT | | HG | | PPT | |
| | β (95% CI) | p-value | β (95% CI) | p-value | β (95% CI) | p-value | β (95% CI) | p-value |
| TMT-A | −0.12 (− 0.55, 0.06) | 0.114 | −0.33 (−2.60, − 1.32) | < 0.001 | −0.33 (− 2.58, − 1.29) | < 0.001 | −0.09 (− 0.47, 0.10) | 0.177 |
| TMT-B | −0.02 (−1.11, 0.84) | 0.782 | − 0.12 (− 4.38, − 0.06) | 0.044 | −0.12 (− 4.38, − 0.04) | 0.046 | −0.01 (− 1.04, 0.90) | 0.888 |
| Digit symbol[a] | 0.02 (− 0.39, 0.31) | 0.827 | 0.30 (1.08, 2.56) | < 0.001 | 0.30 (1.08, 2.56) | < 0.001 | 0.03 (−0.39, 0.28) | 0.751 |

Each of the regressions was performed separately for each independent variable (TMT-A, TMT-B, and digit symbol)
Model 1: includes two hand variables analyzed separately as independent variables and adjusted for age (a continuous variable), sex, years of education, TMIG-Index of Competence, GDS, hypertension, stroke, heart disease, diabetes and MMSE
Model 2: includes two hand variables analyzed together as independent variables and adjusted for the same covariates as Model 1
CI Confidence Interval, HG Handgrip strength, PPT Purdue Pegboard Test
[a]The total number of subjects analyzed was 207

importance of hand dexterity as a measurable hand motor indicator for the early detection of impairment of executive function in high-functioning older adults. However, the findings of the current study need to be interpreted with caution. First, this is a cross-sectional study, and therefore we cannot establish a cause and effect relationship between hand dexterity and executive function; longitudinal studies are needed to elucidate this association. Second, only TMT and Digit symbol tests were used to evaluate executive function; therefore, more executive function tests should be used to provide further support to the association with hand dexterity. Third, the PPT evaluates finger and hand dexterity; however, due to the complexity of fine motor function, it is necessary to include more hand dexterity tests to better understand the association with executive function.

## Conclusions

The present study showed that hand dexterity, not handgrip strength, associates with executive function variables in community-dwelling older adults with intact global cognitive performance, evaluated by MMSE scores. Our results suggest that hand dexterity, which was measured by the Purdue Pegboard Test, is vulnerable to the effects of aging and may be considered a measurable motor indicator for executive function impairment even in high cognitive functioning older adults. The findings provide a reasonable basis for implementing hand dexterity interventions for the prevention of executive function impairment in community-dwelling older adults.

### Abbreviations

ADLs: Activities of daily living; IADLs: Instrumental activities of daily living; MMSE: Mini-Mental State Examination; PPT: Purdue Pegboard Test; TMIG-IC: Tokyo Metropolitan Institute of Gerontology-Index of Competence; TMT-A: Trail Making Test-Part A; TMT-B: Trail Making Test-Part B; WAIS-R: Wechsler Adult Intelligence Test-Revised

### Authors' contributions

Study concept and design: KK, RS, YF, NS, MY. Acquisition of subjects and/or data: NS, MY, RS, HS, SO, KK. Analysis and interpretation of data: KK, RS and HS. Preparation of manuscript: KK, RS, SO and TT. All authors read and approved the final manuscript: KK, RS, YF, HS, TT, NS, MY, SO.

### Competing interests

The authors declare that they have no competing interests.

### Author details

[1]Research Team for Social Participation and Community Health, Tokyo Metropolitan Institute of Gerontology, 35-2 Sakae-cho, Itabashi-ku, Tokyo 173-0015, Japan. [2]Department of Preventive Medicine and Public Health, School of Medicine, Keio University, 35 Shinanomachi, Shinjuku-ku, Tokyo 160-8582, Japan.

### References

1. Greiner PA, Snowdon DA, Schmitt FA. The loss of independence in activities of daily living: the role of low normal cognitive function in elderly nuns. Am J Public Health. 1996;86:62–6.
2. Hebert LE, Bienias JL, McCann JJ, Scherr PA, Wilson RS, Evans DA. Upper and lower extremity motor performance and functional impairment in Alzheimer's disease. Am J Alzheimers Dis Other Demen. 2010;25:425–31.
3. Aggarwal NT, Wilson RS, Beck TL, Bienias JL, Bennett DA. Motor dysfunction in mild cognitive impairment and the risk of incident Alzheimer disease. Arch Neurol. 2006;63:1763–9.
4. Sakurai R, Ishii K, Yasunaga M, Takeuchi R, Murayama Y, Sakuma N, Sakata M, Oda K, Ishibashi K, Ishiwata K, et al. The neural substrate of gait and executive function relationship in elderly women: a PET study. Geriatr Gerontol Int. 2017;17:1873–80.
5. Taekema DG, Gussekloo J, Maier AB, Westendorp RG, de Craen AJ. Handgrip strength as a predictor of functional, psychological and social health. A prospective population-based study among the oldest old. Age Ageing. 2010;39:331–7.
6. Malmstrom TK, Wolinsky FD, Andresen EM, Miller JP, Miller DK. Cognitive ability and physical performance in middle-aged African Americans. J Am Geriatr Soc. 2005;53:997–1001.
7. Bezdicek O, Nikolai T, Hoskovcova M, Stochl J, Brozova H, Dusek P, Zarubova K, Jech R, Ruzicka E. Grooved pegboard predicates more of cognitive than motor involvement in Parkinson's disease. Assessment. 2014;21:723–30.
8. de Paula JJ, Albuquerque MR, Lage GM, Bicalho MA, Romano-Silva MA, Malloy-Diniz LF. Impairment of fine motor dexterity in mild cognitive impairment and Alzheimer's disease dementia: association with activities of daily living. Rev Bras Psiquiatr. 2016;38:235–8.
9. Song C-S. Relationship between visuo-perceptual function and manual dexterity in community-dwelling older adults. J Phys Ther Sci. 2015;27:1871–4.
10. Rodriguez-Aranda C, Mittner M, Vasylenko O. Association between executive functions, working memory, and manual dexterity in young and healthy older adults: an exploratory study. Percept Mot Skills. 2016;122:165–92.
11. Rinne P, Hassan M, Fernandes C, Han E, Hennessy E, Waldman A, Sharma P, Soto D, Leech R, Malhotra PA, Bentley P. Motor dexterity and strength depend upon integrity of the attention-control system. Proc Natl Acad Sci. 2017;
12. Marshall GA, Rentz DM, Frey MT, Locascio JJ, Johnson KA, Sperling RA. Executive function and instrumental activities of daily living in mild cognitive impairment and Alzheimer's disease. Alzheimers Dement. 2011;7:300–8.
13. Kobayashi-Cuya K, Sakurai R, Suzuki H, Ogawa S, Takebayashi T, Fujiwara Y. Observational evidence of the association between handgrip strength, hand dexterity and cognitive performance in community-dwelling older adults: a systematic review. J Epidemiol. 2018; in press
14. Grigsby J, Kaye K, Baxter J, Shetterly SM, Hamman RF. Executive cognitive abilities and functional status among community-dwelling older persons in the San Luis Valley health and aging study. J Am Geriatr Soc. 1998;46:590–6.
15. Sakurai R, Yasunaga M, Murayama Y, Ohba H, Nonaka K, Suzuki H, Sakuma N, Nishi M, Uchida H, Shinkai S, et al. Long-term effects of an intergenerational program on functional capacity in older adults: results from a seven-year follow-up of the REPRINTS study. Arch Gerontol Geriatr. 2016;64:13–20.
16. Braekhus A, Laake K, Engedal K. A low, 'normal' score on the mini-mental state examination predicts development of dementia after three years. J Am Geriatr Soc. 1995;43:656–61.
17. Veale JF. Edinburgh handedness inventory - short form: a revised version based on confirmatory factor analysis. Laterality. 2014;19:164–77.
18. Fleishman EA, Ellison GD. A factor analysis of fine manipulative tests. J Appl Psychol. 1962;46:96–105.
19. Sanchez-Cubillo I, Perianez JA, Adrover-Roig D, Rodriguez-Sanchez JM, Rios-Lago M, Tirapu J, Barcelo F. Construct validity of the trail making test: role of task-switching, working memory, inhibition/interference control, and visuomotor abilities. J Int Neuropsychol Soc. 2009;15:438–50.
20. Crowe SF. The differential contribution of mental tracking, cognitive flexibility, visual search, and motor speed to performance on parts a and B of the trail making test. J Clin Psychol. 1998;54:585–91.
21. Gaudino EA, Geisler MW, Squires NK. Construct validity in the trail making test: what makes part B harder? J Clin Exp Neuropsychol. 1995;17:529–35.
22. Mahurin RK, Velligan DI, Hazleton B, Mark Davis J, Eckert S, Miller AL. Trail

Hand dexterity, not handgrip strength, is associated with executive function in Japanese...

59

making test errors and executive function in schizophrenia and depression. Clin Neuropsychol. 2006;20:271–88.

23. Arbuthnott K, Frank J. Trail making test, part B as a measure of executive control: validation using a set-switching paradigm. J Clin Exp Neuropsychol. 2000;22:518–28.

24. Gibbons LE, Carle AC, Mackin RS, Harvey D, Mukherjee S, Insel P, Curtis SM, Mungas D, Crane PK. A composite score for executive functioning, validated in Alzheimer's disease neuroimaging initiative (ADNI) participants with baseline mild cognitive impairment. Brain Imaging Behav. 2012;6:517–27.

25. Joy S, Fein D, Kaplan E. Decoding digit symbol: speed, memory, and visual scanning. Assessment. 2003;10:56–65.

26. Koyano W, Shibata H, Nakazato K, Haga H, Suyama Y. Measurement of competence: reliability and validity of the TMIG index of competence. Arch Gerontol Geriatr. 1991;13:103–16.

27. Ajit S, Virach P, Celia B, Cornelius K. Screening for depression among geriatric inpatients with short versions of the geriatric depression scale. Int J Geriatric Psychiatry. 1996;11:915–8.

28. Almeida OP, Almeida SA. Short versions of the geriatric depression scale: a study of their validity for the diagnosis of a major depressive episode according to ICD-10 and DSM-IV. Int J Geriatr Psychiatry. 1999;14:858–65.

29. Trzepacz PT, Hochstetler H, Wang S, Walker B, Saykin AJ. Relationship between the Montreal cognitive assessment and mini-mental state examination for assessment of mild cognitive impairment in older adults. BMC Geriatr. 2015;15:107.

30. Nasreddine ZS, Phillips NA, Bedirian V, Charbonneau S, Whitehead V, Collin I, Cummings JL, Chertkow H. The Montreal cognitive assessment, MoCA: a brief screening tool for mild cognitive impairment. J Am Geriatr Soc. 2005; 53:695–9.

31. Warabi T, Noda H, Kato T. Effect of aging on sensorimotor functions of eye and hand movements. Exp Neurol. 1986;92:686–97.

32. Funahashi S, Andreau JM. Prefrontal cortex and neural mechanisms of executive function. J Physiol Paris. 2013;107:471–82.

33. Koch G, Rossi S, Prosperetti C, Codeca C, Monteleone F, Petrosini L, Bernardi G, Centonze D. Improvement of hand dexterity following motor cortex rTMS in multiple sclerosis patients with cerebellar impairment. Mult Scler. 2008;14:995–8.

34. Peters A. The effects of normal aging on myelin and nerve fibers: a review. J Neurocytol. 2002;31:581–93.

35. Metcalf CD, Irvine TA, Sims JL, Wang YL, Su AW, Norris DO. Complex hand dexterity: a review of biomechanical methods for measuring musical performance. Front Psychol. 2014;5:414.

36. Martin JA, Ramsay J, Hughes C, Peters DM, Edwards MG. Age and grip strength predict hand dexterity in adults. PLoS One. 2015;10:e0117598.

37. Royall DR, Palmer R, Chiodo LK, Polk MJ. Declining executive control in normal aging predicts change in functional status: the freedom house study. J Am Geriatr Soc. 2004;52:346–52.

# 7

# A wearable hip-assist robot reduces the cardiopulmonary metabolic energy expenditure during stair ascent in elderly adults: a pilot cross-sectional study

Dong-Seok Kim[1,2†], Hwang-Jae Lee[1,2†], Su-Hyun Lee[1], Won Hyuk Chang[1], Junwon Jang[3], Byung-Ok Choi[4], Gyu-Ha Ryu[5*] and Yun-Hee Kim[1,2*]

## Abstract

**Background:** Stair ascent is one of the most important and challenging activities of daily living to maintain mobility and independence in elderly adults. Recently, various types of wearable walking assist robots have been developed to improve gait function and metabolic efficiency for elderly adults. Several studies have shown that walking assist robots can improve cardiopulmonary metabolic efficiency during level walking in elderly. However, there is limited evidence demonstrating the effect of walking assist robots on cardiopulmonary metabolic efficiency during stair walking in elderly adults. Therefore, the aim of this study was to investigate the assistance effect of a newly developed wearable hip assist robot on cardiopulmonary metabolic efficiency during stair ascent in elderly adults.

**Methods:** Fifteen healthy elderly adults participated. The Gait Enhancing Mechatronic System (GEMS), developed by Samsung Electronics Co., Ltd., Korea, was used in the present study. The metabolic energy expenditure was measured using a K4b$^2$ while participants performed randomly assigned two conditions consecutively: free ascending stairs without the GEMS or robot-assisted ascending stair with the GEMS.

**Results:** There were significant differences in the oxygen consumption per unit mass (ml/min/kg), metabolic power per unit mass (W/kg) and metabolic equivalents (METs) values between the GEMS and NoGEMS conditions. A statistically significant difference was found between the two conditions in net oxygen consumption and net metabolic power, with a reduction of 8.59% and 10.16% respectively in GEMS condition ($p < 0.05$). The gross oxygen consumption while climbing stairs under the GEMS and NoGEMS conditions was equivalent to 6.38 METs and 6.85 METs, respectively.

**Conclusion:** This study demonstrated that the GEMS was helpful for reducing cardiopulmonary metabolic energy expenditure during stair climbing in elderly adults. The use of the GEMS allows elderly adults to climb stairs with less metabolic energy, therefore, they may experience more endurance in stair climbing while using the GEMS.

**Keywords:** Wearable hip assist robot, Elderly adult, Metabolic energy expenditure, Stair ascent

* Correspondence: gyuha.ryu@samsung.com; yunkim@skku.edu;
yun1225.kim@samsung.com
†Dong-Seok Kim and Hwang-Jae Lee contributed equally to this work.
[5]Office of Biomechanical science, Research Center for Future Medicine,
Samsung Medical Center, Sungkyunkwan University, Irwon-ro 81,
Gangnam-gu, Seoul 06351, Republic of Korea
[1]Department of Physical and Rehabilitation Medicine, Center for Prevention
& Rehabilitation, Heart Vascular Stroke Institute, Samsung Medical Center,
Sungkyunkwan University School of Medicine, Irwon-ro 81, Gangnam-gu,
Seoul 06351, Republic of Korea
Full list of author information is available at the end of the article

## Background

Stair walking (ascending and descending stairs) is one of the most important and challenging activities of daily living required to maintain mobility and independence [1]. However, stair walking demands a variety of physical functions such as proper lower limb strength, joint range of motion, kinesthetic intelligence, and visual processing for safe and coordinated locomotion [2, 3]. Furthermore, stair ascent increases the metabolic energy expenditure compared with level walking [4]. According to the metabolic equivalents (METs) that are a physiological measure expressing the energy expenditure of physical activities and are defined as the ratio of metabolic rate during a specific physical activity to resting metabolic rate, normative walking requires 3.3 METs, whereas normative stair ascent and stair ascent while carrying a moderate load require 5 and 8 METs, respectively [5]. Especially for elderly adults who expend an average of 20% more metabolic energy during walking than young adults [6], stair walking is one of the tasks that places a large burden on daily life. The higher metabolic energy expenditure increases the sense of task effort and fatigue and therefore can contribute to increased risk of falls in elderly adults [7]. For the elderly, a reduction in the energy expenditure of level and stair walking is important elements in preventing falls and maintaining quality of life. Hence, in order to improve cardiopulmonary metabolic efficiency of elderly adults, it is essential to develop useful methods such as physical training utilizing resistance and aerobic exercise, balance training, and assistance using robotic devices.

Specifically, various kinds of wearable-type walking assist robots that provide assistance torque around the hip, knee, and ankle joints are being developed. Recently, many studies using walking assist robots have been performed to identify changes in gait function in elderly adults [8–12]. Several positive effects of walking assist robots on gait function such as gait speed and walking parameters in the elderly have been reported by many research companies and institutions [8–10]. A well-known walking assist robot, the Stride Management Assist Device (SMA, Honda R&D Corporation, Japan), improved gait parameters and reduced glucose metabolism in the lower limb muscles in elderly adults [8]. Shimada et al. reported that a 3-month walking intervention program using the SMA device was useful in improving gait function and the efficiency of muscle efforts during walking in elderly adults [9]. In particular, previous studies have examined the effects of robotic assist on metabolic measurements such as oxygen consumption per unit mass, metabolic power per unit mass, and metabolic equivalents. Several studies have also shown that walking assist robots were effective in reducing metabolic energy expenditure during walking in elderly adults [10–12]. Jin et al. reported that a new soft robotic suit reduced net metabolic power by an average of 5.9% in the powered-on condition compared with the powered-off condition in nine elderly adults during walking [11]. Galle et al. reported that bilateral ankle-foot exoskeletons could reduce energy expenditure by 12% in comparison with the powered-off condition in elderly adults. This device also resulted in a 4% reduction in energy expenditure compared to walking in normal shoes [12]. Therefore, metabolic measurement is a very important variable for verifying the assist effect of robotic devices.

Recently, Samsung Advanced Institute of Technology developed the Gait Enhancing Mechatronic System (GEMS, Samsung Electronics Co., Ltd., Korea), which aids the hip joint flexion and extension movement of the wearer during walking. In a previous study, elderly people demonstrated improved gait function, decreased muscle effort, and reduced energy expenditure during walking with the GEMS compared to walking without the GEMS [10, 13].

Most of the studies using walking assist robots for the elderly have been conducted to observe the effect of the robots on gait function and metabolic efficiency in level walking. However, there is limited evidence demonstrating the effect of walking assist robots on gait function and metabolic efficiency in stair walking in elderly adults. Only a few studies on walking assist robots for stair walking have been reported in the literature [14, 15].

Therefore, the aim of this pilot cross-sectional study was to identify the assistance effect of the GEMS as a newly developed wearable hip-assist robot during stair ascent by comparing the energy expenditure of elderly adults with and without the GEMS. We hypothesized that using the GEMS during stair ascent would reduce energy expenditure and improve stair climbing speed compared to stair ascent without GEMS.

## Methods

### Participants

We recruited elderly adults who met the inclusion and exclusion criteria. Fifteen healthy elderly adults participated in the present study [16]. Table 1 shows the characteristics of the participants. Inclusion criteria of this study were as follows: 1) absence of a history of musculoskeletal or central nervous system diseases and 2) physical performance abilities with short physical performance battery scores of 8 or higher (mild and minimal limitations range without any problems in activity of daily living) [17]. Exclusion criteria were as follows: 1) absence of the ability to walk independently due to visual field defects, fractures, or severe muscle weakness, 2) severe dizziness that might lead to falls, and 3) cognitive disorders that might be difficult to understand accurately in this study. All participants provided informed consent before participating in the study. This study protocol was approved by the Samsung Medical Center Institutional Review Board.

**Table 1** Characteristics of the participants

| Characteristic | Value |
| --- | --- |
| Sex (male / female) | 6 / 9 |
| Age, years (mean ± SD) | 74.33 ± 4.56 |
| Height, cm (mean ± SD) | 159.40 ± 5.73 |
| Weight, kg (mean ± SD) | 59.80 ± 9.24 |
| BMI (mean ± SD) | 23.54 ± 3.39 |
| SPPB, points (mean ± SD) | 10.53 ± 1.36 |

*SD* Standard Deviation, *BMI* Body Mass Index, *SPPB* Short Physical Performance Battery

### Wearable hip-assist robot

As show in Fig. 1, the GEMS worn around the waist is composed of a pair of actuators that generate assistance power to the left and right hip joints, a hip brace around the waist, a pair of thigh frames for transmission of assistance torque from the actuators to the thighs, and fabric belts at the ends of the thigh frames. The GEMS is available in two sizes, small (for hip circumferences 70~90 cm) and medium (for hip circumferences 90~100 cm), and each size can be adjusted according to the body size of the individual. Two 70-W brushless DC motors positioned around the hip joints generate assistance torque and deliver the generated torque to each hip joint with a maximum torque of 12 Nm through a 75:1 multi-stage gear system. Each joint has one active degree of freedom for flexion and extension in the sagittal plane by electric actuators and one passive hinge below the active degree of freedom for abduction and adduction in the frontal plane. The range of motion is 120/45 degrees for flexion/extension and 20/20 degrees for abduction/adduction. The battery, CPU, inertial measurement unit (IMU) sensor, and motor driving units are all located on the back of the device. An IMU sensor is used to calculate gait state from the hip joint angles and to determine the assistance torque pattern. The GEMS can work continuously for 1.3 h under normal operating conditions, and its total weight is 2.8 kg.

The assistance strategy of the GEMS for stair ascent utilizes a foot contact event estimated by IMU sensor data and detects user intention as well as reflect user preference [18]. In this strategy, a gait cycle for stair ascent is divided into 4 phases to detect user intention more easily and exactly in real time. The divided gait cycle is as follows: foot contact to pull-up (FC-PU), pull-up to hip crossing (PU-HC), hip crossing to peak joint angle of a swing leg (HC-PJA), and peak joint angle of a swing leg to foot contact (PJA-FC) (Fig. 2). The moments of each events are determined by hip joint angles estimated by two joint angle sensors. Also, this assistance strategy applies criteria for the initiation and termination of assistance torque by recognizing user intention. Pull-up, which is an obvious clue indicating user intention to climb stair, is used as assistance initiation criterion during stair ascent. At the moment of pull-up event detection, the desired assistance durations are determined, and the assistance torques for each stance and swing leg are then generated for a new step. The generated assistance torques are applied to each stance and swing leg in a feedforward manner for the desired assistance duration until the assistance termination criterion is met and are finished at the peak joint angle exploited as assistance termination criterion (Fig. 2). In addition, at the last minute of the peak joint angle event, decay flexion and extension torque profiles are applied to terminate the assistance torque profiles rapidly and smoothly.

### Experimental protocol

The stair ascent trials were conducted at the Samsung Medical Center, Seoul, Korea. Metabolic energy expenditure was measured while participants climb stairs from the first basement level to the fourth floor, a total of 16 flights comprised of 128 steps with each step at 17 cm in height, for a total vertical displacement of 21.76 m.

Prior to initiation of the trials, the physical performance abilities of participants were evaluated through a short physical performance battery test to make sure that they meet the inclusion criteria of scores 8 or higher, and basic physical information (age, gender, height, body weight, waist measurement, leg length, and blood pressure), disease information, and pain information were recorded. In

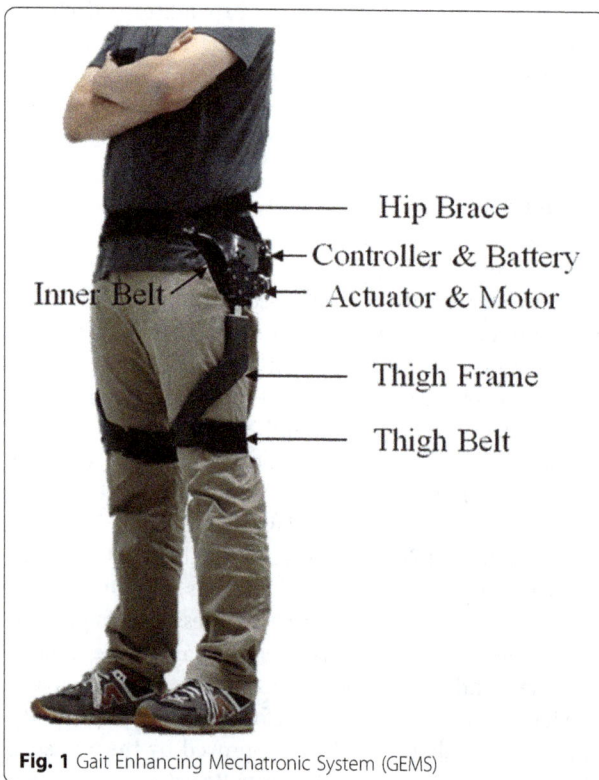

**Fig. 1** Gait Enhancing Mechatronic System (GEMS)

Hip Brace

Controller & Battery

Actuator & Motor

Inner Belt

Thigh Frame

Thigh Belt

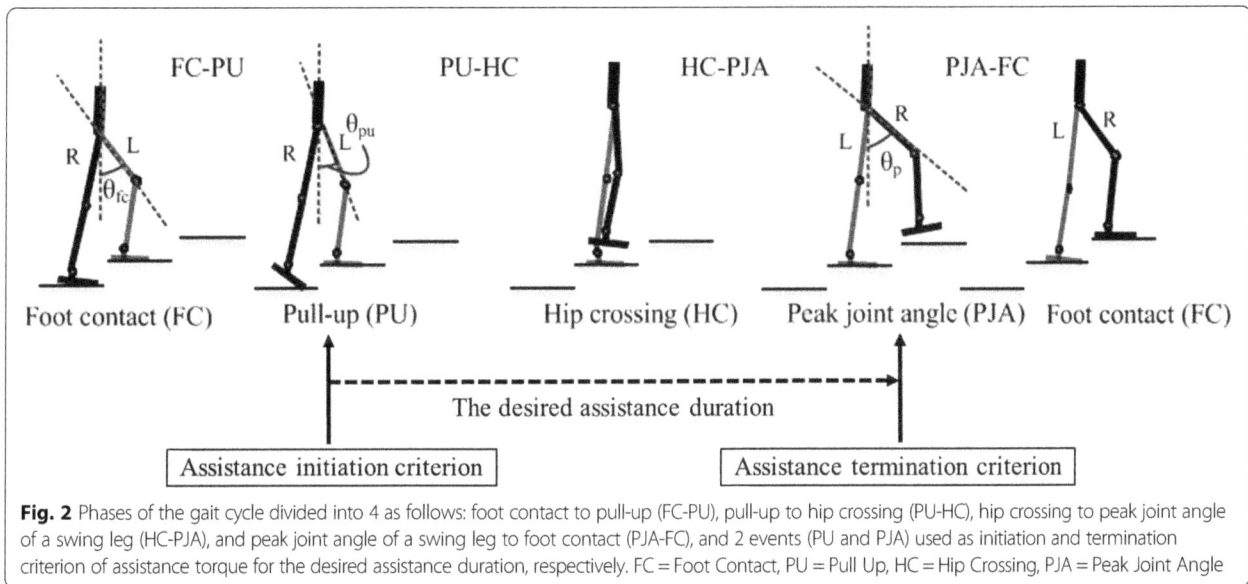

**Fig. 2** Phases of the gait cycle divided into 4 as follows: foot contact to pull-up (FC-PU), pull-up to hip crossing (PU-HC), hip crossing to peak joint angle of a swing leg (HC-PJA), and peak joint angle of a swing leg to foot contact (PJA-FC), and 2 events (PU and PJA) used as initiation and termination criterion of assistance torque for the desired assistance duration, respectively. FC = Foot Contact, PU = Pull Up, HC = Hip Crossing, PJA = Peak Joint Angle

order for participants to wear the GEMS comfortably, the size of the GEMS was adjusted by a researcher. In order to adapt participants to the GEMS and familiarize them with stair ascent with the GEMS, all participants ascended and descended a 6-step custom-made staircase installed in the laboratory for 10 min. While all participants performed stair walking, the assist torque of the GEMS was determined to be the most comfortable level for the individual.

The K4b$^2$ system (Cosmed, Rome, Italy) based on true breath-by-breath technology was used to measure metabolic energy expenditure during stair ascent with and without the GEMS. Before the stair ascent test, all participants were equipped with a K4b$^2$ analyzer unit that was strapped to the chest, and a facial mask connected to an analyzer unit was placed on the nose and mouth. Also, a heart rate monitor (T31 transmitter, POLAR, USA) was strapped around the participant's chest to measure heart rate. Participants were instructed not to talk during the trials.

The stair ascent trials were performed under two different conditions: free ascent without the GEMS (NoGEMS) and robot-assist ascent with the GEMS (GEMS). The experimental protocol of the present study was as follows. All participants stood for 5 min to obtain baseline variables. Participants were then asked to climb stairs from the first basement level to the fourth floor in a step-over-step manner under two different conditions, GEMS and NoGEMS. The GEMS and NoGEMS conditions were conducted in a random order, and just before the second condition, participants stood for 2~3 min to obtain baseline variables once more. Participants rested between the two conditions for 10 min to restore metabolic rate to baseline level. During stair climbing, time

was recorded with a stopwatch to compare the difference in climbing speed between the two conditions.

**Measurement tool**

The K4b$^2$ system, which was worn in a harness on the shoulders, was used to measure metabolic energy expenditure during stair ascent with and without the GEMS. The K4b$^2$ system is a computerized portable system for cardiopulmonary gas exchange measurements based on true breath-by-breath analysis and allows the user to measure the physiological response to exercise without limitations. This device is composed of a facial mask worn over the participant's nose and mouth, a gas sample line, an analyzer unit strapped to the participant's chest, and a battery-operated unit. It is designed to measure the parameters of oxygen consumption, carbon dioxide emission, and ventilation with several sensors. The K4b$^2$ analyzer unit was calibrated before each test for accurate sensor operation. Calibrations of the flow turbine and gas analyzers were performed using a 3-l syringe and gas mixtures, respectively. Heart rate was measured using a heart rate monitor strapped around the participant's chest, and heart rate data were transmitted to a portable device.

**Data analysis**

Metabolic energy expenditure during stair ascent was obtained by the K4b$^2$ system. To estimate the metabolic energy expenditure, we applied net oxygen consumption (ml/min/kg) and net metabolic power (W/kg) computed from VO$_2$ (L/min) and the respiratory exchange ratio (RER) recorded by the K4b$^2$ system because net values give a more direct indication of metabolic efficiency than gross values [19]. The VO$_2$ and RER were computed as the mean values for the last minute of each condition to compare the metabolic energy expenditure consumed for the same time in climbing stairs and were used to calculate the energy cost (kcal/min) of each condition using the regression equation reported by Zuntz [20]. The regression equation which is based on the thermal equivalent of $VO_2$ for non-protein respiratory equivalent was used to calculate the energy cost through mean values of the $VO_2$ and RER for each condition.

$$\text{Energy cost} = VO_2 \times (1.2341 \times RER + 3.8124)$$

Then, energy cost was used to calculate metabolic power of each condition in watts through the conversion factor 69.78 W·kcal/min as follows:

$$\text{Metabolic power} = \text{Energy cost} \times 69.78$$

After that, in order to obtain the net metabolic power of each condition, we subtracted the resting metabolic power form each gross metabolic power [21]. The net metabolic power of each condition was normalized by dividing by body weight (W/kg) and compared with average values.

The average values of the METs, which are a physiological measure expressing the energy expenditure of physical activities, were computed as the average values for the last minute of the GEMS and NoGEMS conditions. The METs intensity during stair ascent with and without the GEMS was calculated by dividing average oxygen consumption (ml/min/kg) by 3.5 ml/min/kg.

### Statistical analysis
Paired t-tests were used to compare significant differences in oxygen consumption, metabolic power, METs values, and stair climbing cadence between the GEMS condition and the NoGEMS condition. Statistical analysis was conducted with Statistical Package for the Social Sciences ver. 22.0 for Windows software (SPSS Inc., Chicago, IL, USA). The statistical significance level for the paired t-tests was set at $p < 0.05$.

### Results
As show in Fig. 3a), we found significant differences between net oxygen consumption per unit mass in the two different conditions. The mean of net oxygen consumption per unit mass with and without the GEMS was $17.43 \pm 4.09$ and $19.07 \pm 4.00$ ml/min/kg, respectively. In addition, the mean of resting oxygen consumption per unit mass obtained before first and second conditions was $4.64 \pm 0.64$ and $5.11 \pm 0.84$ ml/min/kg, respectively. A statistically significant difference was found between the GEMS and NoGEMS conditions in net oxygen consumption per unit mass, with a reduction of 8.59%, corresponding to 1.64 ml/min/kg under the GEMS condition ($p = 0.013$).

Figure 3b) shows that stair ascent with the GEMS required an average of $6.10 \pm 1.15$ W/kg, while stair ascent without the GEMS required an average of $6.79 \pm 1.18$ W/kg of net metabolic power per unit mass. This difference was statistically significant, with a reduction of 10.16%, corresponding to 0.69 W/kg under the GEMS condition ($p = 0.001$). The mean of resting metabolic power per unit mass obtained before first and second conditions was $1.59 \pm 0.17$ and $1.67 \pm 0.24$ W/kg, respectively.

In addition, we calculated the METs to compare the intensity of climbing 128 steps with and without the GEMS. The gross oxygen consumption of climbing stairs under the GEMS and NoGEMS conditions was equivalent to 6.38 METs and 6.85 METs, respectively (Fig. 3c). There was a statistically significant difference in METs value between the two conditions, with a difference of 0.47 METs ($p < 0.05$). Figure 3d) shows the average stair climbing cadence (steps/min) under the GEMS and NoGEMS conditions. The stair climbing with GEMS took an average of 145 s and cadence was an average of $53.25 \pm 4.56$ steps/min. While the stair climbing without GEMS took an average of 144 s and cadence was an average of $53.92 \pm 5.82$ steps/min. There was no significant difference in stair climbing cadence between the two conditions ($p = 0.388$).

In summary, oxygen consumption per unit mass and metabolic power per unit mass were significantly reduced during stair ascent with the GEMS compared to free gait without the GEMS.

### Discussion
The aim of this study was to identify the assistance effect of the GEMS by comparing the energy expenditure between the GEMS and NoGEMS conditions during stair ascent in elderly adults. In the present study, the GEMS was found to reduce oxygen consumption and metabolic power during stair ascent in elderly adults. Furthermore, we demonstrated the assistance effect of the GEMS on stair climbing based on the observation of a significant reduction in energy expenditure in elderly adults with the GEMS.

The gait of the elderly is typically characterized by short step length, slow walking velocity, reduced range of joint motion, and reduced balance [7]. These characteristics increase the risk of falls and unnecessary walking energy expenditure [22]. Metabolic energy expenditure is an important indicator of physical capability because it represents an individual's physiological ability to supply energy to support various physical activities [23]. Previous studies have reported that elderly adults consume 20% more cardiopulmonary metabolic energy than young adults during walking [24, 25]. Furthermore, elderly adults were dependents on the higher metabolic energy expenditure during stair ascent than level walking [26]. Several studies have suggested that degradation in physical function in the elderly, such as decreased sense of balance and loss of muscle strength, might be related to increase in metabolic energy expenditure [24, 27]. Waters et al. reported that elderly

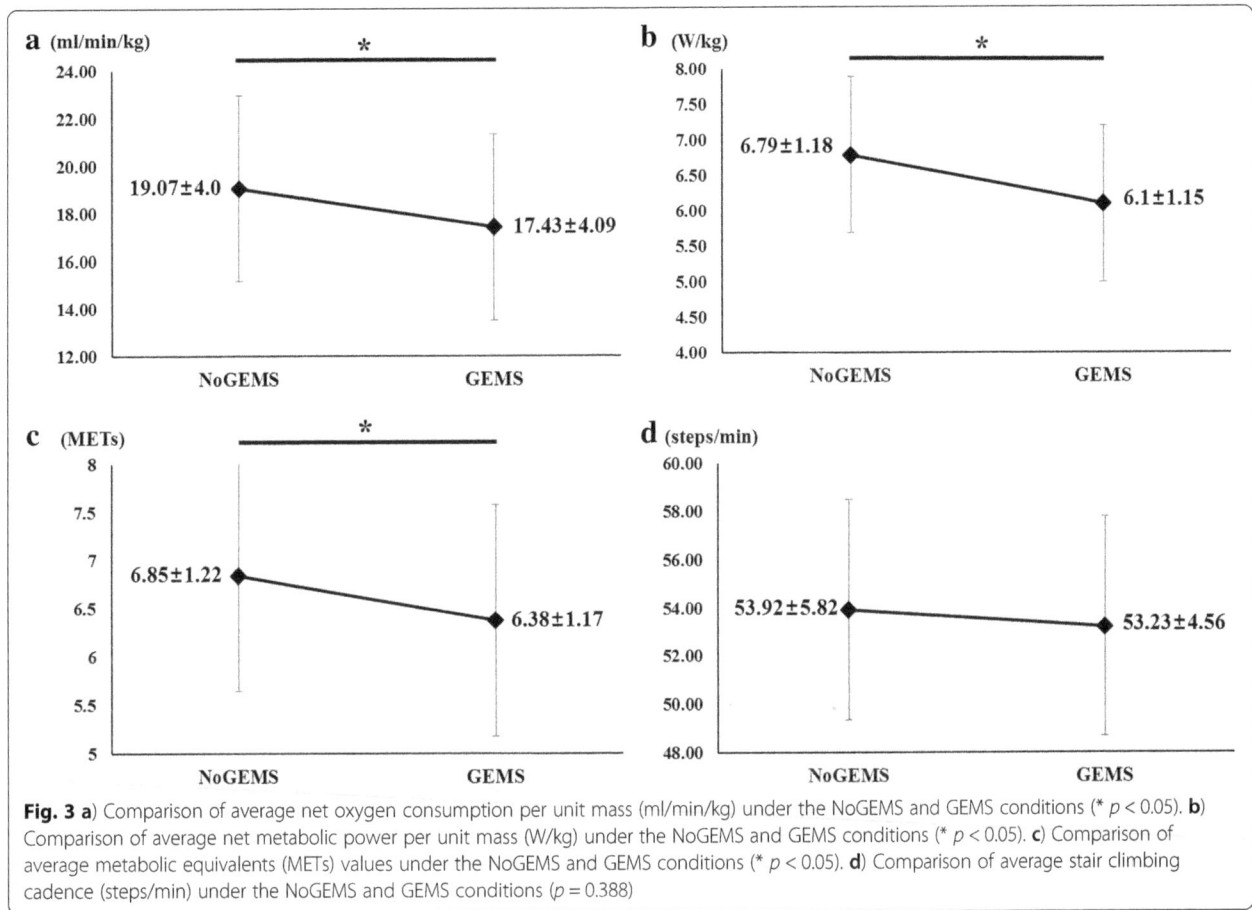

**Fig. 3 a**) Comparison of average net oxygen consumption per unit mass (ml/min/kg) under the NoGEMS and GEMS conditions (* $p < 0.05$). **b**) Comparison of average net metabolic power per unit mass (W/kg) under the NoGEMS and GEMS conditions (* $p < 0.05$). **c**) Comparison of average metabolic equivalents (METs) values under the NoGEMS and GEMS conditions (* $p < 0.05$). **d**) Comparison of average stair climbing cadence (steps/min) under the NoGEMS and GEMS conditions ($p = 0.388$)

with restrictions in range of motion in the lower limb joints expended more metabolic energy expenditure during walking than adults without such restrictions [28]. Also, several studies reported that decline in step length and gait speed contributed to increase in metabolic energy expenditure in elderly adults [24, 29]. As reported several studies, the increase in metabolic energy expenditure in elderly adults is related to gait function. In a previous study utilizing the GEMS, Lee et al. reported the effects of the GEMS on gait speed, cadence, stride length, step width, and muscle effort during level walking and demonstrated that the GEMS improved gait function and cardiopulmonary metabolic efficiency, with a reduction of approximately 7% in oxygen consumption in elderly adults [10]. The result of our study found that the net metabolic energy expenditure reduction was about 10.2% in the GEMS compared to NoGEMS condition. In the other hand, a recent study using hip-assist soft exoskeleton reported reduction of net metabolic energy expenditure by 17.4% during treadmill gait in young adults [30]. Therefore, further studies are needed to directly compare the effect of different robotic devices on metabolic energy expenditure for diverse ADL conditions in elderly adults. Although the GEMS is about 2 kg heavier than the soft

exoskeleton, it is meaningful result that GEMS reduces the metabolic energy expenditure by 10.16% during stair ascent in elderly adults.

Also, this study observed the metabolic power of climbing stairs to compare walking efficiency between assistive gait with the GEMS and free gait without the GEMS. The unit of metabolic power is W (watt) or J/s, indicating how efficiently an individual works per unit time. The calculated net metabolic power, which is based on the measured oxygen consumption ($VO_2$) and carbon dioxide emission ($VCO_2$) values, was 362.13 W under the GEMS condition and 402.93 W under the NoGEMS condition in this study. The present results indicate that the assistance of the GEMS during stair ascent influences walking efficiency, with a reduction of 10.16% in net metabolic power in the elderly. However, as presented in the results, there was no statistically significant difference in stair climbing speed between the GEMS and NoGEMS conditions. Namely, the use of the GEMS allowed elderly adults to perform the same tasks using less energy than without the GEMS. Thus, the GEMS aids elderly adults in using metabolic energy more efficiently during stair ascent. From these results, we suggest that the reduction in metabolic energy expenditure caused by the aid of the GEMS on stair climbing might closely relate to the reduction of muscles activation or improvement of gait function in elderly adults. Recently, various kinds of wearable-type walking assist robots that provide assistance torque around the hip, knee, and ankle joints have been developed for energy-efficient walking and improvement in gait function in elderly adults and patients with gait impairment. Previous studies have reported the effects of other walking assist devices on gait function and metabolic efficiency during walking. Jin et al. reported that a soft robotic suit, which provides an assistive force for hip flexion through winding belts, significantly reduced net metabolic power by an average of 5.9% and increased maximum hip angle by an average of 5.4% during walking in elderly adults [31]. Some energy expenditure effects of the wearable hip assist devices were reported even in young adults. Young et al. (2017) demonstrated that a pneumatic hip exoskeleton improved metabolic efficiency during walking, with a reduction of 9.7% in net metabolic power with the ideal timing of hip flexion [32]. Additionally, Ding et al. showed that soft exosuits, which provide assistance forces to the hip joints, reduced the metabolic power of walking by 4.6%, effectively improving walking efficiency [33]. There are many differences between these previous studies and the present study. The main difference is that previous studies examined level walking, while the present study was conducted while climbing stairs, which requires approximately 30–40% more cardiopulmonary metabolic energy compared with level walking [34, 35]. Also, previous studies compared net metabolic power between power-on and power-off conditions both with the walking assist device attached in order to reduce the advantage of free gait without the device load. The present study compared net metabolic power between stair climbing without the GEMS and stair climbing with the GEMS, which weighs 2.8 kg.

In addition, the METs were observed to compare the physical intensity of climbing 128 stairs with and without the GEMS. The METs are a physiological measure expressing the energy expenditure of physical activities and is defined as the ratio of metabolic rate during a specific physical activity to resting metabolic rate, which is an oxygen consumption at rest of approximately 3.5 ml/min/kg. As such, the physical activity at 3 METs demands three times a resting oxygen consumption of approximately 3.5 ml/min/kg. According to reports from the Compendium of Physical Activities, the METs values during stair climbing while carrying a load of approximately 3 kg and 9 kg were 5 and 6 METs, respectively. The METs values estimated by the Compendium of Physical Activities indicate that, as the load carried increases during stair climbing, the METs values increase. However, our measured results showed that the use of the GEMS during stair climbing decreased the METs values by approximately 0.5 METs, despite the increased device load of 2.8 kg. Therefore, the results from the present study indicate that use of the GEMS has a substantial benefit on reduction in metabolic energy expenditure during stair climbing in elderly adults.

This study has a limitation. Participants of our study had relatively good functional status and elderly people with severe gait disorder were not involved. For this sub-population, who have limitations in muscle power or postural stability for independent walking or stair climbing, further study is needed to assess the clinical effects of the GEMS on efficiency of walking or stair climbing.

## Conclusions

In this study, we found that the GEMS, which is a newly developed wearable hip assist robot designed to improve gait function and metabolic efficiency, is helpful for reducing cardiopulmonary metabolic energy expenditure during stair ascent in elderly adults. Although there was no significant difference in stair climbing speed between the GEMS and NoGEMS conditions, this study demonstrates that the use of the GEMS allows elderly adults to climb stairs with less cardiopulmonary metabolic energy expenditure compared to stair climbing without the GEMS. Therefore, elderly adults may experience more endurance in stair climbing while using the GEMS.

**Abbreviations**
GEMS: Gait Enhancing Mechatronic System; IMU: Inertial measurement unit; METs: Metabolic equivalents; RER: Respiratory exchange ratio

**Funding**
This study was supported by the Samsung Medical Center (PHO0171341) and by a grant from the NRF (NRF-2017M3A9G5083690 and NRF-2016R1A6A3A11930931), which is funded by the Korean government.

**Authors' contributions**
DSK and HJL contributed to experimental design, experimental progress, data analysis and drafting the manuscript. SHL contributed to setting up the experiment and collecting data. WHC contributed to experimental design, data analysis and data interpretation. JWJ contributed to developing the device and the algorithm, and providing device maintenance and repairs. BOC contributed to setting up the experiment and revising the manuscript. YHK and GHR contributed to experimental design, interpreting data and revising the manuscript. Finally, Wearable Hip-assist Robot (GEMS) developed by Samsung Advanced Institute of Technology was provided for this study. All authors read and approved the final manuscript.

**Competing interests**
The authors declare that they have no competing interests.

## Author details
[1]Department of Physical and Rehabilitation Medicine, Center for Prevention & Rehabilitation, Heart Vascular Stroke Institute, Samsung Medical Center, Sungkyunkwan University School of Medicine, Irwon-ro 81, Gangnam-gu, Seoul 06351, Republic of Korea. [2]Department of Health Sciences and Technology, SAIHST, Sungkyunkwan University, Irwon-ro 81, Gangnam-gu, Seoul 06351, Republic of Korea. [3]Samsung Advanced Institute of Technology, Samsung Electronics, 130 Samsung-ro, Yeongtong-gu, Suwon-si, Gyeonggi-do 16678, Republic of Korea. [4]Department of Neurology, Neuroscience Center, Samsung Medical Center, Sungkyunkwan University School of Medicine, Irwon-ro 81, Gangnam-gu, Seoul 06351, Republic of Korea. [5]Office of Biomechanical science, Research Center for Future Medicine, Samsung Medical Center, Sungkyunkwan University, Irwon-ro 81, Gangnam-gu, Seoul 06351, Republic of Korea.

## References
1. Unver B, Ertekin O, Karatosun V. Pain, fear of falling and stair climbing ability in patients with knee osteoarthritis before and after knee replacement: 6 month follow-up study. J Back Musculoskelet Rehabil. 2014;27:77–84.
2. Tiedemann AC, Sherrington C, Lord SR. Physical and psychological factors associated with stair negotiation performance in older people. J Gerontol Ser A Biol Med Sci. 2007;62:1259–65.
3. Bonora G, Carpinella I, Cattaneo D, Chiari L, Ferrarin M. A new instrumented method for the evaluation of gait initiation and step climbing based on inertial sensors: a pilot application in Parkinson's disease. Journal of neuroengineering and rehabilitation. 2015;12:45.
4. Bassett DR, Vachon JA, Kirkland AO, Howley ET, Duncan GE, Johnson KR. Energy cost of stair climbing and descending on the college alumnus questionnaire. Med Sci Sports Exerc. 1997;29:1250–4.
5. Ainsworth BE, Haskell WL, Whitt MC, Irwin ML, Swartz AM, Strath SJ, O Brien WL, Bassett DR, Schmitz KH, Emplaincourt PO. Compendium of physical activities: an update of activity codes and MET intensities. Med Sci Sports Exerc. 2000;32:S498–504.
6. Peterson DS, Martin PE. Effects of age and walking speed on coactivation and cost of walking in healthy adults. Gait & posture. 2010;31:355–9.
7. Hortobágyi T, Finch A, Solnik S, Rider P, DeVita P. Association between muscle activation and metabolic cost of walking in young and old adults. J Gerontology Series A: Biomedical Sciences and Medical Sciences. 2011;66:541–7.
8. Shimada H, Suzuki T, Kimura Y, Hirata T, Sugiura M, Endo Y, Yasuhara K, Shimada K, Kikuchi K, Oda K. Effects of an automated stride assistance system on walking parameters and muscular glucose metabolism in elderly adults. Br J Sports Med. 2008;42:922–9.
9. Shimada H, Hirata T, Kimura Y, Naka T, Kikuchi K, Oda K, Ishii K, Ishiwata K, Suzuki T. Effects of a robotic walking exercise on walking performance in community-dwelling elderly adults. Geriatr Gerontol Int. 2009;9:372–81.
10. Lee H-J, Lee S, Chang WH, Seo K, Shim Y, Choi B-O, Ryu G-H, Kim Y-H. A wearable hip assist robot can improve gait function and cardiopulmonary metabolic efficiency in elderly adults. IEEE Transactions on Neural Systems and Rehabilitation Engineering. 2017.
11. Jin S, Iwamoto N, Hashimoto K, Yamamoto M. Experimental evaluation of energy efficiency for a soft wearable robotic suit. IEEE Transactions on Neural Systems and Rehabilitation Engineering. 2011.
12. Galle S, Derave W, Bossuyt F, Calders P, Malcolm P, De Clercq D. Exoskeleton plantarflexion assistance for elderly. Gait & posture. 2017;52:183–8.
13. Lee S-H, Lee H-J, Chang WH, Choi B-O, Lee J, Kim J, Ryu G-H, Kim Y-H. Gait performance and foot pressure distribution during wearable robot-assisted gait in elderly adults. Journal of neuroengineering and rehabilitation. 2017;14:123.
14. Farris RJ, Quintero HA, Goldfarb M: Performance evaluation of a lower limb exoskeleton for stair ascent and descent with paraplegia. In Engineering in medicine and biology society (EMBC), 2012 annual international conference of the IEEE IEEE; 2012: 1908–1911.
15. Xu F, Lin X, Cheng H, Huang R, Chen Q: Adaptive stair-ascending and stair-descending strategies for powered lower limb exoskeleton. In Mechatronics and Automation (ICMA), 2017 IEEE International Conference on IEEE; 2017: 1579–1584.
16. Foley M, Bowen B. Comparison of metabolic cost and cardiovascular response to stair ascending and descending with walkers and canes in older adults. Arch Phys Med Rehabil. 2014;95:1742–9.
17. Volpato S, Cavalieri M, Sioulis F, Guerra G, Maraldi C, Zuliani G, Fellin R, Guralnik JM. Predictive value of the short physical performance battery following hospitalization in older patients. J Gerontology Series A: Biomedical Sciences and Medical Sciences. 2010;66:89–96.
18. Jang J, Kim K, Lee J, Lim B, Shim Y: Assistance strategy for stair ascent with a robotic hip exoskeleton. In Intelligent Robots and Systems (IROS), 2016 IEEE/RSJ International Conference on. IEEE; 2016: 5658–5663.
19. Brehm MA, Becher J, Harlaar J. Reproducibility evaluation of gross and net walking efficiency in children with cerebral palsy. Developmental Medicine & Child Neurology. 2007;49:45–8.
20. Zuntz N. Ueber die Bedeutung der verschiedenen Nährstoffe als Erzeuger der Muskelkraft. Archiv für die gesamte Physiologie des Menschen und der Tiere. 1901;83:557–71.
21. Griffin TM, Roberts TJ, Kram R. Metabolic cost of generating muscular force in human walking: insights from load-carrying and speed experiments. J Appl Physiol. 2003;95:172–83.
22. DeVita P, Hortobagyi T. Age causes a redistribution of joint torques and powers during gait. J Appl Physiol. 2000;88:1804–11.
23. Wert DM, Brach J, Perera S, VanSwearingen JM. Gait biomechanics, spatial and temporal characteristics, and the energy cost of walking in older adults with impaired mobility. Phys Ther. 2010;90:977–85.
24. Martin PE, Rothstein DE, Larish DD. Effects of age and physical activity status on the speed-aerobic demand relationship of walking. J Appl Physiol. 1992; 73:200–6.
25. Waters R, Lunsford B. Energy expenditure of normal and pathological gait: application to orthotic prescription. Atlas of orthotics. 1985:151–9.
26. Horiuchi M, Endo J, Horiuchi Y, Abe D. Comparisons of energy cost and economical walking speed at various gradients in healthy, active younger and older adults. J Exerc Sci Fit. 2015;13:79–85.
27. Malatesta D, Simar D, Dauvilliers Y, Candau R, Borrani F, Préfaut C, Caillaud C. Energy cost of walking and gait instability in healthy 65-and 80-yr-olds. J Appl Physiol. 2003;95:2248–56.
28. Waters R, Barnes G, Husserl T, Silver L, Liss R. Comparable energy expenditure after arthrodesis of the hip and ankle. JBJS. 1988;70:1032–7.
29. Donelan JM, Kram R. Mechanical and metabolic determinants of the preferred step width in human walking. Proc R Soc Lond B Biol Sci. 2001; 268:1985–92.
30. Zhang J, Fiers P, Witte KA, Jackson RW, Poggensee KL, Atkeson CG, Collins SH. Human-in-the-loop optimization of exoskeleton assistance during walking. Science. 2017;356:1280–4.
31. Jin S, Iwamoto N, Hashimoto K, Yamamoto M. Experimental evaluation of energy efficiency for a soft wearable robotic suit. IEEE Transactions on Neural Systems and Rehabilitation Engineering. 2016.
32. Young AJ, Foss J, Gannon H, Ferris DP. Influence of power delivery timing on the energetics and biomechanics of humans wearing a hip exoskeleton. Frontiers in Bioengineering and Biotechnology. 2017;5.
33. Ding Y, Galiana I, Asbeck AT, De Rossi SMM, Bae J, Santos TRT, de Araujo VL, Lee S, Holt KG, Walsh C. Biomechanical and physiological evaluation of multi-joint assistance with soft exosuits. IEEE Transactions on Neural Systems and Rehabilitation Engineering. 2017;25:119–30.
34. Knaggs JD, Larkin KA, Manini TM. Metabolic cost of daily activities and effect of mobility impairment in older adults. J Am Geriatr Soc. 2011;59:2118–23.
35. Cho KH, Song W, Kim J, Jung EJ, Jang J, Im SH, Kim M. Energy expenditures for activities of daily living in Korean young adults: a preliminary study. Ann Rehabil Med. 2016;40:725–33.

# 8

# Coping with dementia caregiving: a mixed-methods study on feasibility and benefits of a psycho-educative group program

S. Pihet[1,2*] and S. Kipfer[1]

**Abstract**

**Background:** Persons with dementia experience a progressive decline associated with an increasing dependency. Most of the support they require to stay at home comes from their informal caregivers (IC). Dementia informal caregiving imposes high costs on IC's health and quality of life, related to long periods of chronic stress. Based on evidence that more adequate coping strategies can reduce chronic stress and its negative consequences, and that psycho-educative interventions have the broadest effects on IC quality of life, the program "Learning to feel better… and help better" was developed in French-speaking Canada. This group intervention focusing on coping with the daily stress of dementia caregiving showed efficacy in decreasing the behavior problems of the person with dementia and the associated stress reactions in their IC. The objectives of our study were to examine within a one group pre- and post-test design 1) the feasibility of implementing the program in two regions of French-speaking Switzerland, 2) the effects of the program, and 3) the participants' use of the trained strategies in daily life.

**Method:** A mixed-methods concurrent nested design was used to quantitatively evaluate the feasibility, the effects on five core outcomes, and strategy use in daily life. Additional qualitative data documented in depth the acceptability and impact of the intervention.

**Results:** We analyzed 18 complete data sets. Regarding feasibility, qualitative and quantitative results converged towards a very good acceptance of the program and a strong implication of the participants. Regarding effects, the program resulted in substantial and significant improvements in burden ($d = 0.41$, $p < .05$), psychological distress ($d = 0.54$, $p < .05$) and self-efficacy ($d = 0.43$, $p < .05$). The qualitative results emphasized the benefits of a group format: Participants felt understood by peers, could build new social bonds and experienced reduced social isolation. Data regularly collected in daily life showed that participants were using more and more over time the strategies they learned ($\beta_{01} = 0.55$, $p < .001$), particularly reframing.

**Conclusion:** This study expands on the original one conducted by the developers of the program in French-speaking Canada, by showing the feasibility and the very promising effects of this intervention in two regions of French-speaking Switzerland.

**Keywords:** Dementia, Informal caregiver, Psycho-educative intervention, Stress, Coping strategies

* Correspondence: Sandrine.Pihet@heds.ch
[1]School of Health, University of Applied Sciences and Arts Western Switzerland, Fribourg, Switzerland
[2]Haute Ecole de Santé Fribourg, Route des Cliniques 15, 1700 Fribourg, Switzerland

# Background

Dementia is one of the main cause for disability and dependency in older people, with 46.8 million people affected worldwide in 2015. Due to population ageing, in the absence of a cure, we expect 75 million of persons living with dementia in 2030, and 132 million in 2050 [1]. In Switzerland, 148,000 persons were living with dementia in 2016, and this number is expected to double in 2040, due to the Swiss population being among the oldest on the planet [2, 3].

Dementia is associated with a progressive decline in cognitive functions leading the affected person to depend more and more on the assistance, supervision and care of others. In Switzerland, more than half of the persons with dementia live at home (the other half in nursing homes), 43% requiring occasional support, 47% daily support, and 10% continuous support. Informal caregivers of the person with dementia (ICD), often their spouse or adult child, provide most of this support (e.g. [4, 5]). These figures are similar to those of other European countries (e.g. [4]).

The voluntary contribution of ICD is key to the sustainability of most health care systems (e.g. [6]). However taking an IC role is becoming more and more difficult as family size reduces, geographic distance between family members, employment rates of women, and professional pressures increase [7]. The sustainability of ICD contribution is a core public health issue. Supporting ICD is in the interest of the person receiving the care, the health care system and society in general. Describing the support options for IC in Switzerland is a challenge due to the fragmentation of this country composed of 26 states with substantial independence in terms of health politics; Each state further comprises several districts and a large number of municipalities, with some independence in terms of health care organization. Nevertheless, a nationwide evaluation of support options for ICD conducted in 2017 [8] revealed that two thirds of the states had homecare services with expertise in dementia in each of their districts (17, 65%). However only one-third had specialized daycare in each district (9, 35%) or a specialized coordination service (9, 35%), and only one-fourth had specialized night care services in each district (6, 23%). This overview focused primarily on publicly funded support options, while private associations (e.g. Alzheimer Association, Red Cross) also provide valuable offers such as support groups, adapted holidays or home respite, which again vary by state and district. In summary, key support options for IC of persons with dementia are available in most states of Switzerland. However there is a substantial heterogeneity across regions in their density, diversity, and level of coordination.

Despite the rewarding aspects of caregiving, such as maintaining continuity and closeness with the affected person (e.g. [9]), informal caregiving often imposes high demands and costs, particularly for those involved in dementia care. Many ICD experience long periods of chronic stress and heavy burden, reduced quality of life and social isolation, as well as more physical and mental health challenges, compared to their non-caregiving counterparts and to caregivers of persons without dementia (e.g. [5, 10]). ICD burden and health deterioration are core predictors of early institutionalisation [11] and mistreatment [12] of their care recipient.

## Learning to cope better in a psycho-educative group programs for ICD

How can we best prevent ICD exhaustion and protect their quality of life? Focusing on coping strategies with a psycho-educative intervention holds the most promise for countering their chronic stress. A recent meta-analysis of 56 multifactorial studies confirmed that coping strategies and self-efficacy were core and highly stable predictors of burden [13]. Two other meta-analyses showed that psycho-educative interventions have the broadest effects, compared to other forms of ICD support which mostly affect specific domains [14, 15]. Coping with the daily stress of dementia caregiving is the main focus of the psycho-educative program "Learning to feel better... and help better" developed in Quebec, Canada. This group intervention of 15 weekly sessions of 2 h each (for more detail see the methods section) is the sole intervention in French which has already been tested in a randomized controlled trial conducted across six centers. Comparing the 60 participants who received this intervention to 56 control ICD referred to support groups, the program was found more effective in decreasing the frequency of behavior problems of the person with dementia and the associated distress in ICD, with respective effect sizes of $d = 0.09$ and $d = 0.38$ [16]. To the best of our knowledge, such psycho-educative interventions are still seldom available in Switzerland [7]. Based on the above evidence providing support for the dissemination of this program for French-speaking ICD, we aimed to evaluate whether this program could be implemented in a different cultural context, namely French-speaking Switzerland, and to test if the developers' results can be replicated in this new context. As little is yet known about the mechanisms of action of this program, documenting how participants use the strategies they learn in daily life can help gain some understanding of the change processes.

## Aims of the study

We aimed to examine within a one group pre- and post-test design 1) the feasibility of implementing the program in two regions of French-speaking Switzerland, 2) the effects of the program, and 3) the participants' use of the trained strategies in daily life. We favored a mixed-methods approach with a concurrent nested design. We firstly aimed to collect quantitative evidence about feasibility (e.g. dropout rates, acceptability of different components of the program), effects on the five core outcomes considered in the developers' study, and amount of strategy use in daily life. These five outcomes are the frequency of behavior problems of the person with dementia and the reactions of ICDs to these problems, as well as the ICDs' subjective burden, self-efficacy, and psychological distress. In parallel, we aimed to obtain more in-depth qualitative information about the acceptability and impact of the intervention from the point of view of ICDs.

## Methods

In reporting on this quasi-experimental intervention study we follow the TIDieR guidelines [17]. The data presented here were collected from October 2014 to December 2015.

### Sample

We recruited a convenience sample of 26 ICD through service providers in the field of dementia (Alzheimer Association, home care nurses, memory clinics, daycare centers) operating in two regions of the French-speaking part of Switzerland. Participants volunteered for a free psycho-educative intervention focusing on stress management, along with pre- and post-intervention interviews and short reports on a tablet provided twice a week. Inclusion criteria were 1) being the primary caregiver of a person living with a diagnosis of dementia (as reported by the ICD based on a physician evaluation), 2) caring for this person since at least 6 months. Exclusion criteria were 1) insufficient French-language skills, 2) low caregiver burden (score below 10 on the Zarit Burden Interview), and 3) no patient memory and behavioral problems. Participating ICD were mostly women (73%, $N = 19$), spouses of the patient (69%, $N = 18$; others were children: 27%, $N = 7$; and siblings: 4%, $N = 1$), with a median age of 68 years ($Q1 = 60$, $Q3 = 72$, range 37–86). Patients were mostly men (58%, $N = 15$) with a median age of 77 years ($Q1 = 71$, $Q3 = 82$, range 56–94). All had a diagnosis of dementia including 50% ($N = 13$) Alzheimer, 39% ($N = 10$) unspecified or mixed, 4% ($N = 1$) vascular, 4% ($N = 1$) Lewy body, and 4% ($N = 1$) fronto-temporal. ICD predominantly lived in the same household as patients (81%, $N = 21$), had been providing care for a median duration of 3 years ($Q1 = 2$, $Q3 = 5$, range 0.5–10 years), and were currently in charge of the patient for a median of 6 days a week ($Q1 = 4$, $Q3 = 7$, range 1.5–7 days).

### Procedure

The study was performed in accordance with the declaration of Helsinki and approved by the local ethics review board (Commission cantonale (VD) d'éthique de la recherche sur l'être humain, protocol n°175/14). Written informed consent was obtained from each ICD after oral and written information provided by a member of the research team. Figure 1 offers an overview of the study procedure.

Before the intervention, during an individual interview with a trained researcher, participants completed five questionnaires and received training for the daily life reports on the electronic diary. The diary training involved an introduction to the handling of the touchpad (Samsung Galaxy Tab4) on which all daily life questions were answered, and the completion of the first data point with an explanation of each question. Each participant then received a touchpad to take home and was instructed to answer the daily life questions twice a week. By way of an application specifically developed for this study with a focus on usability for elderly, questions were presented one at a time on the screen of the touchpad, written in large characters, along with a slider to give the answer (see Fig. 2).

During the interview, we also discussed whether participants needed a volunteer to care for their loved one with dementia during the intervention, which we could organize with the local Alzheimer Association, our partner in the project. Participants then took part in the intervention described below. After the end of the intervention, participants took part in a second individual interview with the same researcher to complete the five questionnaires again, and report on their experience with the intervention on quantitative and qualitative questions.

### Intervention

The intervention was originally developed by Louise Levesque, Francine Ducharme and their team in the years 2000s based on Lazarus and Folkman transactional theory of stress and coping [18]. The program called "learning to feel better… and help better" aimed at improving the ability of ICD to cope with the stressful demands of caring for a person with dementia living at home [19]. The content of the program focuses on 1) the appraisal of stressful situations, and 2) the coping strategies. Regarding appraisal, participants learn to break down a global situation into specific ones, identify more precisely what is stressful, and distinguish between situations or aspects of it which can be modified and those which cannot. Regarding coping strategies, participants are trained to choose an appropriate strategy depending on whether the situation can be modified or not, use problem solving for modifiable situations (7-step procedure), use reframing for unmodifiable situations (look at things from another angle to reduce painful emotions), and seek for social support (identify precise support needs and best persons to address each of them). In addition, information is provided on how dementia may affect the communication and relational behavior of the affected person, and how ICD may improve their communication skills and prevent tensions. The program uses a combination of 1) information provision, 2) group discussions, 3) work on personal stressful situations, and 4) exercises at home. The content and methods used in program are described in details in Lévesque and co-authors [19].

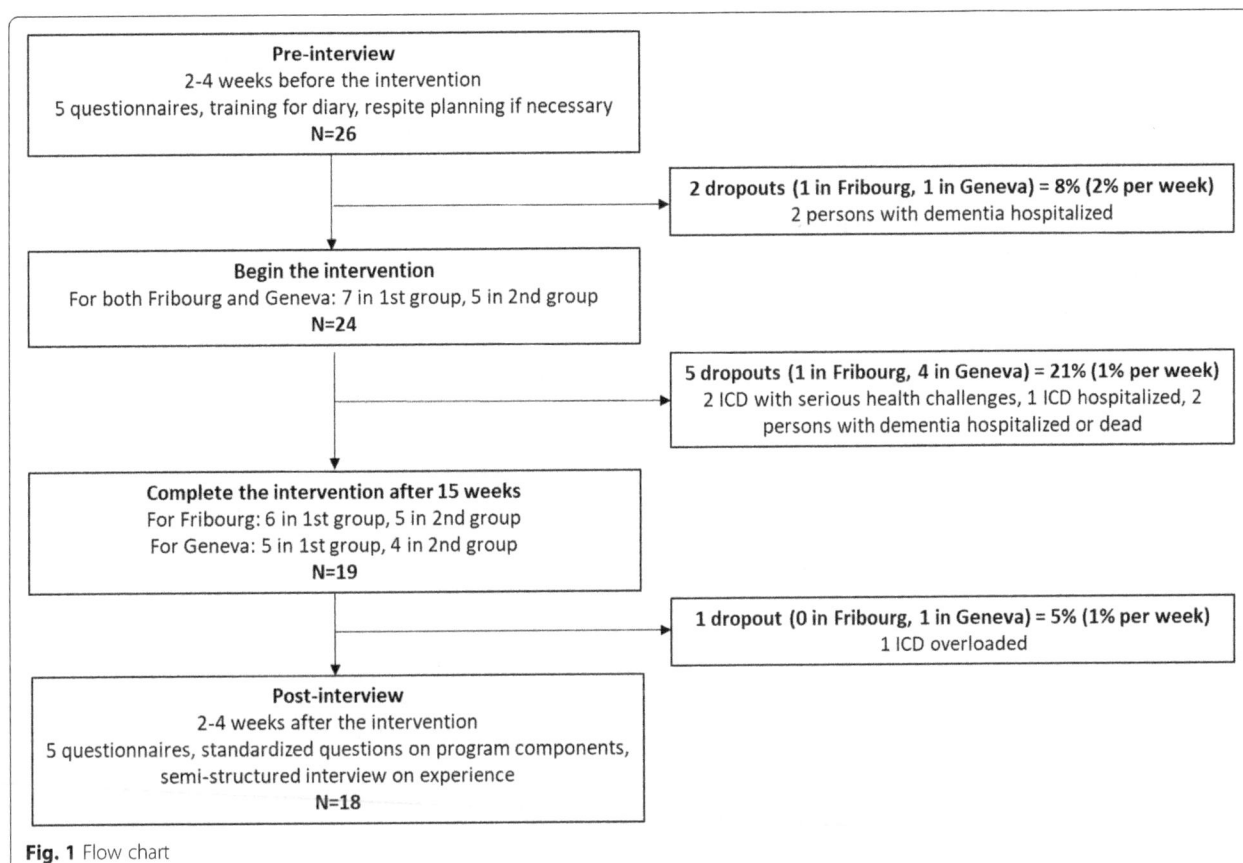

**Fig. 1** Flow chart

Participants receive a booklet containing key information and exercise sheets, and the course leaders provide the intervention according to a detailed manual. The intervention consisted in 15 weekly group sessions of 2 h each, held in a quiet room at the School of Health in Fribourg or at a local daycare center in Geneva. We conducted two consecutive groups in Fribourg, and in Geneva as well. In both sites, 7 participants started the first program session and 5 started the second one. Two nurses with expertise in dementia and work with informal caregivers led the 15 sessions of each intervention group, with 5 different nurses involved across the 4 groups of participants. All nurses had completed a 4-day training to the intervention program and participated in 2 to 3 one-day supervision sessions organized throughout the intervention. The supervision was conducted by a trained psychologist and psychotherapist with extensive experience in psycho-educative group interventions. All sessions were audio-recorded and the adherence to the course manual was assessed as good for 4 randomly selected sessions for each site, by two independent coders who were trained to the program but were not involved in the study.

## Measures

We collected 1) *questionnaire measures* for five outcomes, 2) *daily life reports* for strategy use, and 3)

*quantitative and qualitative post-intervention reports* on the experience in the program.

### Questionnaire measures

**Caregiver's burden** We measured burden with the Zarit Burden Interview [20], a well-validated and widely used 22-items questionnaire. Responses are provided on a scale from 0 (*never*) to 4 (*very often*). Scores above 18 indicating an important burden and scores above 32 a severe one [21].

**Memory and behavioral problems (MBP) and caregiver's MBP-related distress** We measured these two outcomes with the Revised MBP Checklist [22], a questionnaire which measures the frequency of 24 MBP in the preceding week between 0 (*never*) and 4 (*daily*), and the extent to which this problem disturbed or upset the ICD between 0 (*not at all*) and 4 (*extremely*). This questionnaire is in French and has satisfactory psychometric properties: the factor structure is confirmed, the internal consistency is good and the convergent validity is well established [22].

**Caregiver's psychological distress** We used the short version of the Ilfeld Psychiatric Symptoms Index [23], a

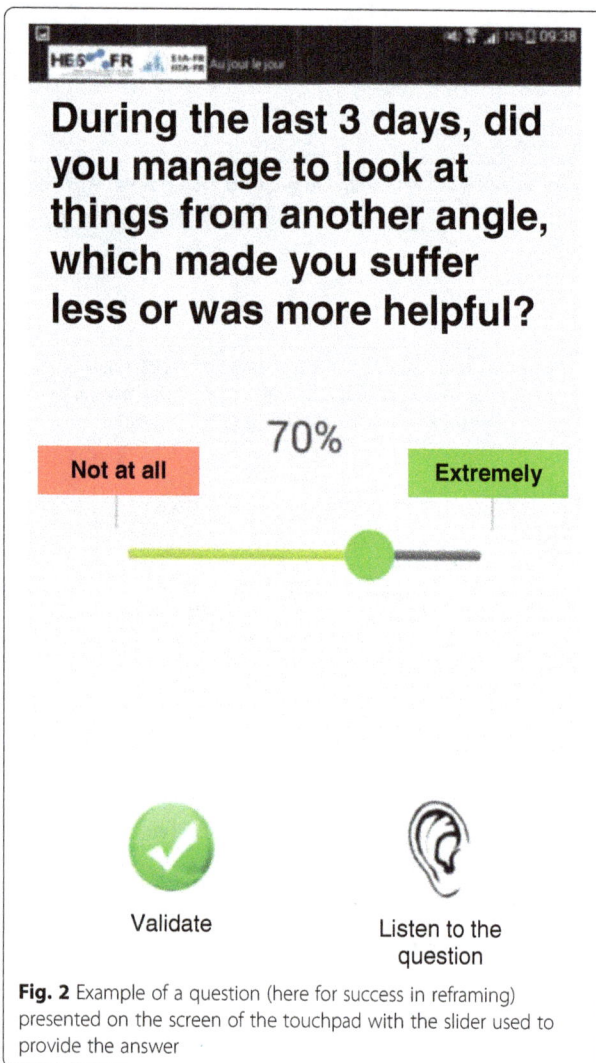

**Fig. 2** Example of a question (here for success in reframing) presented on the screen of the touchpad with the slider used to provide the answer

questionnaire asking participants to rate 14 symptoms related to depression, anxiety, anger and cognitive disturbance, on a 4-point scale from 1 (*never*) to 4 (*very often*). The psychometric properties are satisfactory for the English [23] and French [24] versions.

**Caregiver's self-efficacy** We measured self-efficacy as suggested by Bandura [25], with a visual analogue scale ranging from 0 (*no confidence at all in my ability to assume my caregiver role*) to 10 (*full confidence*).

*Daily life measures*
We collected daily life measures of participants' use of the three strategies taught in the program throughout the 15-week intervention. As is typical in daily life studies, we used a limited number of questions to measure each construct, to prevent overloading the participants and to maintain compliance over time. The following questions were developed specifically for this study, focusing on the

last 3 days, with answers provided on a visual analogue scale yielding a score between 0 (*not at all*) and 100 (*extremely*):

1) *Overall strategy use.* How much did you use the strategies you learned in the program?
2) *Problem solving.* Did you try to solve a problem for which you had no satisfactory solution? Did you manage to solve your problems satisfactorily?
3) *Reframing.* Did you notice some thoughts which made you suffer unnecessarily or exaggeratedly, or which did not help you? Did you try to question these thoughts? Did you manage to look at things from a different angle which made you suffer less or was more helpful?
4) *Support seeking.* Did you feel the need to receive support? Did you receive the support you needed? (An additional question was "Did you ask for the support you needed?", but this piece of data was unusable due to a problem with the answer scale of the question).

*Post-intervention reports on the experience in the program*

**Quantitative** We assessed the perceived usefulness of the 4 strategies taught in the program (communication, modifying unhelpful thoughts, problem solving and support seeking) and the 4 methods used (information provided by the course leaders, working on personal situations, group exchanges, and exercises at home) with 3 items for each: 1) I found it interesting, 2) I found it useful, and 3) It helped me in my daily life. The answers were given on a 5-point scale: 0 *Not at all or very little*, 1 *A little*, 2 *Moderately*, 3 *Very*, 4 *Extremely*. As they were highly correlated (in most cases Spearman's $\rho > .50$) we averaged them. Regarding the 4 strategies, we also asked the two following questions: 1) I found it difficult to understand, 2) I found it difficult to apply, with answers given on the same 5-point scale.

**Qualitative** Qualitative data was collected using semi-structured interviews. The interview guideline focused on the benefits of the program, negative aspects and the extent to which the program met the participants' expectations. Participants were interviews in their homes 2 weeks after the end of the program. The interviews were audio recorded, transcribed word by word and anonymized.

**Data analysis**
*Quantitative*
We used descriptive statistics to provide general information on the study outcomes (means and standard deviations, SD, to allow comparability with the original study, as well as median, Q1, Q3 as the variables showed

some deviations from normality) and to analyze the quantitative post-intervention reports (median, Q1, Q3 and boxplots). The effects of the intervention on the five outcomes were tested with a repeated measures MANOVA, with time (pre versus post) and measure (the 5 questionnaires) as independent variables, and the score as the dependent variable. The effect of the intervention for each outcome was then tested with post hoc paired t-tests (one-tailed), and we computed effect sizes (Cohen's d). Regarding strategy use in daily life, we assessed the mean level at the beginning of the intervention and the linear change over the course of the intervention with multilevel regression with full maximum likelihood estimation (using Hierarchical Linear Modeling, HLM 6; [26]), as the measurement occasions (within-person, Level 1, L1) were nested within the participants (Level 2, L2). Eq. 1 shows our model, where the use of each strategy is predicted by time in days (uncentered, i.e. coded 0 for the first day of the intervention) on L1. In this model $\beta_{00}$ (i.e. the average intercept) indicates the average level of strategy use at the beginning of the intervention. $\beta_{10}$ (i.e. the average slope) is used to test our hypotheses that strategy use increased over time, which is indicated by a positive slope ($p$s are thus one-tailed).

$$\begin{aligned} \text{Level 1}: \text{Strategy use} &= \gamma_0 + \gamma_1 \text{Time} + \text{E} \\ \text{Level 2}: \gamma_0 &= \beta_{00} + R_0 \\ \gamma_1 &= \beta_{10} + R_1 \end{aligned} \qquad (1)$$

## Qualitative
The qualitative data was analysed using the approach from Mayring (2010) for summarizing content analyses with inductive category assignment. This approach is described as very fruitful to allow a true description and understanding of the original material "without bias owing to the preconceptions of the researcher" Mayring, 2014). After the definition of the material a first phase of paraphrasing and generalization of the data was performed. To develop a summarizing coding system, the material was further reduced and abstracted (first and second reduction according to Mayring, 2010). Finally, the summarizing coding system was re-checked with the original material to ensure that the category system matched it well. Findings and discrepancies in the interpretation of the data were regularly discussed in the research group. The analytical software Atlas.ti 7 assisted the analysis process.

## Results
### Feasibility
#### Recruitment process
This study was initiated in partnership with two core service providers in the field of dementia, the largest home care organization in the region of Geneva, and the local Alzheimer Association in the region of Fribourg. The Alzheimer Association also provided volunteers for the supervision of the person with dementia while the ICD attended the program in both regions. Initial efforts of the field partners to recruit through articles in the newsletter of the Alzheimer Association in Fribourg, and through the home care staff (using a flyer) in Geneva, brought only few participants. We then opted for a broader strategy by involving additional service providers (memory clinics, daycare centers, home care services in Fribourg as well) and organizing presentations of the program by the course leaders for each service provider. Regular articles were further published in the newsletters of the Alzheimer Association in Fribourg and the public hospital in Geneva. The main challenges in the recruitment process were: 1) Transporting the specificity of the program to the (often little trained) staff or volunteers involved in the recruitment, who repeatedly saw it as a mere support group; 2) Informing and screening the ICDs contacting us after reading an article or receiving a flyer, which often did not meet our rather stringent inclusion criteria or perceived the requirements of the program as too high in terms of duration, travel, or learning of skills; 3) Providing ICDs with information about the program at the right moment (when they were settled in their role but not yet exhausted), given by a trustworthy person or different independent sources (the memory clinic plus an article plus the home care nurse).

### Dropout rates
Out of the 26 recruited participants, two dropped-out just before starting the program (both due to an unexpected physical illness of the person with dementia requiring hospitalization). Out of the 24 participants who started the program, 19 (79%) completed it. The five participants who dropped out did so within the first 6 sessions, due to hospitalization (after a serious fall, $N = 1$) or death ($N = 1$) of the person with dementia, or the hospitalization (after a serious fall, $N = 1$) or serious illness ($N = 2$) of the ICD. In addition, one participant was unable to complete the follow-up questionnaires due to overload at the time of data collection, so that 18 persons could be included in the final analyses.

### Participation to the program sessions
The average participation rate in the program has been very high (92%). Nearly all participants (94%) took part in more than 12 sessions, to the exception of one ICD who missed 5 sessions due to professional obligations. The few other missed sessions were due to ICD sickness, the death of a relative, or an unavoidable appointment.

## Pre-test questionnaire results: Descriptives

The questionnaires filled in at pre-test ($N = 26$) showed that the ICD burden was overall severe ($M = 39.56$, $SD = 14.21$, median $= 41.25$, $Q1 = 31.00$, $Q3 = 49.25$), with a moderate frequency of patients' MBP ($M = 1.58$, $SD = 0.52$, median $= 1.62$, $Q1 = 1.17$, $Q3 = 1.88$) and caregivers' MBP-related distress ($M = 1.86$, $SD = 0.66$, median $= 1.85$, $Q1 = 1.35$, $Q3 = 2.43$). The ICD reported moderate psychological distress ($M = 26.58$, $SD = 6.88$, median $= 26.50$, $Q1 = 21.50$, $Q3 = 29.00$), and a rather high self-efficacy ($M = 6.90$, $SD = 1.84$, median $= 7.50$, $Q1 = 5.38$, $Q3 = 8.50$). As presented in Table 1, in comparison with the 8 persons who dropped out just before starting or during the program, the 18 completers had more pronounced difficulties on our five outcomes.

## Effects of the program: Changes in questionnaire scores

Comparing pre- and post-intervention scores (see Table 1) with a repeated measures MANOVA, we observed significant effects for time ($F_{(1,17)} = 444.42$, $p < .001$) and the time x measure interaction ($F_{(4,14)} = 152.47$, $p < .001$), indicating the intervention affected our outcomes though not all of them in the same way. Paired t-tests conducted post-hoc confirmed that burden and psychological distress decreased significantly, and self-efficacy increased significantly, with large effect sizes (see Table 1). There was no significant change in the frequency of patients' MBP and caregivers' MBP-related distress. We obtained highly similar results using non-parametric tests.

## Strategy use in daily life

At the beginning of the intervention, overall strategy use was moderate ($\beta_{00} = 41.78$ on a 0 to 100 scale). As hypothesized, overall strategy use increased substantially over time ($\beta_{01} = 0.55$, $p < .001$). Regarding problem solving, at program start, efforts to solve new problems were rather low ($\beta_{00} = 31.35$) however success in solving problems was rather high ($\beta_{00} = 59.48$). We found no significant change over time in efforts ($\beta_{01} = -0.01$, $p = .404$) and a marginal increase in success ($\beta_{01} = 0.10$, $p = .097$). Regarding reframing, at the beginning of the intervention, the identification of unhelpful thoughts was rather low

($\beta_{00} = 34.17$), reframing efforts were moderate ($\beta_{00} = 49.74$), and success in reframing was rather high ($\beta_{00} = 57.26$). In line with expectations, we observed significant increases over time for the identification of unhelpful thoughts ($\beta_{01} = 0.08$, $p = .035$), efforts to reframe ($\beta_{01} = 0.20$, $p = .006$), and success at reframing ($\beta_{01} = 0.25$, $p = .005$). Regarding support seeking, at the beginning of the intervention, the need for support ($\beta_{00} = 44.62$), and success in obtaining it ($\beta_{00} = 43.25$) were moderate. Need for support increased marginally ($\beta_{01} = 0.13$, $p = .062$) while we found no significant change in obtaining support ($\beta_{01} = -0.02$, $p = .394$). In summary, we observed most progresses in the use of reframing, along with a modest improvement in problem solving and a slightly increasing need for social support, but no systematic change in the support received.

## Satisfaction with the diverse methods and contents of the program

As presented in Fig. 3, the median value for the four methods used (information provided by the course leaders, working on personal situations, group exchanges, and exercises at home) was close to 3, corresponding to the answer "very relevant / useful / helpful in daily life". The same was observed for the four types of strategies (communication, modifying unhelpful thoughts, problem solving and support seeking).

Figure 4 presents the results for the two questions exploring whether the participants perceived the four contents as difficult to understand or to apply. For the understanding all medians were at 0 ("Not at all"), and for the application all were between 1 ("A little") and 2 ("Moderately"), the most challenging strategy being the modification of unhelpful thoughts.

## Benefits from and challenges in the program: Qualitative results

The content analysis revealed three main categories: 1) *Sharing experiences and strategies*, which is about participants learning from each other, comparing their situations with others and getting strengthened in their way of handling the situation; 2) *Being in the same boat*, namely feeling

**Table 1** Mean and (SD) for the study variables at pre-test and post-test

| | Pre-test dropouts ($N = 8$) | Pre-test completers ($N = 18$) | Post-test ($N = 18$) | t-test pre-post (df = 17) | Effect size |
|---|---|---|---|---|---|
| Burden (0–88) | 31.63 (17.6) | 43.08 (11.3) | 38.61 (10.7) | 2.13* | 0.41 |
| MBP (0–4) | 1.36 (0.6) | 1.68 (0.5) | 1.67 (0.6) | 0.10 | 0.03 |
| MBP-related distress (0–4) | 1.58 (0.7) | 1.98 (0.6) | 1.98 (0.6) | −0.06 | 0.01 |
| Psychological distress (14–56) | 23.50 (8.3) | 27.94 (5.9) | 25.19 (4.4) | 1.94* | 0.54 |
| Self-efficacy (0–10) | 7.69 (1.6) | 6.56 (1.9) | 7.36 (1.9) | −2.33* | 0.43 |

*Note.* For all the variables listed, higher scores indicate higher levels; *MBP* memory and behavioral problems; * $p < .05$, ** $p < .01$, *** $p < .001$ (one-tailed); for burden, scores above 18 indicate an important burden and scores above 32 a severe one

Coping with dementia caregiving: a mixed-methods study on feasibility and benefits...

75

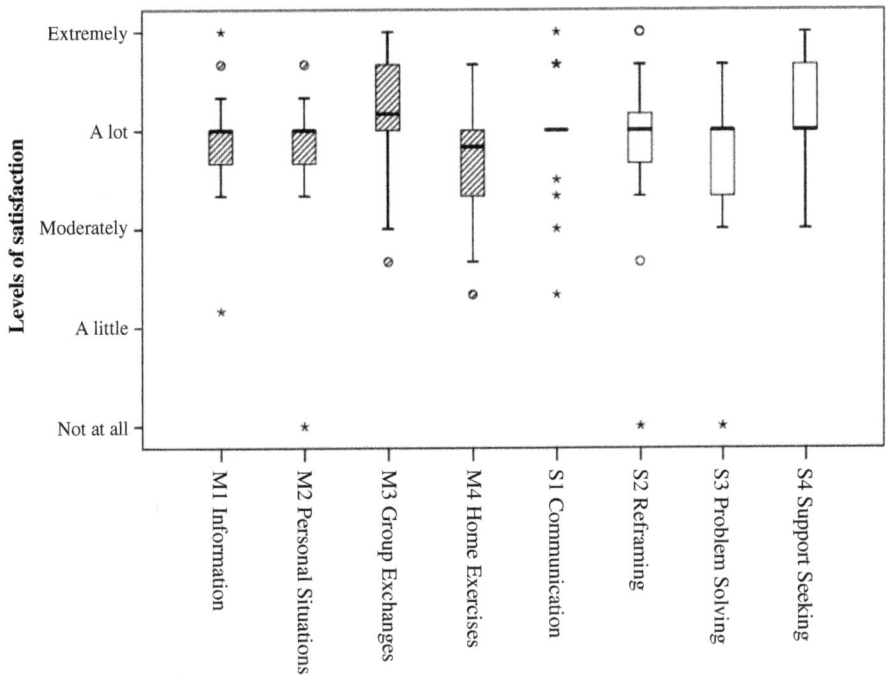

**Fig. 3** Satisfaction with methods (M) and strategies (S)

less alone and feeling understood and connected to the other ICD as they are in similar situations; 3) *Being able to cope*, as the program empowered the participants to develop strategies which helped them managing their challenging situations.

### Sharing experiences and strategies

The participants reported that they learned to talk about their situations and their experiences. For some it was the first time they had the confidence to talk about their difficult situation at home.

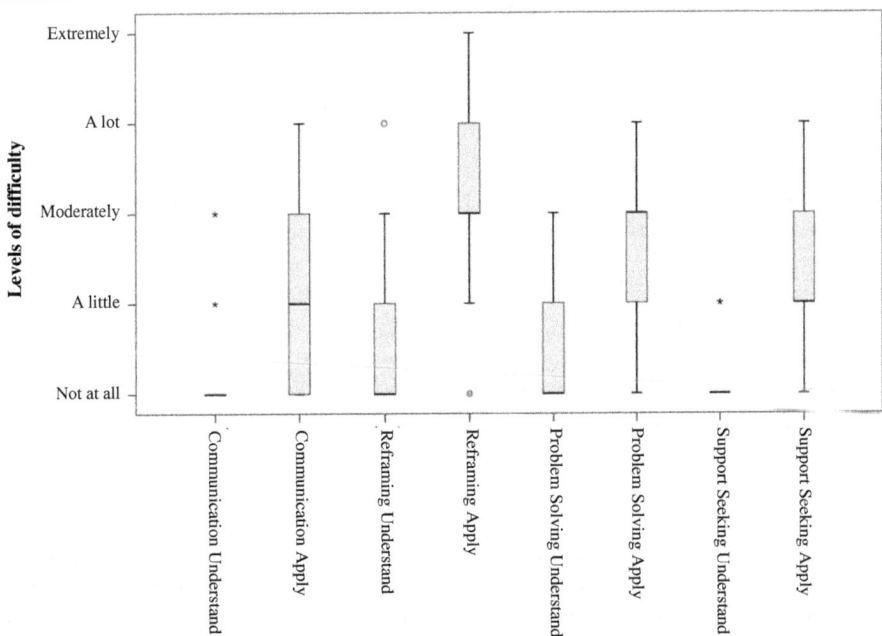

**Fig. 4** Perceived difficulty in understanding or applying the strategies

*«Being able to share and truly being listened to. For me the positive point was finding the confidence to express myself, to say what is going on with my husband. I now speak more often about it, yes, I can express myself more openly.»*

Sharing their experiences allowed them to reflect on their situation, compare it to the situations of others, and learn from each other, especially about helpful strategies.

*«It was a place, where I had room and time to reflect on everyday problems, to which I had no solution. It gave me the opportunity to learn strategies to solve these problems.»*

By comparing their situation with the experiences of other participants they also got encouraged in the way they handle some situations, they learned to appreciate their situation, for example when it was less challenging than those of others, and they got inspired by participants with particular helpful strategies.

*«So it made me finally take account of my situation, yes, it is not easy, there is no-one who wants this life, but I say to myself there are others who really are in much more complicated situations.»*

A participant, who was new to the caregiving role, felt enabled to anticipate and to set limits after listening to the experiences of exhaustion and heavy burden of other participants.

*«All the people who were there, some [people] had more painful and hard circumstances, so I said to myself, this is it, what I can expect for myself [...]. It was very real. A bit too concrete, but this also allowed me to see the limits. How far I can go.»*

Listening to the experiences of others was not always described as an opportunity to learn. Some participants reported getting upset while listening to the burdening stories of others, or finding it painful to imagine they could be facing similar situations in the future.

*«Yes, I had a moment, two or three moments, where it was very hard for me during this course. It was perhaps when there were people who shared too much violent detail, which I wasn't prepared for. That distressed me a bit. And then reality hits you.»*

### Being in the same boat

Being in a group with other ICDs made the participants feel less alone. They realized that others shared the same problems or had similar difficult situations.

*«It brought me a fantastic well-being. Because you feel a bit lonely in the world, when you are like this, but then I saw, there are lots of people with the same problems as me.»*

The participants enjoyed feeling deeply understood by other caregivers with similar experiences or by group leaders with extensive knowledge in this field.

*«We need to talk about our experiences, and to talk to others who know and others who also share the same [experiences], even though they have no solutions, they share. Emotionally they can understand the burden of it, they can understand the degree of isolation that we can feel in this [situation].»*

Participants valued being in a small group, allowing a focus on the specific needs of each participant and discussions on practical issues related their specific situations.

*«It is clear, we were a small group, this also allowed us to develop the things we needed in parallel to the program. Suddenly we were a bit more than a program. It made the work valuable. We could really talk about practical cases [...]. »*

The participants reported that they felt connected to the other participants and described feelings of friendship, empathy and solidarity. They appreciated and underlined the importance of their experience and that of others never being judged. Such a benevolent environment enabled the participants to build supportive relationships, which they expect to persist after the end of the program.

*«Me, I made friendships in the group. [...] It is true, we will stay in contact. So we were not going to go our separate ways, on the contrary we exchanged our telephone numbers and all that and said we are going to meet regularly.»*

### Being able to cope

This category shows the strongest connections to the content of the program and to the aim of empowering the participants. Many of them reported that the program helped them changing their way of thinking by recognizing and modifying unhelpful thoughts.

*«The program gave me a good structure to think about how to approach difficult situations at home and also other things. It gave me a good structure to guide my thoughts, just the basic structure for difficult situations, emotions (...), and me, I had enough structure to hook onto and that immediately meant something to me.»*

Working on unhelpful thoughts also enabled them to see their situation in a less dramatic light and to manage negative emotions.

*« I learned to manage my behavior. I was, before I came, more impatient, I was more aggressive. I am less [aggressive], a lot less. Well, it can still happen at times when I am very tired [...], but I am a lot less aggressive with him now, because before I blew up at every moment. Well anyway, now I have learned [to manage my behavior], this is positive. »*

The importance of taking some distance and taking better care of themselves were mentioned as helpful insights gained during the program.

*«[...] and also to be able to change the things a bit for me. To think a bit more about myself. Doing activities, going to the cinema with my friends a bit more often, to the theatre, and taking some time for myself, that is very important.»*

A deeper understanding of the disease and its symptoms empowered the participants to have more patience, to adapt their communication and to cope better with difficult behaviors of the person with dementia.

*«To say, ok: what do I do? I know he is ill, I know that he doesn't have the capacity anymore, so it is not about me. I have to understand that. It [the program] brought greater understanding about the attitude of my husband [and] his behavior.»*

Information about, and contact details for diverse support organizations were experienced as helpful and facilitating access to support.

*«Then you recognize some openings for getting help. We know where to call, and who to turn to when something happens. This has been very positive.»*

## Discussion

This study aimed at 1) assessing whether the program "Learning to feel better... and help better" could be implemented in French-speaking Switzerland, 2) testing if the effects documented by the developers could be replicated in this new context, and 3) exploring the participants' use of the trained strategies in daily life. Globally, feasibility was very good except for recruitment, and effects were positive and substantial, thus encouraging further dissemination of the program. The group format was a strong asset according to participants, and the use of reframing progressed the most over the course of the intervention.

Regarding feasibility, our qualitative and quantitative results converged towards a very good acceptance of the program and a strong implication of the participants. Recruitment was however challenging. The main barrier was the duration of the program, which discouraged many ICD from participating, as it was too demanding for them, particularly for older persons and those working full-time. Although underuse of diverse support options is very common among ICD and not specific to this program [27], we plan to further explore our recruitment challenges using interviews of the health care professionals and volunteers involved in this process. This information will help use revise the program and/or the recruitment strategy accordingly. Although the dropout rate was moderate, it also raises some issues. Dropouts notably occurred throughout the study and were in nearly all cases related to critical events affecting the ICD or the person with dementia. They therefore seem to be related to the vulnerability of older persons with dementia combined to the heightened risk of health challenges among ICD e.g. [5, 10], rather than to a lack of satisfaction with the program. In this line, reducing the duration of the program could decrease the dropout rate. However, compared to completers, the ICD who dropped out scored more positive at baseline on average (e.g. lower burden, less distress, more self-efficacy). Although these differences were not significant – which is not surprising given our small sample size – they could point to a selection bias towards an under-representation of less burdened individuals in our results. Replication in a larger sample should tell whether less burdened ICD are more likely to drop out from this program or whether this observation was a mere artifact, as is common in small samples.

Regarding effects, the program resulted in substantial improvements in burden, psychological distress and self-efficacy. As in the developers' study [16] conducted in a highly similar sample, the intervention increased ICD quality of life. However the original randomized control trial had smaller effect sizes and found significant effects on different outcomes, namely the frequency of problem behavior of the person with dementia and the associated distress in the ICD. This discrepancy may be related to differences in study design, as a control group takes into account the effects of disease progression, which was not possible in our case. The high self-efficacy observed at the beginning of the program was very similar to the scores in the original validation study of the program (on a 0 to 100 scale, for the control and intervention group respectively, mean = 69.8 and 77.7, SD = 19.4 and 16.7; [16]). These observations indicate that participants in both studies had substantial resources, which is in line with feedbacks from the field professionals supporting us in the recruitment process, who noted that this program requires a significant involvement. Such a program may therefore not cater the primary needs of the most vulnerable ICD, such as those who are exhausted and may benefit in the first line from respite. Additional research is required to clarify the best timing for this intervention and its efficacy according to ICD characteristics. Our modest sample size and the diagnosis of dementia based on ICD report further limit the reliability of our results, which need confirmation within a large-scale randomized control trial including an external assessment of the diagnosis.

The qualitative results emphasized the benefits of a program offered in a group format, in line with results of a meta-analysis showing that psycho-educative interventions in a group format significantly reduced depression in ICD while individual ones did not [28]. Our participants reported reductions in loneliness and social isolation as they felt understood by their peers and could build new strong social bonds, in line with typical positive effects of support groups [15]. Yet, informal contacts with some participants after the end of the program suggested that embedding such a support-group component within a psycho-educational approach made a qualitative difference: Among those who joined the typical local support groups afterwards, many were disappointed about the stronger focus on expressing (negative) emotions than on solving problems, which they experienced as depressing. Further research assessing interventions' efficacy in the area of ICD support should provide more information on the characteristics of the intervention to help disentangle the impact of diverse components.

Openly sharing experiences also facilitated social comparison and anticipation, having both negative and positive aspects. On the positive side, social comparison encouraged participants in their way of handling some situations and invited them to try new options by providing positive examples of management. Hearing others' experiences also helped them get prepared for new challenges in their caregiving. On the negative side, participants were confronted with the painful experiences of others and detailed descriptions of the disease-related decline, which generated strong negative feelings in some of them, for a limited time. These feedbacks highlight some other processes at play beyond the training of coping strategies, many of them related to the complex mourning associated with dementia caregiving [29].

Moreover, the present research used an innovative data collection method to document strategy use. Collecting such information in daily life regularly throughout the intervention proved feasible despite the chronic stress experienced by ICD. These data confirmed that participants were using more and more over time the strategies they learned, and showed that reframing progressed the most. This last finding is in line with the results of a meta-analysis of 11 interventions for ICD comprising this strategy, which documented improvements in anxiety, depression and subjective stress - although no systematic effect was found for coping, subjective burden, reactions to the behaviors of the person with dementia, or institutionalization [30]. Notably, our participants rated reframing as the most challenging strategy to apply, but their qualitative feedbacks underlined how positively this skill affected their caregiving experience by restoring some control over their negative emotions, particularly when facing challenging behaviors of their loved one with dementia. Taken together, these results suggests that learning to reframe one's thoughts is both important and difficult to achieve, and therefore requires specific attention from intervention developers and implementers.

Our less clear results regarding the use of problem solving and support seeking could be due to our questions being too general, as suggested by the high rates of mastery observed already at intervention start. These questions may have failed to capture what our participants did express in their qualitative feedbacks, about having found innovative solutions to their problems, and knowing better where and how to obtain the support they need. Our findings may also be limited by the lack of follow-up data, as some strategies take time to bear fruits, particularly in the area of support seeking. For example, organizing a day-care center for the person with dementia often spans over weeks between the first contact with the institution and the establishment of an adequate routine for all the persons involved. In the same line, managing the difficult behaviors of persons with dementia remains one of the most challenging caregiving task [31]. Therefore, ICDs may require more time to identify the triggers, as well as to develop and test new strategies, so that effects in this area may be better observed at follow-up.

## Conclusion

This study expands on the original one conducted by the developers of the program "Learning to feel better... and help better" in French-speaking Canada, by showing the feasibility and the very promising effects of this program in two regions of French-speaking Switzerland. The original efforts of our study to document the process of the intervention by measuring strategy use in daily life also pave the way for further research aiming to clarify the (most) active components in supporting ICDs. Our next challenge will be to shorten this program and to improve our recruitment procedure in

Coping with dementia caregiving: a mixed-methods study on feasibility and benefits...

79

order to make this helpful program accessible to more informal caregivers of persons with dementia.

## Abbreviations
IC: Informal caregivers; ICD: Informal caregivers of the person with dementia; MBP: Memory and behavioral problems; SD: Standard deviation; TIDieR: Template for Intervention Description and Replication

## Acknowledgements
The authors warmly thank the caregivers who took part in this study and devoted us some of their precious time and energy. This research would not have been possible without the support of the Memory Clinic Fribourg, the homecare nurses in Fribourg and Geneva (imad), the daycare centers in Fribourg, who strongly supported the recruitment. We are also thankful to Christina Moses Passini for her help in the data collection, and to Aurélie Klingshirn, Evelyne Progin, Brigitte Demaurex, Marie-José Walter, and Jorge Azevedo for leading the courses, as well as the Swiss Alzheimer Association – sections Fribourg and Geneva for providing volunteers who cared for the person with dementia during the courses. We are also grateful to Francesco Carrino, Marc Demierre and the HumanTech Institute of the School of engineering and architecture Fribourg for programming the application used to collect the daily life data, and to Alexandre Bischoff, Katia Iglesias, Yoann Uehlinger, Paul Vaucher, and Marika Bana for their valuable comments on earlier drafts.

## Funding
This research is funded by the Leenaards Foundation, Switzerland. The funding body was not involved with the design of the study; or collection, analysis and interpretation of the data; or writing of the manuscript.

## Authors' contributions
SPI designed the study and managed the quantitative and qualitative data collection process as well as the quantitative analysis. SKI performed the qualitative analysis. Both authors contributed substantially to the writing of the manuscript and have read and approved the final version.

## Competing interests
The authors declare that they have no competing interests.

## References
1. Global Observatory for Ageing and Dementia World Alzheimer Report 2015: The Global Impact of Dementia An Analysis of Prevalence, Incidence, Cost and Trends: Alzheimer's Disease International; 2015.
2. OFSP. Stratégie nationale en matière de démence 2014 – 2019. résultats acquis 2014–2016 et priorités 2017–2019. Bern, Switzerland, Office Fédéral de la Santé Publique. p. 2016.
3. Association Alzheimer Suisse. Personnes atteintes de démence en Suisse : chiffres et prévisions [persons with dementia in Switzerland: figures and forecast]: Yverdon-les-Bains, Suisse: association Alzheimer Suisse; 2018.
4. EUROFAMCARE. Services for supporting family carers of older dependent people in Europe: Characteristics, coverage and usage. 2006. Available from: https://www.uke.de/extern/eurofamcare/deli.php#deli9.
5. Perrig-Chiello P, Höpflinger F, Schnegg B. SwissAgeCare: Pflegende Angehörige von älteren Menschen in der Schweiz. 2010. Available from: https://www.spitex.ch/files/CEAAGB6/SwissAgeCare-2010%2D%2D-Schlussbericht.
6. Rudin M, Strub S. Prestations de soins et d'assistance dispensées par les proches : temps investi et évaluation monétaire. 2014. Available from: https://www.spitex.ch/files/ILJD5AG/2014_buero_bass_monetaerebewertung_pflegendeangehoerige_14juli_f_def.pdf.
7. Confédération Suisse. Soutien aux proches aidants: Analyse de la situation et mesures requises pour la Suisse. [Supporting informal caregivers: Situation analysis and required measures for Switzerland] 2014. Available

from: https://www.bag.admin.ch/bag/fr/home/themen/strategien-politik/nationale-gesundheitspolitik/aktionsplan-pflegende-angehoerige.html.
8. Marti S. État des lieux de la prise en charge des personnes atteintes de démence dans les cantons — 2017 [Overview of dementia care in the Swiss states - 2017]. Bern, Switzerland: Conférence suisse des directrices et directeurs cantonaux de la santé; 2017.
9. Motenko AK. The frustrations, gratifications, and well-being of dementia caregivers. The Gerontologist. 1989;29:166–72. http://www.ncbi.nlm.nih.gov/pubmed/2753378
10. Brodaty H, Donkin M. Family caregivers of people with dementia. Dialogues Clin Neurosci. 2009;11:217–28. http://www.ncbi.nlm.nih.gov/pubmed/19585957
11. Gaugler JE, Kane RL, Kane RA, Clay T, Newcomer R. Caregiving and institutionalization of cognitively impaired older people: utilizing dynamic predictors of change. Gerontologist. 2003;43:219–29. http://www.ncbi.nlm.nih.gov/pubmed/12677079
12. Wiglesworth A, Mosqueda L, Mulnard R, Liao S, Gibbs L, Fitzgerald W. Screening for abuse and neglect of people with dementia. J Am Geriatr Soc. 2010;58:493–500. https://doi.org/10.1111/j.1532-5415.2010.02737.x.
13. van der Lee J, Bakker TJ, Duivenvoorden HJ, Droes RM. Multivariate models of subjective caregiver burden in dementia: a systematic review. Ageing Res Rev. 2014;15:76–93. https://doi.org/10.1016/j.arr.2014.03.003.
14. Huis In Het Veld JG, Verkaik R, Mistiaen P, van Meijel B, Francke AL. The effectiveness of interventions in supporting self-management of informal caregivers of people with dementia; a systematic meta review. BMC Geriatr. 2015;15:147. https://doi.org/10.1186/s12877-015-0145-6.
15. Pinquart M, Sorensen S. Helping caregivers of persons with dementia: which interventions work and how large are their effects? International psychogeriatrics / IPA. 2006;18:577–95. https://doi.org/10.1017/S1041610206003462.
16. Hebert R, Levesque L, Vezina J, Lavoie JP, Ducharme F, Gendron C, et al. Efficacy of a psychoeducative group program for caregivers of demented persons living at home: a randomized controlled trial. J Gerontol B Psychol Sci Soc Sci. 2003;58:S58–67. http://www.ncbi.nlm.nih.gov/pubmed/12496309
17. Hoffmann TC, Glasziou PP, Boutron I, Milne R, Perera R, Moher D, et al. Better reporting of interventions: template for intervention description and replication (TIDieR) checklist and guide. BMJ. 2014;348:g1687. https://doi.org/10.1136/bmj.g1687.
18. Lazarus RS, Folkman S. Stress, appraisal, and coping. New York: Springer; 1984. XIII. p. 445.
19. Levesque L, Gendron C, Vezina J, Hebert R, Ducharme F, Lavoie JP, et al. The process of a group intervention for caregivers of demented persons living at home: conceptual framework, components, and characteristics. Aging Ment Health. 2002;6:239–47. https://doi.org/10.1080/13607860220142468.
20. Zarit SH, Orr NK, Zarit JM. The hidden victims of Alzheimer's disease: families under stress. New York: New York University Press; 1985.
21. Hebert R, Bravo G, Preville M. Reliability, validity and reference values of the Zarit burden interview for assessing informal caregivers of community-dwelling older persons with dementia. Canadian Journal on Aging. 2000;19: 494–507. https://doi.org/10.1017/S0714980800012484.
22. Teri L, Truax P, Logsdon R, Uomoto J, Zarit S, Vitaliano PP. Assessment of behavioral problems in dementia: the revised memory and behavior problems checklist. Psychol Aging. 1992;7:622–31. http://www.ncbi.nlm.nih.gov/pubmed/1466831
23. Ilfeld FW. Further validation of a psychiatric symptom index in a normal population. Psychological Reports. 1976;39:1215–28. <Go to ISI>://A1976CU50400039
24. Préville M, Boyer R, Potvin L, Perrault C, Légaré G. Psychological distress: determination of the reliability and validity of the measure used in the Québec health survey. Québec, Canada: Government of Québec, Department of Health and Social Services; 1992.
25. Bandura A. Self-efficacy: toward a unifying theory of behavioral change. Psychol Rev. 1977;84:191 215. http://www.ncbi.nlm.nih.gov/pubmed/847061
26. Bryk AS, Raudenbush SW, Congdon RT. HLM: hierarchical linear modelling with the HLM/2L and HLM/3L programs. Chicago: Scientific Software International; 1994.
27. Brodaty H, Thomson C, Thompson C, Fine M. Why caregivers of people with dementia and memory loss don't use services. Int J Geriatr Psychiatry. 2005; 20:537–46. https://doi.org/10.1002/gps.1322.
28. Thompson CA, Spilsbury K, Hall J, Birks Y, Barnes C, Adamson J. Systematic review of information and support interventions for caregivers of people with dementia. BMC Geriatr. 2007;7:18. https://doi.org/10.1186/1471-2318-7-18.

29. Chan D, Livingston G, Jones L, Sampson EL. Grief reactions in dementia carers: a systematic review. Int J Geriatr Psychiatry. 2013;28:1–17. https://doi.org/10.1002/gps.3795.

30. Vernooij M, Downs M, McCleery J, Draskovic I. Cognitive Reframing for Carers of People with Dementia. Gerontologist. 2011;51:553–4. <Go to ISI>://WOS:000303602003516

31. Black W, Almeida OP. A systematic review of the association between the behavioral and psychological symptoms of dementia and burden of care. Int Psychogeriatr. 2004;16:295–315. http://www.ncbi.nlm.nih.gov/pubmed/15559754

# 9

# Long-term evaluation of the implementation of a large fall and fracture prevention program in long-term care facilities

Patrick Roigk[1]*⏺, Clemens Becker[1], Claudia Schulz[2], Hans-Helmut König[2] and Kilian Rapp[1]

## Abstract

**Background:** Falls and fractures are extremely frequent in long-term care facilities (LTCFs). Therefore, a fall and fracture prevention program was started in nearly 1000 LTCFs in Bavaria/Germany between 2007 and 2010. The components of the program were exercise classes, the documentation of falls, environmental adaptations, medication reviews, the recommendation to use hip protectors and education of staff. The present study aimed to provide a comprehensive evaluation of the implementation process of the program regarding results of the implementation phase and the follow-up of 3–9 years after start of implementation.

**Methods:** Data from numerous sources were used, including data from published studies, statistical data, health insurance claims data and unpublished data from an online questionnaire. To incorporate different aspects, time periods and results, the RE-AIM framework was applied.

**Results:** The program was adopted by 942 of the 1150 eligible LTCFs and reached about 62,000 residents. During the implementation phase exercise classes and recommendation about environmental adaptations were offered in nearly all LTCFs. 13.5% of the residents participated in exercise classes. Hip protectors were available for 9.2% of all residents. In the first implementation wave, femoral fracture rate was significantly reduced by 18% in the first year. At follow-up nearly 90% of all LTCFs still offered exercise classes, which were attended by about 11% of residents. However, only 10% of the exercise classes completely fulfilled the requirements of an effective strength and balance training. Individual advice about environmental adaptations was provided in 74.3% of the LTCFs and nearly all LTCFs claimed to offer hip protectors to their residents. A long-term effect of the program on femoral fractures could not be detected.

**Conclusions:** The program did not affect the femoral fracture rate in the long run. Possible reasons could be a high turn-over of the staff, a reduced fidelity of training components or a shift in daily priorities among the staff.

**Keywords:** Long-term care facilities, Multifactorial fall prevention program, Long-term evaluation, Implementation stage

* Correspondence: patrick.Roigk@rbk.de
[1]Department of Clinical Gerontology, Robert-Bosch-Hospital, Auerbachstrasse 110, 70376 Stuttgart, Germany
Full list of author information is available at the end of the article

# Background

Long-term care facilities (LTCFs) are settings with a particularly high risk for falls. In this setting, the fall rate is reported to be about 2 falls per resident-year [1], which is considerably higher than the fall rate observed in older people living in the community [2]. In LTCFs with 90 beds, for example, a fall can be expected about every other day [3]. Therefore, fall-related injuries such as bruises, lacerations or fractures are common. One of the most serious complications of falls are femoral fractures [4]. They are particularly frequent in residents of LTCFs. In Germany, more than 20% of hip fractures are caused by residents from LTCFs even though their corresponding person-years under observation account only for 4% [5]. Therefore, there is a high interest in measures and programs which reduce the risk of falls and fall-related injuries in residents of LTCFs. At the end of the 1990s two similar cluster-randomized controlled trials from Sweden and Germany demonstrated that a multifactorial approach is able to reduce the fall rate in residents of LTCFs [6, 7]. Motivated by the results of the German trial, a large statutory health insurance company [Allgemeine Ortskrankenkasse Bayern (AOK)] decided to finance the implementation and dissemination of the program in a large number of LTCFs in Bavaria, a federal state with 12.5 million inhabitants in the south of Germany. Compared to the original study, the program components and the implementation plan of the so-called Bavarian fall and fracture prevention program (BF2P2) were somewhat modified and simplified. In total nearly 1000 LTCFs started with the BF2P2 after having signed a contract to participate in the program for at least 3 years [8].

BF2P2 was embedded in daily routine and implemented in a complex setting. To evaluate the public health significance of such an intervention a comprehensive approach which uses different methods and addresses different dimensions at different time periods is needed [9, 10]. Several analyses were published during the implementation phase of the program. They presented results on the process and on the outcome level. In addition, first results of the long-term evaluation were published recently [11]. Each of these analyses addressed only single aspects of the complex intervention. The aim of the present study is to give a comprehensive and holistic overview of the program during the implementation phase and 3–9 years after the start of the implementation by summarizing results from previous studies and by adding new results from the long-term evaluation. The Reach, Effectiveness, Adoption, Implementation and Maintenance (RE-AIM) framework was used to present the various aspects and results in a structured way [12].

# Methods

## Intervention program

The multifactorial BF2P2 aimed to reduce the fall and fracture risk in residents of LTCFs. The components of the program were progressive exercise classes of strength and balance training with weight cuffs, documentation of falls, environmental adaptations, medication reviews and prescription of Vitamin D, recommendation to use hip protectors, education of staff and educational material. Furthermore, a website was provided to present information about fall prevention and a newsletter was sent regularly to the participating LTCFs during the implementation phase [8]. Further description of the components is presented in Table 1. The program components were offered to the residents depending on their individual fall risk and physical and psychological resources.

To implement the BF2P2, change agents and exercise instructors were educated and trained in a one-day session [8]. The health insurance company funded an exercise instructor for each participating LTCF for 6 months to establish the training and to enable the 'co-trainers' (mostly nurses of the care facility) to proceed independently with the strength and balance training after the funded period. The exercise training was carried out according to a manual [13]. Additionally, care representatives of the homes (so-called change agents) served as multipliers in the LTCFs. They were supposed to take responsibility regarding fall prevention in the LTCFs, organize further training and spread their knowledge to the staff of the LTCFs. The participation in the program was voluntary for LTCFs with 35 or more beds and free for all residents irrespective of their health insurance. Each participating LTCF had to sign a contract to ensure the uptake and to implement the components of the program for at least 3 years [8].

The implementation of BF2P2 was coordinated by a statutory health insurance company, the AOK, which covers about 40% of all residents living in LTCFs in Bavaria. The program was implemented successively in four annually time-lagged implementation waves, starting in 2007, 2008, 2009 and 2010, respectively.

## Data source and data analysis

To comprehensively evaluate BF2P2, data from published analyses, data from the federal statistical office, and new and so far not yet published data were used. Data sources are briefly described below for each of the RE-AIM dimensions and also presented in Tables 3 and 4. For a more detailed description we refer to the original publications.

The evaluation of the implementation phase used data from the first and second implementation wave (2007 and 2008). Routine data of the years 2005 through 2013

**Table 1** Components and details of the BF2P2

| Components | Details |
|---|---|
| Exercise classes | Progressive strength training: with dumbbell at 5 different muscles of the upper part of the body and with weight-cuffs at 5 different muscles of the lower part of the body;<br>Progressive balance training: exercises in standing position, gait variations, exercises with aids like balloons, towel or strings;<br>1 h twice a week; groups of 8–10 participants; to qualify for exercise groups, residents had to be able to stand with support; exercises were adapted to each resident's capabilities; exercise instructors for the first 6 months were physiotherapists or sport therapists, supported by a member of the nursing home staff; after 6 months the training was taken over by members of the nursing home staff. |
| Documentation of falls | Compulsory; documentation sheets were sent to the health care insurance (AOK)[a]; regular feedback on fall statistics. |
| Environmental adaptations | Nurses were encouraged to look for person-environment mismatches using an environmental check list which included more than 100 items [41] |
| Medication review, vitamin D | Nurses were encouraged to discuss a regular medication review with the physicians focusing on reduction of inappropriate psychotropic drugs and on the prescription of vitamin D. |
| Hip protectors | Each home received a test kit of 5 hip protectors for demonstration purposes; recommendation of hip protectors was part of the program but they were not reimbursed by most German health care insurance companies. |
| Education and education materials | Change agents received a one-day training course; exercise instructors received a different one-day training course; manual with all contents of the program [13]; material for in-house education; web page with additional information [42]. |

[a]*AOK* Allgemeine Ortskrankenkasse Bayern (health insurance company)

were used for analysis of the long-term effectiveness of BF2P2 on femoral fractures. Additional follow-up evaluations collected data in 2015 (online-questionnaire) and 2016 (observation of exercise classes). Since the LTCFs started with the program in four annually time-lagged implementation waves and the follow-up evaluations took place at different calendar years, the follow-up period differed between different scientific questions and different LTCFs and ranged from 3 to 9 years.

### RE-AIM evaluation model

To present the different aspects and results from the start of the BF2P2 until its long-term evaluation in a

structured way, the RE-AIM framework was applied [12]. This framework is used in order to understand the strengths and weaknesses of the implemented intervention and is appropriate for setting-based and public health interventions. RE-AIM is an acronym for reach (of target population), effectiveness (impact on key outcomes), adoption (among staff and settings), implementation (consistency of the intervention) and maintenance (long-term impact on individual and setting levels). The original RE-AIM definitions and the transfer of these definitions to the BF2P2 (study definitions) are explained in the following sections and presented in Table 2.

**Table 2** Original and for BF2P2 applied study definitions of RE-AIM dimensions; variables and measurement

| Dimension | Original definition | BF2P2<br>Study definition |
|---|---|---|
| Adoption | The absolute number, proportion, and representativeness of settings and intervention agents who are willing to initiate a program. | The proportion of LTCs which participated in BF2P2 |
| Reach | The absolute number, proportion, and representativeness of individuals who are willing to participate in a given initiative | The proportion of residents who benefited from the BF2P2 |
| Implementation | At the setting level, implementation refers to the intervention agents' fidelity to the various elements of an intervention's protocol. This includes consistency of delivery as intended and the time and cost of the intervention. | Availability of components of the BF2P2 in the participating LTCFs during the implementation phase (fall and fracture prevention classes; hip protectors; environmental adaptations; medication) |
| Effectiveness | The impact of an intervention on important outcomes, including potential negative effects, quality of life, and economic outcomes. | Effectiveness and cost-effectiveness of BF2P2 on incident femoral fractures in the first group of LTCFs (implementation wave 1) during the first implementation year (2007) |
| Maintenance | The extent to which a program or policy becomes institutionalized or part of the routine organizational practices and policies. At the individual level, maintenance has been defined as the long-term effects of a program on outcomes after 6 or more months after the most recent intervention contact. | Availability and quality of components of the BF2P2 in the participating LTCFs during follow-up (fall and fracture prevention classes; hip protectors; environmental adaptations; medication); Long-term effect of BF2P2 on incident femoral fractures in all implementation waves between 2007 and 2013 |

## Adoption

The dimension 'Adoption' describes the proportion of LTCFs which participated in BF2P2 and was calculated by dividing the number of participating LTCFs by the number of eligible LTCFs with 35 or more beds. The number of participating LTCFs was obtained from the health insurance company AOK, the number of eligible LTCFs from the federal statistical office [14].

## Reach

The dimension 'Reach' describes the proportion of residents who benefited from the BF2P2. Since BF2P2 aimed to influence the whole setting of the LTCF by its multifactorial approach, all residents of the participating LTCFs were supposed to benefit in one way or another. Therefore, reach was calculated by dividing the number of residents of participating LTCFs by the number of residents of eligible LTCFs with 35 or more beds. The number of residents was estimated using data from the federal statistical office [15].

## Implementation

In our study the dimension 'Implementation' is operationalized by the availability of the following components of the program in the participating LTCFs during the implementation phase: Fall and fracture prevention classes, hip protectors, environmental adaptations and medication. Furthermore, costs of the BF2P2 were assessed.

In 2008, telephone interviews were conducted with change agents (in most cases care managers) from 69 randomly selected participating LTCFs. They were asked about the availability of fall and fracture prevention classes, the acquisition of hip protectors, and if recommendations about environmental adaptations were routinely offered to their residents. This and additional information was used to calculate the incremental costs of the program during the first 18 months of the implementation [16]. At the same time, a nursing scientist visited 48 randomly selected participating LTCFs for 1 day and collected information from 4000 residents about each resident's participation in exercise classes and about each resident's availability and use of hip protectors [17]. The information referred to the previous 4 weeks and was provided by the nursing home staff for each resident. Implemented components are presented as percentages.

## Effectiveness

The dimension Effectiveness was determined by analyzing the effect of the BF2P2 on incident femoral fractures (ICD-10: S72) during the first intervention year (2007; implementation wave 1). Femoral fracture rates were compared between 13,653 residents from 256 LTCFs which

started with BF2P2 during wave 1 (intervention-LTCFs), and 31,668 residents from 893 remaining LTCFs which started during later waves (control-LTCFs). Since LTCFs were not randomized, the selection of LTCFs may have influenced the outcome. Therefore, femoral fracture rates were also calculated for the years before the start of the intervention (2001, 2002, 2003, 2004, 2005, and 2006) and compared between intervention-LTCFs and control-LTCFs. The femoral fracture-related costs and intervention costs were measured from a payer perspective [18]. Claims data provided by AOK served as data source to analyze Effectiveness and Cost-effectiveness.

## Maintenance

The dimension 'Maintenance' is defined as the availability and quality of components of the BF2P2 in the participating LTCFs during follow-up and the Long-term effect of BF2P2 on incident femoral fractures in all implementation waves. The dimension was evaluated during follow-up in three different ways: First, by assessing the availability of fall prevention measures in the long run, second, by analyzing the fidelity of exercise components in the fall and fracture prevention classes according to the initial protocol, and third, by evaluating the long-term effect of the program on incident femoral fractures (ICD-10: S72).

The availability of fall prevention measures was assessed by an online-questionnaire which was sent to the facility managers or care managers of all participating LTCFs in October 2015. As BF2P2 was implemented time-lagged, this time point was 3 to 9 years after implementation for wave 1 to 4, respectively. The questionnaire asked if the initially educated change agents and exercise instructors were still working in the LTCF, if fall and fracture prevention classes were currently available, if hip protectors were currently made available by the LTCFs, if individual advice about environmental adaptations was routinely provided, and if nurses still discussed the residents' medication with the general practitioner (GPs). The response rate to the online questionnaire was 17.7% ($N = 167$). Data from the online-questionnaire have not been published so far.

To evaluate the fidelity of exercise components according to the "Ulmer Modell" a sport scientist visited 40 different classes in 40 randomly selected LTCFs. Each class was visited once between January 2016 and June 2016. The observation of each training session was recorded in a standardized observation sheet and included type, quality and frequency of specific exercise components [19].

To analyze the effect of BF2P2 on incident femoral fractures (ICD-10: S72) from 2005 through 2013, health insurance claims data of 85,148 residents from 802 nursing homes were used. LTCFs of all four implementation waves were incorporated in a comprehensive unbalanced panel data set. For each of the implementation waves, 2 years prior to implementation of BF2P2 were used as baseline and the following 4 years were investigated. The likelihood of a femoral fracture was estimated for every intervention year relatively to the baseline years before BF2P2 started. Fracture rates were standardized to sex, age, and the degree of dependence (care level) [11].

## Results
### Adoption
Of all 1633 Bavarian LTCFs, 1150 LTCFs met the inclusion criterion of having at least 35 beds. Between 2007 and 2010, 942 of the 1150 eligible LTCFs implemented the LTCFs program, which corresponds to a participation rate of more than 80% (Table 3).

### Reach
Since no residents of participating LTCFs were excluded from BF2P2, the program reached about 62,000 (81.9%) residents out of more than 75,000 eligible residents in Bavaria (Table 3).

### Implementation
One of the core components of the program were exercise classes for strength and balance training. Nearly all of the participating LTCFs offered such classes (97.6%). During the implementation period 13.5% of the residents (range 3.4 to 47.8% per LTCF) participated in exercise classes.

Hip protectors were made available for 9.2% of all residents. The availability of hip protectors varied considerably between LTCFs. In 25% of the LTCFs hip protectors were not present at all, whilst in other LTCFs more than 25% of the residents owned hip protectors. However, only 63% of the residents who owned hip protectors actually used them in the 4 weeks prior to the data collection.

Recommendations about environmental adaptations were routinely offered in nearly all LTCFs.

The implementation of the complete program caused additional costs of 6248 EUR (± SD 7340 EUR; pricing year 2008) per LTCF within the first 18 months (Results are displayed in Table 3).

### Effectiveness
During the first intervention year 2007, the femoral fracture rate was significantly reduced by 18% in the first implementation wave compared to the remaining group of LTCFs not yet participating in the program (Table 3).

The incremental cost-effectiveness ratio which was calculated by the difference in mean costs and mean effects at the group level (ICER) was 7481 EUR per year free of femoral fracture. The net benefit turns into a positive value if the willingness-to-pay (WTP) amount reaches around 7500 EUR, which reflects the point estimate of the adjusted cost-effectiveness ratio (ICER) (Table 3).

### Maintenance
During follow-up less than 20% of the initially educated change agents, who were supposed to serve as multipliers in the facilities, were still available. 55.5% of the current exercise instructors had received a specific education regarding the contents of the exercise program during the implementation phase (Table 4).

Nearly 90% of the LTCFs still offered exercise classes and about 11% of the residents from all participating LTCFs which offered exercise classes attended exercise classes at the follow-up assessment. Most of the exercise instructors (62.5%) had a qualification in nursing (registered nurse or nursing assistance), a smaller proportion (37.5%) in physiotherapy or occupational therapy. Components of strength training were a frequent part of the training (Table 1). However, only 30% of the classes used the recommended weight cuffs for the strength training of the lower extremities. Furthermore, balance exercises were only sparsely or not at all performed in many of the classes. The balance exercises were performed more frequently when exercise instructors had a therapeutic qualification. Only 10% of the exercise classes completely fulfilled the requirements of the fall prevention training according to the given standards of the 'Ulmer Modell' (Table 4).

At the follow-up assessment nearly all LTCFs claimed to offer hip protectors to their residents. The percentage of residents for whom hip protectors were made available by the LTCFs was nearly 20% (Table 4). This is clearly higher than the availability during the implementation phase. However, we had no information how many residents actually used hip protectors.

Individual advice about environmental adaptations was provided in 74.3% of the LTCFs (Table 4).

In more than two thirds of the LTCFs (70.9%) nurses discussed the residents' medication frequently with the GP. However, the prescription of Vitamin D was part of the discussion within the ward round only in a few LTCFs (Table 4).

As described above, the femoral fracture rate was significantly reduced in the first intervention year of the first wave. For the same wave, a reduction was also observed in the second and partly in the third year. In the fourth year, which was the first year after the funded implementation phase ended, a reduction

**Table 3** Dimensions Adoption, Reach, Implementation and Effectiveness of the RE-AIM framework of the BF2P2 during the implementation period (2007–2010)

| RE-AIM dimension | Parameters of the RE-AIM dimension | Data source and time period |
|---|---|---|
| Adoption | | |
| All LTCFs in Bavaria, N | 1633 | • Statistic data from the federal statistical office [14] |
| Eligible LTCFs (≥35 beds) among all LTCFs in Bavaria, n (%) | 1150 (70.4) | |
| Participating LTCFs (Adopters) per eligible LTCFs, n (%) | 942 (81.9) | • Claims data by AOK[a] |
| Reach | | |
| Residents living in all LTCFs in Bavaria, N | 107,507 | • Statistic data from the federal statistical office [15] |
| Residents living in eligible LTCFs (≥35 beds), n (%) | 75,685 (70.4) | |
| Residents of participating LTCFs, n (%) | 61,986 (81.9) | |
| Implementation | | |
| Fall and fracture prevention classes | | |
| Interviewed facility- or care manager of participated LTCFs, N | 69 | • Telephone interviews in 69 LTCFs in 2008 [16] |
| LTCFs offering classes, n (%) | 67 (97.6) | |
| Residents in observed LTCFs, N | 4000 | • Field visits in 48 LTCFs in 2008 [8] |
| Residents attending the classes, n (%) | 540 (13.5) | |
| Hip protectors | | |
| Residents in observed LTCFs, N | 3924 | • Field visits in 48 LTCFs in 2008 [17] |
| Residents owning hip protectors, n (%) | 361 (9.2) | |
| Use of hip protector during the last 4 weeks if available, n (%) | 229 (63.6) | |
| Environmental adaptations | | |
| Interviewed facility- or care manager of participated LTCFs, N | 69 | • Telephone interviews in 69 LTCFs in 2008 [16] |
| LTCFs in which individual advice about environmental adaptations was provided regularly, n (%) | 68 (98.6) | |
| Costs | | |
| Additional costs caused by the implementation of the program within the first 18 month, € (SD) | 6248 (±7340) | • Telephone interviews in 69 LTCFs in 2008 [16] |
| Effectiveness | | |
| Risk of femoral fractures (intervention LTCFs vs. control LTCFs) in the first implementation wave in 2007, HR (95%CI) | 0.82 (0.72–0.93) | • Claims data by AOK[a] from 256 LTCFs / 13,653 residents in 2007 [8] |
| Incremental cost-effectiveness ratio (ICER), € per year free of femoral fracture | 7.481 | • Claims data by AOK [A] from 256 LTCFs/ 10,178 residents in 2007 [18] |

*n* number of residents who participated in fall and fracture prevention classes and used hip protectors and number of participated LTCs who offered the program components of the BF2P2, *LTCFs* Long term care facilities (in Bavaria)
[a]*AOK* Allgemeine Ortskrankenkasse Bayern (health insurance company)

of femoral fractures was no longer observable. In contrast, the intervention was not associated with a significant reduction of femoral fractures in any year of the waves 2, 3 and 4. Therefore, only a transient reduction of femoral fractures in only the first implementation wave was observed whilst a long-term effect of BF2P2 in terms of reducing femoral fractures could not be detected (Table 4).

**Discussion**

This paper provides a comprehensive evaluation of the fall and fracture prevention program BF2P2. The majority of all Bavarian LTCFs adopted the program and the majority of residents were reached. Numerous core components of BF2P2 like recommendations about environmental adaptations or exercise classes were implemented. We found a transient reduction of femoral

**Table 4** Maintenance of the BF2P2 fall prevention components, fidelity of the training components and long term results in fracture incidence in participating LTCFs during follow-up

| RE-AIM dimension | Parameters of the RE-AIM dimension | Data source and time period |
|---|---|---|
| Maintenance of the implemented components | | |
| LTCFs in which the primarily educated personnel was still available | | |
| Interviewed facility- or care manager of participated LTCFs, N | 110 | Online questionnaire in 167 LTCFs in 2015 |
| Change agent of the LTCFs, n (%) | 21 (19.1) | |
| Exercise instructor of the LTCFs, n (%) | 61 (55.5) | |
| Fall and fracture prevention classes | | |
| Interviewed facility- or care manager of participated LTCFs, N | 167 | Online questionnaire in 167 LTCFs in 2015 |
| LTCFs offering classes, n (%) | 146 (87.4) | |
| Residents in observed LTCFs, n | 4013 | Structured observation in 40 LTCFs in 2016 [19] |
| Residents attending the classes, n (%) | 432 (10.8) | |
| Fidelity of the training components | | |
| Observed LTCFs, N | 40 | Structured observation in 40 LTCFs in 2016 [19] |
| Classes which used weight cuffs, n (%) | 12 (30.0) | |
| Classes with an appropriate number (≥6) of balance exercises, n (%) | 10 (25.0) | |
| Classes which completely fulfilled the requirements of an effective strength and balance training, n (%) | 4 (10) | |
| Hip protectors | | |
| Interviewed facility- or care manager of participated LTCFs, N | 167 | Online questionnaire in 167 LTCFs in 2015 |
| Number of LTCFs offering hip protectors to their residents, n (%) | 156 (93.4) | |
| Residents in interviewed LTCFs, n | 15,577 | |
| Numbers of residents' for whom hip protectors were made available by the LTCFs, n (%) | 2950 (18.9) | |
| Environmental adaptations | | |
| Interviewed facility- or care manager of participated LTCFs, N | 167 | Online questionnaire in 167 LTCFs in 2015 |
| LTCFs in which individual advice about environmental adaptations was provided regularly, n (%) | 124 (74.3) | |
| Medication | | |
| Interviewed facility- or care manager of participated LTCFs, N/N | 165/146 | Online questionnaire in 167 LTCFs in 2015 |
| Staff talked to GPs about residents' medication 'frequently'[a], n (%) | 117 (70.9) | |
| Staff talked to GPs about Vitamin D prescriptions 'frequently'[a], n (%) | 19 (13.0) | |
| Long-term effectiveness of fracture prevention | | |
| Intervention year, | | |
| Implementation wave 1 | | |
| Two years before the intervention (baseline), OR | 1.00 | Claims data by the AOK[b] from 802 LTCFs/ 85,148 residents from 2005 to 2013 [11] |
| First year of BF2P2, OR (95%CI) | 0,87 (0.75–0.99) | |
| Second year of BF2P2, OR (95%CI) | 0,80 (0.62–1.04) | |
| Third year of BF2P2, OR (95%CI) | 0,92 (0.82–1.02) | |
| Fourth year of BF2P2, OR (95%CI) | 0,99 (0.84–1.18) | |
| Implementation waves 1–4, combined | | |

**Table 4** Maintenance of the BF2P2 fall prevention components, fidelity of the training components and long term results in fracture incidence in participating LTCFs during follow-up *(Continued)*

| RE-AIM dimension | Parameters of the RE-AIM dimension | Data source and time period |
|---|---|---|
| Two years before the intervention (baseline), OR | 1.00 | |
| First year of BF2P2, OR (95%CI) | 0.96 (0.89–1.05) | |
| Second year of BF2P2, OR (95%CI) | 0.96 (0.84–1.10) | |
| Third year of BF2P2, OR (95%CI) | 0.97 (0.91–1.03) | |
| Fourth year of BF2P2, OR (95%CI) | 1.04 (0.95–1.15) | |

*n* number of residents who participated in fall and fracture prevention classes and used hip protectors and number of participating LTC's which offered the program components of the BF2P2, *LTCFs* Long term care facilities (in Bavaria)
*OR (95%CI)* Odds ratio (95% confidence interval)
[a]'frequently' combines the two answer categories 'always' and 'often' of a 5-point Likert scale (always; often; sometimes; seldom; never)
[b]*AOK* Allgemeine Ortskrankenkasse Bayern (health insurance company)

fractures in the first implementation wave, but no effect on femoral fractures in the following waves. Even after a follow-up of 3–9 years, most of the intervention components were still available. However, the initially educated instructors and change agents were often not available any more due to a high turnover of LTCF staff. A long-term effectiveness of BF2P2 over all Bavarian LTCFs could not be detected.

There are only few studies which analyzed the implementation of fall prevention measures in routine care of LTCFs. They usually focused on specific aspects like effectiveness [20, 21], uptake of and adherence to exercise classes [22] or on facilitators and barriers of using hip protectors [23]. To the best of our knowledge the BF2P2 is the so far largest implementation program for fall and fracture prevention in LTCFs and also the first program with such a comprehensive evaluation including different methods, levels and time periods.

More than 80% of all eligible LTCFs in Bavaria implemented the program. The extremely high adoption rate may be attributed to the publication of a new standard for nurses in fall prevention in 2006 [24] which had to be realized in the facilities from 2009 on [§113a SGB XI]. Therefore, the education of change agents and exercise instructors and the financial support of the exercise classes over 6 months by the health insurance company were considered as an opportunity to transfer evidence based knowledge into practice in a structured way. The degree of implementation of most of the components was also high. For example, nearly all LTCFs offered exercise classes and individual environment counsels.

Therefore, it was disappointing that we observed only a transient reduction of femoral fractures in only the first implementation wave whilst a long-term reduction of femoral fractures could not be detected. Since the study was not randomized, the restriction of the transient effect of the intervention to the first implementation wave may be explainable by a higher motivation of those LTCFs starting first with the program. This suggests that the program is in principle able to reduce femoral fractures, if the motivation of the institutions and the staff is high. The transient reduction in the first wave also shows that it seems to be difficult to maintain a high standard in fall and fracture prevention over a period of several years.

Our comprehensive evaluation over several years revealed different reasons for the failure of a long-term reduction of femoral fractures. First, the components of the program affected the residents in different ways and with different intensity. During the implementation phase, for example, only 13.5% of all residents participated in training classes. One reason is that the exercise classes can be only attended if the resident's functional and cognitive status allows at least standing with support and following the instructions of the exercise instructor. However, the participation rate was clearly lower than 25%, which was mentioned in the study by Becker et al [6]. The health insurance company financed only one exercise class per LTCF independently from its size. This may have excluded eligible residents from exercise due to capacity restrictions.

Second, quality and fidelity of the training program was often not sufficient. In addition, the progressive nature of the exercises may often not have been realized. This may be explained by the high turnover [25, 26] of exercise instructors, which means a loss of expertise. Also, the observed heterogeneity of residents' functional and cognitive status in LTCFs [27] may be a reason. This would force exercise instructors to adapt their training to the needs and abilities of participants, who may be more functionally impaired than presumed.

Third, the program recommended hip protectors in high-risk residents but provided only a test-kit of five hip protectors for each LTC. Since hip protectors are not reimbursed by health insurance companies, only a minority of residents owned hip protectors and even a lower percentage (5.8%) used them regularly during the implementation phase. At the time of the follow-up evaluation, most of the LTCFs were able to offer their residents hip protectors from an own pool. This underlines that fall and fracture prevention is still on the facilities' agenda. Unfortunately, the currently available hip protectors in the LTCFs of our study did not have a significant effect on the femoral fracture rate. This contributes to the discussion about the effectiveness of hip protectors in daily routine of long-term care [28, 29]. Possible reasons for a lack of effectiveness of hip protectors in LTCFs may be poor adherence by the residents, differing attitudes of the staff regarding their benefit, and different brands with different biomechanical properties.

Fourth, discussion about the appropriateness of drugs with the GPs was stated to be performed in 70% of the LTCFs at follow-up but we question that it was actually done in 70% of the individuals. On the one hand nurses may feel uncomfortable to discuss a resident's medication with GPs [30, 31], on the other hand the prescription or termination of fall-inducing drugs like neuroleptics or benzodiazepines are often triggered by information given by nurses. Particularly rare was the discussion about the prescription of vitamin D which is known to have a beneficial effect on bone quality and on fall risk in people with low serum levels [32]. We do not know if it was discussed more frequently during the implementation phase since this component was only assessed at follow-up.

Fifth, since the publication of the new standard in fall prevention in 2006 seven additional standards dealing with other topics like nutrition- or pain management and had also to be implemented into daily routine in the LTCFs. This may have lowered priority of fall prevention in long-term care. Furthermore, the promotion of physical activity is also a priority in long-term care [33, 34]. Physical activity has many benefits and may increase autonomy and self-determination but in case of a poor quality of gait or risk taking behaviour it can also interfere with the aim of preventing falls.

The BF2P2 may have had beneficial effects like an increase of social contacts, quality of life or physical function and physical activity. These effects were not measured in the BF2P2 but well known from other fall prevention trials [35, 36]. Nevertheless, our approach failed to give a sustainable solution how the huge burden of fall-related injuries in LTCFs can be reduced on a population level. The one-day training session for the change agents and the exercise instructors may be far too little to change the culture within LTCFs, even though the change agents were supposed to act as multipliers. Therefore, different strategies and an increase of intensity, quantity and repetition of the education over a longer time period may be an approach for the future [37]. This would be associated with a considerable additional investment. Another approach could be to reconsider the measures introduced so far. New generations of LTCFs, which are smaller and differ in architecture and care-concepts from facilities of the past [38], may offer new opportunities for more effective measures. Examples could be architectural solutions for a better supervision of residents at risks, compliant flooring [39] or partnerships with other organizations (e.g. sport associations offering additional exercise classes) [40].

A strength of the current evaluation is our comprehensive approach which analyzed process and outcome variables, included different methods and time periods and used a standardized framework [12] for the reporting of the results in a structured way. It covers a highly relevant topic of the public health sector and evaluates a large program which is included in daily routine. The data are representative and cover a complete federal state.

A weakness of our evaluation is that the availability of some of the program components such as fall and fracture prevention classes or hip protectors were assessed by different instruments during implementation phase and follow-up. This limits the comparability of the results. Furthermore, only 17.7% of the LTCFs completed the online questionnaire at follow-up which could have biased our results. The conditions in LTCFs differ from country to country and from healthcare system to healthcare system. This limits the generalizability of our results.

## Conclusion

In conclusion, the BF2P2 did not affect the femoral fracture rate in the long run. However, we observed a transient reduction of femoral fractures in the first implementation wave. This suggests that the dissemination of an evidence-based program into routine care is principally able to reduce femoral fractures. We identified different reasons which may have limited the effectiveness of the program like a high turn-over of staff, a reduced fidelity of training components or a shift in daily priorities among the staff. Fracture prevention in long-term care remains a challenge. A higher investment to guarantee a sustainable change of the implemented measures and processes in LTCFs or the introduction of completely new measures could be perspectives for the future.

**Abbreviations**
AOK: Allgemeine Ortskrankenkasse; BF2P2: Bavarian fall and fracture prevention program; GP: General Practitioner; ICER: Incremental cost-effectiveness ratio; LTCFs: Long-term care facilities; RE-AIM framework: Reach, Effectiveness, Adoption, Implementation and Maintenance framework; WTP: Willingness-to-pay

**Funding**
This study was funded by the German Federal Ministry of Education and Research (grants 01EL1405A, 01EL1405B). AOK Bayern had no influence on the intervention components but participated in the implementation process. The evaluation of the intervention was not funded, and not influenced, by AOK Bayern.

## Authors' contributions

PR was involved in the development of the questionnaire and the documentation sheet for the follow up online survey and the observation of the exercise classes, respectively. Furthermore he was involved in the analyses and interpretation of the follow-up data and was the major contributor in writing the manuscript. KR was involved in the analyses and interpretation of the data of the prior published studies, analyses of the follow-up data and gave input for the first draft of the manuscript, all subsequent drafts and contributed in writing the manuscript. CB was the major contributor in the study design of BF2P2, involved in the analyses and interpretation of the data of the prior published studies, analyses of the follow-up data and critically revised the manuscript for publication. CS was involved in the analyses and interpretation of the follow-up data and critically reviewed the manuscript. HHK was involved in the analyses and interpretation of the data of the prior published studies, analyses of the follow-up data and critically revised the manuscript for publication.

## Competing interest

The authors declare that they have no proprietary, financial, professional, or other personal competing interests of any nature or kind.

## Author details

[1]Department of Clinical Gerontology, Robert-Bosch-Hospital, Auerbachstrasse 110, 70376 Stuttgart, Germany. [2]Department of Health Economics and Health Services Research, University Medical Center Hamburg-Eppendorf, Hamburg, Germany.

## References

1. Rubenstein LZ, Josephson KR, Robbins AS. Falls in the nursing home. Ann Intern Med. 1994;121(6):442–51.
2. Rubenstein Laurence Z. Falls in older people: epidemiology, risk factors and strategies for prevention. Age Ageing. 2006;35(suppl_2):ii37–41 https://doi.org/10.1093/ageing/afl084.
3. Rapp K, Becker C, Cameron ID, König HH, Büchele G.: Epidemiology of Falls in Residential Aged Care: Analysis of More Than 70,000 Falls From Residents of Bavarian Nursing Homes. J Am Med Dir Assoc 2012;13(2):187.e1–6. doi: https://doi.org/10.1016/j.jamda.2011.06.011. Epub 2011 Aug 4.
4. Dyer SM, Crotty M, Fairhall N, Magaziner J, Beaupre LA, Cameron ID. Sherrington C for the fragility fracture network (FFN) rehabilitation research special interest group: a critical review of the long-term disability outcomes following hip fracture. BMC Geriatr. 2016;16:158. https://doi.org/10.1186/s12877-016-0332-0.
5. Rapp K, Becker C, Cameron ID, Klenk J, Kleiner A, Bleibler F, König HH, Büchele G. Femoral fracture rates in people with and without disability. Age Ageing. 2012;41(5):653–8 https://doi.org/10.1093/ageing/afs044.
6. Becker C, Kron M, Lindemann U, Sturm E, Eichner B, Walter-Jung B, Nikolaus T. Effectiveness of a multifaceted intervention on falls in nursing home residents. J Am Geriatr Soc. 2003;51(3):306–13.
7. Jensen J, Lundin-Olsson L, Nyberg L, Gustafson Y. Fall and injury prevention in older people living in residential care facilities. A cluster randomized trial. Ann Intern Med. 2002;136(10):733–41.
8. Becker C, Cameron ID, Klenk J, Lindemann U, Becker S, König H-H, Rapp K. Reduction of femoral fractures in long-term care facilities: the Bavarian fracture prevention study. PLoS One. 2011;6(8):e24311. https://doi.org/10.1371/journal.pone.0024311 Epub 2011 Aug 30.
9. Hulscher M, Laurant MGH, Grol R. Process evaluation on quality improvement interventions. Qual Saf Health Care. 2003;12(1):40–6.
10. Fixsen DL, Naoom SF, Blase KA, Friedman RM, Wallace F. Implementation research: A synthesis of the literature. Tampa, FL: University of South Florida, Louis de la Parte Florida Mental Health Institute, The National Implementation Research Network; 2005. [FMHI Publication 231]
11. Schulz C, Lindlbauer I, Rapp K, Becker C, König HH. Long-term effectiveness of a multifactorial fall and fracture prevention program in Bavarian nursing homes: an analysis based on health insurance claims

data. J Am Med Dir Assoc. 2017;18(6):552.e7–552.e17. https://doi.org/10.1016/j.jamda.2017.03.012.
12. Glasgow RE, Vogt TM, Boles SM. Evaluating the public health impact of health promotion interventions: the RE-AIM framework. Am J Public Health. 1999;89(9):1322–7.
13. Becker C, Lindemann U, Rissmann U, Warnke A. Sturzprophylaxe. Sturzgefährdung und Sturzverhütung. Heimen: Vincentz Network Hannover; 2006. ISBN 3–87870–131-4
14. Die Gesundheitsberichterstattung des Bundes: Pflegeheime und verfügbare Plätze in Pflegeheimen. Gliederungsmerkmale: Jahre, Region, Art der Einrichtungen/Plätze, Träger. Wiesbaden 2017. http://www.gbe-bund.de/gbe10/pkg_isgbe5.prc_isgbe?p_uid=gast&p_aid=68319353&p_sprache=D.
15. Die Gesundheitsberichterstattung des Bundes: Pflegebedürftige (Anzahl). Gliederungsmerkmale: Jahre, Region, Pflegestufen, Art der Betreuung. Wiesbaden 2017. http://www.gbe-bund.de/gbe10/pkg_isgbe5.prc_isgbe?p_uid=gast&p_aid=68319353&p_sprache=D.
16. Heinrich S, Weigelt I, Rapp K, Becker C, Rissmann U, König H-H. Sturz- und Frakturprävention auf der Grundlage des Nationalen Expertenstandards Sturzprophylaxe Umsetzung und Kosten im Versorgungsalltag im Setting Pflegeheim. Z Gerontol Geriat. 2011. https://doi.org/10.1007/s00391-011-0243-9.
17. Klenk J, Kurrle S, Rissmann U, Kleiner A, Heinrich S, König HH, Becker C, Rapp K. Availability and use of hip protectors in residents of nursing homes. Osteoporos Int. 2011;22(5):1593–8. https://doi.org/10.1007/s00198-010-1366-3 Epub 2010 Aug 4.
18. Heinrich S, Rapp K, Stuhldreher N, Rissmann U, Becker C, König HH. Cost-effectiveness of a multifactorial fall prevention program in nursing homes. Osteoporos Int. 2013;24(4):1215–23. https://doi.org/10.1007/s00198-012-2075-x Epub 2012 Jul 18.
19. Roigk P, Rupp K, Becker C, Schulz C, König HH, Rapp K. Long-term evaluation of the fidelity of a strength and balance training in long-term care facilities. The Bavarian fall and fracture prevention program (BF2P2). Physioscience. 2018;14(01):5–12. https://doi.org/10.1055/s-0044-100543.
20. Cameron ID, Gillespie LD, Robertson MC, Murray GR, Hill KD, Cumming RG, Kerse N. Interventions for preventing falls in older people in care facilities and hospitals. Cochrane Database Syst Rev. 2012;12:CD005465. https://doi.org/10.1002/14651858.CD005465.pub3.
21. Vlaeyen E, Coussement J, Leysens G, Van der Elst E, Delbaere K, Cambier D, Denhaerynck K, Goemaere S, Wertelaers A, Dobbels F, Dejaeger E, Milisen K. Characteristics and effectiveness of fall prevention programs in nursing homes: a systematic review and meta-analysis of randomized controlled trials. J Am Geriatr Soc. 2015;63(2):211–21. https://doi.org/10.1111/jgs.13254 Epub 2015 Feb 2.
22. Hawley-Hague H, Horne M, Skelton DA, Todd C. Older adults' uptake and adherence to exercise classes: instructors' perspectives. J Aging Phys Act. 2016;24(1):119–28. https://doi.org/10.1123/japa.2014-0108 Epub 2015 Jul 23.
23. Korall AM, Feldman F, Scott VJ, Wasdell M, Gillan R, Ross D, Thompson-Franson T, Leung PM, Lin L. Facilitators of and barriers to hip protector acceptance and adherence in long-term care facilities: a systematic review. J Am Med Dir Assoc. 2015;16(3):185–93. https://doi.org/10.1016/j.jamda.2014.12.004.
24. Deutsches Netzwerk für Qualitätsentwicklung in der Pflege (DNQP). Expertenstandard Sturzprophylaxe in der Pflege. [einschließlich Kommentierung und Literaturstudie]. 1. Aktualisierung. Osnabrück: DNQP; Schriftenreihe des Deutschen Netzwerks für Qualitätsentwicklung in der Pflege; 2013.
25. Vlaeyen E, Stas J, Leysens G, Van der Elst E, Janssens E, Dejaeger E, Dobbels F, Milisen K. Implementation of fall prevention in residential care facilities: a systematic review of barriers and facilitators. Int J Nurs Stud. 2017;70:110–21. https://doi.org/10.1016/j.ijnurstu.2017.02.002 Epub 2017 Feb 3.
26. Lee SH, Kim HS. Exercise interventions for preventing falls among older people in care facilities: a meta-analysis. Worldviews Evid-Based Nurs. 2017;14(1):74–80. https://doi.org/10.1111/wvn.12193 Epub 2016 Dec 16.
27. Schäufele M, Köhler L, Hendlmeier I, Hoell A, Weyerer S. Prevalence of dementia and medical Care in German Nursing Homes: a nationally representative survey. Psychiatr Prax. 2013;40(4):200–6. https://doi.org/10.1055/s-0033-1343141 Epub 2013 May 13.
28. Santesso N, Carrasco-Labra A, Brignardello-Petersen R. Hip protectors for preventing hip fractures in older people. Cochrane Database Syst Rev. 2014;3:CD001255. https://doi.org/10.1002/14651858.CD001255.pub5.

29. Milisen K, Coussement J, Boonen S, Geeraerts A, Druyts L, Van Wesenbeeck A, Abraham I, Dejaeger E. Nursing staff attitudes of hip protector use in long-term care, and differences in characteristics between adherent and non-adherent residents: a survey and observational study. Int J Nurs Stud. 2011;48(2):193–203. https://doi.org/10.1016/j.ijnurstu.2010.07.008 Epub 2010 Aug 12.

30. Hibbeler B, Rieser S. Hausbesuche im Heim: Wege zur besseren Versorgung. Dtsch Arztebl. 2012;109(19):A950–4.

31. Brasaite I, Kaunonen M, Suominen T. Healthcare professionals' knowledge, attitudes and skills regarding patient safety: a systematic literature review. Scand J Caring Sci. 2015;29(1):30–50. https://doi.org/10.1111/scs.12136 Epub 2014 Apr 8.

32. Reid IR, Bolland MJ, Grey A. Effects of vitamin D supplements on bone mineral density: a systematic review and meta-analysis. Lancet 2014; 383(9912):146-155.

33. Deutsches Netzwerk für Qualitätsentwicklung in der Pflege (DNQP). Expertenstandard nach § 113a SGB XI Erhaltung und Förderung der Mobilität in der Pflege. Abschlussbericht. 2014. https://www.gkv-spitzenverband.de/media/dokumente/pflegeversicherung/qualitaet_in_der_pflege/expertenstandard/Pflege_Expertenstandard_Mobilitaet_Abschlussbericht_14-07-14_finaleVersion.pdf.

34. Douma JG, Volkers KM, Engels G, Sonneveld MH, Goossens RHM, Scherder EJA. Setting-related influences on physical inactivity of older adults in residential care settings: a review. BMC Geriatr. 2017;17(1):97. https://doi.org/10.1186/s12877-017-0487-3.

35. Netz Y, Wu MJ, Becker BJ, Tenenbaum G. Physical activity and psychological well-being in advanced age: a meta-analysis of intervention studies. Psychol Aging. 2005;20(2):272–84.

36. Stathi A, Simey P. Quality of life in the fourth age: exercise experiences of nursing home residents. J Aging Phys Act. 2007;15(3):272–86.

37. Harvey G, Kitson A. Translating evidence into healthcare policy and practice: single versus multi-faceted implementation strategies – is there a simple answer to a complex question? Int J Health Policy Manag. 2015;4(3):123–6. https://doi.org/10.15171/ijhpm. 2015.54.

38. Kuratorium Dt. Altershilfe Wilhelmine-Lübke-Stift. Die fünfte Generation: KDA-Quartiershäuser: Ansätze zur Neuausrichtung von Alten- und Pflegeheimen; Auflage: 1. 2012. ISBN-13: 978-3940054272.

39. Lachance CC, Jurkowski MP, Dymarz AC, Robinovitch SN, Feldman F, Laing AC, et al. Compliant flooring to prevent fall-related injuries in older adults: a scoping review of biomechanical efficacy, clinical effectiveness, cost-effectiveness, and workplace safety. PLoS One. 2017;12(2):e0171652. https://doi.org/10.1371/journal.pone.0171652.

40. Rapp K, Kampe K, Roigk P, Kircheisen H, Becker C, Lindlbauer I, König HH, Rothenbacher D, Büchele G. The osteoporotic fracture prevention program in rural areas (OFRA): a protocol for a cluster-randomized health care fund driven intervention in a routine health care setting. BMC Musculoskelet Disord. 2016;17:458. https://doi.org/10.1186/s12891-016-1308-0.

41. Marx L, Nußberger J, Ziller A. Barrierefreie Wohnungen. Stuttgart: Leitfaden zu den Planungsgrundlagen. Wirtschaftsministerium Baden-Württemberg; 1994. p. 11–61.

42. Robert-Bosch-Hospital Stuttgart. Available: Accessed 6 Dec 2010.

# 10

# Psychological distress in elderly people is associated with diet, wellbeing, health status, social support and physical functioning- a HUNT3 study

Kjersti Grønning[1]* iD, Geir A. Espnes[1], Camilla Nguyen[1], Ana Maria Ferreira Rodrigues[2,3], Maria Joao Gregorio[2,3], Rute Sousa[2,3], Helena Canhão[2,3] and Beate André[1]

## Abstract

**Background:** The increasing proportion of people growing old, demands expanded knowledge of how people can experience successful aging. Having a good life while growing old is dependent on several factors such as nutrition, physical health, the ability to perform activities of daily living, lifestyle and psychological health. Furthermore, unhealthy food intake is found to be a modifiable risk factor for depression in elderly people. To promote elderly's health and wellbeing, the influence of nutrition, lifestyle, physical functioning, and social support on psychological distress needs exploring. Therefore, the purpose of this present study is to investigate the associations between psychological distress and diet patterns when adjusting for other life style behaviors, wellbeing, health status, physical functioning and social support in elderly people.

**Methods:** The present study is cross sectional, using data from wave three of the Nord-Trøndelag Health Study (2006–2008). Data include psychological distress measured by the Hospital Anxiety and Depression Scale (HADS), sociodemographic information, measurements of lifestyle behaviours (including diet patterns), wellbeing, health status, social support and physical functioning.

**Results:** The sample consisted of 11,621 participants, 65 years or older. Cluster analysis categorized the participants in two food clusters based on similarities in food consumption (healthy $N = 9128$, unhealthy $N = 2493$). Stepwise multivariable linear regression analyses revealed that lesser psychological distress in the elderly was dependent on gender, diet, smoking, better scores on health and wellbeing, social support and less problems performing instrumental activities of daily living.

**Conclusion:** Knowledge about the influence of diet patterns in relation to psychological distress provide valuable insights into how society can promote healthy lifestyles to an ageing population, e.g. by increasing older people's food knowledge.

**Keywords:** Mental health, Life style, Diet, Older adults

* Correspondence: kjersti.gronning@ntnu.no
[1]Department of Public Health and Nursing, Center for Health Promotion Research, Norwegian University of Science and Technology (NTNU), Postbox 8905, 7491 Trondheim, Norway
Full list of author information is available at the end of the article

## Background

The proportion of people older than 65 years is growing faster than any other age group [1]. Recognition of this require expanded knowledge on how this large portion of population can experience successful ageing. Successful ageing is about staying healthy [2] and connected to a diversity of factors, such as psychological resources, life satisfaction, social participation, functioning and personal growth [3]. Wellbeing is also linked to health and age and refers to how people experience the quality of their lives [4], comprising emotional responses, feelings of happiness, sadness, anger, stress, purpose and meaning in life [5]. The process of successful ageing [1] is about extending healthy life expectancy and quality of life for all people as they age, but it is also about optimizing opportunities for health and participation in social, economic, cultural, spiritual and civil matters. Lack of social support has shown to have a negative influence on future quality of life among elderly people [6].

As people grow older, the prevalence of chronic illness is increasing, which challenge the health system to make easily accessible services to meet the growing needs for chronic illness management, risk reduction, promoting healthy lifestyles, and improving the aging population's quality of life [7]. Wellbeing have a protective role in health maintenance for older people [8], where nutrition and diet prevent frailty. Frailty is a continuum of being at risk of losing, or having lost, social and general resources, activities, or abilities that are important for fulfilling one or more basic social needs during the life span [9]. Also, sociodemographic factors, lifestyle, functional impairments [10], higher level of depression, poor self-rated health and negative affect [11] are shown to be significantly associated with frailty. One study found a strong association between depression and incident of frailty in older women [12].

In summary, a 2017 review [11] states that a wide variety of factors, such as sociodemographic, physical, biological, lifestyle, diet, activities of daily living (ADL), and psychological factors (e.g. depressive symptoms) are associated with frailty. A healthy diet includes food types like fruits, vegetables, fish, whole-grain bread and water [13]. Thus, healthy diets also consist of food variety, enabling food components to be met adequately and comprehensively [14]. Several publications have revealed that healthy diets are associated with better quality of life [13, 15, 16]. For instance, studies have shown that individuals with a higher score for adherence to a Mediterranean-style diet [17, 18] and higher consumption of low-fat milk and yogurt [19] have lower odds of developing frailty, while a variety and quality of diets in older people [20] is increased by factors, such as social resources, money and help from friends and neighbors.

To improve quality of life of older persons, it is important to screen and develop interventions targeting frailty components [6]. Moreover, as elderly's psychological status and lifestyle behaviours are associated with frailty, it is important to investigate the influence of life style behaviors and health status variables in relation to psychological distress, in addition to less studied factors such as type of neighborhoods [11]. Therefore, the aim of this study is to investigate the associations between diet patterns and psychological distress in elderly people when adjusting for other life style behaviors, wellbeing, health status, physical functioning and social support by using data from a longitudinal epidemiological observational study in Norway [21].

## Methods

### Sample

The Nord-Trøndelag Health Study (HUNT Study) is one of the largest health studies ever performed, collecting data in four waves, HUNT 1 (1984–1986), HUNT 2 (1995–1997), HUNT 3 (2006–2008) and HUNT 4 (ongoing) [22]. This present study is based on data collected in the HUNT 3 wave (2006–2008). The HUNT3 wave (50,807 participants) contain information on the inhabitants' sociodemographic status, living conditions, life-styles behaviors and health status. In this study, elderly inhabitants are defined as being 65 years or older in 2006 when the HUNT3 data collection started.

### Variables and measures

The outcome variable was psychological distress measured by the Hospital Anxiety and Depression Scale (HADS) [23]. HADS has been translated into Norwegian and is a valid and reliable measure [24] to assess psychological distress. HADS total score range from zero (best) to 42 (worst) as a continuous variable.

The independent variables consist of sociodemographic variables, variables assessing life style behaviors (diet, smoking, alcohol), social support, overall health, wellbeing, and instrumental activities of daily living (1-ADL). Sociodemographic information contained information on sex (male/female) and living situation (cohabitating yes or no). Variables assessing life style behaviors included diet (healthy or unhealthy diet pattern group), current smoking (yes or no) and alcohol consumption (4–7 times a week, 2–3 times a week, about once a week, 2–3 times a month, about once a month, a few times a year, not at all the last year, and never drank alcohol). Food consumption was collected by asking how often of the following foodstuff the participants normally eat. Then, the diet pattern variable was created by re-coding categorical food variables into continuous variables and calculating the average weekly consumption. A healthy diet pattern was characterized as more consumption of fruits, vegetables, boiled potatoes, oily fish, whole-grain bread and water, while the unhealthy diet pattern consisted of larger amount of/consumption of chocolate/candy, pasta, sausages, sugar free and sugary soft drinks, and whole milk, juice, white and semi-grain bread.

Variables assessing social support was assessed by two items from the Social Cohesion and Support Index (SCS) [25], «*do you have friends that can help you when you need them*» and "*do you have friends that you can speak to confidentially*", in addition to one item from the Short Form-8 (SF-8) health survey [26]. The SF-8 question "*to what extent has your physical health or emotional problems limited you in your usual socializing with family or friends during the last 4 weeks*" has the following response alternatives; not at all, very little, somewhat, much or was not able to socialize where lower score indicates less problems. As people's community is relevant for social support, we included three items (network united, network distrust and network welfare) from the HUNT instrument, Local community [22]. The questions were "*I feel a strong sense of community with the people who live here*" (network united), "*we do not trust each other here*" (network distrust) and "*people like living here*" (network welfare), with answers strongly agree, somewhat agree, unsure, somewhat disagree or strongly disagree.

Wellbeing was assessed by a single item "*thinking about your life at the moment, would you say that you by and large are satisfied with life, or are you mostly dissatisfied, which* is found to be a sufficient and valid measure [27]. The response alternatives were very satisfied, satisfied, somewhat satisfied, neither satisfied nor dissatisfied, somewhat dissatisfied, dissatisfied, very dissatisfied. Overall health was measured with the question "*how is your health at the moment*" with the response alternatives poor, not so good, good or very good. We assessed physical functioning by instrumental activities of daily living (I-ADL), defined as problems performing one or more instrumental activities. The activities were preparing hot food, doing light housework, doing heavier housework, washing clothes, paying bills, taking medicine, being able to move outside the house, go shopping and taking a bus without help [28].

## Analyses

The data was analyzed using IBM SPSS Statistics (version 22) [29]. To investigate differences between elderly dependent on diet clusters, we conducted bi-variate analyses where continuous and categorical variables were analyzed with independent t-tests and Pearson's chi-squared test, respectively. To investigate

independent associations between diet patterns and psychological distress when adjusting for other life style behaviors (smoking and alcohol consumption), wellbeing, health status, physical functioning and social support, we created a regression model where groups of variables were added to the model in five steps (Table 2). After each step, we excluded the non-significant variables. Multiple regression analysis are powerful statistical procedures suited to estimate the linear relationship between an outcome variable and one or more predictor variables [30]. Other principal assumptions in addition to linearity that justify the use of linear regression models are statistical independence of the errors, homoscedasticity and normality of the error distribution. In this study, the assumptions of linear regression analyses, values of inter-correlations, the Durbin-Watson and Variance Inflation Factor were not violated. Only cases with valid values for all variables are included in the analyses. In multivariable regression analyses, the standardized beta coefficient (Beta) compares the strength of the association between the independent and dependent variable when adjusting for other independent variables in the model. The level of significance was set to $p < 0.05$. Only cases with valid values for all variables are included in the analyses. Contribution of the independent variables in the model is expressed as explained variance (adjusted $R^2$).

The diet pattern variable was created through K-means cluster analysis [31], which is suitable for data with large sample sizes. Cluster analysis classify individuals with similar traits into separate groups. In this study, we re-coded categorical food variables into continuous variables by calculating the average weekly consumption. Then, we standardized these continuous food variables before running the K-means cluster analysis to make sure that food groups did not influence the clusters with specific frequency [31]. The result from the K-means cluster analyses resulted in two different diet patterns (healthy and unhealthy) which are already published [13]. We created the variable cohabitating by recoding elderly's living situation into a dummy variable. Those registered as married, or living with a registered partner was given value one and those registered as single, separated, divorced, surviving partner, or widower represented the reference category, value zero.

## Results

The sample consisted of 11,621 participants, 65 years or older in 2006. The sample's characteristics are presented in Table 1, showing that the healthy diet group consisted of more females, more elderly living with someone, less smokers and less alcohol consumption. In addition, participants in the healthy diet pattern group had a lower

**Table 1** Descriptive characteristics of elderly dependent on diet pattern group

| Variables | Healthy diet cluster N = 9128 N (%) or mean (SD) | Unhealthy diet cluster N = 2493 N (%) or mean (SD) | P-value |
|---|---|---|---|
| HADS total score (0–42) ↓ | 7.56 (5.1) | 8.75 (5.5) | .000* |
| Sociodemographic information | | | |
| Female | 5119 (56.1) | 1181 (47.4) | .000* |
| Cohabitating | 5872 (64.3) | 1248 (50.1) | .000* |
| Lifestyle style behaviors | | | |
| Ex-smoker | 7282 (83.7) | 1871 (83.1) | .006* |
| Alcohol consumption (1–8) ↓ | 4.82 (1.9) | 5.12 (1.9) | .000* |
| Overall health and wellbeing | | | |
| Life-satisfaction (0–7) ↓ | 2.25 (1.0) | 2.41 (1.0) | .000* |
| Health at the moment (0–4) ↑ | 2.66 (0.6) | 2.56 (0.6) | .000* |
| Social support | | | |
| SCS (friends support) | 7377 (92.2) | 1895 (90.5) | .000* |
| SCS (friends talk) | 7204 (90.6) | 1875 (89.2) | .059 |
| SF-8 (0–5) ↓ | 1.54 (0.9) | 1.69 (1.0) | .000* |
| Network united (1–5) ↓ | 1.78 (0.9) | 1.87 (1.0) | .000* |
| Network distrust (1–5) ↑ | 3.61 (1.4) | 3.36 (1.4) | .000* |
| Network welfare (1–5) ↓ | 1.38 (0.7) | 1.46 (0.8) | .000* |
| I-ADL | | | |
| Can prepare warm meals without help from others (yes = 1) | 5063 (96.1) | 1449 (94.8) | .028* |
| Can do the shopping without help from others (yes = 1) | 5063 (95.5) | 1453 (94.7) | .196 |
| Can go out without help from others (yes = 1) | 5187 (97.8) | 1478 (96.7) | .009* |
| Can do light housework without help from others (yes = 1) | 5168 (98.0) | 1466 (96.3) | .000* |
| Can do heavier housework without help from others (yes = 1) | 4423 (84.3) | 1177 (77.8) | .000* |
| Can do the laundry without help from others (yes = 1) | 4764 (91.5) | 1357 (89.9) | .048* |
| Can pay bills without help from others (yes = 1) | 5073 (95.6) | 1432 (93.7) | .001* |
| Can take medicines without help from others (yes = 1) | 5097 (98.5) | 1453 (97.5) | .009* |
| Can take the bus without help from others (yes = 1) | 4672 (91.4) | 1258 (86.7) | .000* |

↑Higher score is better, ↓lower score is better
HADS = Hospital Anxiety and Depression Scale, SCS = Social Cohesion and Support Index, SF-8 = the Short Form-8 Health Survey, I-ADL = instrumental activities of daily living
*p-value < .05

level of psychological distress, higher scores on well-being, better scores on social support and less problems performing I-ADL's except from being able to do the shopping without help from others. The internal consistency (Cronbach's Alpha) of the HADS in this sample was 0.82.

Table 2 presents the results from the multivariable regression analyses. In step 1, both demographic variables, being male and living with someone were associated with less psychological distress. When adding the variable healthy diet pattern to the model, the analyses showed that there was an independent association between having a healthy diet pattern and less psychological distress. In step three of the analyses, other

lifestyle behaviors like alcohol consumption and smoking were added to the model. The results showed that increased alcohol consumption and smoking were associated with higher psychological distress. In step four, the analyses still showed that having a healthy diet pattern were associated with less psychological distress when adjusting for demographics, other lifestyle behaviors and instrumental activities of daily living. Instrumental activities of daily living as being able to prepare warm meals, go out, do heavier housework do the laundry and pay bills without help from others were associated with lower psychological distress. In the final step of the analyses, we added variables assessing wellbeing, health status and social

**Table 2** Explained variance in psychological distress among elderly > 65 years old

| Independent variables | Psychological distress (HADS) | | | | | | | | | |
|---|---|---|---|---|---|---|---|---|---|---|
| | STEP 1 | | STEP 2 | | STEP 3 | | STEP 4 | | STEP 5 | |
| | Beta | P-value | Beta | P-value | Beta | P-value | Beta | P-value | Beta | P-value |
| Sociodemographic | | | | | | | | | | |
| Cohabitating (yes = 1) | −.029 | .008* | −.015 | .181 | | | | | | |
| Sex (male = 1) | −.072 | .000* | −.083 | .000* | −.078 | .000* | −.096 | .000* | −.081 | .000* |
| Lifestyle style behaviors | | | | | | | | | | |
| Healthy diet cluster (yes = 1) | | | −.097 | .000* | −.089 | .000* | −.075 | .000* | −.048 | .000* |
| Smoker | | | | | .057 | .000* | .073 | .000* | .048 | .000* |
| Alcohol consumption (1–8)↓ | | | | | .044 | .000* | .004 | .771 | | |
| I-ADL | | | | | | | | | | |
| Prepare warm meals | | | | | | | −.063 | .001* | −.056 | .000* |
| Go out | | | | | | | −.066 | .000* | −.025 | .080 |
| Do heavier housework | | | | | | | −.076 | .000* | .039 | .010* |
| Do the laundry | | | | | | | −.035 | .040* | −.023 | .148 |
| Pay bills | | | | | | | −.025 | .155 | | |
| Take medicines | | | | | | | −.003 | .850 | | |
| Do the shopping | | | | | | | .024 | .249 | | |
| Do light housework | | | | | | | .030 | .088 | | |
| Take the bus | | | | | | | −.034 | .057 | | |
| Health and wellbeing | | | | | | | | | | |
| Life-satisfaction (0–7) ↓ | | | | | | | | | .297 | .000* |
| Health at the moment (0–4) ↑ | | | | | | | | | -,119 | .000* |
| Social support | | | | | | | | | | |
| SF-8 (0–5) ↓ | | | | | | | | | .101 | .000* |
| Network distrust (1–5) ↑ | | | | | | | | | −.086 | .000* |
| Network welfare (1–5) ↓ | | | | | | | | | .099 | .000* |
| Network united (1–5) ↓ | | | | | | | | | −.001 | .928 |
| SCS (friends talk) (yes = 1) | | | | | | | | | −.036 | .013* |
| SCS (friends support) (yes = 1) | | | | | | | | | −.008 | .570 |
| Adjusted R² | 0.07% | | 0.16% | | 0.19% | | 4.8% | | 24.3% | |

Multiple linear regression analyses, standardized coefficients = Beta, * p-value < .05
↑ Higher score is better, ↓lower score is better
HADS = Hospital Anxiety and Depression Scale, SCS = Social Cohesion and Support Index, SF-8 = the Short Form-8 Health Survey, I-ADL = instrumental activities of daily living (Can do the following tasks without help from others)

support to the model. The multivariable regression analyses showed that the healthy diet variable still had an independent statistical significant influence on psychological distress when adjusting for the other variables in the model.

Moreover, the final model showed that in addition to a healthy diet, being male, being able to prepare warm meals or do heavier housework without help from others, reporting better health and life satisfaction were positively associated with less psychological distress. In addition, more social support in terms of having friends that they could speak to confidentially, experiencing less problems that limited usual socializing with family or friends, and better scores on the community feelings welfare and distrust were all independently statistically significantly associated with less psychological distress. The model as a whole explained 24.3% of the variance in psychological distress.

## Discussion

The aim of this study was to investigate associations between psychological distress and diet patterns when adjusting for other life style behaviors, wellbeing, health status, physical functioning and social support in elderly people.

Psychological distress in elderly people is associated with diet, wellbeing, health status, social support...

97

## The influence of diet patterns on psychological distress

In a previous HUNT study [13], a significant difference in psychological distress between elderly people with a healthy and unhealthy diet was found, but the study did not adjust for possible confounders. In this study, we performed multiple linear regression analysis and adjusted for other independent variables when studying the association between diet patterns and psychological distress. The regression model showed that having a healthy diet was associated with less psychological distress in the elderly when adjusting for other lifestyle behaviours that in other studies have shown to influence older people's wellbeing [32] and psychological distress [11].

Furthermore, this study confirm findings from other studies showing that sociodemographic determinants are associated with diet quality [33] and social relationships are linked to dietary behavior [34]. Conklin and colleagues [34] found that being single or widowed was associated with lower scores on vegetable variety, and the associations were enhanced when combined with male gender, living alone or infrequent friend contact. Our bi-variate analyses showed that unhealthy diet patterns were more common among males and elderly with fewer supportive friends. These findings confirmed the results from another study [20] showing that varieties and quality of diets in elderly were influenced by social resources and help from friends and neighbors.

Gender differences in food preferences are shown as essential in several studies [33, 35] indicating that females prefer more vegetables and fruits than males [16]. Our analyses found more females in the healthy diet pattern group, and having a healthy diet was associated with less psychological distress. Yet, the multivariable analyses showed that being female in itself were associated with level of psychological distress.

As the design of this study is cross-sectional, it is not possible to establish a causal association saying that psychological distress is the "outcome" and diet the "exposure" since the relationship could be the opposite direction. However, another study found associations between depressive symptoms and having a diet containing more meat, and that a "meat dietary pattern" was most common in males [16]. Hence, the inconsistent findings regarding the associations between depressive symptoms, diet and gender, need to be further studied.

Furthermore, it is also evident that other lifestyle behaviors, besides diet, influence elderly people's psychological health. This study demonstrates that smoking and alcohol consumption are independently associated with higher levels of psychological distress when adjusting for variables assessing wellbeing, health status, physical functioning and social support. As such, this study confirms that several lifestyle behaviors (diet, smoking and alcohol consumption) are important domains to target in relation to promoting elderly people's health and wellbeing. Smoking is for instance found to be more common in elderly with unhealthy diets [16].

However, it is clear that society needs to be aware of several factors, besides diet and other lifestyle behaviors, when aiming for improving elderly people's psychological status. As this study showed, the ability to prepare warm meals without help from others predicted less psychological distress as well as the ability to socializing with family or friends. These findings, along with evidence from other studies [34, 36, 37], indicate that being social and in interaction with family or friends is of great importance, both for eating healthy and maintaining good psychological health. For instance, the United States has established a variety of programs to improve elderly's diet, increase social interaction, and delay loss of independence. Several benefits, such as better health, better nutritional intake and improved social interaction were found from these programs [36].

For society, having knowledge of factors associated with less psychological distress is important to promote elderly's health and detect risk factors [38]. Several health promotion programs are found effective in supporting elderly's social participation and self-management [9]. In this study, self-management in terms of maintaining the ability to perform activities of daily living, such as preparing warm meals, were associated with less psychological distress. As such, nutrition and food intake play a significant role for both, physical and psychological health in older age [15]. There is evidence that healthy dietary patterns rich in fruit, vegetables, fish, whole grains and starchy low-fat staple foods are likely to promote healthy ageing, including life expectancy and lesser risk of cardiometabolic diseases [39].

## Strengths and limitations

The strength of this study is the large sample of elderly inhabitants. Data includes a detailed registration of food intake, in addition to valid and widely used measurements assessing lifestyle behaviors, health status, wellbeing, physical and social functioning. A limitation of the study is that the questionnaires are all based on self-report, and it has no objective measures of food intake or biological data. However, the data make it possible to investigate associations between self-reported information on lifestyle behaviours such as diet or food intake, and variables assessing elderly's psychological distress, health, wellbeing, social support and physical functioning and compare our findings with other studies from different countries. Another limitation in this study is the cross-sectional design. Even though it is possible to detect associations between diet patterns, life style behaviors, wellbeing, health status, physical functioning, social support and psychological distress in this sample of elderly people, it is not possible to establish a causal association between psychological distress and the other variables.

## Conclusion

This study found that elderly inhabitants with a healthy dietary pattern were associated with less psychological distress when adjusting for other life style behaviors, wellbeing, health status, physical functioning and social support. In addition, less psychological distress were independently associated with favorable health behaviors such as non-smoking and lesser alcohol consumption, better health status, higher wellbeing, more social support and less problems performing activities of daily living. Knowledge about the influence of favorable health behaviors, such as eating healthy in relation to psychological distress, provide valuable insights into how society can promote healthy lifestyles to an ageing population. Society should use this knowledge to improve the quality of life of older persons, e.g. by develop interventions that increase older people's food knowledge and knowledge about how to self-manage and promote one's health.

### Abbreviations

The Hunt Study: the Nord-Trøndelag Health StudyWHOWorld Health OrganizationQOLQuality of lifeADLActivities of daily livingHADSthe Hospital Anxiety and Depression ScaleSCSSocial Cohesion and Support IndexSF-8the Short Form-8 Health Survey

### Acknowledgements

We would like to thank all people involved in The Nord-Trøndelag Health Study (The Hunt Study) data collection. The HUNT Study is a collaboration between HUNT Research Centre (Faculty of Medicine and Health Sciences, Norwegian University and Technology (NTNU)), Nord-Trøndelag County Council, Central Norway Regional Health Authority, and the Norwegian Institute of Public Health.
We would also like to thank all our colleagues in the ProFooSe Study group.

### Funding

This paper is funded by the European Economic Area (EEA) Grants, Promoting Food Security in Portugal (ProFooSe Study) Portugal-Norway. The EEA Grants and Norway Grants represent the contribution of Iceland, Liechtenstein and Norway to reducing economic and social disparities and to strengthening bilateral relations with 15 EU countries in Central and Southern Europe and the Baltics (https://eeagrants.org/).

### Authors' contributions

KG, GAE, CN and BA designed the study, KG performed the data analyses, and all authors (KG, GAE, CN, AMFR, MJG, RS, HC and BA) interpreted the data analyses and participated in the manuscript preparation. All authors read and approved the final manuscript.

### Competing interests

The authors have no financial or non-financial competing interest in the design of the study, data collection, and analysis, interpretation of data or in writing the manuscript.

### Author details

[1]Department of Public Health and Nursing, Center for Health Promotion Research, Norwegian University of Science and Technology (NTNU), Postbox 8905, 7491 Trondheim, Norway. [2]CEDOC, EpiDoC Unit, NOVA Medical School, Universidade Nova de Lisboa, Lisbon, Portugal. [3]EpiSaude Association, Evora, Portugal.

### References

1. WHO. Active aging: a policy framework. 2001a. http://apps.who.int/iris/bitstream/10665/67215/1/WHO_NMH_NPH_02.8.pdf. Accessed 27 Feb 2018.
2. Fries JF. Reducing disability in older age. JAMA. 2002;288:3164–6.
3. Bowling A, Dieppe P. What is successful ageing and who should define it? BMJ. 2005;331:1548–51.
4. WHO. Official Records of the World Health Organization. 1946. New York. http://www.who.int/about/mission/en/
5. Diener E, Eunkook SM, Lucas RE, Smith HL. Subjective well-being: three decades of progress. Psychol Bull. 1999;125:276–302.
6. Gobbens RJJ, Van Assen MALM. The prediction of quality of life by physical, psychological and social components of frailty in community-dwelling older people. Qual Life Res. 2014;23:2289–300.
7. Bang KS, et al. Health Status and the Demand for Healthcare among the Elderly in the Rural Quoc-Oai District of Hanoi in Vietnam. Biomed Res Int. 2017; https://doi.org/10.1155/2017/4830968.
8. Steptoe A, Deaton A, Stone AA. Subjective wellbeing, health, and ageing. Lancet. 2015;385:640–8.
9. Bunt S, Steverink N, Olthof J, van der Schans CP, Hobbelen JSM. Social frailty in older adults: a scoping review. Eur J Ageing. 2017;14:323–34.
10. Poli S, et al. Frailty is associated with socioeconomic and lifestyle factors in community-dwelling older subjects. Aging Clin Exp Res. 2017;29:721–8.
11. Feng, et al. Risk factors and protective factors associated with incident or increase of frailty among community-dwelling older adults: A systematic review of longitudinal studies. PLoS One. 2017; https://doi.org/10.1371/journal.pone.0178383.
12. Lakey SL, et al. Antidepressant use, depressive symptoms, and incident frailty in women aged 65 and older from the Women's Health Initiative observational study. J Am Geriatr Soc. 2012;60:854–61.
13. André B, et al. Is there an association between food patterns and life satisfaction among Norway's inhabitants ages 65 years and older? Appetite. 2017;110:108–15.
14. Hollis JH, Henry CJK. Dietary variety and its effect on food intake of elderly adults. J Hum Nutr Diet. 2007;20:345–51.
15. Milte CM, McNaughton SA. Dietary patterns and successful ageing: a systematic review. Eur J Nutr. 2016;55:423–50.
16. Gregorio MJ, et al. Dietary patterns characterized by high meat consumption are associated with other unhealthy life styles and depression symptoms. Front Nutri. 2017; https://doi.org/10.3389/fnut.2017.00025.
17. Talegawkar SA, et al. A higher adherence to a Mediterranean-style diet is inversely associated with the development of frailty in community-dwelling elderly men and women. J Nutr. 2012;142:2161–6.
18. León-Muñoz LM, et al. Mediterranean diet and risk of frailty in community-dwelling older adults. J Am Med Dir Assoc. 2014;15:899–903.
19. Lana A, Rodriguez-Artalejo F, Lopez-Garcia E. Dairy consumption and risk of frailty in older adults: a prospective cohort study. J Am Geriatr Soc. 2015;63:1852–60.
20. Dean M, et al. Factors influencing eating a varied diet in old age. Public Health Nutr. 2009;12(12):2421–7.
21. Krokstad S, Langhammer A, Hveem K, Holmen TL, Midthjell K, et al. Cohort Profile: the HUNT Study, Norway. Int J Epidemiol. 2013;42:968–77.
22. NTNU. https://hunt-db.medisin.ntnu.no/hunt-db/#/instrument/129. Accessed 27 Feb 2018.
23. Zigmond AS, Snaith RP. The hospital anxiety and depression scale. Acta Psychiatr Scand. 1983;67:61–70.
24. Bjelland I, Dahl AA, Haug TT, Neckelmann. The validity of the Hospital Anxiety and Depression Scale An updated literature review. J Psychosom Res. 2002;52:69–77.
25. Sørensen T, Mastekaasa A, Sandanger I, Kleiner R, Moum T, et al. Contribution of local community integration and personal social network support to mental health. Norsk Epidemiol. 2002;12:269–74.

26. Ware JE, Kosinski M, Dewey JE, Gandek B, et al. How to score and interpret single-item health status measures: a manual for users of the SF-8 health survey. Lincoln: Quality Metric Incorporated; 2001.

27. Bowling A. Just one question: If one question works, why ask several? J Epidemiol Community Health. 2005;59:342–5.

28. Grov EK, Fossa SD, Dahl AA. Activity of daily living problems in older cancer. survivors: a population-based controlled study. Health Soc Care Commun. 2010;18:396–406.

29. IBM Corp. Released 2013. IBM SPSS statistics for windows, version 24.0. Armonk: IBM Corp; 2016.

30. Polit DF. Statistics and data analysis for nursing research. Upper Saddle River: Pearson; 2010.

31. Magidson J, Vermun JK. Latent class models for clustering: A comparison with Kmeans. Can J Market Res. 2002;20:37–44.

32. Myint PK, et al. Lifestyle behaviours and quality-adjusted life years in middle and older age. Age Ageing. 2011;40:589–95.

33. Irz X, Fratiglioni L, Kuosmanen N, Mazzocchi M, Modugno L, et al. Sociodemographic.determinants of diet quality of the EU elderly: a comparative analysis in four countries. Public Health Nutr. 2014;17:1177–89.

34. Conklin AI, Forouhi NG, Surtees P, Khaw KT, Wareham NJ, et al. Social relationships. and healthful dietary behaviour: evidence from over-50s in the EPIC cohort, UK. Soc Sci Med. 2014;100:167–75. https://doi.org/10.1016/j.socscimed.2013.08.018.

35. Song HJ, Simon JR, Patel DU. Food preferences of older adults in senior nutrition. programs. J Nutr Gerontol Geriatr. 2014;33:55–67. https://doi.org/10.1080/21551197.2013.875502.

36. Gergerich E, Shobe M, Christy K. Sustaining Our Nation's Seniors through Federal Food. and Nutrition Programs. J Nutr Gerontol Geriatr. 2015;34:273–91. https://doi.org/10.1080/21551197.2015.1054572.

37. Aartsen M, Veenstra M, Hansen T. Social pathways to health: On the mediating role of the social network in the relation between socio-economic position and health. SSM Popul Health. 2017;3:419–26.

38. Markle-Reid M, Browne G, Weir R, Gafni A, Roberts J, et al. Nurse-led health promotion interventions improve quality of life in frail older home care clients: lessons learned from three randomized trials in Ontario, Canada. J Eval Clin Pract. 2013;19:118–31.

39. Kiefte-de Jong JC, Mathers JC, Franco OH. Nutrition and healthy ageing: the key ingredients. Proc Nutr Soc. 2014;73:249–59.

# 11

# Age dependency of risk factors for cognitive decline

N. Legdeur[1]* (ID), M. W. Heymans[2], H. C. Comijs[3], M. Huisman[2,4], A. B. Maier[5,6] and P. J. Visser[1,7]

## Abstract

**Background:** Risk factors for cognitive decline might depend on chronological age. The aim of the study was to explore the age dependency of risk factors for cognitive decline in cognitively healthy subjects aged 55–85 years at baseline.

**Methods:** We included 2527 cognitively healthy subjects from the Longitudinal Aging Study Amsterdam (LASA). Median follow-up was 9.1 (IQR: 3.2–19.0) years. The association of genetic and cardiovascular risk factors, depressive symptoms, inflammation markers and lifestyle risk factors with decline in MMSE and memory function was tested using spline regression analyses.

**Results:** Subjects were on average 70.1 (SD 8.8) years old at baseline. Based on a spline regression model, we divided our sample in three age groups: ≤70 years (young-old), > 70–80 years (old) and > 80 years (oldest-old). The association of LDL cholesterol, homocysteine, hypertension, history of stroke, depressive symptoms, interleukin-6, a1-antichymotrypsin, alcohol use and smoking with cognitive decline significantly differed between the age groups. In general, the presence of these risk factors was associated with less cognitive decline in the oldest-old group compared to the young-old and old group.

**Conclusions:** The negative effect of various risk factors on cognitive decline decreases with higher age. A combination of epidemiological factors, such as the selection towards healthier subjects during follow-up, but also risk factor specific features, for example ensuring the cerebral blood flow in case of hypertension, explain this diminished association at higher age. It is important to take these age differences into account when applying preventive strategies to avert cognitive decline.

**Keywords:** Cognitive decline, Risk factors, Aging, Oldest-old

## Background

Dementia is a growing health problem with an expected number of 115 million cases worldwide in 2050 [1]. The prevalence of dementia increases steeply with age from a prevalence of 2.6% in subjects aged 65–69 years and a prevalence of 43.1% in subjects aged 90 years and older [1]. Insight in the risk factors for cognitive decline is essential in the search for preventive strategies for cognitive impairment and dementia. Former studies identified a range of potential risk factors including the APOE (apolipoprotein E) ε4 allele, cardiovascular risk factors, depressive symptoms, inflammation markers and

lifestyle factors [2–8]. However, whether the effect of risk factors on cognitive decline in cognitively healthy subjects is dependent on age is not clear, as the majority of the previous studies did not discriminate between younger and older subjects and the number of subjects aged 80 years and older in these studies was generally low [8, 9]. Still, there is increasing evidence that the association of risk factors with cognitive decline becomes less strong at higher age and may even have a protective effect [10]. For example, the risk of the APOE ε4 allele on Alzheimer's dementia (AD) decreases after the age of 70 years [11]. In addition, the association of cardiovascular risk factors with cognitive decline might decrease with increasing age [10, 12–14].

The aim of the present study was to explore whether the association of risk factors with cognitive decline in

* Correspondence: n.legdeur@vumc.nl
[1]Alzheimer Center Amsterdam, Department of Neurology, Amsterdam Neuroscience, Vrije Universiteit Amsterdam, Amsterdam UMC, PO Box 7057, 1007, MB, Amsterdam, the Netherlands
Full list of author information is available at the end of the article

cognitively healthy subjects across the age range of 55 to 85 years was dependent on age. We hypothesized that predictive accuracy would change with age for APOE ε4 allele and cardiovascular risk factors based on previous studies and we performed exploratory analyses to test whether age effects were also present for other established risk factors including depressive symptoms, inflammation markers, alcohol use, smoking and physical activity.

## Methods

### Study sample

Data were derived from the on-going Longitudinal Aging Study Amsterdam (LASA) [15]. This is a longitudinal, population-based study in the Netherlands focusing on trajectories of physical, psychological, social and cognitive functioning in subjects aged 55 years and older. In 1992–1993 a random sample of men and women aged 55–85 years, stratified for age and sex, from three geographic areas of the Netherlands (Amsterdam, Zwolle and Oss) was included. Follow-up measurements were conducted about every 3 years. Data collection included a main and medical interview conducted in the homes of the subjects. The main interview was done by trained and supervised interviewers and the medical interview was performed by trained nurses. All subjects gave informed consent and the study was approved by the Ethical Review Board of the VU University Medical Center (VUmc), Amsterdam, the Netherlands and conducted according to the principles of the Helsinki declaration.

At the start of the study in 1992–1993, 3107 subjects were enrolled. To select cognitively healthy subjects at baseline, subjects with an age and education corrected MMSE lower than 27 points were excluded (this cut-off is based on the lowest 10th percentile of the MMSE in the Maastricht Aging Study (MAAS) [16], leaving 2527 subjects at baseline. In 1995–1996, 2545 subjects were re-examined. See for further details about the following cycles of this LASA cohort and for the sample size per risk factor Additional file 1: Table S1 and S2.

### Measurements

#### Biomaterial

The ApoE phenotyping was done either in 1992–1993 or 1995–1996 at the Immunochemisch Laboratorium of the VUmc. The blood samples were frozen at -80 °C until determination in 1997–1998. The method used is described by Havekes et al. (1987) and consisted of iso-electric focusing of delipidated serum samples, followed by immunoblotting [17]. In the analyses, we used the presence of an ApoE ε4 isoform (phenotypes ε2/4, ε3/4, ε4/4) as a dichotomous variable [17]. The ApoE ε4 isoform was used as proxy for the presence of an APOE ε4 allele.

Cholesterol levels (total cholesterol, High-Density Lipoprotein (HDL) cholesterol and Low-Density Lipoprotein (LDL) cholesterol) and homocysteine (in combination with vitamin B12) were determined in morning blood samples collected in 1995–1996 (second LASA cycle). Subjects were allowed to eat toast and drink tea, but no dairy products. The EDTA plasma samples were stored at -80 °C and analyzed by the Department of Clinical Chemistry of the VUmc in 2001/2002 (homocysteine) and 2005 (cholesterol). For determination of total cholesterol and HDL cholesterol enzymatic colorimetric tests were used. LDL cholesterol was calculated as total cholesterol minus HDL-cholesterol minus VLDL-cholesterol; VLDL-cholesterol was calculated as total triglyceride concentration expressed in mmol/L multiplied by 0.456 [18]. This method is less reliable when the triglyceride level is ≥5.0 mmol/L. Therefore, this analysis was only done for triglyceride levels of < 5.0 mmol/L. Total homocysteine was determined with the Abbott IMx analyser which uses fluorescence polarization immunoassay (FPIA) technology. Serum levels of vitamin B12 were determined at the Endocrine Laboratory of the VUmc with a competitive immunoassay luminescence on the automated ACS 180 System (Bayer Diagnostics, Mijdrecht, The Netherlands).

For determination of the inflammation markers (interleukin-6 (IL-6), C-reactive protein (CRP) and a1-antichymotrypsin (ACT)) serum collected in 1992–1993 (only in Amsterdam and Zwolle) was stored at -80 °C until determination in 2002–2004. Sensitive regular immunoassays (ELISA) were used at Sanquin Research (Amsterdam) to determine IL-6, CRP and ACT. CRP was expressed in ug/ml, IL-6 in pg/ml and ACT in % of normal plasma. The normal human plasma pool (% NHP) used as a standard for ACT contained ~ 300 mg ACT per L. For part of the subjects, CRP levels were determined directly after blood sampling.

Both the cholesterol as the inflammation markers, were added to the analyses as continuous variables.

#### Comorbidity

Hypertension was defined as a blood pressure > 140/90 mmHg measured at the upper arm or the use of antihypertensive medication collected in the first follow-up measurement in 1995–1996 (at baseline blood pressure was measured only at the finger). Post-hoc we also analyzed the association of a measured high blood pressure and the use of antihypertensive medication with cognitive decline separately.

The presence of a history of myocardial infarction (MI), DM or stroke was assessed by self-report. The assessment of comorbidity by self-report was found to be comparable with the medical information reported by the general practitioner [19].

Depressive symptoms were assessed using the Center for Epidemiologic Studies Depression scale (CES-D) [20]. The CES-D is a self-report scale containing 20 items describing depressive symptoms. The maximum score is 60 with higher scores indicating more depressive symptoms. In the analyses, the CES-D was used as a continuous variable.

### Lifestyle

The number of alcohol consumptions was categorized into three categories: 0 alcoholic drinks per day ('none' group), 1–2 alcoholic drinks for men and 1 alcoholic drink for women per day ('minimal' group) or > 2 alcohol drinks for men and > 1 alcohol drink for women per day ('moderate' group) [8]. Smoking was dichotomized in 'yes (or stopped within one year)' or 'no'.

For the assessment of physical activity, the LASA Physical Activity Questionnaire (LAPAQ) was used addressing walking outdoors, bicycling, light household, heavy household, and two sports activities [21]. The subjects are asked how often and how long they carried out these activities in the past 2 weeks. In the analyses, total physical activity in minutes per day was used as a continuous variable.

### Cognitive outcome measures

Two different neuropsychological tests were used as outcome measures: The Mini-Mental State Examination (MMSE) and 15 Words Test (15WT). The MMSE is the most used screening instrument for global cognitive dysfunction [22]. The score ranges from 0 to 30 points, with higher scores indicating better cognitive functioning. The 15WT is the Dutch version of the Auditory Verbal Learning Test [23]. Fifteen words have to be learned over five trials. In LASA the 15WT is restricted to three trials due to a limitation in time. In this study we used the maximum immediate recall score and delayed recall score, both ranging from 0 to 15 words. The delayed recall was assessed after 20 minutes of distraction.

### Statistical analyses

#### Spline regression analyses

Former studies, have shown that the association between age and cognition is nonlinear [24]. Linear regression techniques are therefore not sufficient enough to estimate this association and spline regression analyses are indicated to fit the nonlinear longitudinal associations between age and the cognitive outcome measures more precisely (Additional file 2: Spline regression analyses) [25]. To achieve the best fit of the data with a spline regression model, either linear or cubic splines can be used. Based on the likelihood-ratio (LR) test we

determined which of these two types of splines showed a better fit with our data. We examined the positions where the splines join smoothly together, referred to as knots in spline regression analyses. We identified the optimal position of the knots by testing both a model with one and two knots and moving those 5 years up and down. The ages that corresponded to the position of the knots were used to separate our sample into different age groups, to facilitate interpretation of results. Lastly, for all the different risk factors and outcome measures we compared our final model with a linear regression model without splines to test whether the model with splines showed a better fit (based on the LR test).

### Differences between age groups at baseline

Statistically significant differences in baseline characteristics between the age groups were determined by using ANOVA for continuous variables, chi-square for categorical variables and Kruskal-Wallis test for skewed variables. Mixed model analysis was used to determine the difference in cognitive test score change per year in the age groups.

### Association of risk factors with cognitive outcome measures

We performed three different analyses to determine the association of the risk factors (measured at baseline or, for hypertension and some biomaterial measurements, in the second cycle) with the cognitive outcome measures. In all these analyses, splines (determined as described in 2.3.1) were added to the model to estimate the association between age and the cognitive outcome measure. First, we determined the association of the risk factors with the three cognitive outcome measures in the total sample by using a linear mixed model (including a random intercept and fixed slopes). Secondly, we added the interaction of the risk factors with the splines to the analyses to assess the age dependency of the risk factors. Because the splines represent different age groups, a significant interaction means that the association of that risk factor with the cognitive outcome measure is different between age groups. If this interaction was statistically significant for a categorized risk factor, we visualized the association in a figure. Lastly, we determined the association coefficient per age group of the risk factors with the cognitive outcome measures. This last step helps us to interpret the results we found with the interaction analyses (we also performed these analyses for the risk factors that did not show a significant interaction). All the analyses were adjusted for sex and education (in years).

### Selection during follow-up

To determine whether there was a selection towards healthier subjects during follow-up, we determined the *baseline* values of the risk factors and cognitive outcome measures of the subjects that were present in the sample during each LASA cycle. Decreasing baseline values during follow-up would be indicative of selection towards healthier subjects.

### Statistical software
The spline regression analyses were performed with the statistical software R version 3.2.5 (http://www.r-project.org). The statistical significance of the association of the risk factor with cognitive decline per age group was determined with Stata version 15. The differences in baseline characteristics between the three age groups were analyzed with SPSS Statistics version 22. The level of significance was set to $p = 0.05$.

## Results
We included 2527 subjects (51.2% women) who were on average 70.1 (SD: 8.8, range: 54.8–85.6) years at baseline and had 9.1 (SD: 3.4) years of education (Table 1). Median follow-up was 9.1 (IQR: 3.2–19.0) years.

### Determination of the best-fitted spline regression model
For the longitudinal associations between the cognitive outcome measures and age in the total group, a linear spline regression model showed a better fit then a cubic spline regression model. A model with two knots placed at the ages 70 and 80 years showed the best fit for the three outcome measures, dividing the sample in three age groups: ≤70 years (young-old subjects), > 70–80 years (old subjects) and > 80 years (oldest-old subjects) (Fig. 1). The spline regression model showed a better fit then a linear regression model without splines for all the different associations.

### Differences between age groups at baseline
Most characteristics differed between age groups (Table 1). Years of education, follow-up time, scores on the cognitive tests, total and LDL cholesterol levels, alcohol use, smoking and physical activity all decreased with age. The level of homocysteine and inflammation markers and the presence of cardiovascular comorbidities and depressive symptoms increased with age.

### Association of risk factors with cognitive decline in the total sample
In the total sample, the presence of high homocysteine levels, history of stroke and depressive symptoms were associated with more decline in MMSE and the 15WT (Table 2). Alcohol use was associated with less decline in MMSE and the 15WT. The presence of APOE ε4 was associated with more decline in MMSE and a history of DM with more decline in the 15WT. Cholesterol levels, hypertension, history of MI, inflammation markers,

smoking and physical activity were not associated with cognitive decline.

### Age dependency of risk factors
The association of LDL cholesterol, homocysteine, hypertension, history of stroke, depressive symptoms, IL-6, ACT, alcohol use and smoking with cognitive decline differed between the age groups (Table 3 and Fig. 2). The presence of APOE ε4, total and HDL cholesterol level, a history of DM or MI, CRP level and physical activity did not show an age effect. In general, the regression coefficient changed from a negative association in the young-old and old subjects to a positive association in the oldest-old subjects. This means that on top of the decline in MMSE and 15WT as visualized in Fig. 1, the presence of these risk factors was associated with more decline in MMSE or 15WT in the young-old and old subjects and less decline in MMSE or 15WT in the oldest-old subjects. If we determined the association of the age-dependent risk factors with cognitive decline per age group, we found that hypertension, high IL-6 levels, and alcohol use were significantly associated with less cognitive decline in the oldest-old subjects (Table 3 and Additional file 1: Tables S5–S6). Smoking was significantly associated with more memory decline in the young-old subjects and high LDL cholesterol with more MMSE decline in the young-old subjects (Table 3 and Additional file 1: Table S6).

Post-hoc analyses with hypertension defined by the measured high blood pressure only or the use of antihypertensive medication only, yielded similar results (Additional file 1: Table S3).

### Selection during follow-up
Subjects who were retained in the later LASA cycles had a lower age, higher level of education, higher scores on the cognitive outcome measures, higher cholesterol levels, less comorbidities, lower levels of inflammation markers, higher alcohol use, lower levels of smoking and had a higher level of physical activity at baseline compared to subjects who dropped out during follow-up (Additional file 1: Table S4).

## Discussion
This study showed that the association of LDL cholesterol, homocysteine, hypertension, history of stroke, depressive symptoms, IL-6, ACT, alcohol use and smoking with cognitive decline was age-dependent. In general, these risk factors were associated with more cognitive decline in the young-old and old subjects and less cognitive decline in the oldest-old subjects. APOE ε4 genotype and DM were negatively associated with cognitive decline regardless of age.

**Table 1** Baseline characteristics of subjects in the total sample

| Characteristic | Total sample | ≤70 years | > 70–80 years | > 80 years | P-value[b] |
|---|---|---|---|---|---|
| Sample size[a] | 2527 | 1292 | 794 | 441 | |
| Age, y | 70.1 (8.8) | 62.6 (4.2) | 75.5 (2.9) | 82.6 (1.5) | |
| Female, % | 51.2 | 52.3 | 50.0 | 50.3 | 0.48 |
| Education, y | 9.1 (3.4) | 9.5 (3.3) | 8.7 (3.2) | 8.6 (3.7) | < 0.01 |
| Follow-up, y (median, IQR) | 9.1 (3.2–19.0) | 13.3 (8.9–19.2) | 6.2 (3.0–13.0) | 4.9 (3.3–8.9) | < 0.01 |
| MMSE, points (median, IQR) | 28 (27–29) | 29 (26–30) | 28 (24–30) | 27 (24–30) | < 0.01 |
| Change in MMSE per year (SE) | −0.11 (0.00) | − 0.06 (0.00) | − 0.18 (0.01) | − 0.25 (0.02) | < 0.01 |
| 15WT immediate recall, words | 8.1 (2.5) | 8.9 (2.3) | 7.6 (2.4) | 6.3 (2.1) | < 0.01 |
| Change in 15WT immediate recall per year (SE) | −0.11 (0.00) | −0.07 (0.00) | − 0.11 (0.01) | −0.07 (0.02) | < 0.01 |
| 15WT delayed recall, words | 5.3 (2.7) | 6.2 (2.6) | 4.7 (2.5) | 3.5 (2.2) | < 0.01 |
| Change in 15WT delayed recall per year (SE) | −0.11 (0.00) | −0.05 (0.01) | − 0.10 (0.01) | −0.06 (0.02) | < 0.01 |
| APOE ε4, %[c] | 26.3 | 27.8 | 25.2 | 23.6 | 0.29 |
| Total cholesterol, mmol/L | 5.7 (1.0) | 5.9 (1.0) | 5.6 (1.0) | 5.3 (1.1) | < 0.01 |
| LDL cholesterol, mmol/L | 3.7 (1.0) | 3.8 (0.9) | 3.6 (0.9) | 3.4 (1.1) | < 0.01 |
| HDL cholesterol, mmol/L | 1.3 (0.4) | 1.3 (0.4) | 1.4 (0.4) | 1.3 (0.4) | 0.48 |
| Homocysteine, mmol/L | 14.5 (6.1) | 13.5 (5.2) | 14.7 (5.0) | 17.2 (9.2) | < 0.01 |
| Vitamin B12, pMol/L (median, IR) | 266 (212–333) | 268 (219–335) | 264 (213–331) | 249 (196–333) | 0.12 |
| Hypertension, % | 76.7 | 72.9 | 82.2 | 73.7 | < 0.01 |
| Myocardial infarction, % | 8.8 | 6.4 | 11.1 | 11.7 | < 0.01 |
| Diabetes mellitus, % | 7.0 | 4.3 | 8.6 | 12.3 | < 0.01 |
| Stroke, % | 4.4 | 1.6 | 6.7 | 8.7 | < 0.01 |
| CES-D total score (median, IQR) | 5 (2–11) | 5 (2–9) | 6 (3–11) | 7 (3–12) | < 0.01 |
| IL-6, pg/ml (median, IQR) | 1.4 (0.6–2.5) | 1.3 (0.6–2.4) | 1.6 (0.7–2.7) | 1.8 (1.0–3.1) | < 0.01 |
| CRP, ug/ml (median, IQR) | 2.2 (1.0–4.7) | 2.0 (0.9–3.9) | 2.5 (1.3–5.6) | 2.8 (1.4–5.7) | < 0.01 |
| ACT, % of NHP | 173.6 (57.6) | 169.6 (53.0) | 179.3 (66.1) | 177.2 (54.1) | 0.01 |
| Alcohol consumption, % | | | | | |
| None | 20.1 | 15.6 | 25.3 | 24.7 | < 0.01 |
| Minimal[d] | 20.6 | 17.8 | 23.6 | 23.6 | |
| Moderate[e] | 59.4 | 66.6 | 51.1 | 51.7 | |
| Smokers, % | 24.6 | 30.4 | 23.1 | 19.8 | < 0.01 |
| Total physical activity, min per day | 169.2 (114.2) | 188.4 (121.3) | 160.0 (103.7) | 126.8 (95.3) | < 0.01 |

15WT 15 Words Test, ACT a1-antichymotrypsin, APOE apolipoprotein E, CES-D Center for Epidemiologic Studies Depression scale, CRP C-reactive protein, HDL High-Density Lipoprotein, IL-6 interleukin-6, IQR interquartile range, LASA Longitudinal Aging Study Amsterdam, LDL Low-Density Lipoprotein, MMSE Mini-Mental State Examination, NHP normal human plasma, SE standard error
[a]Sample size varies per characteristic (Additional file 1: Table S2). [b]Differences between the three age groups tested with ANOVA for continuous variables, chi-square for categorical variables, Kruskal-Wallis test for non-parametric variables and mixed model analysis for the change in cognitive test scores per year.
[c]Percentage of subjects with an apolipoprotein E ε4 isoform as proxy for an APOE ε4 allele. [d]Women:1 drink/day, men: 1–2 drinks/day. [e]Women: > 1 drink/day, men: > 2 drinks/day. Values are means (SD) unless stated otherwise

Before we discuss these findings in more detail, it should be noted that the baseline age of the subjects with follow-up was lower than that of the subjects who were lost to follow up. The subjects with follow-up also showed a better overall health with less comorbidity. The selection towards younger and healthier subjects at follow-up may explain why the negative impact of the risk factors was strongest in younger subjects. However, it does not explain why these risk factors became

protective at higher age. We reduced the potential selection bias by combining baseline data and follow-up data across the age span in the spline regression model. In this way follow-up data of the selected younger, healthier subjects (Additional file 1: Table S4) were combined with baseline data of the older, less healthy subjects (Table 1).

In addition, most subjects dropped out of the study because of mortality [15]. A comparison of one-year

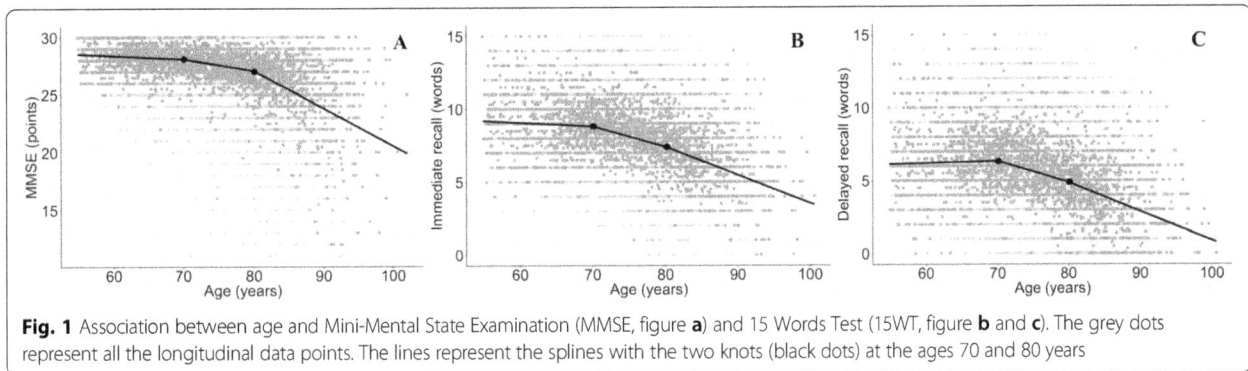

**Fig. 1** Association between age and Mini-Mental State Examination (MMSE, figure **a**) and 15 Words Test (15WT, figure **b** and **c**). The grey dots represent all the longitudinal data points. The lines represent the splines with the two knots (black dots) at the ages 70 and 80 years

mortality rates of LASA subjects with those in the general Dutch population showed that mortality in the LASA subjects was slightly higher than in the general population, but that this difference exceeded 1% only in women aged 80–85 years (unpublished data). Therefore, it may not necessarily affect the generalizability of our findings.

### APOE genotype
Our finding that the APOE ε4 genotype increases the risk for cognitive decline regardless of age is at odds with some earlier studies that reported a decrease of risk for dementia with age [11, 26] but is consistent with others [27]. Differences between studies may be

explained by differences in selection of subjects (normal cognition or MCI) and outcome measure (progression to dementia or cognitive decline).

### Cardiovascular factors
Most cardiovascular factors were associated with less decline at higher age than at younger age, which is in line with previous studies [12, 28]. High cholesterol in late-life can be an indicator of a better nutritional status and a better overall health and therefore associated with less cognitive decline [28, 29]. Additionally, cholesterol synthesis is thought to decrease with aging, but only in AD patients and not in subjects with a normal cognition [30]. The association of low cholesterol with more

**Table 2** The association of risk factors with cognitive decline in the total sample

| Risk factor | MMSE | | | 15WT immediate recall | | | 15WT delayed recall | | |
|---|---|---|---|---|---|---|---|---|---|
| | B | SE | P-value | B | SE | P-value | B | SE | P-value |
| APOE ε4 | −0.25 | 0.24 | < 0.01 | −0.07 | 1.27 | 0.49 | −0.09 | 1.44 | 0.42 |
| Total cholesterol | 0.05 | 0.17 | 0.34 | 0.09 | 1.22 | 0.11 | 0.08 | 1.39 | 0.21 |
| LDL cholesterol | 0.05 | 0.17 | 0.41 | 0.08 | 1.24 | 0.20 | 0.08 | 1.41 | 0.25 |
| HDL cholesterol | 0.16 | 0.16 | 0.20 | 0.23 | 1.21 | 0.08 | 0.07 | 1.42 | 0.67 |
| Homocysteine | −0.05 | 0.12 | < 0.01 | −0.05 | 1.16 | < 0.01 | − 0.06 | 1.33 | < 0.01 |
| Hypertension | 0.13 | 0.28 | 0.26 | −0.02 | 1.26 | 0.88 | −0.03 | 1.43 | 0.85 |
| DM | −0.16 | 0.29 | 0.25 | −0.42 | 1.28 | 0.01 | −0.42 | 1.45 | 0.04 |
| MI | 0.05 | 0.29 | 0.69 | 0.08 | 1.28 | 0.58 | 0.22 | 1.48 | 0.21 |
| Stroke | −0.40 | 0.28 | 0.02 | −0.55 | 1.27 | 0.01 | −0.58 | 1.44 | 0.02 |
| Depressive symptoms | −0.01 | 0.33 | < 0.01 | −0.02 | 1.33 | < 0.01 | −0.02 | 1.50 | < 0.01 |
| CRP | 0.00 | 0.27 | 0.57 | −0.01 | 1.27 | 0.15 | −0.01 | 1.45 | 0.47 |
| IL-6 | 0.01 | 0.26 | 0.46 | 0.01 | 1.27 | 0.72 | 0.02 | 1.44 | 0.42 |
| ACT | 0.00 | 0.27 | 0.68 | 0.00 | 1.27 | 0.74 | 0.00 | 1.45 | 0.87 |
| Alcohol[a]: minimal[b] | 0.27 | 0.10 | < 0.01 | 0.35 | 0.12 | < 0.01 | 0.35 | 0.14 | 0.01 |
| Alcohol[a]: moderate[c] | 0.24 | 0.08 | < 0.01 | 0.41 | 0.10 | < 0.01 | 0.42 | 0.12 | < 0.01 |
| Smoking | −0.09 | 0.25 | 0.26 | −0.16 | 1.27 | 0.09 | −0.03 | 1.46 | 0.77 |
| Physical activity | 0.00 | 0.30 | 0.78 | 0.00 | 1.28 | 0.59 | 0.00 | 1.45 | 0.24 |

B's are determined by linear mixed models in combination with splines and adjusted for sex and education

15WT 15 Words Test, ACT a1-antichymotrypsin, APOE apolipoprotein E, CRP C-reactive protein, DM Diabetes mellitus, HDL High-Density Lipoprotein, IL-6 interleukin-6, LDL Low-Density Lipoprotein, MI Myocardial infarction, MMSE Mini-Mental State Examination

[a]No alcohol use is reference group. [b]Women:1 drink/day, men: 1–2 drinks/day. [c]Women: > 1 drink/day, men: > 2 drinks/day

**Table 3** The association of risk factors with cognitive decline per age group

| Risk factor | MMSE | | | 15WT immediate recall | | | 15WT delayed recall | | |
|---|---|---|---|---|---|---|---|---|---|
| | ≤70 | > 70–80 | > 80 | ≤70 | > 70–80 | > 80 | ≤70 | > 70–80 | > 80 |
| APOE ε4 | 0.72 | **−4.24** | **−10.17** | −0.65 | **−3.85** | **−5.32** | 0.18 | **−4.15** | **−8.52** |
| Total cholesterol | −3.37 | −0.10 | 1.26 | −1.08 | − 1.09 | 1.53 | 0.97 | −1.53 | 1.27 |
| LDL cholesterol | **−5.40*** | 0.66 | 1.83* | −0.18 | −1.92* | 1.96* | 0.68 | **−2.62** | 1.41 |
| HDL cholesterol | 7.35 | −2.17 | −1.07 | − 1.84 | 2.64 | 0.50 | 6.21 | 1.45 | 2.97 |
| Homocysteine | 0.39 | −0.40 | **−0.92** | − 0.39 | − 0.21 | 0.13 | − 0.76* | −0.08 | 0.13* |
| Hypertension | 0.04 | −2.14* | **6.52*** | −5.65* | −0.22 | **5.06*** | −4.04 | 3.54 | 0.43 |
| DM | −0.95 | −0.46 | −9.32 | − 0.11 | −3.49 | −0.29 | −1.68 | −5.44 | 4.90 |
| MI | 2.42 | −1.59 | 2.23 | 0.41 | 1.93 | 5.64 | 4.90 | 0.62 | **10.14** |
| Stroke | 1.25 | −9.16* | 9.16* | 2.60 | −0.34 | 6.70 | 0.79 | −1.58 | −4.30 |
| Depressive symptoms | −0.07 | 0.02 | −0.06 | −0.21 | 0.00 | 0.07 | −0.11* | −0.23 | 0.21* |
| CRP | −0.18 | 0.18 | 0.19 | −0.21 | 0.03 | 0.19 | −0.19 | −0.11 | 0.16 |
| IL-6 | 0.02* | −0.10* | **1.31*** | 0.27 | −0.11 | 0.64 | 0.31 | −0.03 | 0.88 |
| ACT | 0.00 | 0.01 | **0.06** | −0.01 | − 0.01 | 0.03 | − 0.01* | −0.04 | 0.03* |
| Alcohol[a]: minimal[b] | 2.82* | −0.26 | **7.93*** | 3.19 | −3.09 | −0.31 | 5.91 | −3.03 | 0.25 |
| Alcohol[a]: moderate[c] | 0.78 | −0.95 | 3.48 | 2.85 | −3.51 | 1.42 | 3.19 | −0.47 | −0.69 |
| Smoking | −0.30 | −1.05 | −5.15 | **−5.84*** | 0.53* | −1.13 | **−4.52** | −2.88 | −0.61 |
| Physical activity | 0.00 | 0.00 | **0.02** | −0.01 | 0.01 | 0.00 | 0.01 | 0.01 | 0.00 |

Shown are beta's (multiplied by 100) of the associations of a risk factor with cognitive decline within each age group. They show the extra cognitive decline (next to the overall cognitive decline as visualized in Fig. 1) per age group in the presence of a risk factor. A negative beta indicates that a unit increase in the risk factor is associated with more cognitive decline. Bold beta's indicate a significant (*p* < 0.05) association with cognitive decline in that age group (in Additional file 1: Tables S5–S7 we present the standard errors and *p*-values corresponding to the beta's in this table per age group)

*15WT* 15 Words Test, *ACT* a1-antichymotrypsin, *IL-6* interleukin-6, *LDL* Low-Density Lipoprotein, *MMSE* Mini-Mental State Examination

*Association of risk factor with MMSE or 15WT decline is significantly different between these two age groups. In case of three *: difference is significant between ≤70 and > 80 years old group and between > 70–80 and > 80 years old group. Beta's are determined by linear mixed models in combination with splines and adjusted for sex and education

[a]No alcohol use is reference group. [b]Women:1 drink/day, men: 1–2 drinks/day. [c]Women: > 1 drink/day, men: > 2 drink/day

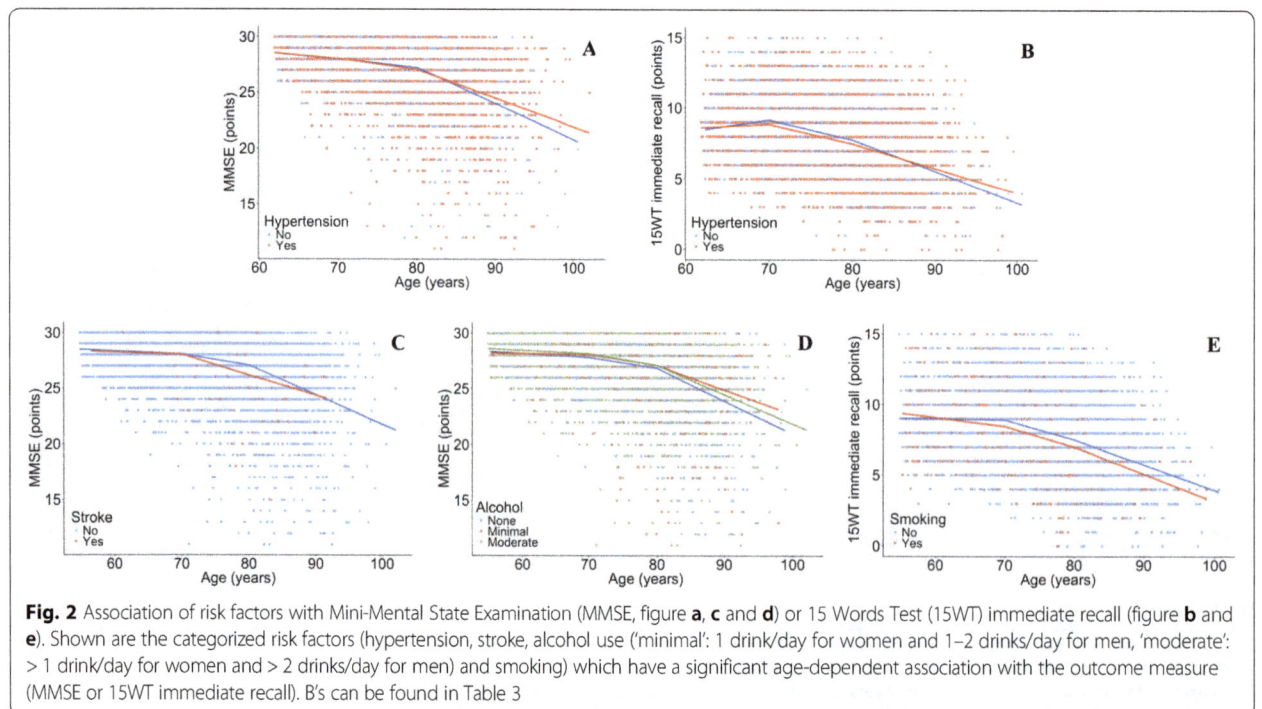

**Fig. 2** Association of risk factors with Mini-Mental State Examination (MMSE, figure **a**, **c** and **d**) or 15 Words Test (15WT) immediate recall (figure **b** and **e**). Shown are the categorized risk factors (hypertension, stroke, alcohol use ('minimal': 1 drink/day for women and 1–2 drinks/day for men, 'moderate': > 1 drink/day for women and > 2 drinks/day for men) and smoking) which have a significant age-dependent association with the outcome measure (MMSE or 15WT immediate recall). B's can be found in Table 3

cognitive decline in the oldest-old subjects might therefore be an expression of underlying AD pathology.

Hypertension may prevent cognitive decline at old age by ensuring the cerebral blood flow [31, 32]. On the other hand, low blood pressure can be a consequence of neurodegenerative disease and therefore an early sign of dementia onset, although this is an aspect which one can also expect in the young-old subjects [33, 34].

### Depressive symptoms

Earlier studies have shown that depressive symptoms are an important risk factor for cognitive decline and dementia, also among the oldest-old subjects [7, 35]. We replicated this finding for the total sample but also found that the association of depressive symptoms with memory decline was less in the oldest-old group than in the young-old group. This may be explained by the fact that older subjects score higher on the CES-D questionnaire for reasons other than depression, such as somatic morbidity [36]. In line with this explanation, earlier cross-domain latent growth models on LASA data demonstrated that delayed recall was associated with increasing levels of depressed affect, but not with depressive somatic symptoms [37].

### Inflammation markers

Inflammation has been described as an important mechanism underlying cognitive decline but most of these studies were performed in younger subjects [38]. We did not find an association of inflammation markers with cognitive decline in the total sample but noted differences between age groups showing that higher IL-6 and ACT levels were associated with less cognitive decline in subjects aged 80 years and older compared to younger subjects. Potentially, higher inflammation markers in older subjects are a sign of a better inflammatory response and therefore related to better overall health and cognitive functioning.

### Lifestyle factors

Minimal and moderate alcohol use were positively associated with decline in MMSE and memory functioning compared to no alcohol use, which is in line with earlier studies [3, 8]. We found that the positive association of alcohol use with cognition was strongest in subjects aged 80 years and older. In this age group, no alcohol use is frequently related to poor physical functioning. Therefore, the negative association of no alcohol use with cognitive decline is potentially an indirect effect [39].

In accordance with our findings, a meta-analysis in 2015 showed that the negative association of smoking with cognitive decline is decreasing with age [40]. Survival bias and the presence of competing risks are probably the most important phenomena to explain this finding [40–42].

In contrast to a meta-analysis of observational studies, we did not find an association between physical activity and cognitive decline [43]. However, a meta-analysis of intervention studies on the effect of aerobic exercise on cognitive decline in cognitively normal subjects did not find an effect [44]. We found that in the oldest age group less physical activity was associated with more cognitive decline, but because the over age interaction effect was not statistically significant, this finding should be interpreted cautiously.

### Cognitive outcome measures

We used different cognitive tests as outcome measure (MMSE, 15WT total and delayed recall) and in the total sample, most variables showed similar findings for the different outcome measures and the course of the tests was very similar with age (Table 2 and Fig. 1). However, we also found different results for the different outcomes, which may be explained by the fact that the tests measure different disease processes; memory decline is presumed to be an early marker of Alzheimer's disease and decline in MMSE can be caused by a broader range of diseases [45].

### Strengths and limitations

This is the first study that analyzes the influence of age on the association of different types of risk factors with cognitive decline in one prospective cohort study. Earlier studies have indicated age differences but never studied the various risk factors in one cohort. Additionally, the use of a nonlinear analyze technique, is an important added value of this study to earlier literature. A limitation of this study is that we did not have data about the presence of cardiovascular risk factors, such as hypertension and high cholesterol, before age 55 years. Therefore, we could not discriminate between a high blood pressure and cholesterol emerging at high age or already present at younger ages. While we tested many risk factors with different outcomes at the same time, this also increased the risk of false-positive findings. However, we decided not to correct for multiple testing given the exploratory nature of the study and the increased risk of missing important findings when applying Bonferroni adjustments (type II errors) [46, 47]. For simplification purposes, we describe our results in relation to cognitive decline, although we only used the MMSE and 15WT to assess cognition. It therefore needs to be noted that these results cannot automatically be extrapolated to other forms of cognition. In addition, the 15WT is a test for verbal episodic memory and does not assess other types of memory such as visual and semantic memory.

## Scientific and clinical implications

With this study we showed that age needs to be taken into consideration when studying risk factors for cognitive decline. It is not only needed to add age as a confounder but especially as an effect modifier to analyses as it changes the relation between a risk factor and cognitive decline. From a clinical perspective, these results suggest that different preventive strategies might be effective in young-old versus oldest-old subjects. Antihypertensive and cholesterol lowering medication might not be appropriate for the oldest-old subjects who develop hypertension and hypercholesterolemia at a high age.

## Conclusions

The associations of LDL cholesterol, homocysteine, hypertension, history of stroke, depressive symptoms, IL-6, ACT, alcohol use and smoking with cognitive decline were different per age group. They were all less strongly associated with cognitive decline in the older subjects compared to younger subjects. Selection towards healthier subjects during follow-up need to be considered as possible explanation but also risk factor specific considerations, such as ensuring the cerebral blood flow in case of hypertension, need to be taken into account. These age differences are important when applying preventive strategies to avert cognitive decline.

## Abbreviations

15WT: 15 Words Test; ACT: A1-antichymotrypsin; AD: Alzheimer's dementia; APOE: Apolipoprotein E; CES-D: Center for Epidemiologic Studies Depression scale; CRP: C-reactive protein; DM: Diabetes mellitus; HDL cholesterol: High-Density Lipoprotein cholesterol; IL-6: Interleukin-6; IQR: Interquartile range; LAPAQ: LASA Physical Activity Questionnaire; LASA: Longitudinal Aging Study Amsterdam; LDL cholesterol: Low-Density Lipoprotein cholesterol; LR: Likelihood-ratio; MAAS: Maastricht Aging Study; MI: Myocardial infarction; MMSE: Mini-Mental State Examination; NHP: Normal human plasma; SD: Standard deviation; SE: Standard error; VLDL cholesterol: Very-low-density lipoprotein cholesterol; VUmc: VU University Medical Center

## Funding

This work has received support from the EU/EFPIA Innovative Medicines Initiative Joint Undertaking EMIF grant agreement no. 115372. The Longitudinal Aging Study Amsterdam (LASA) is primarily funded by the Dutch Ministry of Health, Welfare and Sports and the VU University Amsterdam.

## Authors' contributions

MH and HCC are both involved in the design of the Longitudinal Aging Study Amsterdam and are responsible for the data collection. PJV created the concept for this manuscript. MWH and NL performed the statistical analyses. NL wrote the first and final drafts of the manuscript. MWH, HCC, MH, ABM and PJV contributed to and approved the final version.

## Competing interests

PJV is currently acting as a Section Editor for BMC Geriatrics. The other authors declare that they have no competing interests.

## Author details

[1]Alzheimer Center Amsterdam, Department of Neurology, Amsterdam Neuroscience, Vrije Universiteit Amsterdam, Amsterdam UMC, PO Box 7057, 1007, MB, Amsterdam, the Netherlands. [2]Department of Epidemiology and Biostatistics, Amsterdam Public Health Research Institute, Vrije Universiteit Amsterdam, Amsterdam, the Netherlands. [3]GGZ inGeest / Department of Psychiatry, Amsterdam Public Health Research Institute, Vrije Universiteit Amsterdam, Amsterdam, the Netherlands. [4]Department of Sociology, Vrije Universiteit Amsterdam, Amsterdam, the Netherlands. [5]Department of Medicine and Aged Care, @AgeMelbourne, Royal Melbourne Hospital, University of Melbourne, Melbourne, Australia. [6]Department of Human Movement Sciences, @AgeAmsterdam, Faculty of Behavioural and Movement Sciences, Vrije Universiteit Amsterdam, Amsterdam, the Netherlands. [7]Department of Psychiatry & Neuropsychology, School for Mental Health and Neuroscience, Maastricht University, Maastricht, the Netherlands.

## References

1. World Health Organization and Alzheimer's Disease International. Dementia - A public health priority. 2012.
2. Kramer AF, Colcombe SJ, McAuley E, Scalf PE, Erickson KI. Fitness, aging and neurocognitive function. Neurobiol Aging. 2005;26:124–7. https://doi.org/10.1016/j.neurobiolaging.2005.09.009.
3. Baumgart M, Snyder HM, Carrillo MC, Fazio S, Kim H, Johns H. Summary of the evidence on modifiable risk factors for cognitive decline and dementia: a population-based perspective. Alzheimers Dement. 2015;11:1–9. https://doi.org/10.1016/j.jalz.2015.05.016.
4. Smith RG, Todd S, Passmore PA. Chronic medical disease and cognitive aging: toward a healthy body and brain. Inflammation and Cognitive Decline. Edited by Kristine Yaffe. Can Geriatr J. 2013;16(3):143–44.
5. Bretsky P, Guralnik JM, Launer L, Albert M, Seeman TE. The role of APOE-epsilon4 in longitudinal cognitive decline: MacArthur studies of successful aging. Neurology. 2003;60:1077–81. https://doi.org/10.1212/01.WNL.0000055875.26908.24.
6. Cheng G, Huang C, Deng H, Wang H. Diabetes as a risk factor for dementia and mild cognitive impairment: a meta-analysis of longitudinal studies. Intern Med J. 2012;42:484–91. https://doi.org/10.1111/j.1445-5994.2012.02758.x.
7. Van Den Kommer TN, Comijs HC, Aartsen MJ, Huisman M, Deeg DJH, Beekman ATF. Depression and cognition: how do they interrelate in old age? Am J Geriatr Psychiatry. 2013;21:398–410. https://doi.org/10.1016/j.jagp.2012.12.015.
8. Anstey KJ, Mack HA, Cherbuin N. Alcohol consumption as a risk factor for dementia and cognitive decline: Meta-analysis of prospective studies. Am J Geriatr Psychiatry. 2009;17:542–55. https://doi.org/10.1097/JGP.0b013e3181a2fd07.
9. Anstey KJ, Lipnicki DM, Low L-F. Cholesterol as a risk factor for dementia and cognitive decline: a systematic review of prospective studies with Meta-analysis. Am J Geriatr Psychiatry. 2008;16:343–54. https://doi.org/10.1097/01.JGP.0000310778.20870.ae.
10. Bullain SS, Corrada MM. Dementia in the oldest old. Continuum (Minneap Minn). 2013;19:457–69. https://doi.org/10.1212/01.CON.0000429172.27815.3f.
11. Farrer LA, Cupples LA, Haines JL, Hyman B, Kukull WA, Mayeux R, et al. Effects of age, sex, and ethnicity on the association between apolipoprotein E genotype and Alzheimer disease. A meta-analysis. APOE and Alzheimer disease Meta analysis consortium. JAMA. 1997;278:1349–56. https://doi.org/10.1001/jama.1997.03550160069041.
12. Qiu C, Winblad B, Fratiglioni L. The age-dependent relation of blood pressure to cognitive function and dementia. Lancet Neurol. 2005;4:487–99. https://doi.org/10.1016/S1474-4422(05)70141-1.
13. Harrison SL, Stephan BCM, Siervo M, Granic A, Davies K, Wesnes KA, et al. Is there an association between metabolic syndrome and cognitive function in very old adults? The Newcastle 85+ study. J Am Geriatr Soc. 2015;63:667–75. https://doi.org/10.1111/jgs.13358.
14. van den Berg E, Biessels GJ, de Craen a J, Gussekloo J, RGJ W. The metabolic

syndrome is associated with decelerated cognitive decline in the oldest old. Neurology. 2007;69:979–85. https://doi.org/10.1212/01.wnl.0000271381.30143.75.

15. Huisman M, Poppelaars J, van der Horst M, Beekman ATF, Brug J, van Tilburg TG, et al. Cohort profile: the longitudinal aging study Amsterdam. Int J Epidemiol. 2011;40:868–76. https://doi.org/10.1093/ije/dyq219.

16. Reijs BLR, Ramakers IHGB, Elias-Sonnenschein L, Teunissen CE, Koel-Simmelink M, Tsolaki M, et al. Relation of odor identification with Alzheimer's disease markers in cerebrospinal fluid and cognition. J Alzheimers Dis. 2017;60:1025–34. https://doi.org/10.3233/JAD-170564.

17. Havekes LM, De Knijff P, Beisiegel U. A rapid micromethod for apolipoprotein E phenotyping directly in serum. J Lipid Res. 1987;28:455–63.

18. Friedewald WT, Levy RI, Fredrickson DS. Estimation of the concentration of low-density lipoprotein cholesterol in plasma, without use of the preparative ultracentrifuge. Clin Chem. 1972;18:499–502.

19. Kriegsman DM, Penninx BW, van Eijk JT, Boeke AJ, Deeg DJ. Self-reports and general practitioner information on the presence of chronic diseases in community dwelling elderly. A study on the accuracy of patients' self-reports and on determinants of inaccuracy. J Clin Epidemiol. 1996;49:1407–17. https://doi.org/10.1016/S0895-4356(96)00274-0.

20. Radloff LS, Teri L. Use of the Center for Epidemiological Studies-Depression Scale with older adults. Clin Gerontol. 1986;5:119–36. https://doi.org/10.1007/BF01537606.

21. Stel VS, Smit JH, Pluijm SMF, Visser M, Deeg DJH, Lips P. Comparison of the LASA physical activity questionnaire with a 7-day diary and pedometer. J Clin Epidemiol. 2004;57:252–8. https://doi.org/10.1016/j.jclinepi.2003.07.008.

22. Folstein MF, Folstein SE, McHugh PR. "Mini-mental state". A practical method for grading the cognitive state of patients for the clinician. J Psychiatr Res. 1975;12:189–98. https://doi.org/10.1016/0022-3956(75)90026-6.

23. Rey A. L'examen clinique en psychologie. Paris: Presses Universitaires de France; 1964.

24. Verhaeghen P, Salthouse TA. Meta-analyses of age-cognition relations in adulthood: estimates of linear and nonlinear age effects and structural models. Psychol Bull. 1997;122:231–49. https://doi.org/10.1037//0033-2909.122.3.231.

25. Chen H, Zhao B, Cao G, Proges EC, O'Shea A, Woods AJ, et al. Statistical approaches for the study of cognitive and brain aging. Front Aging Neurosci. 2016;8:1–10. https://doi.org/10.3389/fnagi.2016.00176.

26. Corrada MM, Paganini-Hill A, Berlau DJ, Kawas CH. Apolipoprotein e genotype, dementia, and mortality in the oldest old: the 90+ study. Alzheimers Dement. 2013;9:12–8. https://doi.org/10.1016/j.jalz.2011.12.004.

27. Elias-Sonnenschein LS, Viechtbauer W, Ramakers IHGB, Verhey FRJ, Visser PJ. Predictive value of APOE-ε4 allele for progression from MCI to AD-type dementia: a meta-analysis. J Neurol Neurosurg Psychiatry. 2011;82:1149–56. https://doi.org/10.1136/jnnp.2010.231555.

28. Mielke MM, Zandi PP, Sjögren M, Gustafson D, Ostling S, Steen B, et al. High total cholesterol levels in late life associated with a reduced risk of dementia. Neurology. 2005;64:1689–95. https://doi.org/10.1212/01.WNL.0000161870.78572.A5.

29. Weverling-Rijnsburger AW, Blauw GJ, Lagaay AM, Knook DL, Meinders AE, Westendorp RG. Total cholesterol and risk of mortality in the oldest old. Lancet (London, England). 1997;350:1119–23. https://doi.org/10.1016/S0140-6736(97)04430-9.

30. van den Kommer TN, Dik MG, Comijs HC, Lutjohann D, Lips P, Jonker C, et al. The role of extracerebral cholesterol homeostasis and ApoE e4 in cognitive decline. Neurobiol Aging. 2012;33:622.e17–28. https://doi.org/10.1016/j.neurobiolaging.2011.02.019.

31. Corrada MM, Hayden KM, Paganini-Hill A, Bullain SS, DeMoss J, Aguirre C, et al. Age of onset of hypertension and risk of dementia in the oldest-old: the 90+ study. Alzheimers Dement. 2017;13:103–10. https://doi.org/10.1016/j.jalz.2016.09.007.

32. Kennelly SP, Lawlor BA, Kenny RA. Blood pressure and the risk for dementia-a double edged sword. Ageing Res Rev. 2009;8:61–70. https://doi.org/10.1016/j.arr.2008.11.001.

33. Ruitenberg A, Skoog I, Ott A, Aevarsson O. Blood pressure and risk of dementia: results from the Rotterdam study and the Gothenburg H-70 study. Blood Press. 2001:33–9. https://doi.org/10.1159/000051233.

34. Skoog I, Lernfelt B, Landahl S, Palmertz B, Andreasson LA, Nilsson L, et al. 15-year longitudinal study of blood pressure and dementia. Lancet (London, England). 1996;347:1141–5. https://doi.org/10.1016/S0140-6736(96)90608-X.

35. Spira AP, Rebok GW, Stone KL, Kramer JH, Yaffe K. Depressive symptoms in oldest-old women: risk of mild cognitive impairment and dementia. Am J Geriatr Psychiatry. 2011;19:S56–7.

36. Berkman LF, Berkman CS, Kasl S, Freeman DHJ, Leo L, Ostfeld AM, et al. Depressive symptoms in relation to physical health and functioning in the elderly. Am J Epidemiol. 1986;124:372–88. https://doi.org/10.1093/oxfordjournals.aje.a114408.

37. Brailean A, Aartsen MJ, Muniz-Terrera G, Prince M, Prina AM, Comijs HC, et al. Longitudinal associations between late-life depression dimensions and cognitive functioning: a cross-domain latent growth curve analysis. Psychol Med. 2017;47:690–702. https://doi.org/10.1017/S003329171600297X.

38. Gorelick PB. Role of inflammation in cognitive impairment: results of observational epidemiological studies and clinical trials. Ann N Y Acad Sci. 2010;1207:155–62. https://doi.org/10.1111/j.1749-6632.2010.05726.x.

39. Anstey KJ, Windsor TD, Rodgers B, Jorm AF, Christensen H. Lower cognitive test scores observed in alcohol abstainers are associated with demographic, personality, and biological factors: the PATH through life project. Addiction. 2005;100:1291–301. https://doi.org/10.1111/j.1360-0443.2005.01159.x.

40. Zhong G, Wang Y, Zhang Y, Guo JJ, Zhao Y. Smoking is associated with an increased risk of dementia: a meta-analysis of prospective cohort studies with investigation of potential effect modifiers. PLoS One. 2015;10 https://doi.org/10.1371/journal.pone.0118333.

41. Chang C-CH, Zhao Y, Lee C-W, Ganguli M. Smoking, death, and Alzheimer's disease: a case of competing risks. Alzheimer Dis Assoc Disord. 2012;26:300–6. https://doi.org/10.1097/WAD.0b013e3182420b6e.

42. Hernán MA, Alonso ALG. Cigarette smoking and dementia: potential selection bias in the elderly. Epidemiol (Cambridge, Mass). 2008;19:242–6. https://doi.org/10.1097/EDE.0b013e31816bbe14.

43. Blondell SJ, Hammersley-Mather R, Veerman J. Does physical activity prevent cognitive decline and dementia?: a systematic review and meta-analysis of longitudinal studies. BMC Public Health. 2014;14:1–12. https://doi.org/10.1186/1471-2458-14-510.

44. Young J, Angevaren M, Rusted J, Tabet N. Aerobic exercise to improve cognitive function in older people without known cognitive impairment (review). Cochrane Database Syst Rev. 2015:1–141. https://doi.org/10.1002/14651858.CD005381.pub4. www.cochranelibrary.com

45. Jansen WJ, Ossenkoppele R, Tijms BM, Fagan AM, Hansson O, Klunk WE, et al. Association of cerebral amyloid-β aggregation with cognitive functioning in persons without dementia. JAMA Psychiatry. 2018;75:84–95. https://doi.org/10.1001/jamapsychiatry.2017.3391.

46. Bender R, Lange S. Adjusting for multiple testing - when and how? J Clin Epidemiol. 2001;54:343–9. https://doi.org/10.1016/S0895-4356(00)00314-0.

47. Perneger TV. What's wrong with Bonferroni adjustments. BMJ. 1998;316 https://doi.org/10.1136/bmj.316.7139.1236.

# 12

# Identifying and understanding the health and social care needs of older adults with multiple chronic conditions and their caregivers: a scoping review

Katherine S. McGilton[1,2]*, Shirin Vellani[1], Lily Yeung[1], Jawad Chishtie[2,13], Elana Commisso[3], Jenny Ploeg[4], Melissa K. Andrew[5], Ana Patricia Ayala[6], Mikaela Gray[6], Debra Morgan[7], Amanda Froehlich Chow[7], Edna Parrott[8], Doug Stephens[8], Lori Hale[8], Margaret Keatings[8], Jennifer Walker[9], Walter P. Wodchis[3,10], Veronique Dubé[11], Janet McElhaney[12] and Martine Puts[1]

## Abstract

**Background:** As the population is aging, the number of persons living with multiple chronic conditions (MCC) is expected to increase. This review seeks to answer two research questions from the perspectives of older adults with MCC, their caregivers and their health care providers (HCPs): 1) What are the health and social care needs of community-dwelling older adults with MCC and their caregivers? and 2) How do social and structural determinants of health impact these health and social care needs?

**Methods:** We conducted a scoping review guided by a refinement of the Arksey & O'Malley framework. Articles were included if participants were 55 years or older and have at least two chronic conditions. We searched 7 electronic databases. The data were summarized using thematic analysis.

**Results:** Thirty-six studies were included in this review: 28 studies included participants with MCC; 12 studies included HCPs; 5 studies included caregivers. The quality of the studies ranged from moderate to good. Five main areas of needs were identified: need for information; coordination of services and supports; preventive, maintenance and restorative strategies; training for older adults, caregivers and HCPs to help manage the older adults' complex conditions; and the need for person-centred approaches. Structural and social determinants of health such as socioeconomic status, education and access influenced the needs of older adults with MCC.

**Conclusion:** The review highlights that most of the needs of older adults with MCC focus on lack of access to information and coordination of care. The main structural and social determinants that influenced older adults' needs were their level of education/health literacy and their socioeconomic status.

**Keywords:** Scoping review, Multimorbidity, Older adults, Caregivers, Health care providers, Needs

* Correspondence: kathy.mcgilton@uhn.ca
[1]Lawrence S. Bloomberg Faculty of Nursing, University of Toronto, Toronto, ON, Canada
[2]Toronto Rehabilitation Institute, University Health Network, 550 University Avenue, Toronto, ON M6K 2R7 416 597 3422 (2500), Canada
Full list of author information is available at the end of the article

## Background

Many older adults live with multiple chronic conditions (MCC), also known as multimorbidity [1, 2]. While there are several definitions of multimorbidity, it is defined in this review as the presence of two or more chronic medical conditions which may negatively impact an individual's daily living, particularly with higher numbers of coexisting conditions [3]. Older adults living with MCC often rely on the support of informal caregivers to help them manage their daily lives [4, 5]. Caregiving for older adults, without the appropriate supports, can negatively affect an individual's financial, emotional and psychological wellbeing [6].

Factors related to social and structural determinants of health can further worsen the challenges of managing complex health issues for older adults with MCC [7]. This is especially true for older women, ethno cultural minorities, Indigenous persons, persons with cognitive impairment (CI), persons with lower socioeconomic status (SES), or persons living in rural or remote communities [8, 9]. Currently, not enough is known about the needs of older adults with MCC and their caregivers and how different determinants of health influence their needs as most conceptualizations of multimorbidity focus on the biomedical dimensions of MCC [10].

To date, there are syntheses of existing evidence on the spectrum of multimorbidity and implications for care [11]; occurrence, causes and consequences of multimorbidity [12]; tools to assess patient treatment priorities [13]; interventions to improve outcomes for persons with MCC [14]; and a review of chronic care models to reorganize care for patients with MCC [15]. However, to our knowledge, there is no review on the health and social care needs of community-dwelling older adults with MCC and their caregivers. Therefore, a comprehensive review is needed to inform the development of interventions designed to meet the needs, and hence promote the quality of life, of older adults with MCC and their caregivers.

In light of this gap, we undertook a scoping review to summarize the available research studies on the health and social care needs of community-dwelling older adults with MCC and their caregivers. The review seeks to answer two research questions from the perspectives of older adults with MCC, their caregivers and their health care providers (HCPs):

1) What are the health and social care needs of community-dwelling older adults with MCC and their caregivers?
2) How do social and structural determinants of health – such as gender, socioeconomic status, or level of education – impact the health and social care needs?

The scoping review methodology was chosen because it was 1) flexible in that it allowed for the inclusion of qualitative and quantitative studies [16]; 2) unrestrictive, thus allowing for the exploration of widely varied topics such as patient and caregivers needs, as well as determinants of health [16]; 3) a systematic method for summarizing and identifying gaps in existing literature [16]; and 4) citizen engaged because it includes a stakeholder consultation to inform research and subsequently evidence informed interventions [17].

## Methods

The protocol for our scoping review has been published [18] but is briefly summarized below. The scoping review methods framework outlined by Arksey and O'Malley [16] and refined by Levac et al. [17], Colquhoun et al. [19] and Daudt et al. [20] was used. The framework includes six steps: 1) identifying the research questions (listed above); 2) identifying relevant literature; 3) study selection; 4) charting the data; 5) collating, summarizing and reporting the results; 6) consulting with key stakeholders and translating knowledge. Below we briefly summarize each step.

To identify relevant literature, two academic health sciences librarians (APA and MG) prepared the search strategy in consultation with the research team. The databases searched include OVID Medline (1946 to 2017, including Epub Ahead of Print, and In Process & Other Non-Indexed Citations), OVID Embase (1947 to 2017), OVID PsycINFO (1806 to 2017), OVID Social Work Abstracts (1968 to 2017), EBSCO CINAHL Plus with Full Text (1981 to 2017), EBSCO AgeLine (1966 to 2017), and Cochrane Central. The search strategies were translated using each database platform's command language, controlled vocabulary, and appropriate search fields. MeSH terms, EMTREE terms, APA thesauri terms, CINAHL headings, and text words were used for the search concepts of health and social care needs and priorities, Indigenous populations and multimorbidity.

We applied a modified adult age filter to the Medline strategy [21]. This filter was translated and applied to the other databases. The filters were not validated. Language limits were applied to capture English, French, Dutch, and German articles; and the final searches were completed in May 2017. For the full Medline strategy, see Additional file 1: Table S1. Additionally, we searched the reference lists of included studies. Covidence systematic review software was used to facilitate the review (www.covidence.org).

In terms of preparing the co-authors to assist with the review, the two lead PIs (KM and MP) and the librarian held training sessions with the researchers and stakeholders to ensure they understood definitions of health and social care and were familiar with the inclusion and exclusion criteria and how to use Covidence. During this phase we went through titles and abstracts together ($n = 20$) to ensure they were prepared. Conflicts were decided upon by the two lead PIs, KM and MP. The definition of social care that guided this review was from the WHO world report on Ageing and Health: Social care address the needs associated with performance of the activities of daily living, connection to one's social networks such as family, friends and community; access to social programs for supports in poverty, unemployment, old age and disability to optimize social protection [7].

Studies were selected through a two-step process using the selection criteria below. First, each of the titles and corresponding abstracts were independently reviewed by two team members. Then, two reviewers independently assessed the relevant full text articles (see Fig. 1 PRISMA flow chart). In cases of disagreement between reviewers, one of the two principal investigators (MP and KM) resolved the conflict.

The inclusion criteria included:

- Studies which reported on health and/or social care needs of older adults living with MCC or on health and/or social care needs of caregivers of older adults living with MCC and/or identified needs/areas for improvement.
- Any type of primary study (quantitative, qualitative or mixed methods); involving community dwelling older adults aged $\geq$ 55 years; studies that included a wider age range, but the mean/median age was $\geq$ 55 years; studies which included a sub-group analysis for this population.

In light of the fact that Indigenous persons experience multiple and complex health conditions at younger ages than other populations, we included all literature that focused on persons 55 years of age or older living with MCC, in order to capture relevant literature related to the care needs of ageing Indigenous persons [22].

The exclusion criteria included:

- Expert opinions, editorials, and materials that did not include original data.
- Published in other languages than English, French, Dutch and German

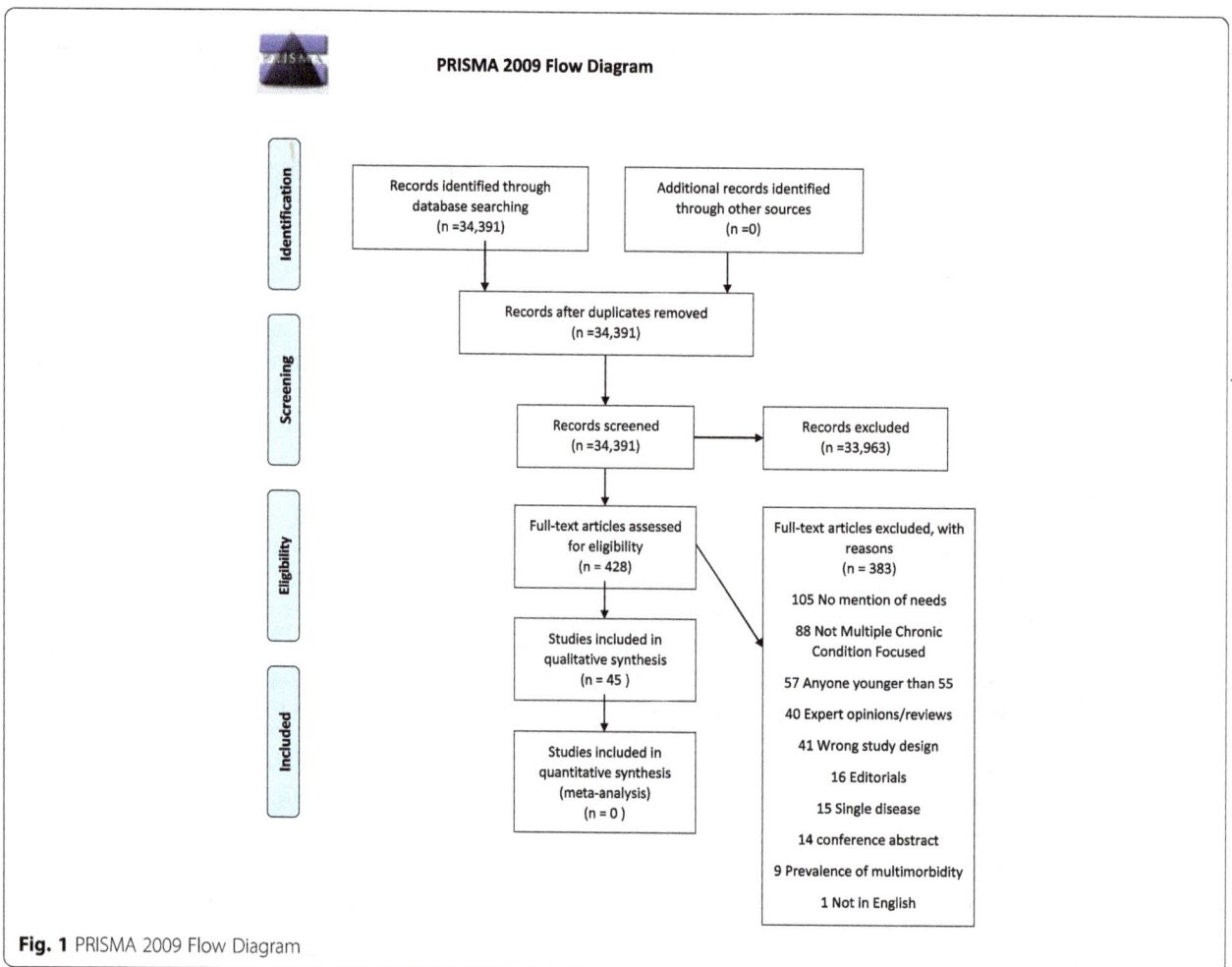

**PRISMA 2009 Flow Diagram**

Identification: Records identified through database searching (n =34,391). Additional records identified through other sources (n =0).

Screening: Records after duplicates removed (n =34,391). Records screened (n =34,391). Records excluded (n =33,963).

Eligibility: Full-text articles assessed for eligibility (n = 428). Full-text articles excluded, with reasons (n = 383): 105 No mention of needs; 88 Not Multiple Chronic Condition Focused; 57 Anyone younger than 55; 40 Expert opinions/reviews; 41 Wrong study design; 16 Editorials; 15 Single disease; 14 conference abstract; 9 Prevalence of multimorbidity; 1 Not in English.

Included: Studies included in qualitative synthesis (n = 45). Studies included in quantitative synthesis (meta-analysis) (n = 0).

**Fig. 1** PRISMA 2009 Flow Diagram

A data abstraction form using Microsoft Excel software was created to guide data extraction. Furthermore, codes representing the World Health Organization's (WHO) definition of structural and social determinants of health [23] were included to map the studies that identified these determinants as important considerations when identifying needs and preferences of older adults with MCC. The data abstraction form was pilot tested and refined by the researchers (KM, MP, JC) to ensure consistency. Two reviewers independently abstracted the relevant information from the studies, with one researcher confirming the information.

During the testing of the data abstraction process it became clear that the studies focused on needs and preferences of Indigenous older adults and how data were collected were conceptually distinct from those studies focusing on groups of non-Indigenous older adults. Thus, considering these differences, it was decided to separate the review results into two papers and results concerning the needs and preferences of Indigenous older adults with MCC will be summarized in a separate paper. Team members who have experience in Indigenous health research took the lead on the other paper (JW, AC).

Data extracted included: details on the study (type of study, aim of study, origin, response rate etc.), study characteristics (study setting), patient and/or caregiver characteristics (age, gender, ethnicity, location, number and types chronic conditions), involvement of caregiver, health and social care needs, and (if categorized) categories/themes used. Since there was substantial heterogeneity among the included studies, the data were summarized using thematic analysis [24]. Using an iterative process, the first author developed descriptive codes, which were grouped together into a smaller number of categories to draw conclusions. The codes were discussed with the entire team until we reached consensus. Once the codes were agreed upon, the codes and their smaller number of categories were shared with a small group of expert qualitative researchers (JP, VD) and they were revised to minimize bias. This process was repeated to find patterns across the three different sub-groups, older adults, caregivers and HCPs. The quality of the research studies was assessed using the Mixed Methods Appraisal Tool (MMAT) [25]. The MMAT allows inclusion of qualitative, quantitative and mixed methods studies with quality criteria relevant to each study design. As we aimed to provide a comprehensive overview of needs, no study was excluded based on the MMAT score alone.

Finally, in accordance with Step 6 of our scoping review framework, we organized a stakeholder consultation meeting on 22 May 2017. We included older adults with MCC (n = 3), caregivers (n = 3), HCPs (n = 3), representatives of provincial organisations (n = 3), and primary care organizations (n = 2) to provide feedback on the findings and to offer suggestions for next steps. For this meeting we presented the results and asked the stakeholders specific questions related to:1) their thoughts, reflection and opinions on the information presented; 2) if there were any unmet health and social care needs, priorities and preferences of older adults with multiple chronic conditions living in the community and their caregivers, that was not highlighted in our presentation; 3) and additional social determinants of health (such as income, social support networks; education; employment/working conditions; gender; and culture) that may have impacted the health and social care needs of older persons with multiple chronic conditions; 4) and their insights about future research ideas to explore in this topic area. Two groups were developed so more sharing could occur and equal representation from both persons living with MCC and their caregivers and HCPs. The groups were facilitated by the two PIs. Notes were taken by two team members, compared, synthesized and then content analyzed. Their comments were summarized and are presented below. Additionally, to ensure we had stakeholder engagement throughout the project, three of the stakeholders who attended this meeting were selected prior to the funding of the research project. In fact one older adult with MCC and one caregiver provided testimonials during the application phase on the importance of this research. They also assisted with reviewing of abstract titles as we provided training and support for them.

## Results

The perspectives of older adults, their caregivers, and their HCPs, were considered when identifying needs of older adults with MCC. The following sections highlight the characteristics of the studies, the details of the study participants across all the studies that were reviewed and the thematic analysis of the findings.

### Characteristics of included studies

In this review 34,391 abstracts were retrieved and reviewed by two independent reviewers (see Table 1). 428 articles were selected for full text review and 45 were retained. Of these 9 were focused on Indigenous older adults so for this review, a total of 36 articles were included. Thirty studies were qualitative studies [26–55], four were cross-sectional studies [56–59], one was mixed method study [60] and one was a secondary qualitative data analysis [61] (Table 1). Twenty two studies were conducted in North America [26, 28–30, 33, 35, 37, 38, 41, 43, 46–52, 55, 57–60], ten in Europe [31, 32, 34, 39, 40, 44, 45, 54, 56, 61] and three in Australia/New Zealand [27, 42, 53].

We sought information from older adults with MCC, their caregivers and health care providers about needs of older adults with MCC and some researchers included more than one perspective in their studies [26, 31, 34, 38,

**Table 1** Characteristics of included studies

| Author and year | Continent | Inclusion criteria | Study design | Data collection methods | Sampling Strategy | Analysis methods used |
|---|---|---|---|---|---|---|
| Adeniji 2015 | Europe | Recruited from 4 large general practices in UK. Identified from registers of long term conditions, have at least two MCC (of COPD, coronary heart disease, diabetes, osteoarthritis, and depression) | Cross Sectional Observational | Mailed questionnaires | Convenience | Descriptive statistics and multivariable regression analysis |
| Ancker 2015 | North American | Adult English speaking patients with MCC, as well as health care providers with experience providing care for patients with MCC | Qualitative | One to one Interviews | Purposive | Grounded theory, thematic analysis |
| Ansari 2014 | Australia | One or more pre-existing comorbidity along with a new diagnosis of COPD in last 24 months; age 40–85; history of smoking; from primary care setting | Qualitative | One to one interview | Purposive | Thematic analysis |
| Bardach 2012 | North America | Physicians from family medicine and internal medicine specialties were recruited from rural and urban practices, community and academic settings 1 obstetrics-gynecology physician was included, as they serve as primary care provider for some women. | Qualitative | One to one, semi structured interviews | Purposive | Content, Thematic analysis |
| Barstow 2015 | North America | OT were identified by those attending an online forum and at a national conference who provided direct care to older adults with low vision > 1 year. Older adults with confirmed low vision from an age-related eye disease, aged 65 years and over, with at least 1 comorbid condition and no more than mild cognitive impairment | Mixed Method (cross sectional observation and qualitative) | Online surveys for OTs; one to one interviews with older adults | Convenience for OTs; Purposive for older adults | Descriptive statistics for surveys. Content analysis for qualitative. |
| Bayliss 2003 | North America | Individuals were recruited through flyers in family medicine practices in Denver for participants who self-identified as having 2 or more chronic illnesses. They screened out those with active terminal illness, HIV, and uncontrolled psychiatric illnesses. | Qualitative | One to one interviews | Purposive | Qualitative comparative analysis |

**Table 1** Characteristics of included studies *(Continued)*

| Author and year | Continent | Inclusion criteria | Study design | Data collection methods | Sampling Strategy | Analysis methods used |
|---|---|---|---|---|---|---|
| Bayliss 2007 | North America | Participants of a health maintenance organization who were 65 years or older and had a diagnosis of diabetes, depression and osteoarthritis for a period of 2 years prior to the study and they were drawn from disease specific registries validated against ICD codes | Cross sectional | Survey | Convenience for survey; random for qualitative interview. | Descriptive statistics, Multivariate linear regression |
| Beverly 2011 | North America | Mentally alert community-dwelling adults, aged 60 years or older, reporting a diagnosis of Type 2 diabetes and the presence of one or more chronic conditions in addition to diabetes | Qualitative | Eight 90 min Focus groups of 2–6 patients | Purposive | Thematic analysis |
| Bunn 2017 | Europe | They recruited purposive samples of people living with dementia and at least one of the following three conditions: diabetes, stroke or vision impairment. They also recruited family carers and healthcare professionals who organise and deliver care for people with stroke, diabetes and VI in primary and secondary care. | Qualitative | Focus groups with HCPs; one to one interviews with patients and caregivers; one to one interviews with HCPs as well. | Purposive | Thematic and ontent analysis informed by theories of continuity of care and access to care. |
| Burton 2016 | Europe | Eligible patients were identified from clinics and support groups but no inclusion criteria reported | Qualitative | One to one interviews | Not clear. | Thematic analysis |
| Cheraghi-Sohi 2013 | Europe | Patients who had osteoarthritis (OA) whose transcript contained narrative of one or more condition in addition to OA and include information pertaining to condition prioritization. | Secondary analysis of qualitative data | Secondary data of one to one qualitative interviews | Purposive | Amplified secondary analysis, content analysis |
| Clarke 2014 | North America | Aged 70 years and older and had at least 3 chronic conditions of which one of them had to be arthritis/ back problems/ cataracts/ glaucoma/ diabetes/ heart disease | Qualitative | One to one interviews | Purposive | Thematic analysis (Marshall and Rossman's (2006) seven key analytic procedure) |
| Coventry 2014 | Europe | To include 5 patients per criterion: age, gender, combination of illnesses and level of deprivation. Socioeconomic | Qualitative | One to one interviews | Convenience- HCP. Purposive- patients | Thematic analysis |

**Table 1** Characteristics of included studies *(Continued)*

| Author and year | Continent | Inclusion criteria | Study design | Data collection methods | Sampling Strategy | Analysis methods used |
|---|---|---|---|---|---|---|
| | | deprivation (defined by Index of Multiple Deprivation), number and type of long term conditions, age and gender. HCP inclusion criteria: Tried to recruit 5 in each criterion: deprivation status of the practice area; role (i.e. salaried family physician, practice nurse); and number of years' experience. | | | | |
| DiNapoli 2016 | North America | Aged 50 years and over with at least a CIRS-G 2 score in three or more organ systems and MMSE> 24 and no deficit in language skills, bipolar disorder or other chronic psychotic disorders or no other neurodegenerative disorders | Qualitative | One to one interview | Purposive | Descriptive statistics, thematic analysis |
| Fortin 2005 | North America | Adult patients without cognitive impairment or uncontrolled illnesses, have at least 4 chronic conditions and not followed by other researchers. | Qualitative | Focus groups | Purposive | Other |
| Fried 2008 | North America | Aged 65 and older and were taking five or more medications daily; undergoing treatment for multiple conditions; English speaking. People with severe hearing loss or cognitive impairment, defined as inability to remember two or more items on a three-item test of short-term recall were excluded | Qualitative | Focus groups | Purposive | Thematic and content analyses using constant comparative method |
| Gill 2014 | North America | Patients: 65 years or older, diagnosed with 2 or more chronic conditions, with an informal caregiver who participated in the patient's healthcare; spoke English as a first language; could provide consent | Qualitative | One to one interviews | Purposive | Inductive thematic analysis with saturation of themes |
| Grundberg 2016 | Europe | Being a district nurse with experience with caring for community-dwelling homebound older adults with MCC | Qualitative | One to one interviews, focus groups | Snowballing | Content analysis |
| Hansen 2015 | Europe | Community dwelling; 3 or more coexisting chronic conditions; being a regular patient of the participating family physician practice; ability to participate in interview (no blindness/ | Qualitative | Focus groups | Purposive | Content analysis |

**Table 1** Characteristics of included studies *(Continued)*

| Author and year | Continent | Inclusion criteria | Study design | Data collection methods | Sampling Strategy | Analysis methods used |
|---|---|---|---|---|---|---|
| | | deafness); ability to speak German; no lethal illness in last 3 months; ability to consent e.g. no dementia; no participation in other studies at the current time; | | | | |
| Kuluski 2013 | North America | 65 years or older; ability to communicate in English; two or more chronic diagnoses; ability to give informed consent; an informal caregiver who agreed to participate in an interview | Qualitative | One to one interview | Purposive | Descriptive statistics; Thematic analysis |
| Lo 2016 | Australia | Patients with diabetes and chronic kidney disease (stages 3–5, eGFR < 60 mL/min/ 1.73 m2) and their carers; capable of giving consent and stable mental state. These patients from Monash health, Alfred health in Melbourne and the royal north shore and concord hospital in Sydney. | Qualitative | Focus groups for patients; semi structured interviews for carers | Purposive | Generic inductive thematic approach |
| Loeb 2003 | North America | Mentally alert community-dwelling adults, aged 55 or older, who reported the presence of at least two chronic conditions | Qualitative | Focus Groups | Purposive | Thematic and content analyses |
| Mason 2016 | Europe | Having advanced multimorbidity defined as having multiple life-limiting illnesses or progressively deteriorating health due to several long-term conditions. Patients with moderate to severe cognitive impairment were excluded. Patients were asked to nominate a family carer who consented separately | Qualitative | One to one interviews. Serial interviews at 8–12 week intervals. Among 87 interviews, 42 with patients alone, 2 with carers alone, 43 were joint interviews | Purposive | Constructivist thematic analysis. |
| McDonnall 2016 | North America | Recruited from a previous study, from the centre for Deaf-Blind youths and adults, and ads and electronic discussion groups. 55 years and older who have dual sensory loss | Cross sectional | Survey | Purposive | Descriptive statistics Open-ended responses were independently coded by two the authors, and discrepancies were discussed until agreement was reached |
| Morales-Asencio 2016 | Europe | Patients experiencing situations with high probability of complexity, such as the coexistence of several chronic diseases impacting quality of life, the frequent interaction with health services, or the | Qualitative | One to one interview with caregiver present | Purposive | Qualitative inductive content analysis |

**Table 1** Characteristics of included studies *(Continued)*

| Author and year | Continent | Inclusion criteria | Study design | Data collection methods | Sampling Strategy | Analysis methods used |
|---|---|---|---|---|---|---|
| | | existence of health/social determinants. Gender was also included as a selection criterion because of the proven differences in significance granted by men and women to their health care events and to their process experience | | | | |
| Naganathan 2016 | North America | 65 years of age or older, and diagnosed with two or more chronic conditions, patient capacity to provide informed consent, presence of informal care-giver and patient English proficiency. | Qualitative | One to one interview | Convenience | Descriptive statistics, thematic analysis |
| Noël 2005 | North America | 8 primary care clinics in 4 regions in the US were selected. The study sites were chosen based on known regional variations in veteran's health and differences in clinic size and organization. Four clinics were in large metropolitan settings and four were in rural areas. 4/8 were based in tertiary care hospitals and the others were free standing community clinics. Patients were invited by primary care physician if they had 2 or more diseases, have no severe cognitive/ mental health illnesses. | Qualitative | Focus groups | Purposive | Thematic analysis |
| Ravenscroft 2010 | North America | Recruitment criteria: (1) adults (19 years or older) with diagnosed stage 1 to 4 Chronic Kidney Disease (CKD), (2) attending a clinic for management of their CKD, (3) coexisting diabetes mellitus and/or Cardiovascular disease, or both, and (4) capable of communicating in English | Qualitative | One to one interviews | Purposive | Thematic analysis |
| Richardson 2016 | North America | Be at least 18 years of age or older, (2) have a diabetes diagnosis, and (3) have at least two other diagnosed chronic conditions. Excluded patients with cognitive deficits, uncontrolled psychiatric illness. | Qualitative | One to one interview, chart review | Purposive | Descriptive statistics, content analysis with naturalistic approach |

**Table 1** Characteristics of included studies (Continued)

| Author and year | Continent | Inclusion criteria | Study design | Data collection methods | Sampling Strategy | Analysis methods used |
|---|---|---|---|---|---|---|
| Roberge 2016 | North America | Clinicians from 3 different university affiliated family health teams in Quebec. Clinicians: 1) provision of services to patients with chronic diseases; 2) at least 12 months of clinical experience; Patients: 1) age 18 years or older, 2) presence of a chronic disease (e.g. diabetes, arthritis, chronic obstructive pulmonary disease); 3) depression or anxiety disorder (panic disorder, agoraphobia, social anxiety disorder or generalized anxiety disorder) in the past 2 years according to clinician's diagnosis; 4) good knowledge of French or English; 5) having a family physician in one of the three clinics. Exclusion criteria for patients were the inability to provide consent, cognitive impairment, and a history of manic episodes or a psychotic disorder. | Qualitative | One to one interview | Purposive | Thematic analysis |
| Roberto 2005 | North America | Women 65 years or older with two or more of heart disease, diabetes or osteoporosis. | Qualitative | One to one interview | Purposive | Thematic analysis- based on life course perspective and trajectory model of chronic illness |
| Ryan 2016 | North America | Those who have high needs (combinations of major chronic conditions, under 65 and disabled, frail elderly with multiple functional limitations; insurance status). | Cross sectional observational | One to one interviews | Random-The 2016 Commonwealth Fund Survey of High-Need Patients was conducted by SSRS from June 22 to September 14, 2016, as a part of SSRS's weekly, nationally representative omnibus survey | Prevalence reported only |
| Schoenberg 2011 | North America | 41 and over; diagnosis of two or more chronic illnesses, have 'just enough money to get by' or 'not enough money to make ends meet'. | Qualitative | One to one interview | Purposive | Thematic and content analyses |
| Sheridan 2012 | New Zealand | Based on ethnicity (Maori, Pacific, Asian, or New Zealand European), 50 years or older, two or more chronic conditions, admitted to hospital two or more times for five or more bed days between Jan and Dec 2008 | Qualitative | One to one interviews | Purposive | Qualitative Descriptive approach |

**Table 1** Characteristics of included studies *(Continued)*

| Author and year | Continent | Inclusion criteria | Study design | Data collection methods | Sampling Strategy | Analysis methods used |
|---|---|---|---|---|---|---|
| Smith 2010 | Europe | Family Physicians who also trained medical trainees were selected from Trinity College Dublin; Pharmacists were selected from pharmacists attending a chronic disease management resource group | Qualitative | Focus groups | Purposive | Thematic analysis |
| Zulman 2015 | North America | Individuals who receive care at an academic medical center or at a Veterans Affair facility in Northern California. eligibility criteria for the focus groups (≥3 chronic conditions and experience using technology to help them care for their health or manage their health care) Did not exclude based on age, health status, functional/cognitive status. | Qualitative | Focus groups | Purposive | Thematic and Content analyses |

*CIRS-G* Cumulative Illness Rating-Geriatrics
*COPD* Chronic obstructive pulmonary disease
*eGFR* estimated Glomerular Filtration Rate
*HCP* Health care provider
*MCC* Multiple Chronic Conditions
*MMSE* Mini Mental State Examination
*OT* Occupational therapist
*SD* Standard deviation

40–42, 44, 46, 50, 53, 60]. Thirty-four studies included participants with MCC [26, 27, 29–38, 40–53, 55–61] and the sample size ranged from 8 [60] to 1274 participants [58] with a total of 3058 participants in the studies. Seven studies included caregivers of older adults with MCC [31, 38, 41, 42, 44–46] and the sample sizes varied from 8 [42] to 33 [31] with a total of 137 participants. In the twelve studies that included health care providers [26, 28, 31, 34, 38–41, 46, 50, 54, 60], the sample sizes ranged from 4 [38, 41] to 59 [60] and a total of 201 HCPs participated. Included papers were published between 2003 and 2017.

### Characteristics of the study participants
The mean age of older adults ranged from 55 to 64 in four studies [26, 35, 52, 55], 65 to 74 in nine studies [27, 34, 36, 42, 43, 45, 56, 57, 61], and 75 to 84 in twelve studies [30–33, 37, 38, 40, 41, 44, 46, 51, 60] (see Table 2). Seven studies reported age ranges [29, 47–50, 53, 59]. Mean age and age ranges of older adults with MCC are presented in Table 1. The percentage of female older adults with MCC ranged from 6% [49] to 100% [51]. Of the 36 studies included in the review, 22 studies included at least 50% females as their study participants [26, 28–30, 32, 33, 36, 37, 39, 43, 45, 48, 50–53, 56–61]. Two studies did not report the proportion of female respondents [34, 54].

MCC was determined mostly (24/32 studies) by health care providers, and/or staff assisting them, or the sample was drawn from clinical data bases and disease trajectories [26, 27, 30–32, 34–36, 38, 40–42, 44–50, 52, 53, 56, 59, 61]. Five studies did not explicitly state how MCC was established for the sample of patients during the recruitment process, although the inclusion criteria mentioned at least two or more conditions and the appropriate age range for older adults [33, 37, 51, 57, 58]. MCC was self-reported by patients in two studies [29, 43]. Frailty was not mentioned as a condition included in the MCCs.

The mean number of chronic conditions ranged from 2 to 4 in six studies [26, 34, 51, 52, 59, 61], from 5 to 7 in ten studies [30, 33, 37, 38, 41, 43, 46, 49, 55, 56], and 8 or more in one study [36]. Three studies reported range of number of chronic conditions [27, 29, 48]. The most reported conditions included hypertension, cardiovascular disease, chronic pain, osteoarthritis, COPD and cancer. Depression and other mental health conditions were also reported. Nineteen studies did not report the mean number of conditions [27–29, 31, 32, 35, 39, 40, 42, 44, 45, 47, 48, 50, 53, 54, 57, 58, 60].

Twenty-two studies reported the ethnicity of the study participants [26, 27, 29–33, 35, 37, 41–43, 47–49, 52, 53, 55, 57–60]. Most study participants were Caucasian or

**Table 2** Characteristics of study participants

| Author and year | Sample size and mean age (age range) | % Female | Diseases | Number of diseases | Ethnicity | SES | Living situation/ Marital status | Education | Other |
|---|---|---|---|---|---|---|---|---|---|
| *Older adult characteristics* | | | | | | | | | |
| Adeniji 2015 | N = 486. mean age 70 (range 31–91) | 52 | COPD, coronary heart disease, diabetes, osteoarthritis, depression | Median: 7; range: 2–20 | Not reported | 13% in paid jobs; no further details. 68% owned cars | Not reported | 60% completed school/GCSE as a minimum level of education | |
| Ancker 2015 | N = 22 mean age = 64 (range 37–89) | 50 | Hypertension, heart disease, chronic pain, depression, asthma, HIV, hepatitis C & diabetes | Mean = 3.5 (SD 1.5). Minimum 2 conditions. | 32% black | 32% had Medicare, 32% had Medicaid & 36% had commercial insurance | 68% not currently married | Not reported | 36% English as second language. > 80% over the age of 55 yrs. |
| Ansari 2014 | N = 17 Mean age 67; (range 43–84) | 47 | High cholesterol, hypertension, depression & smoking, COPD, arthritis | Range 1–7 | Mostly Caucasian | Not reported, sample ranges from student to employed to retired, 11% unemployed and 1 person (5%) volunteer | 65% live with spouse; 30% live alone; 5 (one person) live with a grandchild | 9 had some high school education, the rest higher including 6 university | |
| Barstow 2015 | N = 8. mean age was 79 years (range 66–92). | 75 | Arthritis- 88% hypertension- 62% hypotension- 25% cancer- 50% osteoporosis- 38% hearing impairment- 38% cardiac/circulatory system problems- 51% kidney problems- 37% digestive problems- 25% urinary system problems- 25% pulmonary problems- 13% | It was assessed using the General Health Questionnaire | White | Not reported | Not reported | Not reported | |
| Bayliss 2007 | N = 16 Range 31–70 years. | 66 | Osteoarthritis, depression & diabetes | 38% had 4–9; 62% had 10–16 conditions | Ethnicity: 11% Hispanic/Latino; 88% other. Race: 90% white; 8% other; 2% black African American | 76% less than USD 45,000; 17% more than 45,000. | 53% married; 14% divorced/ separated; 2% never married; 29% widowed. | 35% High-school educated; 10% some high school or less; 31% some college/ 2 year degree; 22% 4 year college degree. | |

122

**Table 2** Characteristics of study participants (Continued)

| Author and year | Sample size and mean age (age range) | % Female | Diseases | Number of diseases | Ethnicity | SES | Living situation/ Marital status | Education | Other |
|---|---|---|---|---|---|---|---|---|---|
| Bayliss 2003 | N = 352 55% in age range of 65–74; 45% were 75 and above | 81 | Hypertension, COPD, chronic bronchitis, emphysema, asthma, musculoskeletal disorders, history of depression, vision problems, coronary arterial disease, migraine, obesity, gastroesophageal reflux, congestive heart failure, depression, osteoarthritis & diabetes, history of depression | Median: 4; range: 2–7 | All white | 7: < 15, 000; 8: > 15,000 ranging up to 60,000 USD | Not reported | At least high school education. High school graduate: 2; Some college: 7; College graduate: 5; Post-college: 2 | |
| Beverly 2011 | N = 32. mean 75.3 ± 7.4; range 60–88 | 56.3 | Hypertension, retinopathy, hypercholesterolemia coronary artery disease neuropathy, cardiac arrhythmia, hypothyroidism, depression, myocardial infarction, asthma, chronic pain, presbycusis, stroke, chronic obstructive pulmonary disease, leukaemia, nephropathy, prostate cancer, insomnia, diabetes, arthritis and cancer | Mean 5.2; Range 3–9 | 100% white | Not reported, 94% retired | 72% married | Mean 14.6 years of education; range 9–20 | |
| Bunn 2017 | N = 28, median age 82.5, range 59–94 | 36 | Alzheimer's disease 56%, mixed dementia 19%, vascular dementia 17%, Parkinson's with dementia 8%, diabetes, stroke, vision impairment | Not reported | 85% white– majority British white | Not reported | 78% patients lived with a carer | Not reported | |
| Burton 2016 | N = 30. Age 65–95 | 53 | Diabetes, arthritis, cancer, stroke, hypertension, high cholesterol, angina, gout, cardiovascular disease | Not reported | All white except one South Asian | Not reported | 15/30 live alone, 13 live with partner and 2 with a family member | Not reported | |
| Cheraghi-Sohi 2013 | N = 30. mean 69; range 55–86 | 60 | Osteoarthritis, cancer, diabetes | Mean 4; Range 2–9 | Not reported | Not reported | Not reported | Not reported | |
| Clarke 2014 | N = 35. Mean age of men 78.6. Mean women 80.3. Range 73–91 | 54 | Back problems/ cataracts/ glaucoma/ heart disease, cancer, diabetes, arthritis | Range: 3–14; average 6 | African 1, Asian/ South Asian 3, European 7, North American 23, South American 1 | < 15,000 4, 15–24,999 4, 25–34,999 7, 35–44,999 3, 45–54,999 6, 55–64 1,65–74 1, 75–84 5 | Participants lived in own home or retirement home. Currently married/ common law 13, divorced/ separated 5, never | College/ University 6, graduate school 7, high school 9, some high school 7, technical school | |

Gerontology and Geriatrics

**Table 2** Characteristics of study participants (Continued)

| Author and year | Sample size and mean age (age range) | % Female | Diseases | Number of diseases | Ethnicity | SES | Living situation/ Marital status | Education | Other |
|---|---|---|---|---|---|---|---|---|---|
| Coventry 2014 | $N = 20$ age Mean age 66.2 (54–88). | Not reported | Depression, COPD, cardiovascular disease, asthma, diabetes, arthritis | Median: 2.55; range: 2–4 | Not reported | Not reported | married 4, widowed 13 | 6 | |
| DiNapoli 2016 | $N = 28$. Mean age 63.4 SD 6.3 | 22 | Not identified on the excel | CIRG score mean 14.1 SD 3.3 & | 64% White, rest not reported | 4/28 working. 1 self-employed, 17 retired, 6 unemployed | 61% non-married, 39% married | High-school educated (education mean: 13.71 ± 2.35) | Not reported |
| Fortin 2005 | $N = 25$. mean 72.7 SD 8.2 | 60 | Diabetes, others not reported | Mean 14.4 SD 4.5 | Not reported | Only 20% had more than 50,000 income, the rest mostly between 10,000 and 40,000 | 48% were married, 32% widowed 8% divorced/ separated and 12% never married | 76% had up to grade 12 education, 16% college and 4% university education | |
| Fried 2008 | $N = 66$. Age 65 and older; > 75+ 6 participants | 67 | Hypertension, diabetes mellitus, ischemic heart disease, congestive heart failure, chronic lung disease, depression, arthritis, falls, urinary incontinence, osteoporosis | Median: 5; range 3–8; | 76% white, 23% white, 1% other, 3% Latino | Not reported | 48% lived alone. 39% married | | |
| Gill 2014 | $N = 28$. mean age: 82.3 (SD 7.7); | 44 | Not reported | Median 5 (SD 2.4) | Not reported | Not reported | 82% of the caregivers were spousal caregivers | Most pts. and caregivers had more than high school education and lived in a single-family home | |
| Hansen 2015 | $N = 21$. mean 77 (70–88) | 47 | Hypertension, lower back pain, diabetes, cancer, arthritis, osteoporosis, cardiac arrhythmias, cerebral ischemia, lower limb varicosities, prostatic hyperplasia, vision reduction, gout, intestinal diverticulosis, psoriasis, atherosclerosis, renal insufficiency, cardiac valve disorders, gallstones, | Not reported | Not reported | Not reported | Married: men 72%; women 40%; Widow: men 9%; women 40%; Divorced: men 9%; women 9%; Never married: men 9% | 7 patients had a low education level; 7 had a medium level, and 6 had a high level | |

**Table 2** Characteristics of study participants (*Continued*)

| Author and year | Sample size and mean age (age range) | % Female | Diseases | Number of diseases | Ethnicity | SES | Living situation/ Marital status | Education | Other |
|---|---|---|---|---|---|---|---|---|---|
| Kuluski 2013 | N = 28. mean age: 82.3 (7.7 SD) | 44 | cardiac insufficiency, anemias, neuropathies, migraine, urinary tract calculi, dizziness, hemorrhoids, gynecological problems | 4.61 (SD 2.43) | 96% Caucasian, 4% other | 85% can support self financially | 70% live in a single-family home; 15% apartment; 7% retirement home. 67% married; 33% other. | 70% greater than high school; 30% high school diploma or less | |
| Lo 2016 | N = 58; median age 67 (range 48–84) | 29 | Chronic kidney disease stage 3–5, depression, diabetes | Not reported | Majority of focus group participants were Caucasian (72.4%), South Asian (13.8%), Asian (10.3%), Pacific Islander (1.7%) or Hispanic (1.7%) | Not reported | Not reported | Not reported | |
| Loeb 2003 | N = 37 older adults. Mean age 72; range 55–88 | 70 | Not reported | Mean 4.5; Range 2–11 | 100% Caucasian | Not reported | 100% independent and community dwelling. | Not reported | |
| Mason 2016 | N = 37. Mean 76; range 55–92 | 38 | Heart, respiratory, liver and renal failure, neurological conditions and mild dementia | Not reported | Not reported | Not reported | Not reported | Not reported | |
| McDonnall 2016 | N = 131. Mean age 69.9 (range of 55 to 99) | 62 | Hearing and vision loss | Not reported | 89% white, 4% African American, 3% American Indian, 1% Hispanic, 1.5% mixed and other unknown | Not reported | Private residence/ living alone 36%; private residence with spouse or others (53%); Retirement or assistive living facility (8%). | Not reported | |
| Morales-Asencio 2016 | N = 18. mean age 73.6 years | 61 | Diabetes, arthritis, cancer, cardiovascular disease, chronic respiratory, congestive heart failure, COPD/ asthma/ renal impairment | Not reported | Not reported | Participants from working class neighborhoods, and in some cases, significantly limited living | Two patients had no family caregiver. Participants lived in working class neighborhoods | Not reported | All were receiving home care |

**Table 2** Characteristics of study participants *(Continued)*

| Author and year | Sample size and mean age (age range) | % Female | Diseases | Number of diseases | Ethnicity | SES | Living situation/ Marital status | Education | Other |
|---|---|---|---|---|---|---|---|---|---|
| | | | | | | conditions | | | |
| Naganathan 2016 | N = 28. Mean 82.3 | 43 | Not reported | Average 5; interquartile range of 3–7 | Not reported | Not reported | 70% lived in a single home. | 70% had higher education | 19% patients reported currently receiving home care; 96% receiving support from family caregiver, 70% from friends and neighbors, 26% from community programs |
| Noël 2005 | N = 60. Age range 30s–80s no mean age provided | 20 | Not reported | Not reported | Majority white; African-Americans and Hispanics | Not reported | 4 urban clinics and 4 rural clinics | Not reported | All veterans |
| Ravenscroft 2010 | N = 20. 30% >74y; 45% 65–74y; 25% 45–64 | 55 | Cardiovascular disease, chronic kidney disease, diabetes | Except one patient, all had 3 or more chronic conditions, majority with 3 or 4 stage chronic kidney disease | Caucasian 90%; black 10% | 20% employed; 70% retired; 10% unemployed. | 55% married; 30% widowed; 15% single. Participants: city - 85%; rural - 15% | 60% beyond high school; 20% high school; 20%; less than high school | Home language - 80% English exclusively; 20% other |
| Richardson 2016 | N = 33. 12% (51–60); 67% (61–70); 12% (71–80); 9% (81–90) | 6 | Diabetes, arthritis, cancer, hypertension, chronic pain, heart disease, | Mean = 6; Range 3–11 | 82% White; 18% black; 3% Hispanic; 97% non-Hispanic | 12% under 10,000; 15% 10,000–19,999; 30% 20,000–39,999; 18% 40,000–49,999; 9% 50,000 +. | 64% married; 33 divorced; 3 widowed | 3% did not complete HS; 18% high school grad; 52% some college; 27% college or higher | |
| Roberge 2016 | N = 10. 5 were 60 years or older. | 50 | Depression; anxiety; cardiovascular diseases; pulmonary conditions & musculoskeletal conditions | Not reported | Not reported | Not reported | 7/10 married or lived with a partner | 7/10 had high school degree or less | |
| Roberto 2005 | N = 17. mean 76.1 (range 69–84) | 100 | Diabetes, heart disease, osteoporosis | mean 4.1; range 2–6 | Not reported | Monthly income: two < 750; six 750–1000; one 1001–1299; Two 1300–1999; One 2000–2999; Two 3000–3900; three not reported. | 11 Widowed; 1 Single; 4 Married; 1 Divorced. 11 lived alone, 1 with son, 1 with daughter, 4 with husband. | 3 greater than high school; 12 high school; 2 < high school | |
| Ryan 2016 | 1805 were qualified as high need; 1274 | 52 | Diabetes | Not reported | White, non-Hispanic: 64; | The high needs population has | The high needs population has | Not reported | The high needs population has |

**Table 2** Characteristics of study participants (*Continued*)

| Author and year | Sample size and mean age (age range) | % Female | Diseases | Number of diseases | Ethnicity | SES | Living situation/ Marital status | Education | Other |
|---|---|---|---|---|---|---|---|---|---|
| | Multiple complex chronic conditions; 379 under 65 disabled; 152 frail elderly. 82% 50 years and older with high needs. | | | | Black, non-Hispanic: 10 & Hispanic: 15 | lower level of income than the general US population | | lower level of education than the general US population | |
| Schoenberg 2011 | N = 20. Mean age 55 | 85% | Heart disease or hypertension; arthritis; type 2 diabetes; cancer; stroke; and other illnesses | Mean of 4 | 95% white | 65% less than $10,000 20% $10,001–15,000 5% $15,001–20,000 10% $20,001–25,000. | 55% married. Most lived with at least one other person | 15% had less than high school 25% attended some high school 55% earned a high school diploma or equivalent 5% had some postsecondary education | All unemployed. Average length of stay in county is 36 years. 70% had no health insurance. Those who did report insurance, indicated Medicaid, Medicare, or disability coverage. |
| Sheridan 2012 | 33 were aged 55–74 and 13 were 75+ | 50 | Cardiovascular, COPD, congestive heart failure, depression, gout, diabetes, arthritis | Most had 3+ chronic conditions | 32/42 were from ethic minority groups: 19 pacific, 12 Samoans, Maori 8 and Asian 3. | Lowest socioeconomic class quintile in Auckland | 33 lived with family, 6 alone and 3 in residential care. 33 lived with family, 6 lived alone, 3 lived in residential care. | Not reported | |
| Zulman 2015 | N = 53. Mean 59 (SD =11) | 26 | Diabetes, arthritis, cancer, hypertension, chronic pain, depression, headaches, PTSD, Lung/ breathing problems, prostate problems | Mean 5 (SD 2) | White, non-Hispanic 81%; Black, non-Hispanic 6%; His-panic 9%; Other, non-Hispanic 13% | <$50,000 43%; $50,001–$75,000 16%; >$75,001 41% | Not reported | High school degree or less 8%; some college + 44%; college degree or more 48% | |

Health care professional characteristics

| Year and author | Sample size and mean age | Type of provider | | | | Years of experience | Other | | |
|---|---|---|---|---|---|---|---|---|---|
| Ancker 2015 | N = 7, no age provided | 2 Nurse Practitioners, 2 internists; 2 family medicine physicians; 1 emergency medicine physician | | | | Not collected | 4/7 Females | | |
| Bardach 2012 | N = 12, age range 31–47. | Family medicine, internal medicine and OB/GYN | | | | 3–22 years | They were all affiliated with a university health system but 5 practices in offsite community locations | | |
| Barstow 2015 | N = 59, no age provided | Occupational therapists | | | | OT experience:< 10 year 25%, 10–20 45% & > 20 | | | |

**Table 2** Characteristics of study participants (Continued)

| Author and year | Sample size and mean age (age range) | % Female | Diseases | Number of diseases | Ethnicity | SES | Living situation/ Marital status | Education | Other |
|---|---|---|---|---|---|---|---|---|---|
| Bunn 2017 | 56 health care providers, no age provided | Family physicians; consultants with specialty in diabetes & VI; Rest not mentioned | | | | 30%; Low vision experience: < 10 68.3%,10–20 | Not reported | | |
| Coventry 2014 | N = 20, no age provided | 16 family physicians and 4 Practice Nurses | | | | 18 (5–36) | | | |
| Gill 2014 | N = 4, no age provided | 4 family physicians from one family health team | | | | Not reported | | | |
| Grundberg 2016 | N = 25, age range 31–83. | Nurses. 2/25 were specialized nurses in mental health care. 4 had BScN degree, 6 MN degree. Most worked full time | | | | range 4 months –34 years | 2 were specialized RNs in mental health care. Most of them completed training in motivational interviewing | | |
| Hansen 2015 | N = 15, mean age 53.4 (range 39–55) | Family physicians | | | | 14.6 years (7–28) | Family physicians treated 500 to 749 patient every 3 months and 35.7% worked in single practices | | |
| Kuluski 2013 | N = 4, no age provided | Family physicians | | | | Mean: 3; 3 practiced for at least 10 years, 1 physician had practiced 1 year. | | | |
| Naganathan 2016 | N = 4, no age provided | 4 family physicians | | | | Not reported | 46% physicians reported that patient currently receiving home care; 93% receiving support from family caregivers; 57% from friends and neighbours; 46% from community programmes. | | |
| Roberge 2016 | N = 18. Ae clinicians half were 30–39 years old | Clinicians (family physician, nurse, psychologist, social worker; n = 18) | | | | 56% had > 10 years' experience | Clinicians felt at ease treating pts. with anxiety and depressive disorders. Sixteen had access to support of other mental health services and they had attended on average 1.7 days of continuing education related to mental health. | | |
| Smith 2010 | | Family physicians | | | | Not reported | | | |

Caregiver characteristics

| Author and year | Sample size | Age | %female | Relationship to older adult | | | Health | Education | Other |
|---|---|---|---|---|---|---|---|---|---|
| Bunn 2017 | N = 33 | Median age 65, range 46–90 | 82% | 64% of carers were a spouse, 14% adult child | | | Not reported | Not reported | Carers: 85% white |
| Gill 2014 | N = 28 | Mean age: 70.5; SD 11.3 | 79% | Spouse | | | Most had more than high school education | Not reported | Lived in a single-family home |

**Table 2** Characteristics of study participants (*Continued*)

| Author and year | Sample size and mean age (age range) | % Female | Diseases | Number of diseases | Ethnicity | SES | Living situation/ Marital status | Education | Other |
|---|---|---|---|---|---|---|---|---|---|
| Kuluski 2013 | N = 28, 70.5 (SD 11.3) | 82% | | | 61% were spouses; 32% child; 3.5% sibling; 3.5% friend | Not reported | Not reported | Not reported | |
| Lo 2016 | N = 8, No description provided except that they were carers of chronic kidney disease Stage 5 patients | Not reported | Not reported | | | Not reported | Not reported | Not reported | |
| Mason 2016 | N = 17, Not reported | Not reported | Not reported | Not reported | | Not reported | Not reported | Not reported | |
| Morales-Asencio 2016 | N = 18, Not reported | Not reported | Not reported | spouse 72%, son/daughter 17% | | | | | |
| Naganathan 2016 | N = 28, 70.5 (SD = 11.3) years of age | 82% | | 61% spousal caregivers | | 64% > high school | | | > 75% lived in a single family home |

*COPD* Chronic obstructive pulmonary disease
*OT* Occupational therapist
*PTSD* Post Traumatic Stress Disorder
*SD* Standard Deviation

white, followed by 'non-Hispanic', Hispanic, black and South Asian populations. Other ethnicities were also reported in smaller proportions. Fourteen studies did not report ethnicity of the study participants [28, 34, 36, 38–40, 44–46, 50, 51, 54, 56, 61].

Nineteen of the 36 studies did not report the socio-economic status of the participants [28, 30–32, 34, 37–40, 42–44, 46, 47, 50, 54, 57, 60, 61]. Four studies included the employment status [27, 35, 48, 56], with most participants being unemployed. Income levels were reported from study participants belonging to varied socio-economic levels. Varied education levels were reported for study participants. Amongst all studies reporting education levels, most participants ranging from 35 to 70%, had high school education or higher [27, 29, 30, 33, 35, 36, 38, 41, 46, 48, 49, 51, 55, 56, 59], except for one study reporting education levels of high need adults being lower than the general population in the US [58]. Sixteen out of the 36 studies did not report education of the participants [26, 31, 32, 34, 37, 39, 42–45, 47, 53, 54, 57, 60, 61].

Living situation was reported with patients living with someone or alone. There was a wide variation in patients with MCC living alone, with a spouse and/or with family. Proportion of persons living with a spouse ranged from 13 to 82% [27, 30, 35, 36, 38, 40, 48–51, 59], while 30 to 50% of participants were living alone [27, 32, 37]. Urban-rural distribution was not reported by most studies, except one mentioning that there were 15% rural participants [48] and another mentioning that 50% of the clinics were rural [47]. No definitions of rurality were given.

The mean age of caregivers ranged from 69 to 71 [31, 38, 41, 46]. Three studies did not report the mean age of caregivers [42, 44, 45]. Eighty-two percent of the caregivers were female. Seventy-two percent were spouses of the older adults while 21% were adult children. In terms of HCPs, 1 study included nurse practitioners [26], physicians were included in 10 studies [26, 28, 31, 34, 38, 40, 41, 46, 50, 54], nurses were included in 4 studies [34, 39, 45, 50], psychologists were included in 1 study [50], pharmacists were included in 1 study [54], social workers in 1 study [50], and occupational therapists were included in 1 study [60]. The HCPs' experience working with patients with MCC ranged from 4 months [39] to 36 years [34]. More detailed characteristics of the participants are presented in Table 2.

## Quality of the included studies
The quality assessment results are presented in Additional file 2: Table S2, available on line. The quality was moderate to good for most studies. We defined good quality as having a yes on all relevant quality criteria ($n = 13$), moderate as having items with no/can't tell and the rest yes for relevant criteria ($n = 23$). There were no

studies ranked as poor, which indicated a no on the majority of relevant quality assessment criteria. This rating scale allowed us to compare the different studies of different quality [62]. The rating scale allowed us to rate studies of different quality. Six studies used convenience samples [34, 39, 46, 56, 59, 60]. It was not always clear how the data were analyzed nor who analyzed the data [26, 29, 31, 61]. Also, it was not always clear how findings were influenced by researchers' interactions with participants [31, 33, 35, 38, 44, 46, 48, 52, 54, 61].

## Thematic analysis of the findings
Five themes emerged from the data and there was convergence on most of the key themes between the older adults, the caregiver and the HCPs (Table 3). They included: 1) Need for information; 2) Need for coordination of services and supports; 3) Need for preventive, maintenance and restorative strategies, 4) Need for training to help manage the older adults' complex conditions, and 5) Need for person-centred approaches. The few discrepancies within the themes will also be discussed.

## Need for information
The need for access to information was a theme that emerged the most often in the studies included in the review [26, 32, 38, 40, 45, 53, 56, 61]. Older persons with MCC spoke about the need for more information about their medical conditions. Specifically, they addressed the need for HCPs to use less technical terms and jargon [40], thorough explanations of diagnoses by specialists [40], comprehensive explanation of treatment options [40], and the rationale as to why certain medications were prescribed to them [56]. Patients believed that having a greater understanding of their conditions would help them better manage their conditions and gain greater control over their lives and be empowered [61]. However, many felt they did not have enough information for disease self-management [45]. Some older adults found that self-care required for one condition could make self-care for another condition difficult, as the advice was sometimes incompatible [29].

Patients also reported lack of timely information and poor communication between multiple HCPs [38], and often did not feel like they were being heard which led to distrust and feeling powerless [53]. Likewise, caregivers commented on the poor communication between HCPs and older adults, and because of the lack of seamless sharing of information between various team members and specialists, caregivers felt they needed to step in [31]. Because of the lack of information family members found themselves taking on an advocacy role, needing to participate in acquiring medical and service information as well as medical decision making [31].

**Table 3** Overview of identified needs

| First Author Publication Year | Actual Needs identified by older adults |
|---|---|
| Adeniji 2015 | The needs which were identified most frequently (50% or higher) included: 'Lack of information about my medical condition' (55%) 'Poor communication between different doctors or clinics' (55%) 'Lack of information about treatment options' (60%) 'Having to wait a long time to get an appointment for specialists (hospital doctors)' (60%) 'Lack of information about why my medication was prescribed to me' (50%) |
| Ancker 2015 | Some patients perceive medical records management as the team's responsibility whereas other perceived it as their own. Patients make judgments about what data is relevant to their health. Managing transfers of medical information to solve problems such as health insurance denials is a tremendous amount of work that goes unrecognized. |
| Ansari 2014 | New COPD diagnosis motivated participants to modify healthcare behaviors such as need to include physical activity and monitor diet; lack of communication between the participants and their physicians; expressed the need individualized plan and support for smoking cessation. The participants found managing MCC challenging due to the need to consume various medications and schedule various appointments, and voiced that after some time, the meds stop working. Participants who were most affected by arthritis and then developed COPD, found it quite challenging due it causing breathing difficulty, an additional problem with arthritis. |
| Barstow 2015 | The patients describe their experiences but did not identify needs |
| Bayliss 2007 | Self-reported health status: 12% excellent/very good; 38% good; 36% fair; 14% poor. Multivariable model was constructed: After adjusting for effects of multimorbidity, psychosocial factors were independently associated with health status and physical functioning. Greater disease burden, persistent depressive symptoms and financial constraints were associated with both lower health status and lower physical functioning. Symptoms and and/or treatments interfere with each other, and combined with a lower income level, were associated with lower physical functioning. Higher levels of patient-provider communication were associated with lower levels of physical functioning. Interactions were found between disease burden and communication, financial constraints, and the compound effect of conditions; additionally, impact of certain barriers may not be constant across the range of morbidity. Other factors that were significantly associated with the outcomes but did not contribute to the final models include: self-efficacy, being overwhelmed by a single condition; knowledge about medications and health literacy. |
| Bayliss 2003 | patients were asked what barriers to their self-management was and the barriers included the self-care required for one condition could make the self-care for another condition difficult, the advice was sometimes incompatible, the symptoms influence each other and the medications can cause symptoms of the other disease worse, lack of knowledge, financial constraints to pay for all treatments, emotional stress of the diseases, need for adequate communication with providers, need for social support, need for understanding conditions and logistical issues dealing with multiple conditions. |
| Beverly 2011 | Prioritizing health conditions: (i) Most patients acknowledge that complications of their diabetes motivated them to pay greater attention to their diabetes to diminish the progression of these complications. (ii) Patients reported prioritizing health conditions and severity or importance. (iii) Patients described feeling frustrated, confused, and overwhelmed in response to conflicting recommendations, particularly for diet, physical activity and medication regimens. |
| Bunn 2017 | Both patients with dementia & caregivers expressed the need for continuity of care and involving them in the decision making process. |
| Burton 2016 | In the interview asking the participant about their health. The participants who all had vision loss indicated challenges to accessing information, being dependent on family and friends to read letters and other information. The family physician was acting as another barrier to information and appointment attendance. Patients want their family physician to better coordinate care for persons with vision loss and other health conditions. |
| First Author Publication Year | Actual Needs identified by older adults |
| Cheraghi-Sohi 2013 | Patient had a need for control and knowledge about their conditions. Patients had fluctuating priorities highlighting the importance of regular assessments during clinician-patient consultation to allow for better treatment planning. Patient priorities shift according to perceptions of control and/or interactions with clinical professionals. Focusing on management of only one single condition can lead to worse self-management. |
| Clarke 2014 | They want their family physician to be thorough, they want to be referred to the expert, and they want their family physician to build a good trusting relationship for them. A third want their family physician to have a more person centered approach to decision making |
| Coventry 2014 | Successful self-management in multimorbidity hinged on the interplay and interdependence between contextual factors related to 1) patients capacity (access to resources), knowhow and confidence and physical and emotional abilities to accomplish self-management activities; 2) Responsibility was successful to self-management - patients had to be responsible for self-management tasks; 3) patients had to be motivated to manage their condition |
| DiNapoli 2016 | Access to providers, asking for preference in provider, wanting their health care provider to build a doctor patient relationship, working together with the patient in a timely matter. To address mental health issues in the treatment for their chronic conditions. Advocate for the use of mental health services, advertise services available |
| Fortin 2005 | Access to the family physician or specialist can be complicated due to automatic telephone messages, long waiting lings or the number of phone calls required. It creates anxiety. Also the waiting times in the ED are long and it is not clear when it is an emergency that they need to go to the ED (lack of capacity to determine the seriousness of the illness). Similarly there are long waiting times to see a specialist and the need for a referral is a barrier to access care. However, utilizing the family |

**Table 3** Overview of identified needs *(Continued)*

| First Author Publication Year | Actual Needs identified by older adults |
|---|---|
| | physician to determine whether ED or a specialist was needed could also speed up the access to care. |
| Fried 2008 | 1) Participants spoke about the concern with competing outcomes - the adverse effects of medications was a competing outcome that influenced their treatment decision making. 2) Participants spoke about global cross-disease outcomes (like preventing a stroke or heart attack) instead of disease specific outcomes (like lower blood pressure); Preference was for the treatment that would achieve the most desired outcome |
| Gill 2014 | Patients reported lack of timely information and poor communication between health care providers and they had difficulty with symptom management and adhering to treatment recommendations. The patients complained about excessive wait times to see specialists. Furthermore, they had difficulty coordinating their care and medical trainees were even not consulting with their supervisor. Patients indicating not know how to prioritize their care and needs. |
| Hansen 2015 | Patients expressed that there is no thorough explanations of the diagnoses by the specialists requiring them to go to their family physicians for clarity; need to have transfer of communication between family physicians and the specialists so family physicians are adequately informed of the patients' MCC; difficulty understanding technical terms/jargons; patients expressed that they want to be seen by their family physicians as a person and not merely a number |
| Kuluski 2013 | 4 main themes:<br>health maintenance; health improvement; behavior change; and preparation for future needs.<br>'-Most patients wanted to prevent aggravating their health and chronic condition; these related to: avoiding inability to perform tasks because of pain;<br>-Improvement matters to resume participating in physical and social activities that they were used to.<br>-Behavior change was expressed as a need for losing weight and exercising, and being able to do more to relieve their caregivers;<br>-Some expressed the need for preparing for the future which meant having home support, transitioning to a long term care facility. This was not always preferred; some wanted to stay and get help at home. |
| First Author Publication Year | Actual Needs identified by older adults |
| Lo 2016 | Both patients and caregivers emphasized the key role of self-management, socio-economic situation and negative experiences as key in their health care as well as 5 health care service level factors empowerment of patient and the caregiver, access to care, poor coordination of care, continuity of care and poor recognition of psychological comorbidities. Being from a non-English speaking background led to difficulties in patient education, and self-management particularly with regard to nutrition. There is an extra financial burden due to due to transportation costs, paying for medication, marking and for maintaining a healthy lifestyle as well as community services that were used. The person who feels not well fatigue and disability impacted special life and relationships in a negative way. Psychiatric comorbidities such as depression make health self-management more difficult. Patients want more education to understand their disease, how to manage and the adverse outcomes. They appreciated support groups and sell-directed eLearning. The information should have been more combined for all diseases; the patient education material can be contradictory. There are problems with the coordination of care due to poor communication between hospital and primary care. Patients experience problems due to specialty boundaries, health care providers were unwilling to provide advice or offer help with problems that were not their scope. Patients experience a lack of continuity in care many different specialists with conflicting opinions. They felt one person should be in charge such as the PCP. Appointments should be scheduled so they don't clash. Lack of access, lack of close by parking, too short consultation time, lack of interpreters, difficulty reaching health care providers, |
| Loeb 2003 | Patients described periods of gaining, losing, and maintain capabilities through their experience of living with multiple chronic conditions. The main need was to maintain current capacity to perform activities of daily living. Following a period of declining capabilities (like a hospitalization); they worked towards a process of regaining capabilities to reestablish their previous health state. Coping strategies used to keep what they have included: relating with health care providers, medicating, exercising, changing dietary patterns, seeking information, relying on spirituality and/or religion, and engaging in life |
| Mason 2016 | Complicated, confusing and sometimes unresponsive services.<br>- Lack of care coordination and continuity among service providers<br>- Attending clinics was physically demanding.<br>- Frequent changes to medication changes cast doubts on their use.<br>- Some perceived their care to be poorer because they are older (experiencing inequity).<br>- Focused on living life to the fullest in the present. Thus, some participants avoided advance planning and only sought help when they were very ill or unable to cope. Deteriorating health was perceive as a manifestation of aging and thus delayed seeking help. Delaying services was furthermore seen as a way to preserve autonomy. |
| McDonall 2016 | communication (understanding and being understood), transportation/mobility issues, access print, communication with health/service providers in the community, and training how to use technology, assistance with errands, information about assistive technologies for hearing, activities to participate in. In terms of the services they would have liked to have included transportation, older blind program, volunteers to assist with daily activities, and a senior center. They also discussed that health care providers should receive education on how to approach persons with a dual sensory impairment to maintain their dignity. |
| Morales-Asencio 2016 | They had limited resources and there lots of barriers, lack of elevator in building, health care providers were not proactive in providing all information. Maintaining lifestyles was difficult. Implementing a treatment was difficult for some patients, and took time and effort. Lack of coordination of care, fragmentation of care. No clear care pathway when issues arise leading to ED visits. Not enough information given by provider for disease self-management. If support is offered it is helpful for |

**Table 3** Overview of identified needs *(Continued)*

| First Author Publication Year | Actual Needs identified by older adults |
|---|---|
| | adaption to the illness and treatment adherence. Health care services are fragmented and not adapted to persons with complex needs. |

| First Author Publication Year | Actual Needs identified by older adults |
|---|---|
| Naganathan 2016 | Patients<br>- Some felt a loss of independence and less in control<br>- Patients emphasized wanting to remain at home and not be institutionalized- echoed by caregivers and physicians.<br>- Sources of tension between patients, caregivers, and HCPs- discordance between patients' perception of their independence and the amount of support are needed. Sometimes leading to caregiver burnout when family refuse help.<br>- highlighted the importance of social networks. |
| Noel 2005 | Illnesses had a significant impact on their daily life activities, work activities, social and family life. Uncertainty about their prognosis and inability to plan the future were important stressors. There were several problems with the health care system: 1) ling waits for referrals; 2) lack of continuity between clinics; 3) access to urgent care was not ideal; 4) poor communication with provider. Physicians had too many patients, were too busy or did not have enough support to provide care they needed. The time allowed for appointments was not long enough to discuss their health care needs. As they had many appointments scheduling was difficult to avoid impacting their work and family life. Patients felt specialists do not take their complaints seriously. |
| Ravenscroft 2010 | -Fragmented care delivery: location of services across multiple locations, even within a single organization; lack of access to patient information leading to duplication of investigations, other problems;<br>-Fragmentation complicated by health care provider's time, information sharing with patients; logistical problems in keeping appointments such as transport, parking, etc.<br>-MCC patients' issues magnified with seemingly small health care issues, as these were repeated, increasing frustration levels, and finding solutions over and over again.<br>Discovering the health system:<br>-Process of ongoing discovery about the social structures within the health care system: patients perceived different parts, and constructed their own theories about it; providers difficult to differentiate between specialties, ranks and roles; regulation of interactions between them and providers; avoidance of MCC patients, referring them to others; reasonable expectations from the system were more often unrealistic;<br>Managing the health care system:<br>-patients strategized navigating the system; monitoring their care; they actively advocated through asking questions, voicing concerns and even 'directing' their providers; building and maintaining connections and relationships with trusted providers, and sought opportunities to end relationships with providers they did not trust; taking advantage of loopholes such as appointment cancellations to. |
| Richardson 2016 | Veterans ranked their prioritization of their conditions according to: 1) perceived role of the condition in the body - that is, how the condition linked with the overall body function; 2) how the individual self-managed their conditions; 3) dealing with pain; 4) health care perception of which condition to prioritize<br>Patients prioritized conditions by family history anticipating the same outcomes; impact on other conditions, daily activities such as mobility; and that have potential serious consequences if unmanaged. They also lacked knowledge about root causes of the conditions.<br>Among self-management tasks, they prioritized conditions which required medical monitoring, felt in control of, activities based on financial costs, newer conditions requiring changes to daily routines.<br>Patients prioritized pain management.<br>Patients did not disclose their priorities to their HCPs. However, according to the patients, their HCPs have suggested which conditions to prioritize. |
| Roberge 2016 | There were time constraints and patients hesitated to talk about their mental health. Not all patients wanted to talk about both their chronic condition and their mental health problem at the same family physician visit. Patients. felt stigmatized because of their mental health problem. Patients felts there are a lack of access to psychotherapy. Patients also reported lack of availability, costs, compatibility, language difficulty accessing services and their clinician's lack of knowledge of available resources. |

| First Author Publication Year | Actual Needs identified by older adults |
|---|---|
| Roberto 2005 | The women identified nine problems associated with their health concerns: pain, falls, functional limitations (e.g., activities of daily living [ADLs], instrumental activities of daily living [IADLs]), sleep disturbances, reduced energy, psychological distress (e.g., stress, worry), financial strain, medications, and compliance with treatment regime. The combination of problems attributed to different conditions increased the magnitude of the effect the women's health had on their daily lives. Pain and a decline in energy frequently interfered with completion of daily activities. To compensate for this, many women reduced and slowed down the pace of activities they performed while emphasizing the importance of maintaining independence Appreciative of support from family members, at times the women received more help and advice than they preferred. Accepting health-related changes was not al-ways easy for the women and often was complicated by the response and intended support of others |
| Ryan 2016 | -Social isolation and unmet social needs: High needs patients showed emotional distress in last 2 years; 37% felt socially isolated, including lack of companionship, feeling left out, lonely and isolated as compared to 15% other adults in the sample. |

**Table 3** Overview of identified needs *(Continued)*

| First Author Publication Year | Actual Needs identified by older adults |
|---|---|
| | -Delaying care: 44% high needs patients reported delaying care due to an access issue- 22% transport as compared to 4% other adults; limited clinic hours; 29% due to inability to get appointments. <br> -95% of high need patients had a regular doctor/clinic; 65% high need and 68% older adults were able to get answers to medical queries; <br> -35% high need patients reported easily accessing care after hours without going to the emergency room, as compared to 53% other adults. <br> --Assistance in managing conditions: <br> -For stress, 43% could access counseling services when wanted; of the 53% high need patients needing multiple providers, 43% had a provider coordinating treatment; Of the 57% having issues with ADLs, 38% had someone to help them; 3/4th of which were relatives; <br> -Insurance was also important: <br> --Patient centered communication: 60% high-need patients had providers who fully engage in patient-centered communication, compared to other adults (52%). However, 82% of high-need adults were less likely to report that providers involve them in treatment decisions vs. 90% of others; 85% vs. 91% would listen carefully to them. |
| Schoenberg 2011 | 1) Participants viewed multimorbidity as more than the sum of its individual conditions. This led to worry over negative health consequences and conflicting and confusing treatment. 2) Community conditions including scarcity of personal resources, in adequate transportation to health care appointments, health care provider shortages, and insufficient healthy choices/resources undermined their self-management. 3) They managed their multimorbidity by settling into a routine that was often at odds with biomedical recommendations, but ones that worked for them. |
| Sheridan 2012 | The visits with their family physician are short, mostly to describe pills, and lack of involved of practice nurses. Many reported feeling lonely, sad and suicidal. Most participants wanted to self-manage their conditions but they needed more information. The patients received conflicting messages from the different clinicians, feel that their provider do not communicate. Patients felt not being heard, there was difficulty in communicating and anger and mistrusts. Patients felt powerless. |
| Zulman 2015 | 3 Major themes <br> 1. Managing a high volume of Information and Tasks: -High volume of records from multiple systems; absence of a comprehensive system in emergencies; Paperwork increases with each encounter with a provider; self-management routines to manage medicines, diets, etc.; -Health information: usually disease specific info available; condition interactions, risk of medication interactions, especially with multiple providers not available. Complicated medication regimes; patient may be the only person aware of it; multiple self-management tasks required throughout the day; multiple appointments to manage. -Communication: Complexity of MCC makes it difficult to seek care from new providers. 2. Coordinating multiple providers: almost no opportunity to involve multiple providers in a single discussion on management. 3. Serving as Expert and advocate: patients find themselves isolated/alone to resolve needs. -Peer support: difficult to find. -Caregivers: get overwhelmed with complexity and number of MCCs. |

| First Author Publication Year | Actual Needs identified by caregivers |
|---|---|
| Bunn 2017 | Family members expressed the need to take charge to aid in getting continuity and access to services for their loved ones with dementia. They need to advocate for services and participate in medical decision making for the person living with dementia. They also played active role in coordinating care and services as well as navigate the healthcare system such as for arranging appointments and associated transportation needs, managing medications and serve as a means of communication between various providers. Caregivers reported formal support for persons living with dementia as inadequate. Lack of seamless sharing of information between various HCPs from different specialties. They identified a gap between the social care and healthcare and expressed the need for collaboration between them. As, this gap increases the risk for adverse events such as hypoglycemia. |
| Gill 2014 | Caregivers also indicated long wait times, poor communication and lack of care coordination. It was difficult managing appointments with their work; they prefer to have a point person to talk to arrange care. Caregivers describe intentional noncompliance by the patient and due to complex city, facing stress from high risk decisions, feeling pressured and hopeless. |
| Kuluski 2013 | 6 themes, of which first 3 were the same as patient goals. For future needs preparation, they wanted the patients' acceptance for services. <br> -Health maintenance: keep up a social network and involved in activities, e.g. through regaining mobility and pain management; having a caregiver to rely on; acceptance of care from outside by the patient. <br> -Doing tasks for the patient. some wanted to continue tasks for the patient, e.g. keeping appointments, medication management, nutrition; <br> -Keeping the patient safe; with dignity so that patients don't feel that they are being treated as invalid; which would also promote acceptance. Safety a major concern for dementia patients. <br> -Helping patients maintain dignity, particularly at the end of life. <br> -Stress management a major concern, to at least 'keep sane.' |
| Mason 2016 | Being a carer was not a choice. <br> - carers experience physical and emotional stress |
| Naganathan 2013 | Caregivers <br> - Sources of tension about disagreement between patients and caregivers about future plans, and how to stay healthy and safe. |

**Table 3** Overview of identified needs *(Continued)*

| First Author Publication Year | Actual Needs identified by older adults |
|---|---|
| | - Emphasized the importance of formal supports for IADLS to alleviate caregiver burden and improve patient-caregiver relationships.<br>- Felt immense burden with navigating healthcare system to obtain sufficient home care services. |

| First Author Publication Year | Actual Needs identified by health care providers |
|---|---|
| Ancker 2015 | Providers need easy access to their patients' information to make the best care decisions. Providers also talked about patient's health literacy - for example patients selective reporting of information. Physicians often recognized that the patients understanding of the health care system influenced the way they shared their medical histories. |
| Bardach 2012 | The physicians believed that their patients lacked the resources to follow prevention recommendations; the lack access to exercise, financial restraints to exercise or buy healthy food, lack of community resources, uninsured patients who have no access to resources. System barriers were also reported, time restraints, lack of reimbursement for preventative counseling. There is also a lack of care coordination particularly in the absence of EMR. |
| Barstow 2015 | The HCPs described how comorbidities increased the number of visits, more visits cancelled and the need to collaborate with the caregivers well as the need for home visits. Nearly 60% identified a need for case coordination and many needs for referrals to other health care providers such as psychologists/counselor, physicians and diabetes educator |

| First Author Publication Year | Actual Needs identified by health care providers |
|---|---|
| Bunn 2017 | HCPs used practices for alleviating the impact of living with dementia by reminding them of upcoming appointments, providing them with longer appointment times and same HCP that saw patient and carer. HCP need structured way of preparing for the progressing dementia and resultant worsening symptoms, which may lead to dropping out of the system leading to increased risk for adverse outcomes such as medication errors, caregiver burnout. HCPs spoke about the importance of personalizing care for the person living with dementia |
| Coventry 2014 | Same needs as identified by patients because patients and HCPs data were analyzed together. |
| Gill 2014 | The family physicians also discussed lack of access to care, poor communication and coordination, long wait times, and challenges with compliance, lack of home care for instrumental activities of daily living limitations, dealing with multiple specialists |
| Grundberg 2016 | Patients often do not actively disclose mental health issues. There needs to be continuity of care and time to engage patients in dialogue about mental health. Common health issues in this population: depression, anxiety, sleeps problems and phobias. Patients need prompt psychiatric consultations. District nurses (DNs) need better teamwork with other HCPs so participants can increase their abilities in assessing and addressing mental health issues. DNs need to be more educated about mental health promotion activities and available resources for the patients. Older people with multimorbidity primarily lived alone and felt lonely which contributes to developing depression (especially affected women). Homebound seniors with few visitors are especially at risk for isolation and worsened mental health. |
| Hansen 2015 | Specialists need to thoroughly inform family physicians about their patients' diagnoses; due to lack of communication on diagnoses, family physicians spend a large sum of time to understand patients' condition on their own and also to explain then to the patient; family physicians find this challenging due to a full waiting room; patients requires diseases to be explained at their level of understanding; patients identifies their issues based on symptoms and not necessarily according to prognosis e.g. vertigo |
| Kuluski 2013 | Family physician goals '4 similar themes:<br>-help maintain patient independence<br>-heal, fix or improve symptoms when possible,<br>-mobilize care for the patient and the caregiver<br>-address safety issues.<br>For the above goals, family physicians focused on preparing both patients and caregivers for worsening of health; maintaining independence; heal, fix or improve symptoms; particularly helping with acute exacerbations of conditions; family physicians emphasized supportive services and infrastructure, such as home care for safety, for both patients and caregivers; patient acceptance of these. For aging caregivers, stress was an important aspect to focus on to keep them healthy. |
| Naganthan 2013 | Family physicians<br>- physician reported a contradiction in that patients and caregivers refused additional support to stay at home when they desire to stay at home.<br>- Caregivers who are heavily or exclusively relied upon by the patients tend to experience higher burden than those who receive support.<br>- Some tension between physicians and families related to safety concerns.<br>- Caregivers are viewed as key in navigating healthcare system and being the patients' advocate |

| First Author Publication Year | Actual Needs identified by health care providers |
|---|---|
| Roberg 2016 | The clinicians reported challenges with adherence as these patients required patient education and regular follow-up, they were often on a complex medication regime and they did not want more medication. Polypharmacy was also a challenge. |

**Table 3** Overview of identified needs *(Continued)*

| First Author Publication Year | Actual Needs identified by older adults |
| --- | --- |
| | The want more training on polypharmacy, more psychiatry rounds and more about different pharmacological options. The physicians reported it was difficult to obtain a consultation from a psychiatry in short term for patients when the pt. was on multiple meds and at risk of interactions but the condition was not deemed urgent. All physicians had difficulty communicating with private practice psychologists and that these psychologists could benefit from a better understanding of the nature and treatment of their pt.'s chronic diseases. The main barriers were the lack of mental health services, the delay accessing specialized services, less than optimal collaboration and communication between professionals, and training needs. For patients it included the burden of care (multiple treatments, frequent consultations) which influenced readiness to access additional services. The health and social service center had long waiting lists, complex pathways, many clinicians and often unspecialized services. |
| Smith 2010 | 5 main themes:<br>1. Multimorbidity and the link to Polypharmacy and ageing. • Multimorbidity a common phenomenon associated mostly with older age. Polypharmacy commonly associated with it, but not being given attention to, and which may add to multimorbidity.<br>• Lack of distinction between multiple conditions and multiple risk factors was linked to the growth in preventive care; also clinical guidelines focused on single diseases which encouraged Polypharmacy.<br>2. Health system issues:<br>-Lack of time for managing complex patients; increased workload;<br>-Poor inter-professional communication, leading to fragmented care; between specialists, family physicians and pharmacists; latter felt isolated<br>3. Individual issues for clinicians: family physicians felt they were the coordinators of care; lacked clinical confidence dealing with complex issues; role of the practice nurse seemed unclear to them in managing MCC patients, since these were too complex for them to manage; making decisions in isolation from specialists; they regarded pharmacists having an important role, esp. for drug interactions;<br>-Pharmacists wanted to be involved but felt overloaded; observed that family physicians don't review medicines; decision making was at the specialist level, where hospital pharmacists could be involved;<br>-Some suggested that specialists/hospitals were pushing their work on to primary care.<br>-Inconsistencies: related to keeping patients under family physicians care, while at the same time wanting access to specialist care.<br>-Clinical uncertainty related to stopping medications by both.<br>-Family physicians felt inadequately managing MMC due to lack of time, and expertise.<br>-Patient issues:<br>Burden of MCC on care givers and patients was acknowledged; with the health system complicating care and patients becoming depressed; cognitive impairment was also an issue; depression and loneliness further burdened caregivers; while some patients took active interest in their care, particularly managing medications.<br>-Potential solutions: Better models of care delivery, with more time for MCC; planning care better proactively; integrating rehabilitation programs; information sharing between providers; clear lines of responsibility. |

*MCC* Multiple chronic conditions

HCPs also found accessing information about the older adult challenging [38]. Not being able to access the information made care decisions challenging [26]. They realized that the information patients shared with them was often related to their level of health literacy so selective reporting occurred [26]. HCPs also described issues related to access to information between fellow HCPs. Family physicians found that specialists did not thoroughly inform them about diagnoses, and hence family physicians spent a lot of time trying to understand the patient's condition on their own and then having to explain it to the patient [40].

From some HCPs and older adults' perspectives, older adults with dementia, mental health conditions and sensory impairments were found to be at higher risk for having needs not met [31, 32, 39]. Older adults with vision impairment indicated that they had additional challenges to accessing information and were dependent on family and friends to read information they received from their HCPs [32]. HCPs also spoke about older adults with mental health issues such as depression, anxiety and phobias experiencing difficulties accessing speciality services [39]. Moreover, HCPs perceived that older adults with dementia required more care such as reminding them about upcoming appointments and longer appointment times [31]. Caregivers for these patients also required more support as HCPs were concerned about caregiver burnout [31].

### Need for coordination of services and supports

Most of the participants reported the lack of coordination of services and supports significantly impacted the daily lives of older adults, caregivers and health care providers. The lack of coordination of services ranged from: lack of access to specialists [35, 36]; long wait times for referrals [56]; conflicting appointments [42]; short appointment time with family physicians [47]; referrals to different specialists with conflicting opinions [42]; duplication of investigations [48]; complicated and unresponsive services [44]; and no opportunity to involve multiple providers in a single discussion [55]. As a result, some patients experienced difficulty with symptom management and adhering to treatment recommendations [38]; and settled into a routine that was at odds with their primary physician's recommendations [52]. Consequently, patients and caregivers became anxious as they were uncertain whether they were making the right choices [58], and they found themselves serving as the expert without the training [55], and felt isolated, frustrated and alone in resolving their issues [30, 58].

Caregivers mentioned that there was a lack of coordinated services in terms of formal support [31], home care services [46] and health maintenance activities [41] available for older adults. Caregivers expressed the preference for having a point person to arrange care [38] and provide continuity. For those caregivers still working, they experienced difficulties managing the care of their family member [38], but they felt they had no other option [31]. Some caregivers found themselves ensuring their family members kept their appointments, took over medication and nutrition management, and were instrumental in ensuring the person maintained their dignity, particularly at the end of life [41]. Taking on this coordinator role was a source of tension between some older adults and their caregivers as they had conflicting ideas about future plans, and how to stay healthy and safe [46].

HCPs [38, 50, 60] also identified the need for better coordinated services and supports and recommended a case coordinator [60]. Physicians identified that older adults with MCC needed to be seen by other specialists such as psychologists, diabetes educators, or mental health specialists and a coordinator could assist with this task [60] because there were often complex pathways to negotiate in order to be seen by these specialists [50]. Also, some family physicians found coordinating with multiple specialists challenging [38]. Fragmented care between specialists, GPs and pharmacists left pharmacists feeling isolated" (Smith et al. 2010).

As found in many of the articles in the review, the lack of coordination of services led to stress for older adults, caregivers and HCPs [31, 38, 44, 46, 48, 55]. Caregivers described that they had experienced their family members being non-compliant because of the complexity they were facing and the high-risk decisions they felt they had to make, which caused them to feel pressured and hopeless [38]. Because systems were so fragmented, many persons with MCC had to repeat their issues to different providers and with this came increasing levels of frustration, as they sought solutions over and over again [48]. Caregivers also became overwhelmed with the complexity and number of chronic conditions their family member had [55], or if their symptoms worsened [31], and they felt burdened by navigating the health care system to obtain services [46], all of which eventually could lead to burnout especially if the family member of older adults refused the help suggested [46]. As

Mason [44] pointed out, being a caregiver was not a choice, and they often experienced physical and emotional stress. Bunn and colleagues (2017) noted a discrepancy between HCPs attempts to coordinate care for older adults with dementia and caregivers' perceptions of these efforts. HCPs perceived they took extra time for older adults and their caregivers, reminding them about their appointments, and preparing for worsening dementia related issues, whilst family members felt more time was required with their HCPs, better coordination was needed as they felt they had to navigate care such as arranging appointments and sharing of information with different HCPs.

### Need for preventive, maintenance and restorative strategies

The need to prevent further deterioration in daily living, maintain current levels of function and restore any lost abilities was articulated by older adults, and echoed by caregivers and HCPs in a few of the studies [27, 41, 45, 46, 49]. Most older adults wanted to prevent the aggravation of their health and chronic conditions [41]. They also articulated the need to maintain current capacity to perform activities of daily living [43] but for many, maintaining lifestyles was difficult [45]. A new diagnosis often motivated older adults to modify their health care behaviors and daily routines [49] such as including physical activity into their daily regime and monitoring their diet [27], however this was difficult for some older adults, and took time and effort [45]. In order to accomplish this modification, a behavior change was often required and if support was offered it was helpful for adoption of the new treatment [45]. For some caregivers, their role included motivating their family member to make these changes, but they struggled with how to do this well and it caused a source of tension between the older adult and their caregiver [46]. Naganathan and colleagues (2016) highlighted discrepancies between caregivers and older adults' future plans on how to stay healthy and remain at home. There was disagreement on how each participant group perceived their independence and how much support was required to live at home. Family physicians were also not sure on how to handle these differences in perceptions as patients and caregivers often refused additional support which raised concerns about remaining safely at home without caregiver burnout resulting as an outcome.

Physicians in a few of the studies knew that their patients lacked the resources to follow prevention recommendations [28]. There was a recognition by HCPs that for some older adults their inability to buy healthy foods, financial restraints to pay for treatments [29], lack of community resources, or being uninsured held many back from participating in prevention [28]. Additionally, physicians also did not receive reimbursement for preventive counselling [28] nor for the longer appointment times required. Family physicians thus aimed to provide guidance by helping with acute exacerbations of conditions and improving symptoms [41]. In addition, they felt their role included emphasizing supportive services, such as home safety so the older adults could maintain function as long as they could, and to prepare both patients and caregivers for worsening of health when the time would come [41]. However, some physicians found some support services lacking such as home care which was essential to maintaining function of older adults [38].

### Need for training to help manage the older adults' complex conditions

A need identified by all three groups was for training to help manage older adults' complex conditions and to plan for the future. Older adults wanted more education to understand their disease, how to manage adverse outcomes and when offered, they appreciated support groups and self-directed eLearning [42]. They also wanted training on how to use technology [57]. Older adults also wanted HCPs to receive education on how to approach persons with dual sensory impairment to maintain their dignity [57]. Both older adults and caregivers, perceived a need for more education and training on health literacy and their medications [59].

Health care providers commented that polypharmacy was a challenge and that they wanted more training on different pharmacological options [50]. In addition, some physicians felt they lacked clinical confidence dealing with multiple complex issues, as clinical guidelines focused on one single condition leading to polypharmacy [54].

### Need for person-centred approaches

The need for more person-centred approaches to service delivery was highlighted in many of the reviewed articles by older adults and their caregivers [31, 33, 40, 48, 53]. Older adults wanted to be seen as a person and not merely as a number [40]. They highlighted the need for patient-centred communication and to be involved in treatment decisions and feel listened to during their interactions with HCPs. Clarke [33] highlighted that the older adults wanted the primary care provider to build a good trusting relationship with them and to have a more person-centred approach to decision making. Older adults wanted to build and maintain connections and relationships with trusted providers and sought to end relationships with providers they did not trust [48]. Many persons felt that they were not being heard, which led to distrust [53] in the relationship and feeling powerless. In only one study reviewed, HCPs did suggest that personalizing care for persons living with dementia was essential [31] and they made sure to

see both the patient and caregiver at each appointment. For those physicians who took a person-centred approach, such as, by taking time and listening to patients, there were repercussions, as often a full waiting room of patients were left in the clinic waiting for their appointments [40].

### Structural and social determinants of health

Structural and social determinants were examined to identify how they influenced needs of older adults (see Table 4). Of the social and structural determinants of health included in the selected studies, twelve mentioned education which is often a proxy for health literacy concerns [26, 27, 38, 43–45, 47, 50–53, 56, 58], nineteen mentioned access issues [27–29, 32, 35, 36, 38, 40, 41, 44–47, 50, 52, 54, 56–58], and fifteen highlighted the impact of socioeconomic status on needs [27–30, 34, 35, 42, 43, 49–53, 58, 59].

In contrast, only three studies cited the link between living circumstances and health and social needs [42, 50, 52]. Some studies mentioned gender [26, 27, 33, 35, 39, 52, 58], ethnicity [30, 42, 48, 50, 53, 58], living situation [27, 31, 35, 39, 42–44, 61] and having a social support network [34, 38, 41, 43, 51–53, 58, 61] in relation to the health and social care needs for older adults with MCC. In summary, it would appear that socioeconomic status, education and access to the health care system were the predominant structural and social determinants of health that influenced the needs of older adults with MCC. Gender, ethnicity, living situation and social support received less attention.

### Stakeholder consultation

All attendees agreed that the identified themes resonated with their experiences. A concern was expressed that few of the studies included older persons over the age of 85 years and emphasized they may have very different needs as they may likely be housebound. Stakeholders pointed out that there needs to be a discussion with patients and caregivers on goals of care in the final years and advanced care planning factoring in advanced age, number of disease conditions, level of function and frailty. They all agreed that access to services and supports were a concern and expressed that older persons with MCC are treated differently in the healthcare system, for example not gaining access to rehabilitation to restore function, which may be suggestive of ageism. Stakeholders felt that the needs of older adults with MCC are much more complex today as compared to several years ago but the level of staff expertise available to them has not kept pace, as care is often provided by unregulated professionals, especially in the community. Stakeholders agreed that caregivers have unique

**Table 4** Overview of Social and structural determinants of Health impacting health and social care needs in older adults with multiple chronic conditions

| Study author and year | SES | Gender | Education | Ethnicity | Living circumstances (rural /urban) | Living situation (alone or not) | Social Support/ network | Access issues |
|---|---|---|---|---|---|---|---|---|
| Adeniji 2015 | | | X | | | | | X |
| Ancker 2015 | | X | X | | | | | |
| Ansari 2014 | X | X | X | | | X | | X |
| Bardach 2012 | X | | | | | | | X |
| Barstow 2015 | | | | | | | | |
| Bayliss 2008 | X | | | | | | | |
| Bayliss 2003 | X | | | | | | | X |
| Beverly 2011 | X | | | X | | | | |
| Bunn 2017 | | | | | | X | | |
| Burton 2016 | | | | | | | | X |
| Cheraghi-Sohi 2013 | | | | | | X | X | |
| Clarke 2014 | | X | | | | | | |
| Coventry 2014 | X | | | | | | X | |
| DiNapoli 2016 | X | x | | | | X | | X |
| Fortin 2005 | | | | | | | | X |
| Fried 2008 | | | | | | | | |
| Gill 2014 | | | X | | | | X | X |
| Grundberg 2016 | | X | | | | X | | |
| Hansen 2015 | | | | | | | | X |
| Kuluski 2013 | | | | | | | X | X |
| Lo 2016 | X | | | X | X | X | | |
| Loeb 2003 | X | | X | | | X | X | |
| Mason 2016 | | | X | | | X | | X |
| McDonnall 2016 | | | | | | | | X |
| Morales-Asencio 2016 | | | X | | | | | X |
| Naganathan 2016 | | | | | | | | X |
| Noël 2005 | | | X | | | | | X |
| Ravenscroft 2010 | | | | x | | | | |
| Richardson 2016 | X | | | | | | | |
| Roberge 2016 | X | | X | X | X | | | X |
| Roberto 2005 | X | | X | | | | X | |
| Ryan 2016 | X | X | X | X | | | X | X |
| Schoenberg 2011 | X | X | | | X | | X | X |
| Sheridan 2012 | X | | X | X | | | X | |
| Smith 2010 | | | | | | | | X |
| Zulman 2015 | | | | | | | | |

needs and there is little regard to their capacity and remuneration for the work, leading to caregiver stress. Finally, one older adult with MCC strongly advocated that we stop applying band-aid solutions (i.e., improving communication between health care providers and older adults) and instead, focus on re-inventing how care is organized and delivered.

## Discussion

Our scoping review highlighted that, of the 36 studies reviewed, there was convergence between needs of older adults from the perspectives of older adults, caregivers and HCPs. The findings from our review revealed that there is a need for access to information, coordination of services and support, strategies for prevention, maintenance and restoration, training and a focus on person-centred approaches. Our findings also suggest that older adults wish to be seen as a person and not merely a collection of disease conditions. Lack of coordination and access to information was prominently highlighted in the studies as well as the stakeholder consultation. The occurrence across various countries and jurisdictions suggests that fragmented services is a prevalent issues warranting further attention.

Specific to structural and social determinants of health, socioeconomic status was one of the main concerns and it was related to older adults' ability to pay for treatments [59], and the extra financial burden that MCC had on the costs of transportation, medication, and maintaining a healthy lifestyle. Access to services was also a major determinant and therefore, coordinating services within and across sectors and considering the needs of all individuals is essential to optimize care. Educational level and health literacy were also highlighted by HCPs as a barrier to effective management of MCC [55]. Gender and ethnicity were also cited, as non-English speaking backgrounds also led to difficulties in patient education and self -management [42]. Similarly, in a recent review by Northwood [10], gender, education, and the health system were found to be most commonly cited determinants of social determinants of health that impact persons with MCC. Less commonly cited were living situation, however, living alone and being homebound with MCC were also seen as contributing to developing depression, especially in women [39]. Furthermore, social isolation was a concern and Ryan [58] found that there was a relationship between social isolation and multiple unmet needs for older adults with MCC. Finally, living in rural areas may result in scarcity of personal resources, lack of family support, inadequate transportation, health care provider and service shortages, and insufficient healthy food choices and resources which could undermine management of MCC in community dwelling older adults.

To a certain degree the findings from this review are in line with priorities for improving care set out in the WHO framework for integrated, people centred health services [63]. This review adds specific details about how needs can be met including service coordination, making sure information goes from provider to provider, continuity, improved access, and assistance navigating the system. In sum, what is required is a restructuring of the health and social care system to incorporate an integrated care approach. This type of approach would result in a HCP responsible for the care coordination of a care plan that has been developed with the older adult and their caregiver to address their priorities and thus, would be more person-centred and tailored to their needs, goals and priorities. In addition, it would involve the interprofessional team across sectors that share

decision-making and communicate to implement the integrated care plan, coordinating the services from different providers and thus reducing the conflicting advice from multiple providers.

Empowering patients and families to self-manage is an important aspect of the care delivery. Promising integrated care models are currently being tested such as the IMPACT clinic [64] and the Guided Care Model [65]. Stakeholder consultation also suggested the presence of discrimination and social injustice due to advanced age. Incorporating patient-centred outcome measures can strengthen governance and accountability to increase the quality of healthcare for older adults with MCC. Finally, there requires a move from hospital-based and curative care to outpatient and preventive care e.g. establishing interprofessional teams and empowering primary care teams through allocating increased healthcare funding to be able to optimize their resources.

In terms of future direction for research, most of the views of the needs of older adults with MCC were consistent with those of their care giver and HCPs and there were few areas of divergence. Practice and research in the future could focus on ensuring the views of older adults and their caregivers are noted by HCPs as this discrepancy most likely influences outcomes. The study by Naganathan et al. (2016) highlighted a key discrepancy about safety concerns at home and supports required to age at home successfully. More research is required to focus on the dignity of risk and how to provide supports to older adults in their homes that are meaningful to them, and may include more social support interventions such as friendly visitor programs versus a focus only on health care needs. In addition, most of the studies in this review were qualitative in nature and thus no relationships between older adults' needs with MCC and outcomes were found, nor predictors of these needs. Finally despite focusing on health and social care needs of older adults, few social care needs were identified. This gap points to a promising area for future research.

The strengths of the scoping review include a comprehensive search of electronic data bases carried out by expert health sciences librarians, two reviewers for data abstractions and multiple checks of the source articles. Given the large number and range of older adults with varying types of multiple chronic conditions included in our selected studies, our findings are fairly representative of persons living with MCC. In addition, the convergence of our findings from the three perspectives which resonated with the stakeholder group helps to validate the results. Due to the number and heterogeneity of the studies retrieved, decisions were made to focus on only the 'needs' of older adults and not their preferences or lived experience.

## Conclusion

Consensus was found among the three perspectives in terms of needs of older adults with MCC. Older adults have needs at the individual, home, and system levels. Issues related to access for information and adequate support and services are pervasive for persons with MCC. Structural and social determinants of health are important to consider when addressing needs and solutions for older adults. Future studies should include developing and testing integrated models of care, and determine if access, information and person-centered approaches utilizing intersectoral strategies can be realized.

### Abbreviations

CI: Cognitive Impairment; HCPs: Health Care Providers; MCC: Multiple Chronic Conditions; MMAT: Mixed Methods Appraisal Tool; SES: Socioeconomic Status; WHO: World Health Organization

### Funding

This work was supported by the Canadian Institutes of Health Research (CIHR) SPOR-PIHCI Knowledge Synthesis grant (Funding Reference Number NKS – 150581). It was also supported by: the Saskatchewan Health Research Fund and the Toronto Rehabilitation Institute.
Dr. Puts is supported by a CIHR New Investigator Award. Dr. McGilton is supported by the Walter and Maria Schroeder Institute for Brain Innovation & Recovery.

### Authors' contributions

All authors have contributed to the manuscript – KM, MP and EC took the lead in the development of the study and in the interpretation of the results, SV, LY, JC, JP, MA, DM, AC, EP, JW, LH, VM and WW assisted with the data abstraction, AA and MG, the librarian scientists contributed to the search, DS, MK contributed to the stakeholder consultation. All authors contributed to the discussion and final review of the manuscript. All authors read and approved the final manuscript.

### Competing interests

The authors declare that they have no competing interests.

### Author details

[1]Lawrence S. Bloomberg Faculty of Nursing, University of Toronto, Toronto, ON, Canada. [2]Toronto Rehabilitation Institute, University Health Network, 550 University Avenue, Toronto, ON M6K 2R7 416 597 3422 (2500), Canada. [3]Institute of Health Policy, Management and Evaluation, University of Toronto, Toronto, ON, Canada. [4]School of Nursing, McMaster University, Hamilton, ON, Canada. [5]Division of Geriatric Medicine, Dalhousie University, Halifax, NS, Canada. [6]Gerstein Information Science Centre, University of Toronto, Toronto, ON, Canada. [7]Canadian Centre for Health and Safety in Agriculture, University of Saskatchewan, Saskatoon, SK, Canada. [8]The Change Foundation, Toronto, ON, Canada. [9]Laurentian University, Sudbury, ON, Canada. [10]Institute for Better Health, Trillium Health Partners, Mississauga, ON, Canada. [11]Faculty of Nursing, Université de Montréal, Montreal, Quebec, Canada. [12]Health Sciences North Research Institute and Northern Ontario School of Medicine, Sudbury, ON, Canada. [13]Rehabilitation Sciences Institute, University of Toronto, Toronto, ON, Canada.

### References

1. Marengoni A, Rizzuto D, Wang HX, Winblad B, Fratiglioni L. Patterns of chronic multimorbidity in the elderly population. J Am Geriatr Soc. 2009; 57(2):225–30.
2. Pefoyo AJ, Bronskill SE, Gruneir A, Calzavara A, Thavorn K, Petrosyan Y, Maxwell CJ, Bai Y, Wodchis WP. The increasing burden and complexity of multimorbidity. BMC Public Health. 2015;15:415.
3. Wallace E, Salisbury C, Guthrie B, Lewis C, Fahey T, Smith SM. Managing patients with multimorbidity in primary care. BMJ : British Medical Journal. 2015;350.
4. Fortin M, Mercer SW, Salisbury C: Introducing multimorbidity. In: ABC of Multimorbidity. Edited by Mercer SW, Salisbury C, Fortin M, First edition edn. West Sussex: UK John Wiley & Sons, Ltd. ; 2014: 1–25.
5. Ploeg J, Matthew-Maich N, Fraser K, Dufour S, McAiney C, Kaasalainen S, Markle-Reid M, Upshur R, Cleghorn L, Emili A. Managing multiple chronic conditions in the community: a Canadian qualitative study of the experiences of older adults, family caregivers and healthcare providers. BMC Geriatr. 2017;17(1):40.
6. Duggleby W, Williams A, Ghosh S, Moquin H, Ploeg J, Markle-Reid M, Peacock S. Factors influencing changes in health related quality of life of caregivers of persons with multiple chronic conditions. Health Qual Life Outcomes. 2016;14(1):81.
7. World Health Organization. World report on ageing and health. Luxembourg: World Health Organization; 2015.
8. Guruge S, Birpreet B, Samuels-Dennis JA. Health status and health determinants of older immigrant women in Canada: a scoping review. Journal of Aging Research. 2015;2015:12.
9. Kuwornu JP, Lix LM, Shooshtari S. Multimorbidity disease clusters in aboriginal and non-aboriginal Caucasian populations in Canada. Chronic Diseases and Injuries in Canada. 2014;34(4):218–25.
10. Northwood M, Ploeg J, Markle-Reid M, Sherifali D. Integrative review of the social determinants of health in older adults with multimorbidity. J Adv Nurs. 2018;74(1):45–60.
11. Lefevre T, d'Ivernois JF, De Andrade V, Crozet C, Lombrail P, Gagnayre R. What do we mean by multimorbidity? An analysis of the literature on multimorbidity measures, associated factors, and impact on health services organization. Rev Epidemiol Sante Publique. 2014;62(5):305–14.
12. Marengoni A, Angleman S, Melis R, Mangialasche F, Karp A, Garmen A, Meinow B, Fratiglioni L. Aging with multimorbidity: a systematic review of the literature. Ageing Res Rev. 2011;10(4):430–9.
13. Mangin D, Stephen G, Bismah V, Risdon C. Making patient values visible in healthcare: a systematic review of tools to assess patient treatment priorities and preferences in the context of multimorbidity. BMJ Open. 2016;6.
14. Smith SM, Wallace E, O'Dowd T, Fortin M. Interventions for improving outcomes in patients with multimorbidity in primary care and community settings. Cochrane Database Syst Rev. 2016;3.
15. Boehmer KR, Abu Dabrh AM, Gionfriddo MR, Erwin P, Montori VM. Does the chronic care model meet the emerging needs of people living with multimorbidity? A systematic review and thematic synthesis. PLoS One. 2018;13(2):e0190852.
16. Arksey H, O'Malley L. Scoping studies: towards a methodological framework. Int J Soc Res Methodol. 2005;8(1):19–32.
17. Levac D, Colquhoun H, O'Brien KK. Scoping studies: advancing the methodology. Implement Sci. 2010;5(1):69.
18. Commisso E, McGilton KS, Ayala AP, Andrew MK, Bergman H, Beaudet L, Dubé V, Gray M, Hale L, Keatings M, et al. identifying and understanding the health and social care needs of older adults with multiple chronic conditions and their caregivers: a protocol for a scoping review. BMJ Open. 2017;7(12):e018247.
19. Colquhoun HL, Levac D, O'Brien KK, Straus S, Tricco AC, Perrier L, Kastner M, Moher D. Scoping reviews: time for clarity in definition, methods, and reporting. J Clin Epidemiol. 2014;67(12):1291–4.
20. Daudt HM, van Mossel C, Scott SJ: Enhancing the scoping study methodology: a large, inter-professional team's experience with Arksey and O'Malley's framework. BMC Med Res Methodol 2013, 13(1):48.
21. Kastner M, Wilczynski NL, Walker-Dilks C, McKibbon KA, Haynes B. Age-specific search strategies for Medline. J Med Internet Res. 2006;8(4):e25.
22. LoGiudice D. The health of older aboriginal and Torres Strait islander peoples. Australasian Journal on Ageing. 2016;35(2):82–5.
23. Solar O, Irwin A. A conceptual framework for action on the social determinants of health. Social Determinants of Health Discussion Paper. 2010;2(Policy and Practice):79.
24. Braun V, Clarke V. Using thematic analysis in psychology. Qual Res Psychol. 2006;3(2):77–101.

25. Pluye P, Gagnon M-P, Griffiths F, Johnson-Lafleur J. A scoring system for appraising mixed methods research, and concomitantly appraising qualitative, quantitative and mixed methods primary studies in mixed studies reviews. Int J Nurs Stud. 2009;46(4):529–46.

26. Ancker JS, Witteman HO, Hafeez B, Provencher T, Van de Graaf M, Wei E. The invisible work of personal health information management among people with multiple chronic conditions: qualitative interview study among patients and providers. J Med Internet Res. 2015;17(6):e137.

27. Ansari S, Hosseinzadeh H, Dennis S, Zwar N. Patients' perspectives on the impact of a new COPD diagnosis in the face of multimorbidity: a qualitative study. NPJ primary care respiratory medicine. 2014;24:14036.

28. Bardach SH, Schoenberg NE. Primary care physicians' prevention counseling with patients with multiple morbidity. Qual Health Res. 2012;22(12):1599–611.

29. Bayliss EA, Steiner JF, Fernald DH, Crane LA, Main DS. Descriptions of barriers to self-care by persons with comorbid chronic diseases. Ann Fam Med. 2003;1(1):15–21.

30. Beverly EA, Wray LA, Chiu CJ, Weinger K. Perceived challenges and priorities in co-morbidity management of older patients with type 2 diabetes. Diabetic medicine : a journal of the British Diabetic Association. 2011;28(7):781–4.

31. Bunn F, Burn AM, Robinson L, Poole M, Rait G, Brayne C, Schoeman J, Norton S, Goodman C. Healthcare organisation and delivery for people with dementia and comorbidity: a qualitative study exploring the views of patients, carers and professionals. BMJ Open. 2017;7(1):e013067.

32. Burton AE, Gibson JM, Shaw RL. How do older people with sight loss manage their general health? A qualitative study. Disability & Rehabilitation. 2016;38(23):2277–85.

33. Clarke LH, Bennett EV, Korotchenko A. Negotiating vulnerabilities: how older adults with multiple chronic conditions interact with physicians. Canadian Journal on Aging. 2014;33(1):26–37.

34. Coventry PA, Fisher L, Kenning C, Bee P, Bower P. Capacity, responsibility, and motivation: a critical qualitative evaluation of patient and practitioner views about barriers to self-management in people with multimorbidity. BMC Health Serv Res. 2014;14(1):536.

35. DiNapoli EA, Cinna C, Whiteman KL, Fox L, Appelt CJ, Kasckow J. Mental health treatment preferences and challenges of living with multimorbidity from the veteran perspective. International Journal of Geriatric Psychiatry. 2016;31(10):1097–104.

36. Fortin M, Maltais D, Hudon C, Lapointe L, Ntetu AL. Access to health care: perceptions of patients with multiple chronic conditions. Canadian family physician Médecin de famille canadien. 2005;51:1502–3.

37. Fried TR, McGraw S, Agostini JV, Tinetti ME. Views of older persons with multiple morbidities on competing outcomes and clinical decision-making. J Am Geriatr Soc. 2008;56(10):1839–44.

38. Gill A, Kuluski K, Jaakkimainen L, Naganathan G, Upshur R, Wodchis WP. "where do we go from here?" health system frustrations expressed by patients with multimorbidity, their caregivers and family physicians. Healthcare policy = Politiques de sante. 2014;9(4):73–89.

39. Grundberg A, Hansson A, Hilleras P, Religa D. District nurses' perspectives on detecting mental health problems and promoting mental health among community-dwelling seniors with multimorbidity. J Clin Nurs. 2016;25(17–18):2590–9.

40. Hansen H, Pohontsch N, van den Bussche H, Scherer M, Schafer I. Reasons for disagreement regarding illnesses between older patients with multimorbidity and their GPs - a qualitative study. BMC Fam Pract. 2015;16:68.

41. Kuluski K, Gill A, Naganathan G, Upshur R, Jaakkimainen RL, Wodchis WP. A qualitative descriptive study on the alignment of care goals between older persons with multi-morbidities, their family physicians and informal caregivers. BMC Fam Pract. 2013;14.

42. Lo C, Ilic D, Teede H, Cass A, Fulcher G, Gallagher M, Johnson G, Kerr PG, Mathew T, Murphy K, et al. The perspectives of patients on health-Care for co-Morbid Diabetes and Chronic Kidney Disease: a qualitative study. PLoS One. 2016;11(1):e0146615.

43. Loeb SJ, Penrod J, Falkenstern S, Gueldner SH, Poon LW. Supporting older adults living with multiple chronic conditions. West J Nurs Res. 2003;25(1):8–23.

44. Mason B, Nanton V, Epiphaniou E, Murray SA, Donaldson A, Shipman C, Daveson BA, Harding R, Higginson IJ, Munday D, et al. My body's falling apart.' understanding the experiences of patients with advanced

45. Morales-Asencio JM, Martin-Santos FJ, Kaknani S, Morilla-Herrera JC, Cuevas Fernandez-Gallego M, Garcia-Mayor S, Leon-Campos A, Morales-Gil IM. Living with chronicity and complexity: lessons for redesigning case management from patients' life stories - a qualitative study. J Eval Clin Pract. 2016;22(1):122–32.

46. Naganathan G, Kuluski K, Gill A, Jaakkimainen L, Upshur R, Wodchis WP. Perceived value of support for older adults coping with multi-morbidity: patient, informal care-giver and family physician perspectives. Ageing Soc. 2016;36(9):1891–914.

47. Noël PH, Frueh BC, Larme AC, Pugh JA. Collaborative care needs and preferences of primary care patients with multimorbidity. Health Expect. 2005;8(1):54–63.

48. Ravenscroft EF. Navigating the health care system: insights from consumers with multi-morbidity. Journal of Nursing & Healthcare of Chronic Illnesses. 2010;2(3):215–24.

49. Richardson LM, Hill JN, Smith BM, Bauer E, Weaver FM, Gordon HS, Stroupe KT, Hogan TP. Patient prioritization of comorbid chronic conditions in the veteran population: implications for patient-centered care. SAGE Open Medicine. 2016;4:2050312116680945.

50. Roberge P, Hudon C, Pavilanis A, Beaulieu M-C, Benoit A, Brouillet H, Boulianne I, De Pauw A, Frigon S, Gaboury I, et al. A qualitative study of perceived needs and factors associated with the quality of care for common mental disorders in patients with chronic diseases: the perspective of primary care clinicians and patients. BMC Fam Pract. 2016;17:1–14.

51. Roberto KA, Gigliotti CM, Husser EK. Older women's experiences with multiple health conditions: daily challenges and care practices. Health care for women international. 2005;26(8):672–92.

52. Schoenberg NE, Bardach SH, Manchikanti KN, Goodenow AC. Appalachian residents' experiences with and management of multiple morbidity. Qual Health Res. 2011;21(5):601–11.

53. Sheridan NF, Kenealy TW, Kidd JD, Schmidt-Busby JIG, Hand JE, Raphael DL, McKillop AM, Rea HH. Patients' engagement in primary care: powerlessness and compounding jeopardy. A qualitative study. Health expectations : an international journal of public participation in health care and health policy. 2015;18(1):32–43.

54. Smith SM, O'Kelly S, O'Dowd T. GPs' and pharmacists' experiences of managing multimorbidity: A 'Pandora's box'. Br J Gen Pract. 2010;60(576): e285–94.

55. Zulman DM, Jenchura EC, Cohen DM, Lewis ET, Houston TK, Asch SM. How can eHealth technology address challenges related to multimorbidity? Perspectives from patients with multiple chronic conditions. J Gen Intern Med. 2015;30(8):1063–70.

56. Adeniji C, Kenning C, Coventry PA, Bower P. What are the core predictors of 'hassles' among patients with multimorbidity in primary care? A cross sectional study. BMC Health Serv Res. 2015;15:255.

57. McDonnall MC, Crudden A, LeJeune BJ, Steverson A, O'Donnell N. Needs and challenges of seniors with combined hearing and vision loss. Journal of Visual Impairment & Blindness. 2016;110(6):399–411.

58. Ryan J, Abrams MK, Doty MM, Shah T, Schneider EC. How High-Need Patients Experience Health Care in the United States. Findings from the 2016 Commonwealth Fund survey of high-need patients. Issue brief (Commonwealth Fund). 2016;(43):1–20.

59. Bayliss EA, Ellis JL, Steiner JF, Bayliss EA, Ellis JL, Steiner JF. Barriers to self-management and quality-of-life outcomes in seniors with multimorbidities. Ann Fam Med. 2007;5(5):395–402.

60. Barstow BA, Warren M, Thaker S, Hallman A, Batts P. Client and therapist perspectives on the influence of low vision and chronic conditions on performance and occupational therapy intervention. Am J Occup Ther 2015; 69(3):p1 8.

61. Cheraghi-Sohi S, Bower P, Kennedy A, Morden A, Rogers A, Richardson J, Sanders T, Stevenson F, Ong BN. Patient priorities in osteoarthritis and comorbid conditions: a secondary analysis of qualitative data. Arthritis Care & Research. 2013;65(6):920–7.

62. Proposal: A mixed methods appraisal tool for systematic mixed studies reviews [http://mixedmethodsappraisaltoolpublic.pbworks.com/w/file/fetch/84371689/MMAT%202011%20criteria%20and%20tutorial%202011-06-29updated2014.08.21.pdf].

63. World Health Organization. Framework on integrated, people-centred health services. In: Sixty-ninth world health assembly; 2016.

# 13

# Technology-based cognitive training and rehabilitation interventions for individuals with mild cognitive impairment

Shaoqing Ge[1]* ⓘ, Zheng Zhu[2,3], Bei Wu[4,5] and Eleanor S. McConnell[1,6]

## Abstract

**Background:** Individuals with mild cognitive impairment (MCI) are at heightened risk of developing dementia. Rapid advances in computing technology have enabled researchers to conduct cognitive training and rehabilitation interventions with the assistance of technology. This systematic review aims to evaluate the effects of technology-based cognitive training or rehabilitation interventions to improve cognitive function among individuals with MCI.

**Methods:** We conducted a systematic review using the following criteria: individuals with MCI, empirical studies, and evaluated a technology-based cognitive training or rehabilitation intervention. Twenty-six articles met the criteria.

**Results:** Studies were characterized by considerable variation in study design, intervention content, and technologies applied. The major types of technologies applied included computerized software, tablets, gaming consoles, and virtual reality. Use of technology to adjust the difficulties of tasks based on participants' performance was an important feature. Technology-based cognitive training and rehabilitation interventions had significant effect on global cognitive function in 8 out of 22 studies; 8 out of 18 studies found positive effects on attention, 9 out of 16 studies on executive function, and 16 out of 19 studies on memory. Some cognitive interventions improved non-cognitive symptoms such as anxiety, depression, and ADLs.

**Conclusion:** Technology-based cognitive training and rehabilitation interventions show promise, but the findings were inconsistent due to the variations in study design. Future studies should consider using more consistent methodologies. Appropriate control groups should be designed to understand the additional benefits of cognitive training and rehabilitation delivered with the assistance of technology.

**Keywords:** Technology, Cognition, Cognitive training, Cognitive rehabilitation, Systematic review

## Background

Due to the aging of the world's population, the number of people who live with dementia is projected to triple to 131 million by the year 2050 [1, 2]. Development of preventative strategies for individuals at higher risk of developing dementia is an international priority [3, 4]. Mild cognitive impairment (MCI) is regarded as an intermediate stage between normal cognition and dementia [5, 6]. Individuals with MCI usually suffer with significant cognitive complaints, yet do not exhibit the functional impairments required for a diagnosis of dementia. These people typically have a faster rate of progression to dementia than those without MCI [5], but the cognitive decline among MCI subjects has the potential of being improved [7, 8]. Previous systematic reviews of cognitive intervention studies, both cognitive training and cognitive rehabilitation, have demonstrated promising effects on improving cognitive function among subjects with MCI [3, 7, 9, 10].

Recently, rapid advances in computing technology have enabled researchers to conduct cognitive training and rehabilitation interventions with the assistance of

* Correspondence: shaoqing.ge@duke.edu
[1]Duke University School of Nursing, 307 Trent Drive, Durham, NC, USA
Full list of author information is available at the end of the article

technology. A variety of technologies, including virtual reality (VR), interactive video gaming, and mobile technology, have been used to implement cognitive training and rehabilitation programs. Potential advantages to using technology-based interventions include enhanced accessibility and cost-effectiveness, providing a user experience that is immersive and comprehensive, as well as providing adaptive responses based on individual performance. Many computerized cognitive intervention programs are easily accessed through a computer or tablet, and the technology can objectively collect data during the intervention to provide real-time feedback to participants or therapists. Importantly, interventions delivered using technology have shown better effects compared to traditional cognitive training and rehabilitation programs in improving cognitive function and quality of life [11–13]. The reasons for this superiority are not well-understood but could be related to the usability and motivational factors related to the real-time interaction and feedback received from the training system [13].

Three recent reviews of cognitive training and rehabilitation for use with individuals with MCI and dementia suggest that technology holds promise to improve both cognitive and non-cognitive outcomes [14–16]. The reviews conducted by Coyle, et al. [15] and Chandler, et al. [14] were limited by accessing articles from only two databases, and did not comprehensively cover available technologies. Hill, et al. [16] limited their review to papers published until July 2016 and included only older adults aged 60 and above. More technology-based intervention studies have been conducted since then, and only including studies with older adults 60 and above could limit the scope of the review given that adults can develop early-onset MCI in their 40s [17]. Therefore, the purpose of this review is to 1) capture more studies using technology-based cognitive interventions by conducting a more comprehensive search using additional databases 2) understand the effect of technology-based cognitive interventions on improving abilities among individuals with MCI; and 3) examine the effects of multimodal technology-based interventions and their potential superiority compared to single component interventions.

## Methods

### Search strategy

PRISMA guidelines were followed for conducting this systematic review [18]. Based on the research aims and key words, an experienced librarian searched five databases: PubMed (Medline), PsychoINFO (EBSCO*host*), CINAHL (EBSCO*host*), Embase, and Cochrane Library (Wiley). The search strategy used a combination of subject headings and key words for these main concepts: technology, MCI, training, and rehabilitation. The full

search strategy is available in Additional file 1. The literature search was limited to empirical studies among human subjects. We did not set boundaries on age since MCI can occur among middle aged to older adults. The literature search was completed on December 1, 2017.

### Inclusion and exclusion of publications

Two authors (SG and ESM) independently reviewed the list of articles found in the literature search. Inclusion criteria were: 1) participants were diagnosed with MCI; 2) a technology-based cognitive training or rehabilitation intervention was evaluated; and 3) an empirical study was conducted. Exclusion criteria were: 1) the effect of the intervention on MCI participants could not be extracted from effects among healthy or dementia participants, and 2) the publication was not in English.

Titles were first reviewed for obvious exclusions. Then, for those retained from the first-round title screening, abstracts were screened. A third-round of full-text screening was then conducted. Any uncertainties or discrepancies between the two authors (SG and ESM) were discussed and resolved.

### Quality assessment

The quality of studies identified as relevant was assessed by two independent reviewers (SG and ZZ) using the Joanna Briggs Institute (JBI) critical appraisal checklist for randomized controlled trials (RCT) and JBI checklist for quasi-experimental studies [19]. Any disagreements that arose were resolved through discussion, or with a third reviewer (BW). The studies were generally methodologically sound with some variations in quality across studies (see Additional file 1: Table S2 and S3).

### Data extraction and synthesis

Two reviewers (SG and ZZ) independently extracted information from each article into the Tables 1 and 2. Disagreements on data extraction were resolved by consensus with the assistance of a third author. A meta-analysis of the 26 articles was inappropriate due to the large variability between the study designs, intervention contents, outcomes measured, and population samples across different studies [20, 21]. We selectively calculated effect sizes for a pair of studies that used the same intervention materials [22, 23]. All data syntheses were conducted by using Revman 5.3 [24]. The forest plot is presented in Additional file 1: Figure S1.

### Results

Based on the strategy and criteria described above, 26 of 411 studies identified were deemed eligible for review. The PRISMA flowchart in Fig. 1 presents the decision pathway for final inclusion of studies.

**Table 1** Sample characteristic of included studies

| First author | Year of publication | Location | Setting/context | Sample size[a] | Age[b] (year) | MCI Criteria | Baseline cognitive characteristic[b] |
|---|---|---|---|---|---|---|---|
| Cipriani, 2006 [29] | 2006 | Italy | Dayhospital | 10(AD) + 10(MCI) | 70.6 | Not specified | MMSE: 28.0 |
| Rozzini, 2007 [40] | 2007 | Italy | Medical centers | 59 | 63–78 | Petersen criteria | MMSE: IG1:26.4 IG2:26.0 CG:26.8 |
| Talassi, 2007 [36] | 2007 | Italy | Community-dwelling | 37(MCI) + 29(AD) | IG:76.2 CG:76.1 | Not specified | MMSE: IG:27.5 CG:26.9 |
| Barnes, 2009 [22] | 2009 | US | Medical centers | 47 | IG:74.1 CG:74.8 | IWG criteria | BRANS: IG:85.2 CG:87.8 |
| Finn, 2011 [25] | 2011 | Australia | Medical center | 27 | IG:69.00 CG:76.38 | IWG criteria | MMSE: IG:28.5 CG:27.5 |
| Rosen, 2011 [23] | 2011 | US | Community-dwelling | 12 | IG:70.67 CG:78.00 | IWG criteria | MMSE: IG:29.33 CG:27.83 |
| Gagnon, 2012 [43] | 2012 | Canada | Medical centers | 24 | IG:68.42 CG:67.00 | Petersen criteria | MMSE: IG:27.83 CG:28.08 |
| Herrera, 2012 [42] | 2012 | France | Medical center | 22 | IG:75.09 CG:78.18 | Petersen criteria | MMSE: IG:27.36 CG:27.18 |
| Man, 2012 [13] | 2012 | Hong Kong | Community service setting | 44 | IG:80.30 CG:80.28 | Petersen criteria | MMSE: IG:21.05 CG:23.00 |
| Gonzalez-Palau, 2014 [33] | 2014 | Spain | Community centers | 39(HE) + 11(MCI) | 74.60 | Petersen criteria | MEC 35: 29.61 |
| Han, 2014 [30] | 2014 | Korea | Medical center | 10 | 72.1 | IWG criteria | MMSE: 26.7 |
| Hughes, 2014 [45] | 2014 | US | Community setting | 20 | IG:78.5 CG:76.2 | MYHAT Cognitive Classification | MMSE: IG:27.2 CG:27.1 |
| Fiatarone Singh, 2014 [26] | 2014 | Australia | Community-dwelling | 100 | 70.1 | Petersen criteria | ADAS-Cog: IG1:8.79 IG2:8.29 IG3:8.02 CG:8.09 |
| Manera, 2015 [32] | 2015 | France | Medical Center and research unit | 9(MCI) + 12(AD) | 75.8 | National Institute on Aging and Alzheimer Association group clinical criteria | MMSE: 27.2 |
| Styliadis, 2015 [34] | 2015 | Greece | Medical facility | 70 | IG1:71.21 IG2:70.42 IG3:72.71 CG1:71.07 CG2:67.64 | Petersen criteria | MMSE: IG1:25.85 IG2:26.21 IG3:25.14 CG1:26.21 CG2:25 |
| Barban, 2016 [39] | 2016 | Italy, Greece, Norway and Spain | Medical centers | 114(HE) + 106(MCI) + 81(AD) | IG:74.4 CG:72.9 | Petersen criteria | MMSE: IG:27.3 CG:28.1 |
| Gooding, 2016 [35] | 2016 | US | Medical center | 74 | 75.59 | Petersen criteria | mMMSE: IG1:51.25 IG2:50.29 CG:50.39 |
| Heyer, 2016 [28] | 2016 | US | Community-dwelling | 68 | IG:75.1 CG:75.2 | IWG criteria | MMSE: 26 |
| Klados, 2016 [37] | 2016 | Greece | Not specified | 50 | IG:69.60 CG:67.92 | Petersen criteria | MMSE: IG:26.04 CG:25.64 |

**Table 1** Sample characteristic of included studies *(Continued)*

| First author | Year of publication | Location | Setting/context | Sample size[a] | Age[b] (year) | Sample size[a] (detail) | MCI Criteria | Baseline cognitive characteristic[b] |
|---|---|---|---|---|---|---|---|---|
| Lin, 2016 [44] | 2016 | US | Community-dwelling | 24 | IG:72.9 CG:73.1 | | Albert criteria | MoCA: IG:24.4 CG:25.6 |
| Vermeij, 2016 [31] | 2016 | Netherlands | Community setting | 25(HE) + 22(MCI) | 68.4 | | Petersen criteria | MMSE > 27.1 Not specified |
| Bahar-Fuchs, 2017 [27] | 2017 | Australia | Community-dwelling | 9(MCI) + 11(MrNPS) + 25(MCI+MrNPS) | 74.8 | | National Institute on Aging and Alzheimer Association group clinical criteria | GDS: 2.9 |
| Delbroek, 2017 [47] | 2017 | Belgium | Residential care center | 20 | IG:86.9 CG:87.5 | | Not specified | Moca: IG:17.5 CG:16.3 |
| Hagovská, 2017 [12] | 2017 | Slovakia | Outpatient psychiatric clinics | 60 | IG:67.8 CG:68.2 | | Albert criteria | MMSE: IG:25.6 CG:24.9 |
| Mansbach, 2017 [38] | 2017 | US | Community-dwelling | 38 | 78.08[c] | | Petersen criteria | BCAT[c]: IG:38.65 CG:35.72 |
| Savulich, 2017 [41] | 2017 | UK | Research and medical center | 42 | IG:75.2 CG:76.9 | | Albert criteria | MMSE: IG:26.6 CG:26.8 |

*IG* Intervention group, *CG* Control group

[a]*HE* Healthy elderly with no history of neurological or psychiatric deficits, *MrNPS* Mood-related neuropsychiatric symptoms

[b]Data only included elderly with MCI

[c]Demographic data included both MCI and AD

**Table 2** Overview of included studies

| First author and year | Study design | Intervention and Technology | Control | Technology description | Sessions/ Duration | Follow-up | Cognitive outcome measures | Other outcome measures | Key findings |
|---|---|---|---|---|---|---|---|---|---|
| Cipriani, 2006 [29] | Pre-post study | Computer based-Cognitive Rehabilitation (cb-CR) programs | NA | TNP software: delivers individualized cognitive rehabilitation exercises in the following cognitive domains: attention, memory, perception, visuospatial cognition, language, and non-verbal intelligence | 2 * 16 * 13–45 min sessions for 8 weeks | 3 months | MMSE Attention: Visual search; Executive function: Trail Making test A and B; Behavioral Memory: RBMT; Psychomotor learning: digit symbol test; Verbal fluency: phonemic and semantic verbal fluency | Depression (GDS); Anxiety: STAI-X1, STAI-X2; ADL: AADL; QOL: SF-12 | MCI: Only significantly improved in memory (RBMT) |
| Rozzini, 2007 [40] | RCT | TNP + ChEIs | CG1: ChEIs CG2: No treatment | TNP Software | 20 * 1 h/ session, five days/week for four weeks | 1 yr | MMSE Memory: Short story recall; Executive function: Rey's figure copy and recall, Raven's colored matrices; Verbal fluency: Letter verbal fluency; Semantic verbal fluency | Mood: depression: GDS; anxiety, apathy Behavioral disturbances: NPI Activities of daily living: BADL | IG: significant improvement in memory, abstract reasoning, and depression CGi: no improvements on any cognition but benefit in depression CG2: no improvement in any outcome measures |
| Talassi, 2007 [36] | CCT | TNP + OT + BT | PR + OT + BT | TNP Software | 30–45 min/ session, 4 days/week for 3 weeks | Intervention end | MMSE Working memory: forward and backward digit span; Executive function: Rey's figure copy; Verbal fluency: phonemic and semantic verbal fluency; CDT; Episodic Memory: episodic memory subset of RBMT; Verbal fluency: Phonemic and semantic verbal fluency; Attention: visual search, processing speed: digit symbol test | Mood: depression GDS; anxiety (Stai-Y1,Stai-Y2; ADL: BADL, IADL, PPT; | MCI subjects in IG improved in executive function, visuospatial memory, anxiety, depression, and PPT but not IADL MCI subjects in CG: no improvements |
| Barnes, 2009 [22] | RCT | cb-CT | Passive computer activities | Computer-based cognitive training software developed by Posit Science Corporation (San Francisco, CA), involving seven exercises including primary and working auditory memory tasks to improve processing speed and accuracy in the auditory cortex | IG: 100 min/ day five days/ week for 6 weeks CG: 90 min/day, 5 days/week for 6 weeks | Intervention end | Global cognitive function: RBANS total score, 5 RBANS index score Memory: CVLT-II Language: COWAT, BNT Executive function: California Trail Making Test Attention: Design Fluency test; Working memory: Spatial Span test | Mood: depression (GDS) | IG showed greater improvement on RBANS total scores but no significant between group difference. Effect sizes for verbal learning and memory measures tended to favor IG. Effect sizes for language and visuospatial function measures tended to favor CG (control group). |

**Table 2** Overview of included studies (Continued)

| First author and year | Study design | Intervention and Technology | Control | Technology description | Sessions/ Duration | Follow-up | Cognitive outcome measures | Other outcome measures | Key findings |
|---|---|---|---|---|---|---|---|---|---|
| Finn, 2011 [25] | RCT | Computerized Cognitive Training Package | No intervention | Lumosity software on a computer contains four or five cognitive exercise that targeted four cognitive domains | 30 sessions, 4–5 sessions/ week | Intervention end | Executive function: IED; Attention: RVP Subjective memory impairment: MFQ Visual memory: PAL | Mood: Depression Anxiety and Stress Scale | IG had significant improvement in visual attention but not processing speed, visual memory, nor mood |
| Rosen, 2011 [23] | RCT | cb-CT | listening to audio books, reading online newspapers, and playing a visuospatial oriented computer game | Computer-based cognitive training software developed by Posit Science Corporation | IG: 24 sessions, 100 mins/day, 5 days/week CG:24 sessions, 90 min/day, 5 days/week | Intervention end | Global cognitive function: RBANS Neuroimaging: fMRI | Not specified | IG > CG: improvement in verbal memory and left hippocampal activation CG: declined in VM |
| Gagnon, 2012 [43] | RCT | Computer-based VP | AC: Computer-based FP | Computer-based divided attention dual-task training: VP: performing both tasks concurrently and varying allocation priorities across the series of blocks, feedbacks are provided; FP: perform both tasks concurrently and to allocate 50/50 attentional resources to each task, no feedbacks provided | 6 * 1 h/ session, 3 times/week for two weeks | Intervention end | Attention: dual task (digit span task, visual detection task); Executive subtest of TEA Attention: Trail Making Test A; Executive function: Trail Making Test B; | QOL: Well-Being Scale Divided attention: Divided Attention Questionnaire | VP showed significant advantage over FP in improving accuracy and reaction time FP and VP both produced improvements on focused attention, speed of processing, and switching abilities No reliable advantage for VP over FP |
| Herrera, 2012 [42] | RCT | Computer –based Memory and attention training | Stimulating Cognitive activities | Computer-based cognitive training that involved a memory task and an attention task | 24 * 60 min/ session twice/week for 12 weeks. | 6 months | MMSE-recall; Memory: the forward and backward digit span test, BEM-144 12-word-list recall, the 16-item free and cued reminding test, sub-score recall of the MMSE, visual recognition subtest from the Doors and People memory battery, the DMS48 test; executive function: Rey–Osterrieth Complex Figure recall test | N/A | Significant improvement in memory, both episodic recall and recognition |
| Man, 2012 [13] | CCT | VR-based memory training program | Therapist-led program | VR: participants use either the joystick or the direction buttons of the keyboard to control the navigation action and give responses to a memory task | 10 sessions, 30 min/ session 2–3 times/week | Intervention end | Memory: MMQ; Episodic Memory: FOME | ADL: Lawton IADL | VR: significant improvement in total encoding, total recall, delayed recall and MMQ-strategy Therapist-led: significant improvement in total recall, delayed recall and MMQ-contentment |

**Table 2** Overview of included studies (Continued)

| First author and year | Study design | Intervention and Technology | Control | Technology description | Sessions/Duration | Follow-up | Cognitive outcome measures | Other outcome measures | Key findings |
|---|---|---|---|---|---|---|---|---|---|
| | | | | | | | | | VR > therapist in improving objective memory; Therapist > VR in subjective memory |
| Gonzalez-Palau, 2014 [33] | Pre-post study | LLM included CTC and PTC | NA | CTC: Gradior Software: a multi-domain cognitive training program including attention, perception, episodic memory and working memory tasks. Principles of feedback and difficulty adaptation are used PTC: FFA: an innovative, low-cost game platform. Work our intensity gradually increases | CTC: 40/ session, three times/week for 12 weeks PTC: one-hour session of FFA, three times/week for 12 weeks | Intervention end | Global cognitive function: The Mini Examen Cognitivo (MEC 35) Memory: Logical Memory subtests of the WMS III Attention: The Color Trail Test 1 and 2 Verbal learning and memory: HVLT-R | Mood: depression(GDS) | For MCI subjects: Significant improvement in global cognitive function, verbal memory,episodic memory, and decrease in symptoms of depression. |
| Han, 2014 [30] | Pre-post study | Ubiquitous Spaced Retrieval-based Memory Advancement and Rehabilitation Training USMART Program | NA | USMART program app on IPad | 24 face-to-face sessions | Intervention end | CERAD-K-N including: verbal fluency: the Categorical Fluency test, the Modified BNT; MMSE; memory: WLMT, WLRT, the Word List Recognition Test, CRT; visuospatial: Constructional Praxis Test; Attention: Trail Making Test A; executive function: Trail Making Test B | N/A | Significantly improved only in memory (WLMT); number of training sessions correlated with WLMT scores |
| Hughes, 2014 [45] | RCT | Interactive video games (Wii) | Healthy aging education program | Nintendo Wii gaming console for interactive video gaming (bowling, golf, tennis, and baseball) | 24 * 90 min, 1 session/ week for 24 weeks | 1 year | Global cognition: CAMCI; Processing speed/ Attention: Tracking A; Executive function: Tracking B; Subjective cognitive ability | Mood/social functioning: CSRQ-25; ADL: TIADL | IG: No significant improvement in any of the outcome measures. Medium effect size estimates were found for global cognition, subjective cognition, executive function, and gait speed |
| Fiatarone Singh, 2014 [26] | RCT | IG1: CT + Sham exercise IG2: PRT + Sham cognitive intervention IG3: CT + PRT | Sham exercise + Sham cognitive intervention | COGPACK program: computer-based multi-modal and multi-domain exercises targeting memory, executive function, attention, and speed of information processing, including 14 progressively more difficult exercises | CG: 60 min IG: 75 min PRT/CT groups, 100 min combined 2–3 days/ week for 6 months | 18 months | Global cognition: ADAS-Cog Executive Function: WAIS-III; Verbal fluency: COWAT, animal naming; Memory: BVRT-R, auditory Logical Memory I and II, subsets of WMS-III, List Learning subsection of ADAS-Cog; Attention: SDMT | ADL: B-IADL | CT prevented memory decline only up until 6 months PRT improved global and executive function until 18 months; PRT was better than CT + PRT in improving global and executive function |

**Table 2** Overview of included studies (Continued)

| First author and year | Study design | Intervention and Technology | Control | Technology description | Sessions/Duration | Follow-up | Cognitive outcome measures | Other outcome measures | Key findings |
|---|---|---|---|---|---|---|---|---|---|
| Manera, 2015 [32] | Pre-post Study | 'Kitchen and Cooking' Game | NA | Computerized Kitchen and Cooking' serious game which challenges attention, executive function, and praxis | 4 weeks | Intervention end | Attention: Trail Making Test A; Visual Memory: the Visual Association Test; Executive function: the Victoria Stroop Test | ADL: IADL, ADL | Significant improvement in executive function. Improvement in MCI > AD. Longer time played correlated with better executive function |
| Styliadis, 2015 [34] | CCT | IG1: Long-Lasting Memories (LLM) Intervention combined cognitive training (CT) and physical training (PT); IG2: CT alone; IG3: PT alone | CG1: Active Control (AC) (documentaries viewing); CG2: Passive Control | LLM training system CT and PT as follows: CT: Greek adaptation of Brain Fitness Software: 6 self-paced exercises focused on categories: Attention and Auditory Processing Speed. PT: FFA game platform incorporating Nintendo WII balance games | 8 weeks; LLM group: Up to 10 h/week; PT group: Up to 5 h/week; CT group: Up to 5 h/week; AC group: Up to 5 h/week | Intervention end | Electroencephalogram (EEG) measures of Cortical activity for delta, theta, beta 1 and beta 2 bands | N/A | A significant training effect was identified in the LLM group revealed by EEG measures but no training effects on the MMSE |
| Barban, 2016 [39] | RCT | IG1: Process-based-Cognitive Training (pb-CT) plus reminiscence therapy (RT) + rest | Reminiscence therapy (RT) + pb-CT | SOCIABLE software on a touch screen computer containing 27 games designed to improve function in 7 cognitive domains: attention, executive function, memory, logical reasoning, orientation, language, and constructional Praxis | 24 * 1 h treatment sessions, 2 sessions/week for a about 3 months | Intervention end | MMSE; Memory: RAVLT; Executive function: Rey–Osterreith Complex Figure Test, Phonological Verbal Fluency Test; Executive function: Trail Making Test | IADL | pb-CT: Significant training effects on memory in MCI subjects and the effect was maintained after reminiscence period; Significant training effect on MMSE was not maintained during reminiscence period; Medium effect sizes |
| Gooding, 2016 [35] | CCT | IG1: Computer based Cognitive Training (cb-CT); IG2: Cognitive Vitality Training (CVT: cb-C + Neuropsychological and Educational Approach to Remediation (NEAR) | Active Control Group (ACG) | cb-CT: Brain Fitness: repeated drill-and-practice exercises involving memory, attention, and executive functions within domain-specific training modules that allow for adaptive training with titrated difficulty levels. Same CT exercises delivered within a framework that allows for personalization, individual control, and contextualization of exercises | 30 * 60 min/session, twice/week for 16 weeks | 4 months | Intellectual functioning: WRAT-3; mMMSE; Verbal learning and Memory: the BSRT, the WMS-R LM I and II subtests; Visual learning and memory: the WMS-R Visual Reproductions (VR) I and II subtests | Mood: depression (BDI-II) | CVT and cb-CT groups had improvements in global cognition, verbal learning, and verbal memory; CVT and cb-CT had significantly greater improvements than ACG in global cognition, verbal memory, and verbal learning; No significant difference between cb-CT and CVT; Largest mood improvement in CVT, significant difference between CVT and ACG but not between CVT and cb-CT |

**Table 2** Overview of included studies (Continued)

| First author and year | Study design | Intervention and Technology | Control | Technology description | Sessions/ Duration | Follow-up | Cognitive outcome measures | Other outcome measures | Key findings |
|---|---|---|---|---|---|---|---|---|---|
| Hyer, 2016 [28] | RCT | Computerized CT program | Sham cognitive training | Cogmed computer training program: Uses multiple rotating exercises daily that are designed to train working memory. | 25 * 40 min /day for over 5 to 7 weeks | 3 months | Working Memory: WMS-III Span Board subtest, WAIS-III Letter Number Sequencing subtest; Attention: Trail Making Test Part A: Executive function: Trail Making Test Part B); Subjective memory: CFQ | ADL: the Functional Activities Questionnaire | Significant improvement of executive function, verbal and non-verbal working memory in both CG and IG; Significant improvement of subjective memory in IG but not CG. Significant between group difference in working memory (Span Board) and in adjustment (FAQ) |
| Klados, 2016 [37] | CCT | Long Lasting Memories (LLM) Intervention (Cognitive Training (CT) + Physical Training (PT)) | Active Control (AC): watching documentary and answering questionnaire | Brain Fitness Software FitForAll | CT: 1 h/day, 3–5 days/ week for 8 weeks PT: 1 h/day, 3–5 sessions/ week for 8 weeks for 8 weeks | Intervention end | Cortical Activity, Cortical Functional Connectivity: beta band | Not specified | IG showed beta band functional connectivity of MCI patients |
| Lin, 2016 [44] | RCT | VSOP | MLA | Software INSIGHT: online program designed by Posit Science, included five training tasks: eye for detail, peripheral challenge, visual sweeps, double decision, and target tracker | 1 h/day 4 days/week for 6 weeks | Intervention end | Processing speed: The Useful Field of View Executive function: The EXAMINER | ADL: TIADL Neuroimaging data: magnetic resonance imaging | IG > CG: improvement in trained (processing speed and attention) and untrained (working memory) cognitive domains, IADL, CEN and DMN |
| Vermeij, 2016 [31] | Pre-post study | WM training program | NA | Cogmed computer program | 25 sessions, 45 min per session for 5 weeks | 3 months | Working memory: WAIS-III Digit Span forward and backward, WMS-III Spatial Span forward and backward; Verbal memory: Dutch equivalent of RAVLT; Figural Fluency: RFFT; Cognitive impairment: CFQ | N/A | IG: Significant improvement in trained verbal and visuospatial working memory tasks as well as executive function. Training gain was larger in the healthy elderly (HE) and was only maintained among HEs. Improvements in non-trained near-transfer tasks, maintained after 3 months follow-up |

**Table 2** Overview of included studies (Continued)

| First author and year | Study design | Intervention and Technology | Control | Technology description | Sessions/Duration | Follow-up | Cognitive outcome measures | Other outcome measures | Key findings |
|---|---|---|---|---|---|---|---|---|---|
| Bahar-Fuchs, 2017 [27] | RCT | home-based individually-tailored and adaptive cb-CT | AC | CogniFit Software: a computer-based program involving 33 tasks designed to train a broad range of cognitive abilities | 2 sessions/day, 3 days/week, for 8-12 weeks | 12 weeks | Composite score global cognition Memory: L'Hermitte Board, Logical Memory, RAVLT Verbal fluency: SydBat Processing speed: the Trails A and B tasks Self-reported cognitive function | Mood | MCI in IG: greater improvement in memory, learning, and global cognition. No training effect in mood, self-reported memory Training gains in MCI (including ADL) were consolidated over time large effect sizes of intervention at the follow-up assessments in learning, delayed memory, and global cognitive function, medium effect size in non-memory composite |
| Delbroek, 2017 [47] | RCT | VR dual task training with the BioRescue | No intervention | BioRescue Software: nine exercises to train balance, weight bearing, memory, attention and dual tasking. Led by a therapist, participants stand on a platform, adjustable difficulties based on performances | Gradually increased from 18 min in week 1 to 30 min in week 5 | Intervention end | The Dutch version of MoCA | Motivation: The Dutch version of IMI emotions: OERS | IG significantly improved on balance, but not on global cognitive function or cognitive-motor dual tasking or gait performance |
| Hagovská, 2017 [12] | RCT | Cb-CT | Classical group-based cognitive training | CogniPlus program: on a computer, includes five sub-programs that involved everyday activities that are similar to everyday activities, targets attention, working memory, long-term memory, planning of everyday activities, and visual-motor abilities. | 20*30 min, 2 sessions/week for 10 weeks | 10 weeks | Self-reported functional activities: FAQ Global cognition: ACE Attention: The Stroop Test | QOL: Spitzer QOL index Functional activities: The Functional Activities Questionnaire | IG demonstrated larger improvements in QoL and attention than CG. The transfer to functional activities was the same between groups |
| Mansbach, 2017 [38] | CCT | cb-CR | No intervention | Memory Match online cognitive rehabilitation module: designed to improve attention and visual memory, requires the participant to visually pair "matching pictures" by remembering their location | 9*30 min/session | Intervention end | Global cognitive functioning: BCAT AD8 Dementia Screening Interview, KPT | Attitudes about their cognitive abilities: SRI Mood: depression: GDS-SF | IG > CG in global cognition at post-intervention assessment |

**Table 2** Overview of included studies *(Continued)*

| First author and year | Study design | Intervention and Technology | Control | Technology description | Sessions/ Duration | Follow-up | Cognitive outcome measures | Other outcome measures | Key findings |
|---|---|---|---|---|---|---|---|---|---|
| Savulich, 2017 [41] | RCT | CT | No intervention | Game Show on iPad: a novel learning and memory game, target to improve episodic memory | 8 sessions, 1 h/session | Intervention end for 4 weeks | MMSE; Episodic memory and new learning: CANTAB PAL; Visual/ spatial abilities: BVMT-R; Processing speed: CAN-TAB CRT | GDS-SF Anxiety and depression: HADS; Apathy: AES | IG > CG: significantly better performance in episodic memory, visuospatial abilities, MMSE, and less apathy |

Pb-CT = Process-based cognitive training, Cb-CR = computer-based cognitive rehabilitation, Cb-CT = computer-based cognitive training, TNP = Neuropsychological Training, WLMT = memory Word List Memory Test, USMART = Ubiquitous Spaced Retrieval-based Memory Advancement and Rehabilitation Training, MSS = Memory Support System, PT = Physical training, CT = cognitive training, LLM = long lasting memories, CCT = clinical controlled trials, or, computerized cognitive training, WM = working memory, ACG = Active Control Group, CVT = Cognitive Vitality Training, NEAR: motivational therapeutic milieu based on Neuropsychological and Educational Approach to Remediation (NEAR) model, FFA = FitForAll, PRT = Progress resistance training, VSOP = Vision-based speed-of-processing, MLA = mental leisure activities, TIADL = the Timed Instrumental Activities of Daily Living, training, ChEIs = cholinesterase inhibitors, VP = Variable Priority, FP = Fixed Priority, VSOP = Vision-based speed-of-processing, MLA = mental leisure activities, TIADL = the Timed Instrumental Activities of Daily Living, QOL-AD = The Quality of Life-AD, PTC = physical training component, CAMCI = The Computerized Assessment of Mild Cognitive Impairment, CSRQ-25 = Cognitive Self-Report Questionnaire-25, RAVLT = the Rey Auditory Verbal Learning Test, AADL = advanced activity of daily living, RBMT = Rivermead behavioral memory test, CERAD-K-N the Korean version of the CERAD Neuropsychological Assessment Battery, DRS-2 = Dementia Rating Scale-2, E-Cog = The Everyday Cognition, WAIS-III = Wechsler Adult Intelligence Scale-Third Edition, WMS-III = Wechsler Memory Scale-Third Edition, CFQ = Cognitive Failures Questionnaire, RFFT = the Ruff Figural Fluency Test, SCWT the Stroop Color-Word Task, IADL = Instrumental Activities of Daily Living scale, ADL = the Independence in Activity of Daily Living index, WRAT-3 = Wide Range Achievement Test-3rd Edition, BSRT = Buschke Selective Reminding Test, MFQ = Memory Functioning Questionnaire, IED = Intra-/extra-dimensional set shifting, RVP = a mea Rapid visual information processing, MFQ = Memory Functioning Questionnaire, PAL Paired-associates learning, SDMT = Symbol Digit Modalities Test, BVRT-R = Benton Visual Retention Test-Revised 5th Edition, B-IADL Bayer Activities of Daily Living, ADAS-Cog = Alzheimer's Disease Assessment Scale-cognitive subscale, MoCA = the Montreal Cognitive Assessment, IMI = Intrinsic Motivation Inventory, OERS = Observed Emotion Rating Scale, NPI = Neuropsychiatric Inventory, BADL = Basic Activities Daily Living, CDT = clock-drawing test, PPT = physical performance test, TEA = Test of Everyday Attention, GDS = Geriatric Depression Scale, GAI = Geriatric Anxiety Scale, AES = Apathy Evaluation Scale, MMQ Multifactorial Memory Questionnaire, FOME = Fuld Object Memory Evaluation, CVLT-II = California Verbal Learning Test – II, COWAT = Controlled Oral Word Association Test, BNT = Boston Naming Test, BCAT = The Brief Cognitive Assessment Tool, FAQ = Functional Activities Questionnaire, ACE = Addenbrooke's Cognitive Examination, EXAMINER = Executive Abilities: Measures and Instruments for Neurobehavioral Evaluation and Research, BCAT = The Brief Cognitive Assessment Tool, SRI = self-rating inventory of Cognitive Ability, KPT = Kitchen Picture Test of Practical Judgment, GDS-SF = Geriatric Depression Scale-Short Form, CANTAB PAL = Cambridge Neuropsychological Test Automated Battery Paired Associates Learning, BVMT-R = Brief Visuospatial Memory Test-Revised, CANTAB CRT = Cambridge Neuropsychological Test Automated Battery Choice Reaction Time, AES = Apathy Evaluation Scale, HADS = Hospital Anxiety and Depression Scale, CEN = central executive network, WLRT = Word List Recall Test, MN = mode network, CRT = Constructional Recall Test, VTA = Visual Association Test

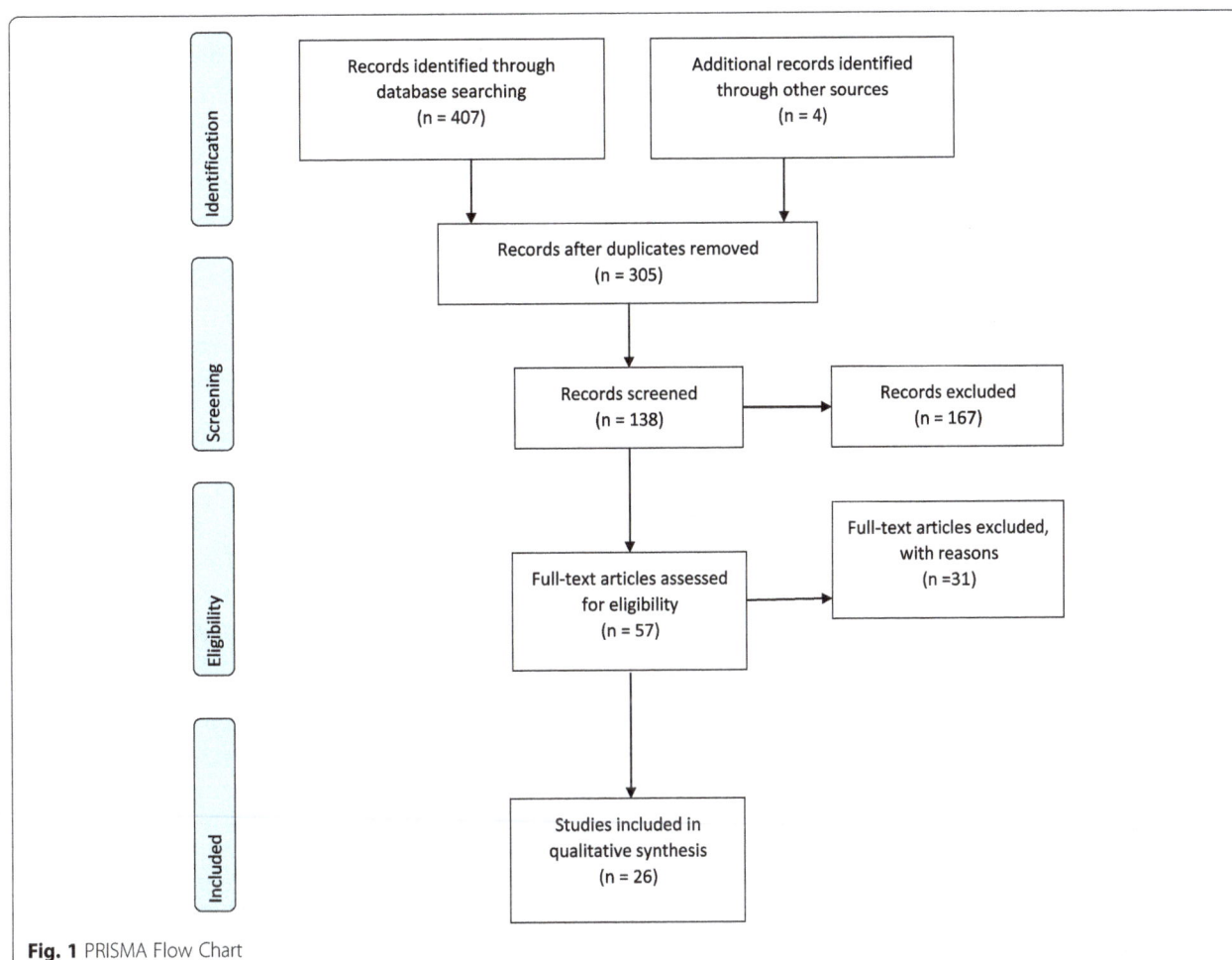

**Fig. 1** PRISMA Flow Chart

## Quality of the studies

Additional file 1: Tables S2 and S3 summarize the quality assessment of the 26 eligible studies using the JBI criteria, which included both randomized controlled trials and quasi-experimental studies. Of these, 15 were randomized controlled trials (Table 2), 6 were controlled clinical trials, 5 were pretest-posttest studies (Table 2).

Among the RCT studies, only four articles [12, 25–27] reported the procedure for randomization. Two studies allocated the participants by utilizing computer-generated random numbers [26, 27], while the other two studies [12, 25] randomized participants by having an independent person use sealed envelopes. The remaining 11 articles did not report the randomization procedure used for allocating participants. Only three studies [26–28] reported that they were double-blinded sham-control trials.

In the quasi-experimental studies, five studies [29–33] utilized pretest-posttest design. The convenience samples and limited sample sizes ($n = 10$; $n = 10$; $n = 22$; $n = 9$; $n = 11$) restricted their generalizability. Six studies utilized a controlled clinical trial design [13, 34–38]. All the studies lacked external validity due to use of convenience samples or sampling methods that were not clearly described. Quasi-experimental studies which lacked randomization also were limited by a potential allocation bias.

## Sample characteristics of the included studies

The sample and design characteristics of each study are summarized in Table 1. More than 40% of the included studies were published from 2016 to 2017 ($n = 11$). Studies were conducted in different countries: United States ($n = 7$), Italy ($n = 3$), Australia ($n = 3$), France ($n = 2$), Greece ($n = 2$), Canada ($n = 1$), Hong Kong ($n = 1$), United Kingdom ($n = 1$), Belgium ($n = 1$), Slavonia ($n = 1$), Spain ($n = 1$), South Korea ($n = 1$), and Netherlands ($n = 1$). Only one study [39] reported recruitment across multiple countries.

The total number of the participants with MCI included in this systematic review was 1040. Seven studies included both participants living with MCI and those with other cognitive statuses (either individuals who were cognitively normal or individuals who had dementia), and reported intervention effects for groups of MCI individuals. The mean age ranged from 67.8 and 87.5. All but three studies reported the criteria used to diagnose MCI. Peterson criteria were used in 12 studies, International Working Group (IWG) criteria were used in five studies, Albert criteria were used in three studies, National Institute on Aging and Alzheimer Association workgroup clinical criteria were used in two studies, and Monongahela-Youghiogheny Healthy Aging Team (MYHAT) Cognitive Classification criteria were used in one study.

## Characteristics of interventions
### Single-component interventions
The majority of the studies ($n = 18$, or 69%) involved single-component technology-based cognitive interventions (Table 2). Characteristics of the interventions varied widely. Seventeen different interventions were utilized in the cognitive training programs studied (see details in Table 2).

### Multimodal interventions
Eight studies utilized multimodal interventions (Table 2). One approach was cognitive training combined with different types of therapies [35, 36, 39, 40]; another approach was cognitive training combined with physical training [26, 33, 34, 37].

**Cognitive training plus therapy** Four studies combined the technology-based cognitive training with other therapies as intervention, specifically reminiscence therapy [39], Neuropsychological and Educational Approach to Remediation (NEAR) [35], occupational therapy [36], and medications (cholinesterase inhibitors (ChEIs)) [40]. Two types of software were involved in the cognitive intervention component, including SOCIABLE [39], and NeuroPsychological Training (TNP) [36, 40]. The training sessions lasted for a minimum of 3 weeks [36] to a maximum of 16 weeks [35].

**Cognitive training combined with physical training** Four studies examined the combined effects of technology-based cognitive and physical training. Two studies used the Long-Lasting Memories (LLM) intervention to provide integrated cognitive and physical training [34, 37], and the physical component was delivered using the FitForAll platform. Gonzalez-Palau, et al. [33] also used the FitForAll platform to provide physical training, but used Gradior program to deliver the cognitive training. Singh and colleagues used Pneumatic resistance machines (Keiser Sports Health Equipment, Ltd) to provide progressive resistance training [26]. The length of these physical trainings lasted from 6 weeks [34] to 6 months [26].

## Overview of technologies
The studies reviewed used the following types of technologies: traditional keyboard computers ($n = 16$), touch screen computers ($n = 4$), gaming consoles or platforms ($n = 5$), and tablets ($n = 3$). Gonzalez-Palau, et al. [33] and Styliadis [34] used both computer and gaming platforms in their interventions. Since 2014, technologies that are more interactive and immersive (virtual reality, gaming console, exergaming platform) have been introduced in cognitive intervention studies.

Compared to traditional therapist-led or pen and paper cognitive interventions, technologies are "smarter" in tracking participants' performances and adjusting the intervention difficulty. By applying technologies as a delivery method, researchers were able to record the participants' performance throughout the intervention process. Thirteen studies tracked participants' performance as one of the outcome variables. Twelve studies used intervention programs that could adjust the intervention difficulties to keep challenging the participants' abilities, as well as avoid distressing them with too many training failures.

## Effects of interventions
### Cognitive outcomes
**Global cognitive function** Twenty-two studies assessed the effects of the interventions on global cognitive function (Table 2). Various instruments were used, including MMSE, Repeatable Battery for Assessment of Neuropsychological Status (RBANS), Computerized Assessment of Mild Cognitive Impairment (CAMCI), Alzheimer's Disease Assessment scale-cognitive subscale (ADAS-Cog), Brief Cognitive Assessment Tool (BCAT), Addenbrooke's Cognitive Examination (ACE), Montreal Cognitive Assessment (MoCA), Spanish version MMSE (MEC35), and composite score from measured cognitive domains.

Out of the 22 studies, eight studies found their intervention significantly improved global cognitive function among individuals with MCI. These studies used different cognitive interventions, all but one [20] of them were interventions targeting multiple cognitive domains. Five studies used an active control group, and three of them found a significant between-group difference in global cognition improvement. Barban, et al. [39] reported a significant treatment effect of a computerized multi-domain process-based cognitive training combined with reminiscence therapy in MMSE mean scores (Cohen's $d = 0.44$). Gonzalez-Palau, et al. [33] reported a significant improvement in global cognitive function (MEC35) among MCI individuals who went through a multi-domain cognitive training program including both cognitive and physical training components. Gooding, et al. [35] compared the computerized cognitive training and cognitive vitality training to an active control group, and reported significantly larger improvements in both intervention groups than the active control group in mMMSE mean score [$F$ (2, 71) = 11.56, $p < 0.001$, $\eta_p^2 = 0.25$] with a medium effect size (Cohen's $d = 0.30 - 0.53$). However, this training effect was not maintained at 3-month follow-up. Bahar-Fuchs, et al. [27] reported a significantly greater improvement in global cognition composite score in the training group than the active control with a large effect size (Cohen's $d = 0.80$). On the other hand, Barnes, et al. [22] found significant RBANS total score improvement in the intervention group after an auditory processing speed and accuracy training, but the between-group difference compared to the active controls was not significant (SD = 0.33). All the other three studies that did not use an active control found significant between-group differences in changes in global cognitive function [26, 38, 41].

Two studies that compared the computer-based cognitive training with listening to audio books, reading online newspapers, and playing a visuospatially-oriented computer game met the requirement for meta-analysis [22, 23]. The design of study, content of intervention, duration and length of follow-up were similar. A total of 59 individuals were included in the meta-analysis. In Additional file 1: Figure S1, the pool weighted standard mean difference score of RBANS total score was 1.62 (95% CI: -1.63 - 4.87). This result indicated that there was no significant difference in the effectiveness for computer-based cognitive training in improving RBANS total score for individuals with MCI after intervention.

**Attention and working memory** Eighteen studies assessed the effects of technology-based cognitive training or rehabilitative programs on attention/working memory, which are required for storage of new information. The most commonly used measures were the digit span test. Other measures included the spatial span test, Trail Making Test A and B, visual search, spanboard, dual task (digit span task + visual detection task), subscale of Addenbrooke's Cognitive Examination, and Symbol Digit Modalities Test (SDMT).

Out of 18 studies, eight studies reported significant improvement in attention/working memory. Two studies compared computerized training programs (Cogmed Software) with no intervention or a sham cognitive intervention [28, 31]. Significant improvements on spanboard ($p = .01$) [28], digit span ($p < .01$) [31], and spatial span ($p < .05$) [31] performance were observed at a 3-month follow-up in the intervention group. Other interventions included memory and attention training, variable

priority training, and vision-based speed-of-processing training. Significant improvements were found in digit span forward ability ($\eta_p^2 = .14$, $p < .05$) [42], accuracy ($p = 0.001$), reaction time ($p < .01$) [43], spatial span ($p = .003$) [22] and working memory ($\eta_p^2 = .28$, $p = .01$) [44]. However, three other studies that measured attention using digit span did not report significant results [23, 33, 36].

In terms of technologies used among the eight studies, all of them applied computerized programs to deliver the interventions. Specifically, they all used a keyboard, not a touch screen, to record the test responses.

**Executive function** Sixteen studies assessed the effect of technology-based cognitive intervention on executive function. Among them, six studies used the Trail Making Task B, six studies used the phonemic and semantic fluency test, four studies used the Rey-Osterreith Complex Figure Test. Other measures included: WAIS Matrices, Ruff Figural Fluency Test, Test of Everyday Attention (TEA), the intra–/extra-dimensional set shifting, and Executive Abilities: Measures and Instruments for Neurobehavioral Evaluation and Research (EXAMINER).

Out of the 16 studies, nine studies reported significant improvement in executive function [22, 26–28, 31, 32, 36, 40, 44]. The interventions used in these studies included both multi-domain cognitive training, specific training tasks, and gaming. The length of interventions ranged from 3 [36] to 24 weeks [26]. Interestingly, three studies used TNP software as an intervention component [29, 36, 40]; although the intervention length varied, two out of the three studies found significant improvement in executive function but used different measures [36, 40]. Talassi [36] found that TNP integrated with occupational therapy and behavioral therapy had a significant improvement in the Rey-Osterreith Complex Figure Test. Rozzini and Costardi [40] found that MCI individuals receiving cognitive training and ChEIs reported significant improvements in Ravens Coloured Progressive Matrices post-intervention ($p < 0.02$). This beneficial effect was not found when using TNP only [29]. However, both Talassi [36] and Rozzini [40] failed to report an effect size for their intervention effect. Other studies that demonstrated significant improvements in executive function varied greatly in terms of sample size, intervention content, total intervention time, and executive function measures.

**Memory** Nineteen studies assessed memory. Sixteen out of the 19 studies found a significant effect on memory. The measures of memory varied greatly. Major measures included the Wechsler Memory Scale (WMS) and Rey Auditory Verbal Learning Test (RAVLT). Four studies used the WMS-III and three out of the four studies found significant improvements in memory after intervention. The intervention used in the three studies included Cogmed computer program [31], Game show on iPad [41], and LLM including both cognitive and physical training components [33]. The intervention period ranged from 5 to 12 weeks and significant improvement in memory was reserved until end of the three months' follow-up [31]. The other study used GOPACK multi-domain cognitive training program to conduct a 6-month intervention but did not find a significant improvement in memory measured by subsets of WMS-III [26]. Three studies used RAVLT to measure verbal memory and all of them found significant benefit of the cognitive interventions being used [27, 31, 39]. The interventions included SOCIABLE, Cogmed, and CogniFit software programs, with the intervention lengths ranged from 5 to 12 weeks and follow-up period up to 3 months [27, 31]. Among the three training software programs, Cogmed targeted on working memory, while the other two targeted on multiple cognitive domains.

Other studies that studied memory as an outcome variable each used various measures including the 12-word-list recall test from the BEM-144 memory battery, the 16-item free and cued reminding test, Buschke Selective Reminding Test, Hopkins Verbal Learning Test, Auditory Logical Memory, Short story recall, WMS-R Visual Reproductions I and II subtests, Pattern recognition memory, Benton Visual Retention Test, short story recall, Rivermead behavioral memory test, and Brief Visuospatial Memory Test-Revised. The interventions of these studies lasted for 3 [36] to 16 weeks [35] with the follow-up time up to 6 months. All but one [32] of these studies demonstrated significant improvements in memory. Manera et al. [32] found the 4-week "kitchen and cooking game" intervention had no significant effect on improving memory.

In terms of technologies, all but two studies used computer to deliver the interventions and used keyboard to collect the data. Only two studies used iPad [41] and VR technology [38] to deliver their memory training programs.

### Non-cognitive outcomes

**Mood** Nine studies assessed depression. The most commonly used measures were Geriatric Depression Scale (GDS) and its short form GDS-SF [22, 29, 33, 36, 38, 40, 41], other inventory used included Beck's Depression Inventory [35] and Depression Anxiety and Stress Scale [25]. Four studies reported significant reduction of depression among individuals with MCI [33, 35, 36, 40]. None of these studies reported effect sizes for their interventions reducing depression. Two

out of these four studies used a multimodal intervention that also integrated physical trainings [33, 36].

Five studies assessed anxiety [25, 29, 36, 40, 41]. The most often used measure was the State Trait Anxiety Inventory (STAI) [29, 36] used in two studies. Only one study showed a significant reduction in anxiety for individuals with MCI. Talassi used a multimodal intervention including cognition, behavioral, and occupational training compared to its control group that had physical rehabilitation, occupational, and behavioral training, and found that the intervention group had significant decrease in anxiety but not the control group participants [36].

**ADL** Eleven studies assessed ADL as a secondary outcome. The Basic Advanced and Instrumental Activities of Daily Living scales were used in 5 studies [29, 36, 40, 44, 45]. Other measures included the Functional Activities Questionnaire [28], B-IADL scale [26], and HK Lawton IADL [13]. Two out of nine studies reported a statistically significant improvement in ADL [27, 44]. However, only one study found a significant between-group difference with a small to medium effect size ($\eta^2 = 0.21$) [44].

**Quality of life** Three studies assessed quality of life [12, 29, 43]. Measures included SF-12 [29], Well-Being Scale [43] and Spitzer-QOL [12]. Only one study reported significant results. Hagovská, et al. [12] found that technology-based cognitive training produced a larger improvement in QoL than classical group-based cognitive training with a medium effect size ($r = 0.69$).

### Discussion

In the past decade, technology-based cognitive interventions have gained increased research interest worldwide. Almost half (42%) of the studies reviewed were published in 2016 and 2017, suggesting the growth in the importance of technology-based interventions. The vast majority of the studies were conducted in developed countries, which may be associated with the limited availability of and familiarity with technology among older adults in lower income countries.

The types of technology used varied across studies and included computers, tablets, VR, and gaming consoles. Computers were the most widely used technology with 77% using computers to assist delivery of cognitive interventions. The majority utilized commercially available software or programs, with only nine of the studies used training programs developed by the study researchers for the specific study purpose. Therapists or coaches were used to teach, assist, or even supervise the use of technologies along the intervention process. In nearly half of studies ($n = 12$) therapists provided instructions at the beginning of the intervention, or provided help throughout the intervention. All but two studies were conducted using only one type of technology, so no conclusions can be drawn regarding the effect of different types of technology on intervention results. Comparing effects of technology across studies was not possible due to the variability among interventions. With the rapid development of technologies, we can anticipate new types of technologies being utilized to assist cognitive training and rehabilitation interventions in the future.

Overall, technology-based cognitive training and rehabilitation have demonstrated promising beneficial effects on various domains of cognition with moderate to large effect sizes. Most studies (e.g., [28, 31, 44]) assessed participants on different cognitive domains that were not limited to the trained task, but also in other non-trained tasks and other cognitive domains, suggesting a transferable beneficial effect of cognitive training and rehabilitation. For example, Hyer, et al. [28] found that working memory training also improved executive function among trained MCI participants, and the impact was preserved until the end of the 3-month follow-up. This transferability is consistent with previous systematic reviews [14, 15]. However, the training gain and transferability of the training gain varied by intervention (e.g., [22]) and delivery method (e.g., [13]). Therefore, future studies are still needed to understand which intervention would benefit various cognitive domains most efficiently.

Only one study included in this review examined whether applying technology as the delivery method would have a stronger effect on the intervention outcomes, in comparison to the use of a traditional manual delivery. Man, et al. [13] compared the training effect of a memory training program delivered with a non-immersive VR-based system versus with color-print images that matched the VR images. This study found that the VR group showed greater improvement in objective memory but the non-VR group reported greater contentment with memory performance, highlighting the potential importance of receiving verbal and emotional support from training therapists on improving participants' satisfaction with their memory performance. This study shows that depending on the outcomes that an intervention targets, technology-based and manual trainings may have their own strengths and weaknesses. No conclusions can be made whether one type of intervention is generally more effective than the other.

The effect of the same technology-based cognitive intervention seems to vary between groups with different level of cognitive decline. Some but still limited evidence suggested that participants without cognitive impairment seem to obtain a larger cognitive improvement from technology-based cognitive interventions than

those with MCI. Vermeij, et al. [31] found that healthy participants had a larger gain in both trained working memory tasks and untrained executive function tasks than those with cognitive impairment. However, the findings are not conclusive. Barban, et al. [39] found that process-based cognitive training improved verbal memory among MCI participants and improved executive function among healthy participants. On the other hand, participants with MCI seem to gain a larger cognitive benefit than those with Alzheimer's disease (AD). Cipriani, et al. [29] fount that the TNP program significantly improved memory and global cognition among participants with MCI, but only improved memory among those with AD. Similarly, Manera, et al. [32] found that the serious cooking game significantly improved executive function among participants with MCI but not those with AD.

Measures of physical function and mood were used in most studies, but unfortunately most of these were used to ensure non-biased randomization assignment at baseline rather than as outcome measures, so we have limited understanding of the effects of technology-based cognitive interventions on these outcomes. Nine studies evaluated mood (e.g., depression, anxiety) as an outcome, and eleven studies included ADL as an outcome variable. Among these, four studies found technology-based cognitive interventions had beneficial effect on mood and two studies found beneficial effect on functional activity. Technology-based cognitive training studies included in this review may have limited impact on mood and functional activity.

Two studies of technology-based cognitive training and one study of technology-based cognitive rehabilitation examined the effect of their interventions on quality of life [12, 29, 43]. However, only one of the four studies reported significant result. Hagovská, et al. [12] found that technology-based cognitive training produced a larger improvement in QoL than classical group-based cognitive training. This lack of effect of cognitive intervention on QoL is consistent with previous systematic review on the efficacy of cognitive interventions on QoL [14]. However, each study used a different QoL instruments, and various research designs (e.g., types of interventions, lengths of follow-up, and types of control groups). Given the limited number of studies conducted, future studies using comparable designs are still needed to further understand the effectiveness of the intervention on quality of life.

A previous systematic review suggested that multimodal cognitive inventions were a promising research area [15]. In our review, we found eight studies that applied multimodal interventions combining technology-based cognitive training and physical exercise or other therapeutic methods. We expected to see the findings of these studies would provide support for speculation that multimodal cognitive interventions would produce a greater impact on improving cognitive function as well as mood and functional abilities. However, the eight reviewed articles provided insufficient evidence to support this conjecture. Five out of the eight studies were not designed to compare the efficacy of multimodal cognitive intervention compared to cognitive intervention alone [33, 34, 36, 37, 39], and it was difficult to draw any conclusions from the remaining three studies remained due to the great variability in the designs across studies. According to one study, customized technology-based cognitive training produced additional benefit, and technology-based cognitive intervention plus ChEIs was superior to ChEIs alone [35]. Interestingly, Fiatarone-Singh, et al. [26] found that progressive resistance training produced more improvement in executive function and global cognition than both cognitive training and multimodal intervention including cognitive training and progressive resistance training. Findings from this study suggest that physical exercise may particularly benefit executive function, but that implementing multimodal cognitive and physical interventions may be too challenging for people with MCI. Previous systematic review on the efficacy of combined cognitive and exercise intervention in older adults with and without cognitive impairment did not find sufficient evidence to confirm the beneficial effect among older adults with cognitive impairment [46]. Taken together, more studies are needed to understand the advantages of a multimodal cognitive intervention in individuals with MCI. Future studies should design appropriate control groups to understand the additional value produced by a multimodal cognitive intervention than a single model intervention. Additionally, researchers should also bear in mind the possibility that older adults with MCI may not be able to manage the cognitive challenge associated with multimodal interventions.

The studies reviewed generally had small sample sizes, ranged widely from 10 [13] to 301 participants [39]. The average sample size across studies was 54; 39% of the studies had sample sizes of less than 30. The small sample sizes may be related to the complicated diagnostic criteria of MCI, the ethical challenges of conducting intervention studies in older adults with MCI, and the limited availability of some technology-based cognitive intervention programs. More importantly, potential beneficial effects of an intervention could be diminished due to a small sample size.

The measures applied varied greatly across studies, which created challenges in the comparison and generalizability of the study findings. Future studies should consider using measures that have been shown to have good validity and reliability as well as have been

frequently used among the MCI population (e.g., CES-D, MMSE, QOL-AD, etc.). Neuroimaging techniques have emerged to be more widely used to obtain information on how technology-based cognitive interventions would affect neural connectivity [37], activation [23], and brain atrophy [31].

We conducted a comprehensive search of literature on the topic area using five major databases. However, this systematic review should be considered in light of its limitations. We only reviewed articles in English language. There may be other relevant studies that were published in other languages. We also need to be aware that technology is developing rapidly so that promising technology-based cognitive training and rehabilitation programs may exist that have not yet been published due to concerns about protecting participants.

## Conclusion

The findings from this systematic review suggest that technology-based cognitive training and rehabilitation programs show promise for improving cognitive function, with some interventions showing moderate to large effect sizes. Computers, tablets, gaming consoles and platforms, and VR systems were the common types of technologies used. Both general and domain-specific cognitive training have led to improved cognition, primarily in memory, but with some evidence that executive function may also be positively affected. Studies that examined the impact of cognitive training on improving mood and functional abilities, have generated less convincing evidence. Multimodal intervention programs integrated technology-based cognitive intervention and other therapies have produced inconsistent findings on the superiority over only applying technology-based single model cognitive intervention. Overall, technology-based cognitive training and rehabilitation are promising intervention methods to improve cognitive function. Future studies should put effort to clarify whether the added benefits of implementing multimodal interventions exist, and carefully consider the potential extra burden caused to individuals with MCI. Additionally, future studies should aim to lessen the variabilities in intervention design and measures applied.

## Abbreviations

ACE: Addenbrooke's Cognitive Examination; AD: Alzheimer's disease; ADAS-Cog: Alzheimer's Disease Assessment scale-cognitive subscale; BCAT: Brief Cognitive Assessment Tool; CAMCI: Computerized Assessment of Mild Cognitive Impairment; ChEIs: cholinesterase inhibitors; GDS: Geriatric Depression Scale; GDS-SF: Geriatric Depression Scale short form; IWG: International Working Group; JBI: Joanna Briggs Institute; LLM: Long-Lasting Memories; MMSE: Mini-mental state examination; MoCA: Montreal

Cognitive Assessment; MYHAT: Monongahela-Youghiogheny Healthy Aging Team; NEAR: Neuropsychological and Educational Approach to Remediation; RAVLT: Rey Auditory Verbal Learning Test; RBANS: Repeatable Battery for Assessment of Neuropsychological Status; RCT: randomized controlled trial; SDMT: Symbol Digit Modalities Test; STAI: State Trait Anxiety Inventory; TEA: Test of Everyday Attention; TNP: Neuropsychological Training; VR: virtual reality; WMS: Wechsler Memory Scale

## Authors' contributions
SG designed and conducted the study, abstracted data, interpreted the results, and played a major role in writing the manuscript. ZZ provided methodological support, helped abstracted data, appraised quality, and helped wrote a certain section of the manuscript. BW helped conceive the study and edited the manuscript. ESM helped conceive the study, screened citations and full-text articles, and edited the manuscript. All authors read and approved the final manuscript.

## Competing interests
The authors declare that they have no competing interests.

## Author details
[1]Duke University School of Nursing, 307 Trent Drive, Durham, NC, USA. [2]Fudan University School of Nursing, Shanghai, China. [3]Fudan University Center for Evidence-Based Nursing, a Joanna Briggs Institute Center of Excellence, Shanghai, China. [4]New York University Rory Meyers College of Nursing, New York, NY, USA. [5]Hartford Institute for Geriatric Nursing, New York University, New York, NY, USA. [6]Geriatric Research, Education and Clinical Center (GRECC) of the Department of Veterans Affairs Medical Center, Durham, NC, USA.

## References
1. Alzheimer's Disease International: World Alzheimer Report 2016. In.; 2016.
2. Prince M, Guerchet M, Prina M. The epidemiology and impact of dementia: current state and future trends. Geneva: World Health Organization; 2015.
3. Gates NJ, Sachdev PS, Singh MAF, Valenzuela M. Cognitive and memory training in adults at risk of dementia: a systematic review. BMC Geriatr. 2011;11(1):55.
4. The White House Office of the Press Secretary: FACT SHEET: the white house conference on Aging 2015. In.; 2015.
5. Petersen RC. Mild cognitive impairment as a diagnostic entity. J Intern Med. 2004;256(3):183–94.
6. Feldman HH, Jacova C. Mild cognitive impairment. Am J Geriatr Psychiatry. 2005;13(8):645–55.
7. Jean L, Bergeron M-È, Thivierge S, Simard M. Cognitive intervention programs for individuals with mild cognitive impairment: systematic review of the literature. Am J Geriatr Psychiatry. 2010;18(4):281–96.
8. Zheng G, Xia R, Zhou W, Tao J, Chen L. Aerobic exercise ameliorates cognitive function in older adults with mild cognitive impairment: a systematic review and meta-analysis of randomised controlled trials. Br J Sports Med. 2016;50(23):1443.
9. Belleville S. Cognitive training for persons with mild cognitive impairment. Int Psychogeriatr. 2008;20(1):57–66.
10. Reijnders J, van Heugten C, van Boxtel M. Cognitive interventions in healthy older adults and people with mild cognitive impairment: a systematic review. Ageing Res Rev. 2013;12(1):263–75.
11. Faucounau V, Wu Y-H, Boulay M, De Rotrou J, Rigaud A-S. Cognitive intervention programmes on patients affected by mild cognitive impairment: a promising intervention tool for MCI? J Nutr Health Aging. 2010;14(1):31–5.
12. Hagovská M, Dzvoník O, Olekszyová Z. Comparison of two cognitive training programs with effects on functional activities and quality of life. Res Gerontol Nurs. 2017;10:172–80.
13. Man D, Chung J, Lee G: Evaluation of a virtual reality-based memory training programme for Hong Kong Chinese older adults with questionable dementia: a pilot study. 2012.

14. Chandler MJ, Parks AC, Marsiske M, Rotblatt LJ, Smith GE. Everyday impact of cognitive interventions in mild cognitive impairment: a systematic review and meta-analysis. Neuropsychol Rev. 2016;26(3):225–51.
15. Coyle H, Traynor V, Solowij N. Computerized and virtual reality cognitive training for individuals at high risk of cognitive decline: systematic review of the literature. Am J Geriatr Psychiatr. 2015;23(4):335–59.
16. Hill NT, Mowszowski L, Naismith SL, Chadwick VL, Valenzuela M, Lampit A. Computerized cognitive training in older adults with mild cognitive impairment or dementia: a systematic review and meta-analysis. Am J Psychiatr. 2017;174(4):329–40.
17. Visser PJ, Kester A, Jolles J, Verhey F. Ten-year risk of dementia in subjects with mild cognitive impairment. Neurology. 2006;67(7):1201–7.
18. Moher D, Liberati A, Tetzlaff J, Altman DG, Group P. Preferred reporting items for systematic reviews and meta-analyses: the PRISMA statement. PLoS Med. 2009;6(7):e1000097.
19. Tufanaru C, Munn Z, Aromataris E, Campbell J, Hopp L: Chapter 3: Systematic reviews of effectiveness. In: *Joanna Briggs Institute Reviewer's Manual The Joanna Briggs Institute, 2017*. Edited by Aromataris E, Munn Z; 2017.
20. Nordmann AJ, Kasenda B, Briel M. Meta-analyses: what they can and cannot do. Swiss Med Wkly. 2012;142:w13518.
21. Greco T, Zangrillo A, Biondi-Zoccai G, Landoni G. Meta-analysis: pitfalls and hints. Heart, lung and vessels. 2013;5(4):219.
22. Barnes DE, Yaffe K, Belfor N, Jagust WJ, DeCarli C, Reed BR, et al. Computer-based cognitive training for mild cognitive impairment: results from a pilot randomized, controlled trial. Alzheimer Dis Assoc Disord. 2009;23:205–10.
23. Rosen AC, Sugiura L, Kramer JH, Whitfield-Gabrieli S, Gabrieli JD. Cognitive training changes hippocampal function in mild cognitive impairment: a pilot study, vol. 2; 2011. p. 617–25.
24. RevMan. Copenhagen: the Nordic Cochrane Centre, the Cochrane collaboration. 5.3 ed; 2014.
25. Finn M, McDonald S. Computerised cognitive training for older persons with mild cognitive impairment: a pilot study using a randomised controlled trial design. Brain Impairment. 2011;12(3):187–99.
26. Fiatarone Singh MA, Gates N, Saigal N, Wilson GC, Meiklejohn J, Brodaty H, et al. The study of mental and resistance training (SMART) study—resistance training and/or cognitive training in mild cognitive impairment: a randomized, double-blind, double-sham controlled trial. J Am Med Dir Assoc. 2014;15(12):873–80.
27. Bahar-Fuchs A, Webb S, Bartsch L, Clare L, Rebok G, Cherbuin N, et al. Tailored and adaptive computerized cognitive training in older adults at risk for dementia: a randomized controlled trial. J Alzheimers Dis. 2017;60(3):889–911.
28. Hyer L, Scott C, Atkinson MM, Mullen CM, Lee A, Johnson A, et al. Cognitive training program to improve working memory in older adults with MCI. Clinical Gerontologist: The Journal of Aging and Mental Health. 2016;39(5):410–27.
29. Cipriani G, Bianchetti A, Trabucchi M. Outcomes of a computer-based cognitive rehabilitation program on Alzheimer's disease patients compared with those on patients affected by mild cognitive impairment. Archives of Gerontology & Geriatrics. 2006;43(3):327–35.
30. Han JW, Oh K, Yoo S, Kim E, Ahn KH, Son YJ, et al. Development of the ubiquitous spaced retrieval-based memory advancement and rehabilitation training program. Psychiatry investigation. 2014;11(1):52–8.
31. Vermeij A, Claassen JA, Dautzenberg PL, Kessels RP. Transfer and maintenance effects of online working-memory training in normal ageing and mild cognitive impairment. Neuropsychol Rehabil. 2016;26(5–6):783–809.
32. Manera V, Petit PD, Derreumaux A, Orvieto I, Romagnoli M, Lyttle G, et al. 'Kitchen and cooking,' a serious game for mild cognitive impairment and Alzheimer's disease: a pilot study. Front Aging Neurosci. 2015;7:24.
33. Gonzalez-Palau F, Franco M, Bamidis P, Losada R, Parra E, Papageorgiou SG, et al. The effects of a computer-based cognitive and physical training program in a healthy and mildly cognitive impaired aging sample. Aging Ment Health. 2014;18(7):838–46.
34. Styliadis C, Kartsidis P, Paraskevopoulos E, Ioannides AA, Bamidis PD. Neuroplastic effects of combined computerized physical and cognitive training in elderly individuals at risk for dementia: an eLORETA controlled study on resting states. Neural plasticity. 2015;2015:172192.
35. Gooding AL, Choi J, Fiszdon JM, Wilkins K, Kirwin PD, van Dyck CH, et al.

Comparing three methods of computerised cognitive training for older adults with subclinical cognitive decline. Neuropsychol Rehabil. 2016;26(5/6):810–21.

36. Talassi E, Guerreschi M, Feriani M, Fedi V, Bianchetti A, Trabucchi M. Effectiveness of a cognitive rehabilitation program in mild dementia (MD) and mild cognitive impairment (MCI): a case control study. Arch Gerontol Geriatr. 2007;44:391–9.

37. Klados MA, Styliadis C, Frantzidis CA, Paraskevopoulos E, Bamidis PD. Beta-band functional connectivity is reorganized in mild cognitive impairment after combined computerized physical and cognitive training. Front Neurosci. 2016;10:55.

38. Mansbach WE, Mace RA, Clark KM. The efficacy of a computer-assisted cognitive rehabilitation program for patients with mild cognitive deficits: a pilot study. Exp Aging Res. 2017;43:94–104.

39. Barban F, Annicchiarico R, Pantelopoulos S, Federici A, Perri R, Fadda L, et al. Protecting cognition from aging and Alzheimer's disease: a computerized cognitive training combined with reminiscence therapy. Int J Geriatr Psychiatry. 2016;31(4):340–8.

40. Rozzini L, Costardi D, Chilovi BV, Franzoni S, Trabucchi M, Padovani A. Efficacy of cognitive rehabilitation in patients with mild cognitive impairment treated with cholinesterase inhibitors. International Journal of Geriatric Psychiatry: A journal of the psychiatry of late life and allied sciences. 2007;22(4):356–60.

41. Savulich G, Piercy T, Fox C, Suckling J, Rowe JB, O'Brien JT, et al. Cognitive training using a novel memory game on an iPad in patients with amnestic mild cognitive impairment (aMCI). Int J Neuropsychopharmacol. 2017;20:624–33.

42. Herrera C, Chambon C, Michel BF, Paban V, Alescio-Lautier B. Positive effects of computer-based cognitive training in adults with mild cognitive impairment. Neuropsychologia. 2012;50(8):1871–81.

43. Gagnon LG, Belleville S. Training of attentional control in mild cognitive impairment with executive deficits: results from a double-blind randomised controlled study. Neuropsychol Rehabil. 2012;22(6):809–35.

44. Lin F, Heffner KL, Ren P, Tivarus ME, Brasch J, Chen DG, et al. Cognitive and neural effects of vision-based speed-of-processing training in older adults with amnestic mild cognitive impairment: a pilot study. J Am Geriatr Soc. 2016;64:1293–8.

45. Hughes TF, Flatt JD, Fu B, Butters MA, Chang CCH, Ganguli M. Interactive video gaming compared with health education in older adults with mild cognitive impairment: a feasibility study. Int J Geriatr Psychiatry. 2014;29(9):890–8.

46. Law LL, Barnett F, Yau MK, Gray MA. Effects of combined cognitive and exercise interventions on cognition in older adults with and without cognitive impairment: a systematic review. Ageing Res Rev. 2014;15:61–75.

47. Delbroek T, Vermeylen W, Spildooren J. The effect of cognitive-motor dual task training with the biorescue force platform on cognition, balance and dual task performance in institutionalized older adults: a randomized controlled trial. Journal of physical therapy science. 2017;29(7):1137–43.

# 14

# Depression, malnutrition, and health-related quality of life among Nepali older patients

Saruna Ghimire[1]* ⓘ, Binaya Kumar Baral[2], Buddhi Raj Pokhrel[2], Asmita Pokhrel[2], Anushree Acharya[3], Dipta Amatya[1], Prabisha Amatya[1] and Shiva Raj Mishra[4]

## Abstract

**Background:** Little is known about the health, nutrition, and quality of life of the aging population in Nepal. Consequently, we aimed to assess the nutritional status, depression and health-related quality of life (HRQOL) of Nepali older patients and evaluate the associated factors. Furthermore, a secondary aim was to investigate the proposed mediation-moderation models between depression, nutrition, and HRQOL.

**Methods:** A cross-sectional survey was conducted from January–April of 2017 among 289 Nepali older patients in an outpatient clinic at Nepal Medical College in Kathmandu. Nutritional status, depression and HRQOL were assessed using a mini nutritional assessment, geriatric depression scales, and the European quality of life tool, respectively. Linear regression models were used to find the factors associated with nutritional status, depression, and HRQOL. The potential mediating and moderating role of nutritional status on the relationship between depression and HRQOL was explored; likewise, for depression on the relationship between nutritional status and HRQOL.

**Results:** The prevalence of malnutrition and depression was 10% and 57.4% respectively; depression-malnutrition comorbidity was 7%. After adjusting for age and gender, nutritional score ($\beta = 2.87$; BCa 95%CI = 2.12, 3.62) was positively associated and depression score ($\beta = -1.23$; BCa 95%CI = $-1.72, -0.72$) was negatively associated with HRQOL. After controlling for covariates, nutritional status mediated 41% of the total effect of depression on HRQOL, while depression mediated 6.0% of the total effect of the nutrition on HRQOL.

**Conclusions:** A sizeable proportion of older patients had malnutrition and depression. Given that nutritional status had a significant direct (independently) and indirect (as a mediator) effect on HRQOL, we believe that nutritional screening and optimal nutrition among the older patients can make a significant contribution to the health and well-being of Nepali older patients. Nonetheless, these findings should be replicated in prospective studies before generalization.

**Keywords:** Nutritional assessment, MNA, Depression, Quality of life, Elderly, Nepal, Mediation, Moderation

## Background

The population of older adults, 60 years and above, in Nepal has increased from 1.5 million to 2.2 million in recent years [1, 2]. The 3.5% population growth rate of the older adults from 2001 to 2011 is higher than the population growth rate (2%) of the overall country [1–3], which hints at a slowly shifting demographic structure in Nepal concomitant with overall gains in life expectancy.

Notably, this growth in life expectancy (10 years gain in the last 20 years) carries a disease burden. Malnutrition and depression are known major problems amongst senior citizens, contributing significantly to decreased health-related quality of life (HRQOL) [4, 5]. Yet, little is known about the health, nutrition, and HRQOL of Nepali older adults.

The national prevalence of malnutrition among Nepali older adults is entirely unknown, although one study conducted in rural Nepal found an estimated 24% prevalence of malnutrition among older adults [6]. The

---

* Correspondence: sarunaghimire@gmail.com
[1]Agrata Health and Education (AHEAD)-Nepal, Kathmandu, Nepal
Full list of author information is available at the end of the article

current study, conducted among urban older patients, will supplement the previous nutritional assessment in rural Nepal [6] to provide more comprehensive knowledge on this important issue. Previous studies examining the prevalence of depression among segments of Nepal's older population found estimates ranging from 47 to 53% [7, 8]. In the absence of large nationally representative studies, small studies conducted in diverse settings, such as the current and previous studies [7, 8], can serve to provide valuable baseline information on depression status and its correlates among the older patients. Aging is one of the most important causes of decreasing HRQOL and wellbeing due to biological senescence and socio-psychological changes [9]. Although HRQOL indicators have played a major role in the development of health services globally [10], this is relatively uncommon in Nepal. Moreover, studies assessing the HRQOL of the burgeoning older population in Nepal are lacking. One previous study reported low HRQOL among older adults [11]; however, the study used a relatively homogenous study population: predominantly female visually impaired nursing home residents, reducing the generalizability of their findings.

In 2010, a comprehensive review by the Nepal Geriatric Centre [3] for the Ministry of Health and Population in Nepal highlighted the lack of studies on the health, nutritional state, and overall HRQOL of older adults in Nepal. They recommended continued research to fill these gaps in knowledge in order to effectively be able to plan programs and interventions that maximize the HRQOL of the older population in Nepal. Therefore, our primary aim was to assess the status of nutrition, depression, and HRQOL among

Nepali older patients and identify factors that are associated with these outcomes.

Our secondary aim was to evaluate the depression-nutrition-HRQOL triad in mediation-moderation models (Figs. 1 and 2). We hypothesized that both depression and malnutrition would have a significant negative impact on HRQOL among the older patients in Nepal. In addition to finding a bidirectional link between nutritional status and depression [4, 12, 13], previous studies have shown that depression and nutrition independently contribute to decreased HRQOL among older adults [4, 5]. Therefore, based on the literature, it is plausible that additional moderating or mediating effects may be present in the nutrition-depression-HRQOL triad; studies exploring such mediation-moderation effects are lacking. Exploring these pathways and determining which pathway is more plausible will enrich our understanding of the HRQOL of the older adults. More importantly, it will aide in devising effective interventions to promote HRQOL and healthy aging among the older adults.

## Methods
### Study procedure
This study, abbreviated as NepEldQOL I, supplements our previous study, NepEldQOL II [14]; together these studies provide the most comprehensive portrayal of the well-being of Nepal's older population to date. The current study was conducted in January–April of 2017 in the outpatient department (OPD) of Nepal Medical College and Teaching Hospital (NMCTH) in Kathmandu, Nepal. According to hospital administration data, NMCTH had a total of 138,684 outpatient

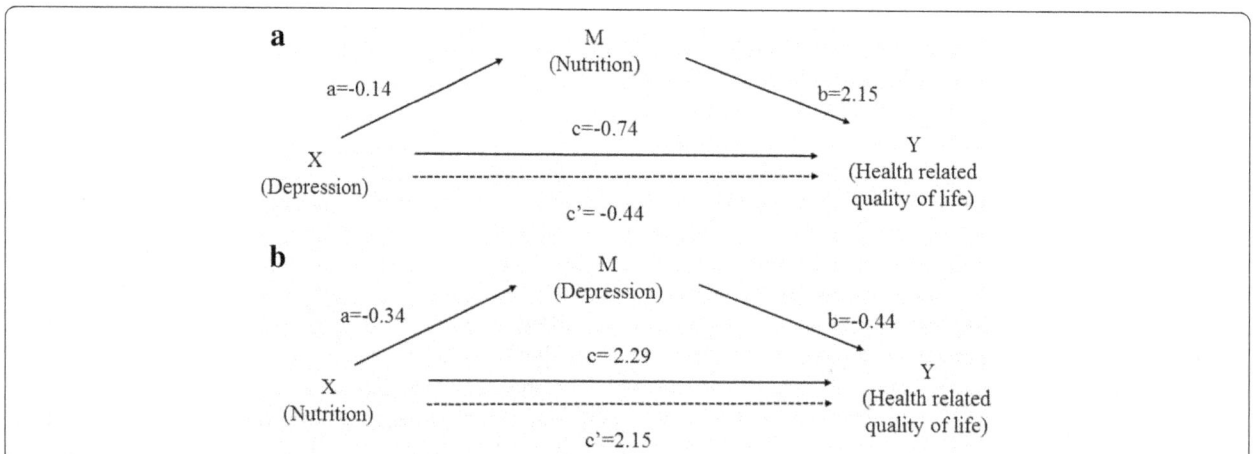

**Fig. 1** Mediation model **a** for the association between depression and health related quality of life, mediated by nutrition; **b** for the association between nutrition and health related quality of life, mediated by depression. X: independent variable; Y: outcome variable; M: mediator variable; a: association between independent variable (X) and potential mediator (M); b: association between potential mediator (M) and outcome variable (Y), controlling for independent variable (X); c: total effect of the independent variable (X) on outcome variable (Y); c': direct effect (unmediated) of independent variable (X) on outcome variable (Y). Model is adjusted for age, sex, ethnicity, marital status, smoking, alcohol use, educational status, perception of negligence/hatred, perceived health status compared to others

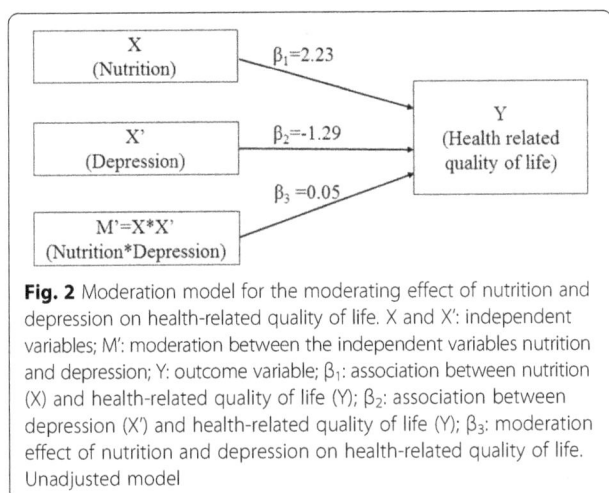

**Fig. 2** Moderation model for the moderating effect of nutrition and depression on health-related quality of life. X and X': independent variables; M': moderation between the independent variables nutrition and depression; Y: outcome variable; $\beta_1$: association between nutrition (X) and health-related quality of life (Y); $\beta_2$: association between depression (X') and health-related quality of life (Y); $\beta_3$: moderation effect of nutrition and depression on health-related quality of life. Unadjusted model

visits in 2016–2017; of these, 16,567 visits were among patients aged 60 years and above.

The required sample size of 289 was calculated by using StatCalc in Epi Info 7 based on a 24% prevalence of malnutrition among Nepali older adults [6], 5% alpha or Type I error and a 5% margin of error. Surveyors were graduate students in medicine and public health who were provided with a one-day extensive orientation on the study tools, sampling strategy, and data collection techniques. Each day, participants were selected by systematic random sampling from the daily "first-come first served" OPD sign-in lists, since NMCTH, like most health service facilities in Nepal, uses only a walk-in appointment system for all new or revisiting patients. The daily OPD record (updated continuously throughout the day) served as the population sample reference frame for each day of data collection, which took place during normal business hours from January to mid-April, when the required sample size was achieved. Surveyors identified patients ages 60 and above from the OPD list, and subsequently approached every third patient to screen for eligibility. Eligible participants were 60 years or older and present in the OPD one on the data collection days. Those too frail physically or mentally to respond, and/or with hearing or speech impairment were excluded. Consent to participate was requested from all eligible patients. If the approached patient was deemed incligible or if s/he refused to participate, the next eligible patient from the OPD list was approached. Of the 297 patients approached, eight eligible patients refused to participate; the remainder granted consent.

## Data collection and variables
Individual face-to-face interviews were conducted with patients in the waiting area of the OPD. The survey tools

were translated from English to Nepali by the second author and then verified by back-translation to English by another author, following the protocol for translations [15]. Any disagreement on translation was resolved by adjudication by a third author and mutual consensus between the three authors.

### Nutritional assessment
Nutritional status was assessed using the Short Form Mini Nutritional Assessment (MNA), validated previously among Nepali older adults [6]. For the measurement of BMI, the surveyors measured each participant's height with a mechanical stadiometer (Prestige HM 007) and weight with a digital weighing scale (SECA GMBH & Co Model: 874). BMI was calculated as weight in kg/(height in m)$^2$ which was categorized as per instructions in the MNA guide [16]. The cumulative MNA score ranges from 0 to 14. A score of less than 8 indicates malnourishment, a score between 8 and 11 points indicates that the subject is at risk of malnutrition and a score of 12 or higher indicates a normal nutritional status. Details on the MNA tool are provided elsewhere [16]; briefly, the MNA short form consists of six items: decline in food intake, involuntary weight loss, mobility, psychological stress, neuropsychological problems and body mass index (BMI). While the World Health Organization defines malnutrition as "deficiencies, excesses, or imbalances in a person's intake of energy and/or nutrients" [17], we use the words "nutritional status" and "malnourished" throughout the manuscript to reflect only deficient nutritional status in order to be consistent with the MNA tool. The Cronbach's Alpha, which is the measurement of scale reliability, for the MNA scale in the current study was 0.59.

### Depression assessment
The Geriatric Depression Scale Short Form (GDS) was used to measure depression [18]. The GDS has been described in detail elsewhere [18]; briefly, it is a 15-item instrument with responses in "Yes/No" format. Of the 15 items, 10 indicate the presence of depression when answered positively while the other five are indicative of depression when answered negatively (reverse coded for cumulation). A cumulative score of 5 or more suggests depression [19]. The validity and reliability of GDS to measure depression among community-dwelling Nepali older adults has been established by a previous study [20]. The Cronbach's Alpha for the GDS was 0.81 in the current study.

### Health-related quality of life
HRQOL was assessed using the European quality of life tool (EQ-5D) [21]. The Nepali versions of the EQ-5D tools have been validated in a previous study [22]. The EQ-5D allows participants to classify their health status

in five different dimensions (i.e., mobility, self-care, usual activities, pain/discomfort and anxiety/depression) and within a three-level response (no problems, moderate problems, and severe problems) [21]. The five dimensions of the ED-5D are then converted into a single index value, called EQ-5D index, by using the "EQ-5D-3L crosswalk index value calculator" [23], using United Kingdom (UK) weights as the reference. The EQ-5D index ranges from 0 to 1, where 0 indicates severely ill, and 1 indicates perfect health. Perfect health is represented by no problems across all five dimensions; severely ill corresponds to severe problems on all five dimensions of EQ-5D.

Additionally, EQ-5D has a vertically calibrated scale called the EuroQol visual analytic scale (EQVAS), which allows participants to rate their overall health on a scale ranging from 0 to 100, where 0 and 100 signify the worst and the best imaginable health state level, respectively. Participants rated their overall health in EQVAS at the level they felt best described their health on the study day. For this study, the Cronbach's Alpha of the EQ-5D scale was 0.79.

### Sociodemographic variables

Sociodemographic variables were self-reported and included age, gender, ethnicity, religion, marital status, educational status, occupation, monthly family income, family structure, smoking, and alcohol use. For ethnicity, the Nepal Health Management Information System's 'caste/ethnic groupings' were used [24]. Due to sparsity in certain categories, related categories were combined to form three categories: Upper caste, Janjatis, and Dalit/other minorities. Education status was categorized into three groups: illiterate; informal (no formal schooling, some literacy); and formal education (any years of formal schooling). Occupation indicated the primary occupation of the participant in the past or the current occupation if currently employed ($n = 27$). Adequate rest was defined as sleeping for more than six hours daily. Information on primary caretakers was collected through open-ended questioning and recoded into two categories: son and daughter-in-law as the first; others as the second.

### Statistical analyses

Statistical analyses were performed in IBM SPSS v22. Numerical variables are expressed as a mean and standard deviation (SD); categorical variables as frequency and percentage. Comparisons of means between the groups were made by independent t-tests or analysis of variance, while frequency distributions were evaluated by Pearson's chi-square ($\chi^2$) test. The Spearman correlation coefficient ($\varrho$) was calculated to estimate the correlation of EQVAS with total MNA and GDS scores.

The factors associated with nutritional status, depression, and HRQOL were assessed by three separate linear regression models, each adjusted for age and sex, using the total score of MNA, GDS, and EQVAS as the dependent variable, respectively. To account for nonnormally distributed outcome variables and a relatively small sample size, bootstrap models with 5000 replications were used for calculating stable estimates of correlates and their bias accelerated and corrected (BCa) 95% confidence intervals.

Two different mediating models were developed for the depression-nutrition-HRQOL triad (Fig. 1): the first uses total MNA score, or nutritional status, as the mediator (Fig. 1a) while the second uses total GDS score, or depression status, as the mediator (Fig. 1b). For moderation analyses (Fig. 2), an interaction between depression and nutritional score was added to a base regression model with depression and nutritional score as independent factors; EQVAS was used as the outcome. The PROCESS macro for SPSS was used for the mediation-moderation analyses. The mediation analyses were first run without any covariates (Model 1); then adjusted for age and sex (Model 2); then further adjusted for ethnicity, marital status, smoking, alcohol use, educational status, perception of negligence/hatred, and perceived health status compared to peers (Model 3). For all statistical tests, two-tailed $p$-values< 0.05 were considered statistically significant.

## Results
### Demographic profile of the participants

Detailed characteristics of the study participants can be found in Table 1. A total of 170 males and 119 females participated. The mean age of participants was 68.5 years, with a range from 60 to 90 years old. Most were Upper caste (46%) or Janjatis (46%), Hindu (76%), married (80%), illiterate (39%), and lived in a joint family (70.6%). The primary past occupation among males was farming (39%); among females it was household chores (48%). Many participants were reluctant to reveal their monthly family income; among respondents ($n = 167$), the mean monthly family income was $205. Only a small proportion (10%) were actively involved in earnings; over half of the participants were taken care by their son and daughter-in-law. The mean (±SD) BMI, EQVAS, MNA, and GDS scores of the participants were 24.9 ± 3.5, 65.2 ± 16.8, 10.9 ± 2.5, and 5.9 ± 3.8, respectively (Table 1).

### Prevalence and correlates of nutritional status

Appendix Table 5 provides the detailed characteristics of participants based on nutritional status categories as defined by MNA. The mean MNA score was 11.0 and ranged from 2 to 14. Only about half of the participants had adequate nutritional status; 10% were malnourished,

**Table 1** The subjects' characteristics according to sex

| | Total (n = 289) n (%) | Male (n = 170) n (%) | Female (n = 119) n (%) | p value |
|---|---|---|---|---|
| Age, (mean ± SD) | 68.5 ± 6.5 | 69.5 ± 6.6 | 67.1 ± 6.1 | **0.002**[a] |
| Gender | | | | |
| Male | 170 (58.8) | | | |
| Female | 119 (41.2) | | | |
| Ethnicity | | | | |
| Upper caste | 134 (46.4) | 84 (49.4) | 50 (42.0) | 0.429 |
| Janjatis | 134 (46.4) | 75 (44.1) | 59 (49.6) | |
| Dalit and minorities | 21 (7.3) | 11 (6.5) | 10 (8.4) | |
| Religion | | | | 0.656 |
| Hindu | 220 (76.1) | 131 (77.1) | 89 (74.8) | |
| Non-Hindu | 69 (23.9) | 39 (22.9) | 30 (25.2) | |
| Marital status | | | | 0.138 |
| Married | 231 (79.9) | 141 (82.9) | 90 (75.6) | |
| Separated/Widow/Single | 58 (20.1) | 29 (17.1) | 29 (24.4) | |
| Educational status | | | | **< 0.001** |
| Illiterate | 112 (38.8) | 46 (27.1) | 66 (55.5) | |
| Informal | 97 (33.6) | 66 (38.8) | 31 (26.1) | |
| Formal | 80 (27.7) | 58 (34.1) | 22 (18.5) | |
| Past Occupation | | | | **< 0.001** |
| Agriculture | 114 (39.4) | 73 (42.9) | 41 (34.5) | |
| Homemaker | 57 (19.7) | – | 57 (47.9) | |
| Business/job | 93 (32.2) | 75 (44.1) | 18 (15.1) | |
| Others | 25 (8.7) | 22 (12.9) | 3 (2.5) | |
| Monthly family income (n = 167), $, (mean ± SD) | 205.3 ± 90.1 | 206.8 ± 88.8 | 203.1 ± 92.7 | 0.799[a] |
| Family Structure | | | | **0.013** |
| Nuclear | 47 (16.3) | 21 (12.4) | 26 (21.8) | |
| Joint | 204 (70.6) | 120 (70.6) | 84 (70.6) | |
| Extended | 38 (13.1) | 29 (17.1) | 9 (7.6) | |
| Smoking | | | | 0.102 |
| Yes | 155 (53.6) | 98 (57.6) | 57 (47.9) | |
| No | 134 (46.4) | 72 (42.4) | 62 (52.1) | |
| Alcohol use | | | | 0.397 |
| Yes | 98 (33.9) | 61 (35.9) | 37 (31.1) | |
| No | 191 (66.1) | 109 (64.1) | 82 (68.9) | |
| Self-rated health status | | | | 0.380 |
| Better | 69 (23.9) | 40 (23.5) | 29 (24.4) | |
| Similar | 139 (48.1) | 87 (51.2) | 52 (43.7) | |
| Worse | 81 (28.0) | 43 (25.3) | 38 (31.9) | |
| Adequate rest | | | | **0.042** |
| Yes | 81 (28.0) | 40 (23.5) | 41 (34.5) | |
| No | 208 (72.0) | 130 (76.5) | 78 (65.5) | |

**Table 1** The subjects' characteristics according to sex *(Continued)*

|  | Total (n = 289) n (%) | Male (n = 170) n (%) | Female (n = 119) n (%) | p value |
|---|---|---|---|---|
| Working currently |  |  |  | **0.012** |
| Yes | 27 (9.3) | 22 (12.9) | 5 (4.2) |  |
| No | 262 (90.7) | 148 (87.1) | 114 (95.8) |  |
| Caretaker |  |  |  | **0.004** |
| Son and daughter in law | 153 (52.9) | 78 (45.9) | 75 (63.0) |  |
| Others | 136 (47.1) | 92 (54.1) | 44 (37.0) |  |
| Ignored/hated for being old |  |  |  | **0.005** |
| Yes | 45 (15.6) | 18 (10.6) | 27 (22.7) |  |
| No | 244 (84.4) | 152 (89.4) | 92 (77.3) |  |
| BMI, kg/m$^2$, (mean ± SD) | 24.9 ± 3.5 | 24.8 ± 3.5 | 24.9 ± 3.7 | 0.837[a] |
| MNA score, (mean ± SD) | 10.9 ± 2.5 | 11.2 ± 2.5 | 10.7 ± 2.5 | 0.099[a] |
| GDS Score, (mean ± SD) | 5.9 ± 3.8 | 5.9 ± 3.9 | 5.8 ± 3.7 | 0.827[a] |
| EQVAS, (mean ± SD) | 65.2 ± 16.8 | 66.4 ± 17.3 | 63.6 ± 16.1 | 0.179[a] |

[a]*p*-value from independent t-test test; all others are chi-square. 1$ = 100 Nepalese rupees

Abbreviation: *SD* standard deviation, *BMI* body mass index, *MNA* mini nutritional assessment short form cumulative score, *GDS* Geriatric depression scale short form cumulative score, *EQVAS* European quality of life visual analytical scale

and 38% were at risk of malnutrition. Comorbidity between depression and malnutrition was prevalent among 6.9% of the participants (Appendix Table 5). In the regression analysis adjusted for age and sex (Table 2), age (β = – 0.07; BCa 95%CI = – 0.12, – 0.01), male gender (β = – 0.65; BCa 95%CI = – 1.25, – 0.07), depression score (β = – 0.18; BCa 95%CI = – 0.26, – 0.10), perception of worsened health (β = – 1.04; BCa 95%CI = – 1.73, – 0.33) and perception of ignorance/hatred due to old age (β = – 1.92; BCa 95%CI = – 2.73, – 1.09) were inversely associated with the nutritional score from the MNA. Likewise, having formal education (β = 0.81; BCa 95%CI = 0.18, 1.47) as well as higher quality of life scores on both the EQ-5D index (β = 2.98; BCa 95%CI = 1.51, 4.30) and the EQVAS (β = 0.06; BCa 95%CI = 0.05, 0.08) were associated with a higher nutritional score on the MNA.

### Prevalence and correlates of depression

Appendix Table 6 provides the detailed characteristics of participants based on depression status as defined by GDS. More than half (57%) of the participants met the criteria of depression (GDS score ≥ 5). In the regression analysis adjusted for age and sex (Table 2), higher age (β = 0.10; BCa 95%CI = 0.03, 0.17), perception of worsened health (β = 1.68; BCa 95%CI = 0.74, 2.60) and perception of ignorance/hatred due to old age (β = 1.58; BCa 95%CI = 0.32, 2.82) were associated with a higher depression score. Compared to illiterate individuals, those having an informal education (β = 1.06; BCa 95%CI = 0.16, 1.96) scored higher on the depression scale whereas those having a formal education (β = – 1.43; BCa 95%CI = – 2.43, – 0.40) scored lower. A higher depression score

on the GDS was associated with a lower score on the nutrition scale (β = – 0.41; BCa 95%CI = – 0.59, – 0.23) and lower quality of life scores: EQ-5D index (β = – 2.49; BCa 95%CI = – 4.61, – 0.48) and EQVAS (β = – 0.06; BCa 95%CI = – 0.09, – 0.03).

### Health-related quality of life and its correlates

The responses of participants in the five dimensions of EQ-5D are provided in Appendix Table 7. The mean EQVAS score and the EQ-5D index were 65.2 and 0.8 respectively; scores were significantly lower among participants meeting the criteria for malnutrition or depression. Thirty-six different health statuses were represented in the EQ-5D (Appendix Table 7).

EQVAS scores were positively correlated with MNA scores (ϱ = 0.44, *p* < 0.001) and negatively correlated with GDS scores (ϱ = – 0.28, *p* < 0.001). In the regression analysis adjusted for age and sex using EQVAS as the outcome (Table 2), a positive association was observed between the EQVAS QOL score and being married (β = 6.57; BCa 95%CI = 1.75, 11.37), having a formal education (β = 5.54; BCa 95%CI = 0.92, 9.99), working currently (β = 11.60; BCa 95%CI = 4.57, 18.07), better perceived health status (β = 11.06; BCa 95%CI = 7.34, 15.03), and higher MNA score (β = 2.87; BCa 95%CI = 2.12, 3.62). Likewise, an inverse association was observed between the EQVAS QOL score and perception of worsen health status (β = – 18.20; BCa 95%CI = – 22.34, – 13.94), perception of being ignored/hated for old age (β = – 8.63; BCa 95%CI = – 13.61, – 3.80), and the depression score (β = – 1.23; BCa 95%CI = – 1.72, – 0.72).

**Table 2** Factors associated with nutritional status, depression, and health-related quality of life

| | MNA | | GDS | | EQVAS | |
|---|---|---|---|---|---|---|
| | β | BCa 95% CI | β | BCa 95% CI | β | BCa 95% CI |
| Age | **−0.07** | **− 0.12, − 0.01** | **0.10** | **0.03, 0.17** | − 0.20 | − 0.54, 0.11 |
| Gender (Reference = Male) | **− 0.65** | **−1.25, − 0.07** | 0.14 | − 0.74, 1.03 | −3.18 | −7.35, 0.82 |
| Ethnicity (Reference = Upper caste) | | | | | | |
| Janjatis | − 0.02 | − 0.60, 0.56 | 0.39 | − 0.46, 1.24 | 0.03 | − 3.82, 3.87 |
| Dalit and minorities | − 0.78 | − 1.97, 0.41 | 1.55 | − 0.10, 3.19 | −2.37 | − 10.67, 5.37 |
| Marital status (Reference = Separated/Widow/single) | 0.48 | − 0.24, 1.18 | −0.48 | − 1.61, 0.62 | **6.57** | **1.75, 11.37** |
| Education (Reference = Illiterate) | | | | | | |
| Informal | 0.50 | −0.09, 1.07 | **1.06** | **0.16, 1.96** | −0.37 | −4.48, 3.61 |
| Formal | **0.81** | **0.18, 1.47** | **−1.43** | **−2.43, −0.40** | **5.54** | **0.92, 9.99** |
| Smoking (Reference = No) | 0.10 | −0.47, 0.65 | −0.08 | − 0.97, 0.76 | −2.29 | −6.20, 1.49 |
| Alcohol use (Reference = No) | −0.06 | − 0.63, 0.48 | −0.04 | − 0.95, 0.89 | 0.39 | −3.64, 4.27 |
| Adequate rest everyday (Reference = No) | 0.17 | −0.56, 0.88 | −0.28 | −1.27, 0.71 | 0.01 | −4.92, 4.89 |
| Family type (Reference = Joint) | | | | | | |
| Nuclear | −0.31 | −1.16, 0.51 | 0.52 | −0.68, 1.73 | −4.89 | −10.24, 0.45 |
| Extended | 0.19 | −0.63, 0.94 | 0.94 | −0.30, 2.20 | −3.01 | −8.97, 2.50 |
| Currently working (Reference = No) | 0.75 | −0.35, 1.77 | −0.90 | −2.32, 0.62 | **11.60** | **4.57, 18.07** |
| Care taker (Reference = Son) | 0.36 | −0.25, 0.96 | −0.38 | −1.27, 0.51 | 0.18 | −3.68, 4.08 |
| Self-perceived health status (Reference = Similar) | | | | | | |
| Better | 0.21 | −0.48, 0.88 | −0.37 | −1.39, 0.70 | **11.06** | **7.34, 15.03** |
| Worse | **−1.04** | **−1.73, −0.33** | **1.68** | **0.74, 2.60** | **−18.20** | **−22.34, − 13.94** |
| Ignored/hated for being old (Reference = No) | **− 1.92** | **−2.73, − 1.09** | **1.58** | **0.32, 2.82** | **−8.63** | **−13.61, −3.80** |
| MNA | – | | **−0.41** | **−0.59, −0.23** | **2.87** | **2.12, 3.62** |
| GDS | **−0.18** | **−0.26, − 0.10** | – | | **−1.23** | **− 1.72, − 0.72** |
| EQ-5D Index | **2.98** | **1.51, 4.30** | **−2.49** | **−4.61, − 0.48** | **33.86** | **25.41, 42.61** |
| EQVAS | **0.06** | **0.05, 0.08** | **−0.06** | **−0.09, − 0.03** | – | |

β: Unstandardized coefficient; BCa: Bias-corrected and accelerated
Adjusted for age and sex
Number of bootstrap samples for bias-corrected bootstrap confidence intervals: 5000
Statistically significant associations are highlighted in bold
Abbreviation: *MNA* mini nutritional assessment short form cumulative score, *GDS* Geriatric depression scale short form cumulative score, *EQVAS* European quality of life visual analytical scale

## Mediation-moderation analysis

### Nutrition as a mediator of the depression – health-related quality of life association

Table 3 and Fig. 1a present the findings from mediation analysis, exploring the depression-nutrition-HRQOL pathway using the MNA score as the mediator. In the unadjusted analysis, the ratio of depression's indirect effect to the total effect through nutrition was 40%. In the final adjusted model (Model 3), nutritional score mediated 41% of the total effect of depression on HRQOL (Table 3).

### Depression as a mediator of the nutrition – health-related quality of life association

Table 4 and Fig. 1b present the findings from the mediation analysis exploring the nutrition- depression-HRQOL

pathway with depression as the mediator. In the unadjusted analysis, depression score mediated 11% of the total effect of nutritional score on HRQOL; this dropped to 6.0% in the final adjusted model (Model 3).

**Moderation analyses** In an unadjusted moderation analysis (Fig. 2), the interaction between MNA and GDS (β = 0.05; BCa 95%CI = − 0.16, 0.26) was not significantly associated with HRQOL.

## Discussion

In this study, we assessed the nutrition status, depression status, and HRQOL of Nepalese community-dwelling older patients in urban Kathmandu. We also explored the differential effects of nutrition, depression, and HRQOL by mediation and moderation analyses. A sizeable

**Table 3** Mediation analysis for the association between depression and health-related quality of life, mediated by nutrition

| | Model 1 | | Model 2 | | Model 3 | |
|---|---|---|---|---|---|---|
| | β | BCa 95% CI | β | BCa 95% CI | β | BCa 95% CI |
| Total effect, c | −1.25 (0.25) | −1.75, − 0.75 | −1.23 (0.26) | − 1.74, − 0.72 | −0.74 (0.24) | −1.20, − 0.28 |
| Direct effect, c' | −0.74 (0.25) | −1.23, − 0.26 | −0.76 (0.25) | −1.25, − 0.28 | −0.44 (0.23) | − 0.88, 0.01 |
| Indirect effect, ab | −0.50 (0.14) | − 0.83, − 0.27 | −0.47 (0.14) | − 0.77, − 0.24 | −0.31 (0.11) | − 0.56, − 0.12 |
| Ratio of indirect to total effect mediated | 0.40 | | 0.38 | | 0.41 | |
| Ratio of indirect to direct effect | 0.68 | | 0.61 | | 0.70 | |

Model 1: Unadjusted mediational model
Model 2: Adjusted for age, and sex
Model 3: Adjusted for age, sex, ethnicity, marital status, smoking, alcohol use, educational status, perception of negligence/hatred, perceived health status compared to others
Number of bootstrap samples for bias-corrected bootstrap confidence intervals: 5000
β: Unstandardized coefficient; BCa: Bias-corrected and accelerated

proportion of our study population had prevalent malnutrition and depression.

In the current study, nutritional and depression were inversely related to each other; many malnourished individuals were depressed and vice versa. Although studies quantifying the relationship between nutrition and depression in older adults in Nepal are lacking, studies from Iran [4, 12], Norway [25], and Brazil [26] support our findings. The link between poor nutrition and depression is biologically plausible [27, 28]: multiple pathways such as inflammation, oxidative and nitrosative stress, as well as a decrease in antioxidant levels [27, 28] support the underlying role of several nutrients in explaining the mechanism of depression.

Our mediation analyses suggested that in the depression-nutrition-HRQOL triad, both nutrition and depression partially mediate each others association with HRQOL; however, nutritional status mediated a greater proportion of the total effect on HRQOL in comparison to depression. Not only did poor nutritional status have a significant direct effect on HRQOL, but it also partially explained the relationship between depression and HRQOL. Patients with depression are more likely to exhibit loss of appetite, decreased food intake, meal skipping, and

disordered eating; which can lead to poor nutritional outcomes and vice-versa [29]. Likewise, in previous studies, nutritional risk was found to be a significant factor associated with HRQOL [4, 30]; nutritional well-being can influence HRQOL by affecting functional ability, muscle mass, and formation and transportation of proteins and hormones [31]. In previous studies, depressive symptoms and impaired nutritional status were independently associated with lower HRQOL scores among the older adults [4, 5]. Our previous study, NepEldQOL II [14], also suggested a potential mediating role of depression in the relationship between nutrition and life-satisfaction. The current study provided preliminary evidence to support the role of nutritional status in maintaining optimal HRQOL among the older patients. Public health interventions for optimizing HRQOL should consider screening for depression and nutritional status simultaneously. Prospective studies, including those that consider healthy adults at baseline, will be needed to confirm these preliminary findings.

A sizeable proportion of study participants had prevalent malnutrition and depression; findings were not unexpected. Older adults are more vulnerable to

**Table 4** Mediation analysis for the association between nutrition and health-related quality of life, mediated by depression

| | Model 1 | | Model 2 | | Model 3 | |
|---|---|---|---|---|---|---|
| | β | BCa 95% CI | β | BCa 95% CI | β | BCa 95% CI |
| Total effect, c | 2.90 (0.35) | 2.20, 3.60 | 2.87 (0.36) | 2.16, 3.58 | 2.29 (0.34) | 1.62, 2.97 |
| Direct effect, c' | 2.58 (0.37) | 1.86, 3.30 | 2.56 (0.37) | 1.83, 3.29 | 2.14 (0.35) | 1.45, 2.84 |
| Indirect effect, ab | 0.32 (0.13) | 0.12, 0.62 | 0.31 (0.12) | 0.12, 0.60 | 0.15 (0.09) | 0.02, 0.38 |
| Ratio of indirect to total effect mediated, (ab/c) | 0.11 | | 0.11 | | 0.06 | |
| Ratio of indirect to direct effect, (ab/c') | 0.13 | | 0.12 | | 0.07 | |

Model 1: unadjusted mediational model
Model 2: Adjusted for age, and sex
Model 3: Adjusted for age, sex, ethnicity, marital status, smoking, alcohol use, educational status, perception of negligence/hatred, perceived health status compared to peers
Number of bootstrap samples for bias-corrected bootstrap confidence intervals: 5000
β: Unstandardized coefficient; BCa: Bias-corrected and accelerated

malnutrition due to age-associated changes in metabolism and/or physiological function which may cause anorexia, loss of appetite, deficits in taste and shifts in dietary choices and eating habits [32]. A previous study from rural Nepal found higher prevalence, (24% compared to our 10%) of malnutrition than this current study [6]. We had expected that the older populations in urban Nepal would have better nutritional status because households in rural areas are more likely to be food deficient [33] with higher overall poverty rates [34]. Additionally, older age, female gender, low literacy and lower family income were also associated with poor nutritional status, findings consistent with a previous study [6]. Moreover, the prevalence of depression found in our study, over 50%, is consistent with a previous hospital-based study from Kathmandu, Nepal where depression, as defined by GDS, was found among 53.2% of the older patients [8].

The mean EQVAS score and the EQ-5D index were 65.2 and 0.8 respectively. Scores were significantly lower among participants meeting the criteria for malnutrition or depression. These findings were expected among older adults given that age is the strongest predictor of HRQOL [4, 5]. Aging is characterized by a gradual and lifelong accumulation of molecular and cellular damage that subsequently leads to a decrease in physiological functions, increased vulnerability to diseases, and a general decline in the capacity of the individual [35, 36]. Furthermore, the impact of depression and poor nutrition may aggravate HRQOL among the older adults who are already susceptible to poor QOL due to their senescence.

### Strengths, limitations, and future research directions

We present a pioneer study that quantifies the HRQOL among urban Nepali older patients, filling gaps and advancing knowledge about the prevalence of and factors contributing to depression and malnutrition among Nepali older patients. Moreover, we explore the relationship between depression, nutritional status, and HRQOL, three important aspects of aging, in the Nepalese context. To our knowledge, the mediation and moderation effects of depression and nutrition with the outcome of HRQOL among the older adults have not been previously explored in any context. HRQOL, looking at health from an individual's perspective, is truly multi-faceted as seen in this study. Simple measures to detect and treat depression among the older adults to improve their overall HRQOL should also examine nutritional wellbeing. Further prospective studies are needed to identify the direction of the relationship between depression and nutrition.

Nonetheless, this study is subject to some limitations, including a relatively small sample size. Due to our cross-sectional study design, no inferences can be made regarding the causal relationships between nutritional status, depression, and HRQOL. Future studies should determine if nutritional risk is associated with QOL over time among older adults. This study recruited participants from outpatient clinics in an urban setting; the nutritional status, depression, and HRQOL of the general population in an urban area and/or those in a rural setting may be different, thus limiting the generalizability of our findings. Exclusion of older patients who were too frail physically or mentally to respond may have resulted in a selection bias that underestimated or biased our findings towards the null. In the current study, the internal consistency of GDS and EQ-5D was high but that of the MNA scale was relatively low (Cronbach's $\alpha = 0.59$); omission of any MNA component score did not substantially increase the alpha value (data not shown). Given that the MNA has already been validated in various settings [37] as well as among Nepali older adults [6], we nonetheless believe it to be a valid tool to assess nutritional status among the older adults. The use of UK's general population weights as reference values in the calculation of the EQ-5D index is not ideal; however, no such reference weights exist for Nepal and the same technique was used in the original study validating the Nepali version of EQ-5D [22] as well as another study from Nepal [38]. We defined adequate rest as sleeping for more than six hours daily; however, the National Sleep Foundation recommends 7–8 h of sleep for older adults [39]; thus we may have overestimated the prevalence of adequate rest. Moreover, sleep hours were self-reported. Increasing age is associated with multi-morbidity that may limit functional capacity and reduce the HRQOL [40]; presence of comorbidities were not assessed in this study. Future studies should look at the possible mediating and bi-directional relationship of multiple morbidities, nutritional status and HRQOL. Lastly, the possibility of residual confounding due to unmeasured covariates cannot be ruled out.

### Conclusions

Both malnutrition and depression were associated with HRQOL among our study population. Given that nutritional status had a significant direct and indirect (as a mediator) effect on HRQOL, we believe that nutritional screening and optimal nutrition among older patients can make a significant contribution to the overall HRQOL for older patients in Nepal. The depression management protocol should account for nutritional wellbeing as well as overall HRQOL in this population. Although we are cautious to make any causal interpretation of the findings, our study lends support to the role of optimal nutritional status and mental health in maintaining the overall health and well-being of older patients in Nepal.

# Appendix

**Table 5** Participant's characteristics by nutritional status

| | Malnourished, n (%) | At risk of malnutrition, n (%) | Normal nutritional status, n (%) | p-value |
|---|---|---|---|---|
| Total (Prevalence) | **30 (10.4)** | **109 (37.7)** | **150 (51.9)** | |
| 95% CI for prevalence | 6.9–13.9 | 32.3–43.4 | 46.2–57.6 | |
| Age, years, (mean ± SD) | 69.6 ± 7.4 | 69.6 ± 7.1 | 67.5 ± 5.6 | **0.021**[a] |
| Gender | | | | **0.028** |
| Male | 17 (10.0) | 54 (31.8) | 99 (58.2) | |
| Female | 13 (10.9) | 55 (46.2) | 51 (42.9) | |
| Ethnicity | | | | 0.157 |
| Upper caste | 13 (9.7) | 43 (32.1) | 78 (58.2) | |
| Janjatis | 13 (9.7) | 56 (41.8) | 65 (48.5) | |
| Dalit and minorities | 4 (19.0) | 10 (47.6) | 7 (33.3) | |
| Religion | | | | 0.270 |
| Hindu | 22 (10.0) | 78 (35.5) | 120 (54.5) | |
| Non-Hindu | 8 (11.6) | 31 (44.9) | 30 (43.5) | |
| Marital status | | | | **0.003** |
| Married | 26 (11.3) | 76 (32.9) | 129 (55.8) | |
| Separated/Widow/Single | 4 (6.9) | 33 (56.9) | 21 (36.2) | |
| Educational status | | | | **< 0.001** |
| Illiterate | 19 (17.0) | 55 (49.1) | 38 (33.9) | |
| Informal | 8 (8.2) | 33 (34.0) | 56 (57.7) | |
| Formal | 3 (3.8) | 21 (26.2) | 56 (70.0) | |
| Past Occupation | | | | **0.008** |
| Agriculture | 15 (13.2) | 56 (49.1) | 43 (37.7) | |
| Homemaker | 4 (7.0) | 21 (36.8) | 32 (56.1) | |
| Business/job | 8 (8.6) | 24 (25.8) | 61 (65.6) | |
| Others | 3 (12.0) | 8 (32.0) | 14 (56.0) | |
| Monthly family income (n = 167), $, (mean ± SD) | 164.4 ± 81.3 | 185.8 ± 92.0 | 222.6 ± 87.0 | **0.007**[a] |
| Family Structure | | | | 0.659 |
| Nuclear | 7 (14.9) | 18 (38.3) | 22 (46.8) | |
| Joint | 18 (8.8) | 79 (38.7) | 107 (52.5) | |
| Extended | 5 (13.2) | 12 (31.6) | 21 (55.3) | |
| Smoking | | | | 0.606 |
| Yes | 14 (9.0) | 57 (36.8) | 84 (54.2) | |
| No | 16 (11.9) | 52 (38.8) | 66 (49.3) | |
| Drinker | | | | 0.432 |
| Yes | 7 (7.1) | 38 (38.8) | 53 (54.1) | |
| No | 23 (12.0) | 71 (37.2) | 97 (50.8) | |
| Self-rated health status | | | | **0.014** |
| Better | 7 (10.1) | 28 (40.6) | 34 (49.3) | |
| Similar | 8 (5.8) | 48 (34.5) | 83 (59.7) | |
| Worse | 15 (18.5) | 33 (40.7) | 33 (40.7) | |
| Adequate rest | | | | 0.727 |
| Yes | 9 (11.1) | 33 (40.7) | 39 (48.1) | |
| No | 21 (10.1) | 76 (36.5) | 111 (53.4) | |

**Table 5** Participant's characteristics by nutritional status *(Continued)*

| | Malnourished, n (%) | At risk of malnutrition, n (%) | Normal nutritional status, n (%) | p-value |
|---|---|---|---|---|
| Working currently | | | | 0.047 |
| Yes | 1 (3.7) | 6 (22.2) | 20 (74.1) | |
| No | 29 (11.1) | 103 (39.3) | 130 (49.6) | |
| Care taker | | | | 0.168 |
| Son and daughter in law | 20 (13.1) | 60 (39.2) | 73 (47.7) | |
| Others | 10 (7.4) | 49 (36.0) | 77 (56.6) | |
| Ignored/hated for being old | | | | **< 0.001** |
| Yes | 13 (28.9) | 20 (44.4) | 12 (26.7) | |
| No | 17 (7.0) | 89 (36.5) | 138 (56.6) | |
| Depression | | | | **< 0.001** |
| Yes | 20 (12.0) | 78 (47.0) | 68 (41.0) | |
| No | 10 (8.1) | 31 (25.2) | 82 (66.7) | |
| BMI, kg/m$^2$, (mean ± SD) | 22.1 ± 3.1 | 24.2 ± 3.8 | 25.9 ± 3.0 | **< 0.001**[a] |
| MNA, (mean ± SD) | 5.7 ± 1.2 | 9.7 ± 1.2 | 12.9 ± 0.8 | **< 0.001**[a] |
| GDS Score, (mean ± SD) | 7.8 ± 4.0 | 6.8 ± 3.6 | 4.8 ± 3.5 | **< 0.001**[a] |
| EQVAS, (mean ± SD) | 49.7 ± 16.3 | 62.5 ± 16.6 | 70.4 ± 14.7 | **< 0.001**[a] |

Statistically significant p-value are highlighted in bold

[a]p-value from analysis of variance; all others are from Pearson's chi-square test

Abbreviation: *SD* standard deviation, *BMI* body mass index, *MNASF* mini nutritional assessment short form cumulative score, *GDS* Geriatric Depression scale short form cumulative score, *EQVAS* European quality of life visual analytical scale

**Table 6** Participant's characteristics by depression status

| | Depression, n (%) | No Depression, n (%) | p value |
|---|---|---|---|
| Total (Prevalence) | 166 (57.4) | 123 (42.6) | |
| 95% CI for prevalence | 51.7–63.0 | 37.0–48.3 | |
| Age, years, (mean ± SD) | 69.3 ± 6.6 | 67.5 ± 6.3 | **0.020**[a] |
| Gender | | | 0.876 |
|   Male | 97 (57.1) | 73 (42.9) | |
|   Female | 69 (58.0) | 50 (42.0) | |
| Ethnicity | | | **0.045** |
|   Upper caste | 67 (50.0) | 67 (50.0) | |
|   Janjatis | 84 (62.7) | 50 (37.3) | |
|   Dalit and minorities | 15 (71.4) | 6 (28.6) | |
| Religion | | | 0.134 |
|   Hindu | 121 (55.0) | 99 (45.0) | |
|   Non-Hindu | 45 (65.2) | 24 (34.8) | |
| Marital status | | | 0.091 |
|   Married | 39 (67.2) | 19 (32.8) | |
|   Separated/Widow/Single | 127 (55.0) | 104 (45.0) | |
| Educational status | | | **0.007** |
|   Illiterate | 66 (58.9) | 46 (41.1) | |
|   Informal | 65 (67.0) | 32 (33.0) | |
|   Formal | 35 (43.8) | 45 (56.3) | |
| Past Occupation | | | 0.202 |
|   Agriculture | 72 (63.2) | 42 (36.8) | |
|   Homemaker | 35 (61.4) | 22 (38.6) | |
|   Business/job | 47 (50.5) | 46 (49.5) | |
|   Others | 12 (48.0) | 13 (52.0) | |
| Monthly family income (n = 167), $, (mean ± SD) | 185.8 ± 72.2 | 228.7 ± 103.4 | **0.003**[a] |
| Family Structure | | | 0.268 |
|   Nuclear | 30 (63.8) | 17 (36.2) | |
|   Joint | 111 (54.4) | 93 (45.6) | |
|   Extended | 25 (65.8) | 13 (34.2) | |
| Smoking | | | 0.639 |
|   No | 75 (56.0) | 59 (44.0) | |
|   Yes | 91 (58.7) | 64 (41.3) | |
| Drinker | | | 0.942 |
|   No | 110 (57.6) | 81 (42.4) | |
|   Yes | 56 (57.1) | 42 (42.9) | |
| Self-rated health status | | | **0.025** |
|   Better | 33 (47.8) | 36 (52.2) | |
|   Similar | 77 (55.4) | 62 (44.6) | |
|   Worse | 56 (69.1) | 25 (30.9) | |
| Adequate rest | | | 0.900 |
|   Yes | 47 (58.0) | 34 (42.0) | |
|   No | 119 (57.2) | 89 (42.8) | |

**Table 6** Participant's characteristics by depression status *(Continued)*

| | Depression, n (%) | No Depression, n (%) | p value |
|---|---|---|---|
| Working currently | | | **0.024** |
| Yes | 10 (37.0) | 17 (63.0) | |
| No | 156 (59.5) | 106 (40.5) | |
| Care taker | | | 0.223 |
| Son and daughter in law | 93 (60.8) | 60 (39.2) | |
| Others | 73 (53.7) | 63 (46.3) | |
| Ignored/hated for being old | | | **0.019** |
| Yes | 33 (73.3) | 12 (26.7) | |
| No | 133 (54.5) | 111 (45.5) | |
| Nutritional status | | | **< 0.001** |
| Malnourished | 20 (66.7) | 10 (33.3) | |
| At risk of malnutrition | 78 (71.6) | 31 (28.4) | |
| Normal nutritional status | 68 (45.3) | 82 (54.7) | |
| BMI, kg/m$^2$, (mean ± SD) | 24.9 ± 3.5 | 24.9 ± 3.6 | 0.957[a] |
| QOL EQVAS, (mean ± SD) | 61.8 ± 16.4 | 69.9 ± 16.4 | **< 0.001**[a] |
| MNASF, (mean ± SD) | 10.5 ± 2.6 | 11.5 ± 2.3 | **0.001**[a] |
| GDS Score, (mean ± SD) | 8.5 ± 2.6 | 2.3 ± 1.3 | **< 0.001**[a] |

Statistically significant p-value are highlighted in bold
[a]p-value from independent t-test; all others are from Pearson's chi-square test
Abbreviation: *SD* standard deviation, *BMI* body mass index, *MNASF* mini nutritional assessment short form cumulative score, *GDS* Geriatric Depression scale short form cumulative score, *EQVAS* European quality of life visual analytical scale

**Table 7** Participants health related quality of life by nutritional and depression status

| | Total | Malnourished | At risk of malnutrition | Normal nutritional status | p-value | Depression | No Depression | p-value |
|---|---|---|---|---|---|---|---|---|
| | n (%) | n (%) | n (%) | n (%) | | n (%) | n (%) | |
| Mobility | | | | | **0.001** | | | **0.003** |
| No Problem | 214 (74.0) | 16 (53.3) | 74 (67.9) | 124 (82.7) | | 112 (67.5) | 102 (82.9) | |
| Some Problem | 75 (26.0) | 14 (46.7) | 35 (32.1) | 26 (17.3) | | 54 (32.5) | 21 (17.1) | |
| Self-Care | | | | | **< 0.001** | | | **0.002** |
| No Problem | 238 (82.4) | 18 (60.0) | 81 (74.3) | 139 (92.7) | | 127 (76.5) | 111 (90.2) | |
| Some Problem | 51 (17.6) | 12 (40.0) | 28 (25.7) | 11 (7.3) | | 39 (23.5) | 12 (9.8) | |
| Usual Activities | | | | | **< 0.001** | | | 0.059 |
| No Problem | 217 (75.1) | 14 (46.7) | 73 (67.0) | 130 (86.7) | | 116 (69.9) | 101 (82.1) | |
| Some Problem | 56 (19.4) | 11 (36.7) | 28 (25.7) | 17 (11.3) | | 39 (23.5) | 17 (13.8) | |
| Unable | 16 (5.5) | 5 (16.7) | 8 (7.3) | 3 (2.0) | | 11 (6.6) | 5 (4.1) | |
| Pain/Discomfort | | | | | **< 0.001** | | | 0.110 |
| No pain | 163 (56.4) | 13 (43.3) | 51 (46.8) | 99 (66.0) | | 85 (51.2) | 78 (63.4) | |
| moderate pain | 111 (38.4) | 10 (33.3) | 56 (51.4) | 45 (30.0) | | 72 (43.4) | 39 (31.7) | |
| extreme pain | 15 (5.2) | 7 (23.3) | 2 (1.8) | 6 (4.0) | | 9 (5.4) | 6 (4.9) | |
| Anxiety | | | | | **< 0.001** | | | 0.160 |
| None | 172 (59.5) | 12 (40.0) | 55 (50.5) | 105 (70.0) | | 93 (56.0) | 79 (64.2) | |
| Moderate | 117 (40.5) | 18 (60.0) | 54 (49.5) | 45 (30.0) | | 73 (44.0) | 44 (35.8) | |
| EQVAS, (mean ± SD) | 65.2 ± 16.8 | 49.7 ± 16.3 | 62.5 ± 16.6 | 70.4 ± 14.7 | **< 0.001**[a] | 61.8 ± 16.4 | 69.9 ± 16.4 | **< 0.001**[b] |
| EQ-5D Index, (mean ± SD) | 0.8 ± 0.2 | 0.6 ± 0.4 | 0.7 ± 0.2 | 0.8 ± 0.2 | **< 0.001**[a] | 0.7 ± 0.3 | 0.8 ± 0.2 | **0.019**[b] |
| No of health status in EQ5D | 36 | 16 | 26 | 22 | | 30 | 20 | – |
| Complete health status (11111) | 88 (30.4) | 7 (23.3) | 23 (21.1) | 58 (38.7) | | 44 (26.5) | 44 (35.8) | – |

Statistically significant p-value are highlighted in bold
[a]p-value from analysis of variance; [b]p-value from independent t-test; all others are from Pearson's chi-square test
Abbreviation: *SD* standard deviation, *EQVAS* European quality of life visual analytical scale, *EQ-5D* European Quality of Life five dimension

### Abbreviations
BCa: Bias Accelerated and Corrected; BMI: Body Mass Index; CI: Confidence Intervals; EQ-5D: European Quality of Life Tool; EQVAS: European Quality of Life Visual Analytic Scale; GDS: Short Form of Geriatric Depression Scale; HRQOL: Health-Related Quality of Life; MNA: Short Form of Mini Nutritional Assessment; NMCTH: Nepal Medical College and Teaching Hospital; OPD: Outpatient Department; QOL: Quality of Life; SD: Standard Deviation

### Authors' contributions
Conceived and designed the study: SG and BKB. Tool translation to Nepali: BRP, and AA. Facilitated data collection in the field: BKB, BRP, AP, AA, DA, and PA. Analyzed the data: SG and SRM. Drafted the manuscript: SG, BKB and SRM. Critical revision of the manuscript: SG, BKB, BRP, AP, AA, DA, PA and SRM. Approval of the final version of the manuscript: SG, BKB, BRP, AP, AA, DA, PA and SRM.

### Acknowledgements
We would like to thank the participants, without whom this study would not have been possible. We would also like to appreciate the efforts of Prescott Cheong and Karen Callahan, School of Community Health Sciences, University of Nevada, Las Vegas, in proof reading our work.

### Competing interests
The authors declare that they have no competing interests.

## Author details

[1]Agrata Health and Education (AHEAD)-Nepal, Kathmandu, Nepal.
[2]Department of Biochemistry, Nepal Medical College and Teaching Hospital, Kathmandu, Nepal. [3]Department of Nutrition and Dietetics, College of Applied Food and Dairy Technology, Purbanchal University, Kathmandu, Nepal. [4]Nepal Development Society, Bharatpur-10, Nepal.

## References

1. Central Bureau of Statistics. Nepal - National Population Census 2001, Tenth census. Kathmandu: National Planning Commission Secretariat, Government of Nepal; 2001.

2. Central Bureau of Statistics. National Population and Housing Census 2011 (National Report). Kathmandu: National Planning Commission Secretariat, Government of Nepal, National Planning Commission Secretariat; 2012.

3. Geriatric Center Nepal. Status Report on Elderly People (60+) in Nepal on Health, Nutrition and Social Status Focusing on Research Needs. Kathmandu: Geriatric Center Nepal and Ministry of Health and Population, Government of Nepal; 2010. Available at: http://ageingnepal.org/wp-content/uploads/2015/05/Status-of-older-people-Nepal.pdf.

4. Keshavarzi S, Ahmadi SM, Lankarani KB. The impact of depression and malnutrition on health-related quality of life among the elderly Iranians. Glob J Health Sci. 2014;7(3):161–70.

5. Shmuely Y, Baumgarten M, Rovner B, Berlin J. Predictors of improvement in health-related quality of life among elderly patients with depression. Int Psychogeriatr. 2001;13(1):63–73.

6. Ghimire S, Baral BK, Callahan K. Nutritional assessment of community-dwelling older adults in rural Nepal. PLoS One. 2017;12(2):e0172052.

7. Ranjan S, Bhattarai A, Dutta M. Prevalence of depression among elderly people living in old age home in the capital city Kathmandu. Health Renaissance. 2014;11(3):213–8.

8. Khattri JB, Nepal MK. Study of depression among geriatric population in Nepal. Nepal Med Coll J. 2006;8(4):220–3.

9. Charles ST, Carstensen LL. Social and emotional aging. Charles S, Carstensen LL. Social and emotional aging. Annu Rev Psychol. 2010;61:383–409.

10. U.S. Department of Health and Human Services. Healthy People 2010. 2nd ed. With Understanding and Improving Health and Objectives for Improving Health. 2 vols. Washington, DC: U.S. Government Printing Office; 2000. Available at: http://www.healthequityks.org/download/Hlthy_People_2010_Improving_Health.pdf.

11. Dev MK, Paudel N, Joshi ND, Shah DN, Subba S. Psycho-social impact of visual impairment on health-related quality of life among nursing home residents. BMC Health Serv Res. 2014;14:345.

12. Ahmadi SM, Mohammadi MR, Mostafavi SA, Keshavarzi S, Kooshesh SM, Joulaei H, et al. Dependence of the geriatric depression on nutritional status and anthropometric indices in elderly population. Iran J Psychiatry. 2013;8(2):92–6.

13. Bhat RS, Chiu E, Jeste DV. Nutrition and geriatric psychiatry: a neglected field. Curr Opin Psychiatry. 2005;18(6):609–14.

14. Ghimire S, Baral BK, Karmacharya I, Callahan K, Mishra SR. Life satisfaction among elderly patients in Nepal: associations with nutritional and mental well-being. Health Qual Life Outcomes. 2018;16(1):118.

15. World Health Organization. Management of substance abuse Research Tools: Process of translation and adaptation of instruments Geneva; 2016. Available from: http://www.who.int/substance_abuse/research_tools/translation/en/.

16. Kaiser MJ, Bauer JM, Ramsch C, Uter W, Guigoz Y, Cederholm T, et al. Validation of the mini nutritional assessment short-form (MNA-SF): a practical tool for identification of nutritional status. J Nutr Health Aging. 2009;13(9):782–8.

17. Malnutrition: Key facts. World Health Organization 2018. Available at: http://www.who.int/news-room/fact-sheets/detail/malnutrition.

18. Yesavage JA, Sheikh JI. 9/geriatric depression scale (GDS) recent evidence and development of a shorter version. Clin Gerontol. 1986;5(1–2):165–73.

19. McDowell I. Measuring health: a guide to rating scales and questionnaires. New York: Oxford University Press; 2006.

20. Gautam R, Houde S. Geriatric depression scale for community-dwelling older adults in Nepal. Asian J Gerontol Geriatr. 2011;6(2):93–9.

21. Rabin R, de Charro F. EQ-5D: a measure of health status from the EuroQol group. Ann Med. 2001;33(5):337–43.

22. Bhattarai P, Niessen L, Shrestha N, Samir K. Health related quality of life of adults in Nepal with respiratory symptoms using WHOQOL and EQ-5D. 2005.

23. van Hout B, Janssen MF, Feng YS, Kohlmann T, Busschbach J, Golicki D, et al. Interim scoring for the EQ-5D-5L: mapping the EQ-5D-5L to EQ-5D-3L value sets. Value Health. 2012;15(5):708–15.

24. Lynn B, Dahal DR, Govindasamy P. Caste, ethnic and regional identity in Nepal: further analysis of the 2006 Nepal demographic and health survey Calverton. Maryland: Macro International Inc.; 2008.

25. Kvamme JM, Gronli O, Florholmen J, Jacobsen BK. Risk of malnutrition is associated with mental health symptoms in community living elderly men and women: the Tromso study. BMC Psychiatry. 2011;11:112.

26. Cabrera MA, Mesas AE, Garcia AR, de Andrade SM. Malnutrition and depression among community-dwelling elderly people. J Am Med Dir Assoc. 2007;8(9):582–4.

27. Maes M, Galecki P, Chang YS, Berk M. A review on the oxidative and nitrosative stress (O&NS) pathways in major depression and their possible contribution to the (neuro)degenerative processes in that illness. Prog Neuro-Psychopharmacol Biol Psychiatry. 2011;35(3):676–92.

28. Maes M, Yirmyia R, Noraberg J, Brene S, Hibbeln J, Perini G, et al. The inflammatory & neurodegenerative (I&ND) hypothesis of depression: leads for future research and new drug developments in depression. Metab Brain Dis. 2009;24(1):27–53.

29. Gibson EL. Emotional influences on food choice: sensory, physiological and psychological pathways. Physiol Behav. 2006;89(1):53–61.

30. Keller HH, Ostbye T, Goy R. Nutritional risk predicts quality of life in elderly community-living Canadians. J Gerontol A Biol Sci Med Sci. 2004;59(1):68–74.

31. Amarantos E, Martinez A, Dwyer J. Nutrition and quality of life in older adults. J Gerontol A Biol Sci Med Sci. 2001;56 Spec No 2:54–64.

32. Wakimoto P, Block G. Dietary intake, dietary patterns, and changes with age: an epidemiological perspective. J Gerontol A Biol Sci Med Sci. 2001;56 Spec No 2:65–80.

33. Nepal Thematic Report on Food Security and Nutrition: National Planning Commission, Central Bureau of Statistics, World Food Program, World Bank, AusAID,UNICEF 2013. Available at: http://documents.wfp.org/stellent/groups/public/documents/ena/wfp256518.pdf

34. Asian Development Bank. Country Poverty Analysis (Detailed) Nepal. Kathmandu, Nepal, 2013. Available at: https://www.adb.org/sites/default/files/linked-documents/cps-nep-2013-2017-pa-detailed.pdf.

35. Kirkwood TB. A systematic look at an old problem. Nature. 2008;451(7179):644–7.

36. Steves CJ, Spector TD, Jackson SH. Ageing, genes, environment and epigenetics: what twin studies tell us now, and in the future. Age Ageing. 2012;41(5):581–6.

37. Vellas B, Villars H, Abellan G, Soto ME, Rolland Y, Guigoz Y, et al. Overview of the MNA--its history and challenges. J Nutr Health Aging. 2006;10(6):456–63. discussion 63-5

38. Ghimire S, Pradhananga P, Baral BK, Shrestha N. Factors associated with health-related quality of life among hypertensive patients in Kathmandu. Nepal Front Cardiovasc Med. 2017;4:69.

39. Hirshkowitz M, Whiton K, Albert SM, Alessi C, Bruni O, DonCarlos L, Hazen N, Herman J, Adams Hillard PJ, Katz ES, et al. National Sleep Foundation's updated sleep duration recommendations: final report. Sleep Health. 2015;1(4):233–43.

40. Ory MG, Cox DM. Forging ahead: linking health and behavior to improve quality of life in older people. Soc Indic Res. 1994;33:89–120.

# 15

# Exercise patterns in older adults instructed to follow moderate- or high-intensity exercise protocol – the generation 100 study

Line Skarsem Reitlo[1,2], Silvana Bucher Sandbakk[1,3], Hallgeir Viken[1], Nils Petter Aspvik[4], Jan Erik Ingebrigtsen[4], Xiangchun Tan[5], Ulrik Wisløff[1,6] and Dorthe Stensvold[1*]

## Abstract

**Background:** Making older adults exercise and keeping them in exercise programs is a major challenge. Understanding how older adults prefer to exercise may help developing tailored exercise programs and increase sustained exercise participation in ageing populations. We aimed to describe exercise patterns, including frequency, intensity, type, location and social setting of exercise, in older adults instructed to follow continuous moderate-intensity training (MCT) or high-intensity interval training (HIIT) over a one-year period.

**Methods:** Frequency, intensity, type, location and social setting (alone vs. together with others) of exercise were assessed using exercise logs from 618 older adults (aged 70–77 years) randomized to MCT or HIIT. All participants completed exercise logs after each exercise session they performed during one year. Pearson Chi-square tests were run to assess the association between intensity, type, location and social setting of exercise with training group.

**Results:** Both groups performed 2.2 ± 1.3 exercise sessions per week during the year. Walking was the most common exercise type in both groups, but MCT had a higher proportion of walking sessions than HIIT (54.2% vs. 41.1%, $p < 0.01$). Compared to MCT, HIIT had a higher proportion of sessions with cycling (14.2% vs. 9.8%, $p < 0.01$), combined endurance and resistance training (10.3% vs. 7.5%, $p < 0.01$), jogging (6.5% vs. 3.2%, $p < 0.01$) and swimming (2.6% vs. 1.7%, $p < 0.01$). Outdoors was the most common exercise location in both training groups (67.8 and 59.1% of all sessions in MCT and HIIT, respectively). Compared to MCT, HIIT had a higher proportion of sessions at a gym (21.4% vs. 17.5%, $p < 0.01$) and sports facility (9.8% vs. 7.6%, $p < 0.01$). Both groups performed an equal amount of sessions alone and together with others, but women had a higher proportion of sessions together with others compared to men (56% vs. 44%, $p < 0.01$).

**Conclusion:** This is the first study that has followed older adults instructed to perform MCT or HIIT over a one-year period, collected data from each exercise session they performed and provided important knowledge about their exercise patterns. This novel information may help researchers and clinicians to develop tailored exercise programs in an ageing population.

**Keywords:** Aging, Aged, Exercise, High-intensity interval training

* Correspondence: dorthe.stensvold@ntnu.no
[1]K.G. Jebsen Center of Exercise in Medicine at Department of Circulation and Medical Imaging, Faculty of Medicine and Health Sciences, Norwegian University of Science and Technology, Trondheim, Norway
Full list of author information is available at the end of the article

# Background

The world population is ageing and the number of older adults with chronic health conditions and physical limitations is expected to increase. This, in turn, could lead to an increased burden on healthcare services [1]. Regular physical activity is an important component of successful ageing and reduces the risk of developing several age- and lifestyle related diseases such as cardiovascular disease, dementia and type 2 diabetes [2–7]. However, making older adults exercise and keeping them in exercise programs is a major challenge [8]. Understanding how older adults prefer to exercise may help developing tailored exercise programs and increase sustained exercise participation in ageing populations.

Many exercise interventions have been conducted under controlled laboratory conditions [9], but we do not know how older adults prefer to exercise when they are not under controlled settings and are free to choose type, location and social setting (e.g. alone vs. together with others) of exercise. Furthermore, it has been shown that high-intensity interval training (HIIT) can induce superior changes in health-related markers compared to continuous moderate-intensity training (MCT) [10–13], also in older adults [14, 15]. The scientific interest in HIIT has greatly increased during recent years [9], but larger and longer studies under free-living conditions are needed to investigate whether HIIT is feasible as a public health strategy among older adults [9, 16]. Therefore, detailed information about older adults exercise patterns with MCT versus HIIT outside laboratory conditions is of particular interest.

Furthermore, exercise initiatives should include strategies that will appeal to various subgroups of older adults. Disparities in physical activity levels between older women and men exist [17, 18], and sex differences are therefore an important consideration when examining exercise patterns.

The aim of this study was to describe exercise patterns, including frequency, intensity, type, location and social setting of exercise, in older adults instructed to follow MCT or HIIT over a one-year period. We also aimed to describe sex differences in exercise patterns in older adults.

# Methods
## Study participants

Between August 2012 and June 2013, all men and women born between years 1936 to 1942 (aged 70–77 years), with a permanent address in the municipality of Trondheim, Norway, were invited to participate in a randomized controlled trial, the Generation 100 study. The primary aim of Generation 100 is to determine the effect of five years of exercise training on morbidity and mortality. The Generation

100 study protocol and study sample characteristics have been published previously [19].

In total, 1567 participants (790 women) met the inclusion criteria, fulfilled baseline testing and were randomized 1:1 into an exercise training group or to a control group. The exercise training group was further randomized 1:1 to either MCT or HIIT. Participants in the exercise groups were instructed to fill in exercise logs after each exercise session they performed. Data in the present study is based on the exercise logs from the first year of the intervention. Therefore, only participants in the exercise groups were included in the present study ($n = 787$). Dropouts in the exercise groups during the first year ($n = 123$) and those with no exercise logs ($n = 46$) were excluded. A total of 618 participants (291 women) were included in the analyses (Fig. 1). The study was approved by the Regional Committee for Medical Research Ethics (REK sør-øst B: 2015/945) and all participants gave their written informed consent before participation.

## Exercise intervention

The MCT group was prescribed two weekly exercise sessions of 50-min continuous activity at 70% of peak heart rate, or approximately 13 on the Borg 6–20 rating of perceived exertion (RPE) scale [20]. The HIIT group was prescribed two exercise sessions a week with 10-min warm-up followed by $4 \times 4$ min intervals at 85–95% of peak heart rate, or approximately 16 on the Borg 6–20 RPE scale. The participants were given individual oral and written information about the training methods, including information about frequency, duration, intensity and examples of exercise sessions. The participants were free to exercise individually, with an exercise type and at a location of their own choosing. Every sixth week the participants met for a supervised spinning session where they exercised with a heart rate monitor. These exercise sessions gave the participants an opportunity to control their intensity during exercise. In addition, organized group exercise was offered twice per week for motivational purposes. Attendance to these exercises was voluntary and the activity performed varied between indoor and outdoor activities such as walking, jogging and aerobics [19]. Besides the two prescribed exercise sessions, the participants were free to exercise as desired.

## Assessment of exercise patterns

Exercise was defined as planned, structured activities, for instance going for walks, skiing, swimming and doing sports, but also as unplanned activities that the participants experienced as exercise. The participants were asked to fill in exercise logs immediately after each exercise session they performed throughout the year and send them to the research center either in prepaid envelopes monthly, or to use internet-based forms following

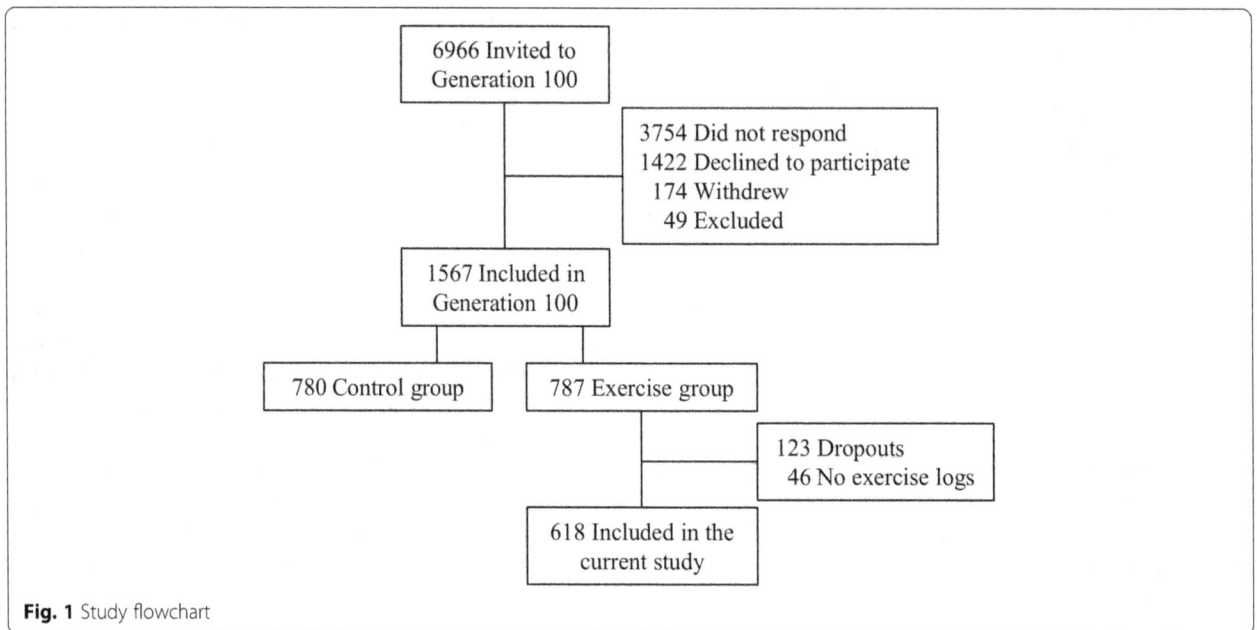

**Fig. 1** Study flowchart

each exercise session [21]. Exercise frequency was calculated as the mean number of sessions reported per week during the year. To assess intensity of exercise the participants reported their subjective RPE on a Borg scale ranging from 6 to 20 [20]. The participants were asked to report the mean intensity level during the exercise session. Ratings from 6 to 10 were classified as low intensity, 11 to 14 as moderate intensity, and 15 to 20 as high intensity. Duration of exercise was measured with a 4-point scale: less than 15 min, 15–29 min, 30 min to 1 h, and more than 1 h. Less than 15 min and 15–29 min was combined due to a low response rate on these response options (1.1 and 8.7% of the total number of exercise sessions, respectively).

To measure exercise type the participants were instructed to choose from the following response options: walking, jogging, cycling, dancing, cross-country skiing, swimming, golf, resistance training and an open-ended response option. Answers in the open-ended response option were categorized into: combined endurance and resistance training, other type of endurance training (e.g. treadmill, aerobic), domestic activities (e.g. housework, gardening), and other (e.g. bowling, horseback riding). Golf was categorized as "other" due to a low response rate (0.5% of the total number of exercise sessions).

The question used to assess location of exercise had the following response options: home, outdoor in nearby area, nature, gym, indoor- and outdoor sports facility. Indoor- and outdoor sports facility was categorized as "sports facility" due to a low response rate on the outdoor sports facility option (1%). For social setting of exercise, the response options were: exercised alone, exercised together with others, and organized by Generation 100.

### Demographics and health characteristics

The baseline testing included clinical examinations, physical tests and questionnaires about health and lifestyle. Age and sex were obtained from the National Population Registry. A previously described questionnaire provided information on physical activity level and sedentary time at baseline [19]. Detailed protocol for assessment of body weight (kg), body height (cm) and body mass index (BMI; $kg/m^2$) is described elsewhere [19]. Testing of peak oxygen uptake ($VO_{2peak}$; mL/kg/min) was performed either as walking on a treadmill or cycling on a stationary bike. The test started with 10 min at a chosen warm-up speed. Approximately every two minutes, either the incline of the treadmill was increased by 2%, or the speed was increased by 1 km/h. The test protocol ended when participants were no longer able to carry a workload due to exhaustion or until all the criteria for a maximal oxygen uptake were reached [22].

### Statistical procedures

Sample characteristics are presented as mean ± standard deviation for continuous variables and proportions for categorical variables. Pearson Chi-square test and independent samples t-test were used to assess potential sex differences. For BMI and weight, a non-parametric test (Mann-Whitney U) was conducted due to the lack of normal distribution. Data from the exercise logs are presented as proportions of the total number of exercise logs. Pearson Chi-square tests were run to assess the associations between frequency, intensity, type, location and social setting of exercise with sex and training group. The results were considered statistically significant if the p-value was less than 0.05. All statistical analyses were performed with SPSS 22 (Statistical Package for Social Science, Chicago, IL, USA).

## Results

The baseline characteristics of the study participants are presented in Table 1. No differences between the training groups existed at study entry. In both groups, men spent more hours in sedentary behavior and had significantly higher weight, height, and $VO_{2peak}$ compared to women. Contrary, more women than men performed at least 30 min of daily physical activity (Table 1). The included participants had higher $VO_{2peak}$ (11%) compared to those with no exercise logs. They also had higher $VO_{2peak}$ (17%) and height (1.7%) compared to dropouts, but a lower BMI (3.7%) ($p < 0.05$). A higher proportion of the included participants performed 30 min of daily physical activity compared to the dropouts (77.3% vs. 66.1%, $p < 0.05$).

### Frequency and intensity of exercise

The participants completed in total 69 492 exercise logs (33 608 HIIT group) during the year, of which 39 075 were received in prepaid envelopes and 30 417 in internet-based forms. Both groups performed $2.2 \pm 1.3$ exercise sessions per week. Almost 80% of the sessions in the MCT group were actually performed with moderate intensity (11–14 on the Borg scale), while almost 60% of the sessions in the HIIT group were performed with high intensity ($\geq 15$ on the Borg scale) (Fig. 2). In the MCT group, women had a significantly higher proportion of sessions with moderate intensity compared to men (81.7% vs. 74.9%, $p < 0.01$). In the HIIT group, men had a higher proportion of sessions with high intensity compared to women (63.7% vs. 52.3%, $p < 0.01$) (Fig. 2). In the MCT group, 9.6, 43 and 47.4% of the sessions had a duration of < 30 min, 30 min to 1 h, and more than 1 h, respectively. The corresponding percentages in the HIIT group were 10.1, 45 and 44.9%.

### Exercise type

Walking was the most common exercise type in both training groups (Fig. 3). Compared to HIIT, MCT had a significantly higher proportion of sessions with walking and resistance training. Contrary, compared to MCT,

HIIT had a higher proportion of sessions with cycling, combined endurance and resistance training, other types of endurance training (e.g. aerobic, treadmill), jogging, swimming and dancing. There were no group differences regarding cross-country skiing and domestic activities (e.g. housework, gardening) (Fig. 3).

In both groups, men had a higher proportion of cycling, cross-country skiing and jogging sessions compared to women (Fig. 4). Men also had a higher proportion of sessions with combined endurance and resistance training and domestic activities than women. In contrast, women had a higher proportion of walking, swimming and dancing sessions than men. There were no sex differences in resistance training and other types of endurance training (Fig. 4).

### Location of exercise

Both groups exercised most frequently outdoors in nearby area and in nature (Fig. 5). Additional analyses showed that outdoors was the most frequently reported exercise location in both warmer (April–October) and colder (November–March) months. The MCT group had a significantly higher proportion of sessions outdoors than the HIIT group. Contrary, compared to the MCT group, HIIT had a higher proportion of sessions at a gym, sports facility and at home (Fig. 5).

In both groups, men had a significantly higher proportion of sessions at a gym compared to women (Fig. 6). Contrary, women had a higher proportion of sessions at a sports facility compared to men. In the MCT group, men had a significantly higher proportion of sessions outdoors compared to women, while the opposite was observed in the HIIT group (Fig. 6).

### Social setting of exercise

Both groups performed an equal proportion of exercise sessions alone (MCT: 50%, HIIT: 49.6%) and together with others (MCT: 50%, HIIT: 50.4%). In both groups, women had a significantly higher proportion of sessions together with others compared to men (56% vs. 44%, $p < 0.01$). The

**Table 1** Sample characteristics of the 618 study participants

| | MCT | | | HIIT | | |
|---|---|---|---|---|---|---|
| | All (n = 313) | Women (n = 152) | Men (n = 161) | All (n = 305) | Women (n = 139) | Men (n = 166) |
| Age (years) | 72.3±1.9 | 72.2±1.8 | 72.5±2.0 | 72.4±2.0 | 72.5±1.9 | 72.2±2.0 |
| Height (cm) | 170.6±8.9 | 163.4±5.0 | 177.4±5.8* | 170.6±8.9 | 163.2±5.2 | 176.9±6.0* |
| Weight (kg) | 75.6±12.9 | 68.2±10.3 | 82.7±11.1* | 75.6±14.0 | 66.5±9.9 | 83.3±12.3* |
| BMI (kg/m²) | 25.9±3.6 | 25.6±3.8 | 26.3±3.4 | 25.8±3.5 | 25.0±3.5 | 26.6±3.3* |
| Sedentary time (h/d) | 5.9±2.2 | 5.3±1.9 | 6.5±2.3* | 5.6±2.1 | 5.0±1.7 | 6.0±2.3* |
| PA >30min/day (yes %) | 77.8 | 83.3 | 72.5* | 77.5 | 82.6 | 73.2* |
| $VO_{2peak}$ (mL/kg/min) | 29.3±6.6 | 26.4±5.1 | 32.0±6.7* | 29.9±6.3 | 27.3±4.5 | 32.1±6.7* |

Data are presented as mean ± standard deviation or proportions (%). *BMI* body mass index, *PA* physical activity, $VO_{2peak}$ peak oxygen uptake
*Significantly different from women within the same training group ($p<0.05$)

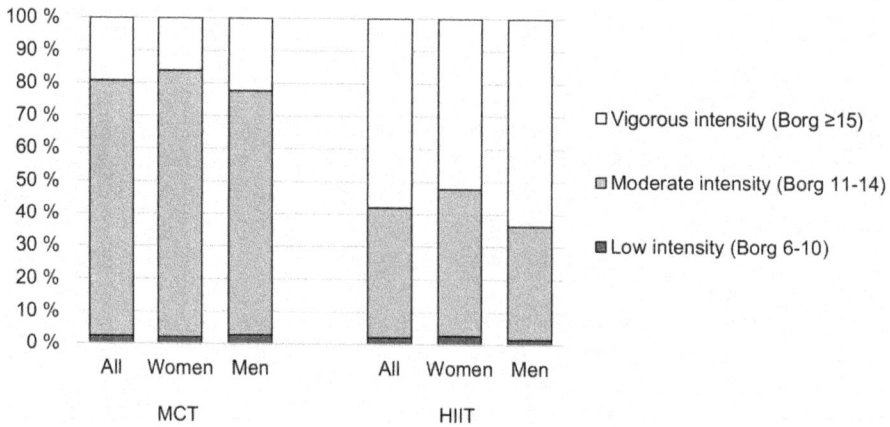

**Fig. 2** Exercise intensity. Data are presented as proportions of the total number of exercise sessions

HIIT group had a significantly higher proportion of sessions organized by Generation 100 compared to the MCT group (8.1% vs. 5.9%, $p < 0.01$).

## Discussion

This is the first study that has followed older adults instructed to perform MCT or HIIT over a one-year period, collected data from each exercise session they performed and provided descriptive data on their exercise patterns. The main finding is that both groups to a large degree exercised with the prescribed intensity. MCT had a higher proportion of walking sessions than HIIT, while HIIT had a higher proportion of jogging sessions than MCT. In addition, HIIT had a higher proportion of sessions with cycling, combined endurance and resistance training, swimming and dancing. Both groups exercised

more frequently outdoors than indoors and performed an equal amount of sessions alone and together with others.

### Frequency and intensity of exercise

Evidence from HIIT studies conducted under controlled laboratory conditions has provided proof-of-concept of efficacy [9]. However, it has been argued that HIIT has high efficacy but low effectiveness [16], and long-term exercise interventions carried out under free-living conditions have been asked for to investigate whether HIIT is feasible as a public health initiative among older adults [9, 16]. Our data showed that both training groups reported on average more than two exercise sessions per week throughout the year. Approximately 60% of the sessions in the HIIT group were performed with a self-reported high-intensity (≥15 Borg scale), indicating that older adults are able to perform HIIT over a long time-period without strict

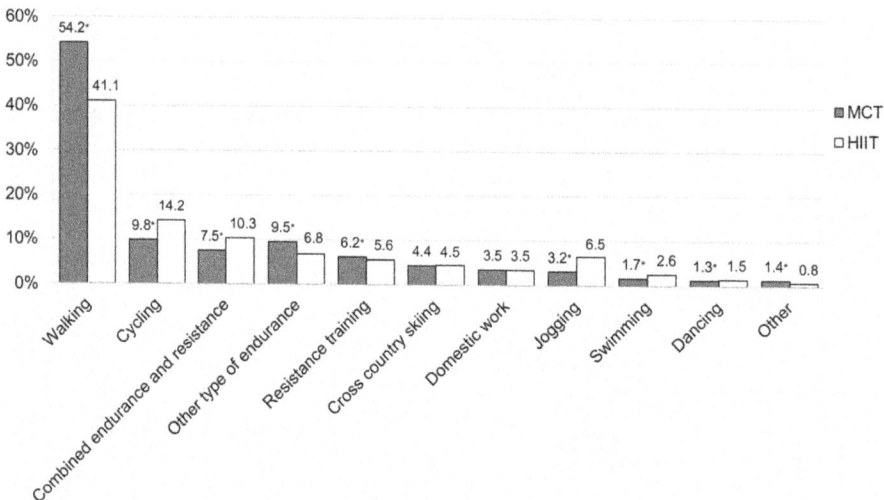

**Fig. 3** Association of exercise type with training group. Data are presented as proportions of the total number of exercise sessions. Other type of endurance; treadmill, cross trainer, aerobics etc., Domestic activities; housework, gardening etc., Other; golf, bowling, horseback riding etc. *Significantly different from the HIIT group ($p < 0.05$)

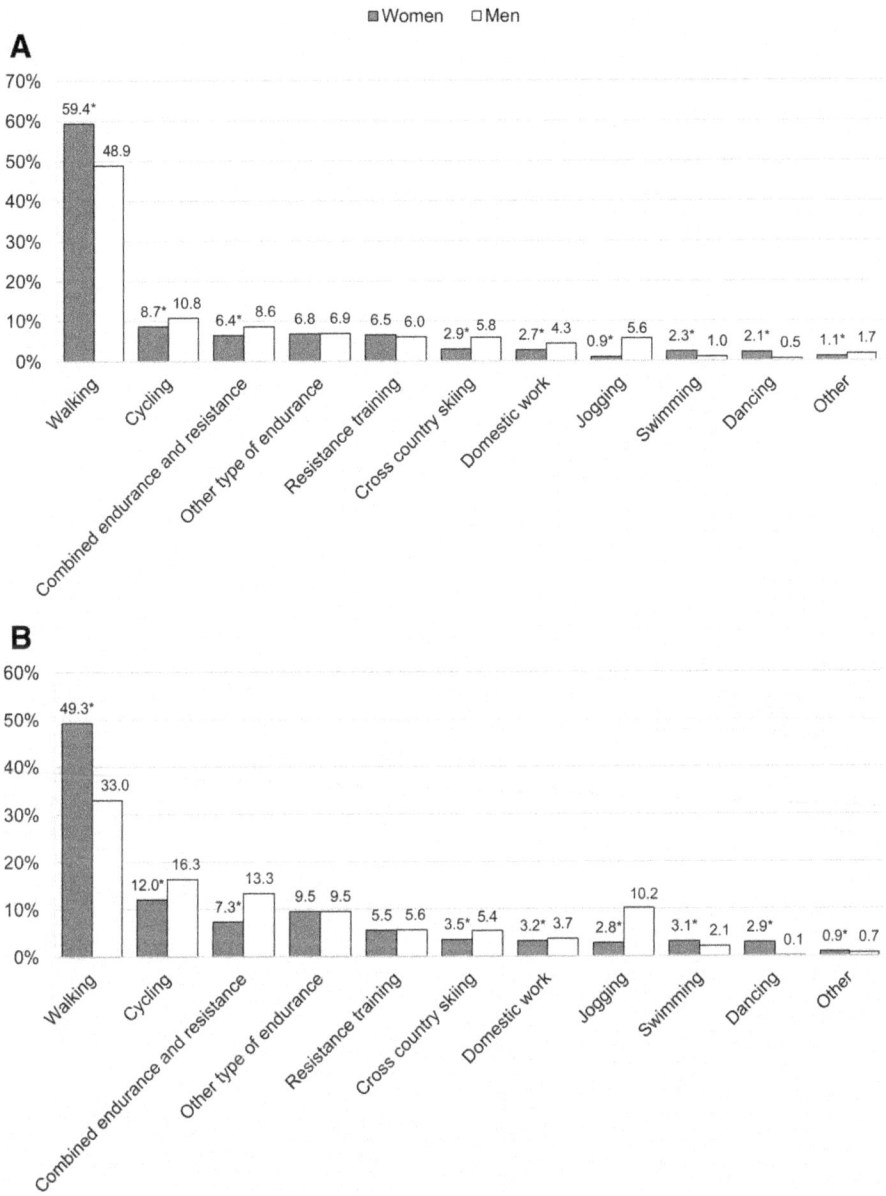

**Fig. 4** Association of exercise type with sex in the MCT (**a**) and HIIT (**b**) groups. Data are presented as proportions of the total number of exercise sessions. Other type of endurance; treadmill, cross trainer, aerobics etc., Domestic activities; housework, gardening etc., Other: golf, bowling, horseback riding etc. *Significantly different from men (*p* < 0.05)

supervision. However, women had a lower proportion of sessions with high-intensity exercise compared to men. This result is in line with previous findings that women (aged 60–67 years) are less likely than men to prefer vigorous physical activity [23].

### Exercise type
In line with the previous literature, our study showed that walking was the most common exercise type among older adults [24, 25]. This result is not surprising as walking is among the most cost effective and accessible means of exercise [26]. In addition, walking has been identified as a

relatively safe exercise alternative to older adults [25]. We found that walking was the most common exercise type in both training groups. However, the MCT group had a higher proportion of walking sessions than the HIIT group, while the HIIT group had a higher proportion of sessions with for instance jogging and cycling. This might indicate that some older adults in the HIIT group feel that it is easier to achieve a high-intensity level when performing jogging and cycling compared to walking. Absolute workload at a given intensity varies greatly among individuals with different levels of cardiorespiratory fitness (CRF) [27], so that e.g. walking at 5 km/h corresponds to

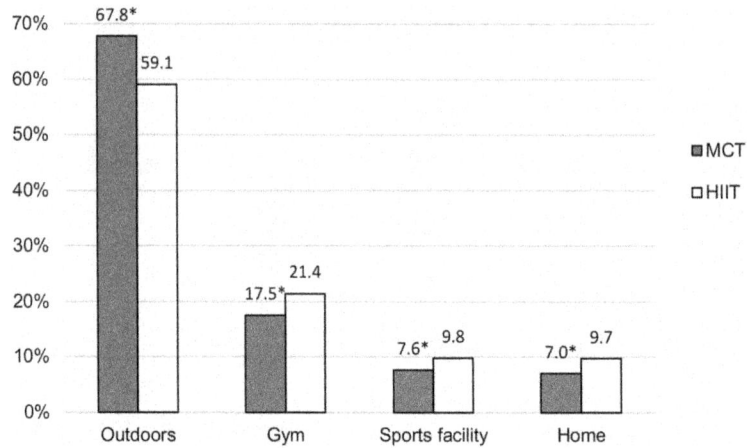

**Fig. 5** Association of exercise location with training group. Data are presented as proportions of the total number of exercise sessions. *Significantly different from the HIIT group (p < 0.05)

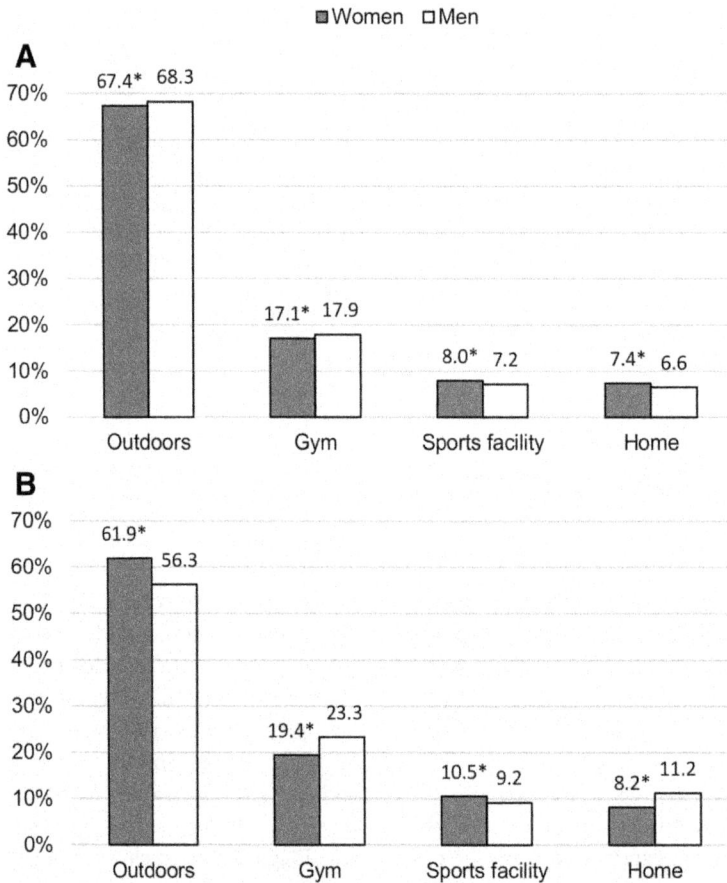

**Fig. 6** Association of exercise location with sex in the MCT (**a**) and HIIT (**b**) groups. Data are presented as proportions of the total number of exercise sessions. *Significantly different from men (p < 0.05)

moderate intensity for an individual with relatively high CRF level, while the same speed exhibits near-maximal intensity for an individual with low CRF. Therefore, the type of exercise an individual need to perform in order to achieve a feeling of high intensity varies from one individual to another [27]. Since ageing often results in CRF decline [28], it is likely that many older adults will reach a feeling of high-intensity when walking. However, those with a high CRF level might need to perform other exercise types, for instance jogging and cycling, to reach the same intensity level during their workout session.

In line with Martin and colleagues [29] we found that women more often engaged in walking, swimming and dancing compared to men, while men more often performed jogging, cycling and winter sports. Our data also showed that men performed a higher amount of sessions with domestic activities and combined endurance and resistance training compared to women. The sex differences were the same in both training groups, indicating that disparities in type of exercise between older women and men are independent of the exercise intensity they are instructed to perform.

### Location of exercise

Outdoors in nearby area and in nature was the most frequently reported exercise location in both training groups. This finding is in line with previous studies reporting that older adults prefer to exercise close to home [23, 30] and outdoors [23]. Interestingly, outdoors was the most common exercise location in both warmer and colder months despite the fact that colder months in Norway consist of more snow, higher prevalence of ice and relatively fewer hours of daylight compared to warmer months. The HIIT group had a higher proportion of sessions at a gym and sport facility compared to the MCT group. This finding is likely related to the fact that the HIIT group reported a higher proportion of sessions with exercise types commonly performed at these locations (e.g. swimming and other types of endurance training) compared to the MCT group. Some older adults might feel that it is easier to reach a high-intensity level with activities located at a gym and sports facility compared to outdoors.

### Social setting of exercise

Our results showed that both the MCT and HIIT group performed an equal amount of exercise sessions alone and together with others, suggesting that both individual and group-related exercise intervention strategies may be attractive to older adults. However, women exercised more frequently together with others than men. This result is in line with previous findings that women aged 60–67 years are less likely than men to prefer physical activity that can be done alone [23], and that more women than men express a need for social support to maintain an exercise program [31].

Altogether, our findings showed that older adults engage in a variety of exercise types, especially when instructed to perform HIIT, suggesting that future exercise interventions might profit of giving older adults the choice of different exercise types instead of offering only one. Our findings also suggest that interventions to promote exercise in older adults should focus on both indoor and outdoor environments. The popularity of exercising outdoors in both colder and warmer months highlight the importance of facilitating outdoors areas such as hiking trails. Furthermore, our findings show that sex differences in exercise patterns exist and need to be taken into consideration when designing exercise programs targeting older men and women. Given the increasing number of older adults [1] and the health benefits associated with exercise [32], information on how to get older adults to exercise and maintain their exercise behavior is important. The results of the present study can help clinicians and researchers to develop exercise programs targeting older adult's interests and in that way improve long-term participation.

### Strengths and limitations

The main strength of this study is the large data material on exercise patterns. Most research on exercise pattern has used a cross-sectional design whereas we followed older adults over a one-year period and collected data from each exercise session they performed. Furthermore, this is the first study to assess differences in exercise patterns between older adults instructed to follow MCT versus HIIT.

Since our data is self-reported, we do not know for sure if we have data from all exercise sessions performed throughout the year. Furthermore, subjective measures are susceptible to recall bias, especially among older adults [17, 18]. However, our results are based on nearly 70000 exercise logs, which is the largest data material on exercise patterns in older adults. In addition, exercise logs have an advantage over the widely employed exercise questionnaires where the subject is asked to recall exercise performed in the past as opposed to recording the exercise right after the moment of occurrence, as is the case with exercise logs.

Selection bias may limit generalizability to other populations of older adults since the included participants in the Generation 100 study were healthier, more educated and more physically active than nonparticipants [19]. However, our study population was diverse and included both healthy as well as older adults with comorbidities, and both inactive and very active older adults were included. The findings in the present study are based on a very large data material, and represent the most comprehensive data material on exercise patterns among older adults to date.

## Conclusions

Our findings show that older adults are able to perform both MCT and HIIT without strict supervision. Furthermore, older adults randomized to MCT versus HIIT have different patterns of exercise type and location of exercise, while there are no differences in social setting of exercise. The observed sex differences were the same in both training groups. Clinicians and researchers might capitalize on our findings when planning future exercise interventions targeting older adults. Our findings may also provide important information for future public health initiatives in order to provide tailored exercise recommendations.

## Abbreviations

BMI: Body mass index$VO_{2peak}$peak oxygen uptake; CRF: Cardiorespiratory fitness.; HIIT: High-intensity interval training; MCT: Continuous moderate-intensity training; RPE: Rating of perceived exertion

## Acknowledgements

The testing of $VO_{2peak}$ was performed at the core facility NeXt Move, Norwegian University of Science and Technology (NTNU). The measurements of body height, body weight and BMI were performed at the Clinical Research Facility, St. Olavs University Hospital.

## Funding

This study was supported by grants from the Liaison Committee for education, research and innovation in Central Norway, The K.G Jebsen Foundation for medical research and the Research Council of Norway. The funding organizations had no role in the design and execution of the study, in the collection, analysis, and interpretation of the data, or in the preparation, review or approval of the submitted manuscript.

## Authors' contributions

LSR, SBS, HV, NPA, JEI, UW and DS contributed to the conception and design of the study. LSR, SBS, HV and DS were responsible for the collection of the Generation 100 data in cooperation with colleagues at the Cardiac Exercise Research Group at the Norwegian University of Science and Technology, Norway. LSR, SBS and XT provided the data for analysis. LSR undertook the data analysis and drafted the manuscript. All authors provided critical insight and revisions to the manuscript. All authors read and approved the final version of the manuscript submitted for publication.

## Competing interests

The authors declare that they have no competing interests.

## Author details

[1]K.G. Jebsen Center of Exercise in Medicine at Department of Circulation and Medical Imaging, Faculty of Medicine and Health Sciences, Norwegian University of Science and Technology, Trondheim, Norway. [2]Department of Cardiology, St Olavs Hospital, Trondheim University Hospital, Trondheim, Norway. [3]Norwegian National Advisory Unit on Exercise Training as Medicine for Cardiopulmonary Conditions, St. Olav's Hospital, Trondheim, Norway. [4]Department of Sociology and Political Science, Faculty of Social and Educational Sciences, Norwegian University of Science and Technology, Trondheim, Norway. [5]Department of Neuroscience and Movement Science, Faculty of Medicine and Health Sciences, Norwegian University of Science and Technology, Trondheim, Norway. [6]School of Human Movement & Nutrition Sciences, University of Queensland, Brisbane, Australia.

## References

1.  WHO. U.S. Department of health and human services. Global health and ageing. 2011.
2.  Smith SC Jr, Allen J, Blair SN, Bonow RO, Brass LM, Fonarow GC, et al. AHA/ACC guidelines for secondary prevention for patients with coronary and other atherosclerotic vascular disease: 2006 update: endorsed by the National Heart, Lung, and Blood Institute. Circulation. 2006;113:2363–72.
3.  Knoops KT, de Groot LC, Kromhout D, Perrin AE, Moreiras-Varela O, Menotti A, et al. Mediterranean diet, lifestyle factors, and 10-year mortality in elderly European men and women: the HALE project. JAMA. 2004;292:1433–9.
4.  Blondell SJ, Hammersley-Mather R, Veerman JL. Does physical activity prevent cognitive decline and dementia?: a systematic review and meta-analysis of longitudinal studies. BMC Public Health. 2014;14:510.
5.  Aune D, Norat T, Leitzmann M, Tonstad S, Vatten LJ. Physical activity and the risk of type 2 diabetes: a systematic review and dose-response meta-analysis. Eur J Epidemiol. 2015;30:529–42.
6.  Brown WJ, McLaughlin D, Leung J, McCaul KA, Flicker L, Almeida OP, et al. Physical activity and all-cause mortality in older women and men. Br J Sports Med. 2012;46:664–8.
7.  Taylor AH, Cable NT, Faulkner G, Hillsdon M, Narici M, Van Der Bij AK. Physical activity and older adults: a review of health benefits and the effectiveness of interventions. J Sports Sci. 2004;22:703–25.
8.  Hawley-Hague H, Horne M, Campbell M, Demack S, Skelton DA, Todd C. Multiple levels of influence on older adults' attendance and adherence to community exercise classes. Gerontologist. 2014;54:599–610.
9.  Gray SR, Ferguson C, Birch K, Forrest LJ, Gill JM. High-intensity interval training: key data needed to bridge the gap from laboratory to public health policy. Br J Sports Med. 2016;50:1231–2.
10. Swain DP, Franklin BA. Comparison of cardioprotective benefits of vigorous versus moderate intensity aerobic exercise. Am J Cardiol. 2006;97:141–7.
11. Wisloff U, Stoylen A, Loennechen JP, Bruvold M, Rognmo O, Haram PM, et al. Superior cardiovascular effect of aerobic interval training versus moderate continuous training in heart failure patients: a randomized study. Circulation. 2007;115:3086–94.
12. Helgerud J, Hoydal K, Wang E, Karlsen T, Berg P, Bjerkaas M, et al. Aerobic high-intensity intervals improve VO2max more than moderate training. Med Sci Sports Exerc. 2007;39:665–71.
13. Tjonna AE, Lee SJ, Rognmo O, Stolen TO, Bye A, Haram PM, et al. Aerobic interval training versus continuous moderate exercise as a treatment for the metabolic syndrome: a pilot study. Circulation. 2008;118:346–54.
14. Molmen HE, Wisloff U, Aamot IL, Stoylen A, Ingul CB. Aerobic interval training compensates age related decline in cardiac function. Scand Cardiovasc J. 2012;46:163–71.
15. Hwang CL, Yoo JK, Kim HK, Hwang MH, Handberg EM, Petersen JW, et al. Novel all-extremity high-intensity interval training improves aerobic fitness, cardiac function and insulin resistance in healthy older adults. Exp Gerontol. 2016;82:112–9.
16. Biddle SJ, Batterham AM. High-intensity interval exercise training for public health: a big HIT or shall we HIT it on the head? Int J Behav Nutr Phys Act. 2015;12:95.
17. Hallal PC, Andersen LB, Bull FC, Guthold R, Haskell W, Ekelund U. Global physical activity levels: surveillance progress, pitfalls, and prospects. Lancet. 2012;380:247–57.
18. Sun F, Norman IJ. While AE. Physical activity in older people: a systematic review. BMC Public Health. 2013;13:449.

Exercise patterns in older adults instructed to follow moderate- or high-intensity exercise...

185

19. Stensvold D, Viken H, Rognmo O, Skogvoll E, Steinshamn S, Vatten LJ, et al. A randomised controlled study of the long-term effects of exercise training on mortality in elderly people: study protocol for the generation 100 study. BMJ Open. 2015;5(2):e007519.

20. Borg GA. Psychophysical bases of perceived exertion. Med Sci Sports Exerc. 1982;14:377–81.

21. LimeSurvey: Training Logs Generation 100. https://survey.medisin.ntnu.no/limesurvey/index.php?sid=54583. Accessed 10 Jan 2018.

22. Stensvold D, Sandbakk SB, Viken H, Zisko N, Reitlo LS, Nauman J, et al. Cardiorespiratory reference data in older adults: the generation 100 study. Med Sci Sports Exerc. 2017;49:2206–15.

23. van Uffelen JGZ, Khan A, Burton NW. Gender differences in physical activity motivators and context preferences: a population-based study in people in their sixties. BMC Public Health. 2017;17:624.

24. Ory MG, Towne SD Jr, Won J, Forjuoh SN, Lee C. Social and environmental predictors of walking among older adults. BMC Geriatr. 2016;16:155.

25. Mobily KE. Walking among older adults. World Leis J. 2014;56:130–40.

26. Notthoff N, Carstensen LL. Positive messaging promotes walking in older adults. Psychol Aging. 2014;29:329–41.

27. Karlsen T, Aamot IL, Haykowsky M, Rognmo O. High intensity interval training for maximizing health outcomes. Prog Cardiovasc Dis. 2017;60:67–77.

28. Fleg JL, Morrell CH, Bos AG, Brant LJ, Talbot LA, Wright JG, et al. Accelerated longitudinal decline of aerobic capacity in healthy older adults. Circulation. 2005;112:674–82.

29. Martin KR, Cooper R, Harris TB, Brage S, Hardy R, Kuh D. Patterns of leisure-time physical activity participation in a British birth cohort at early old age. PLoS One. 2014;9(6):e98901.

30. Burton NW, Khan A, Brown WJ. How, where and with whom? Physical activity context preferences of three adult groups at risk of inactivity. Br J Sports Med. 2012;46:1125–31.

31. King AC. Interventions to promote physical activity by older adults. J Gerontol A Biol Sci Med Sci. 2001;56 Spec No 2:36–46

32. Hamer M, Lavoie KL, Bacon SL. Taking up physical activity in later life and healthy ageing: the English longitudinal study of ageing. Br J Sports Med. 2014;48:239–43.

# 16

# Dementia as a predictor of care-related quality of life in informal caregivers: a cross-sectional study to investigate differences in health-related outcomes between dementia and non-dementia caregivers

Nina Karg[1*], Elmar Graessel[1], Ottilie Randzio[2] and Anna Pendergrass[1]

## Abstract

**Background:** The objectives of this study with a large sample of informal caregivers (CG) were a) to compare health-related outcomes of CGs caring for a patient with dementia and those caring for a relative with another chronic disease and b) to check whether dementia is a predictor of CG's care-related quality of life (QoL) in CarerQoL-7D.

**Methods:** This cross-sectional study involved self-reported data from 386 informal CGs who applied for an initial grade or upgrade of the care level of the care recipient at the Medical Service of Compulsory Health Insurance Funds of Bavaria (Germany). By obtaining data this way, systematic biases often associated with the acquisition of CGs were prevented. Bivariate and multiple analyses were conducted using a univariate covariance model (ANCOVA).

**Results:** Bivariate analyses showed significantly higher levels of subjective burden and lower QoL in the dementia group. No significant differences were found in terms of physical health and depressiveness, though there was a tendency suggesting higher levels of depressiveness in dementia CGs. Multiple analysis explaining QoL by dementia status after controlling for CG's sex, age and employment status revealed a significant effect of dementia, suggesting caregiving for a dementia patient was associated with lower QoL.

**Conclusions:** Results of the study suggest that caring for a relative with dementia is associated with poorer health, i.e. greater levels of subjective burden and depressiveness, and predicts lower QoL in CGs. These findings emphasize the importance of specific interventions aiming to support informal CGs of dementia patients.

**Keywords:** Home care, Informal caregivers, Dementia, Caregiver health, Care-related quality of life

## Background

In 2013, 71% of all care recipients (CR) legally classified as dependent on long-term care in the Federal Republic of Germany lived in private households and in 92% of the cases they received daily assistance from private individuals providing informal care on a non-professional base [1, 2]. By accepting the responsibility for a care-dependent family member, informal caregivers (CGs) are faced with a variety of new challenges that transform the individual life. Numerous studies have examined the effects of caregiving on CG's health and demonstrated that CGs are at higher risk of jeopardizing both their physical and mental health compared to non-caregiving subjects of the same age and population (e.g. [3, 4]). Pinquart and Sörensen [4] found significantly higher levels of perceived strain in CGs compared to non-caregivers, which is associated with greater physical health problems and a higher likelihood of

* Correspondence: nina.karg@uk-erlangen.de
[1]Department of Psychiatry and Psychotherapy, Center for Health Service Research in Medicine, Friedrich-Alexander-University Erlangen-Nuremberg, Schwabachanlage 6, D-91054 Erlangen, Germany
Full list of author information is available at the end of the article

developing psychological and psychiatric morbidities, as well as higher mortality rates [5–7].

CGs of dementia patients are often called "the invisible second patients" [8], because dementia caregiving often exceeds the demands associated with caregiving for solely physically impaired CRs. Caregiving for a person with dementia is associated with several stressors that are specific to dementia and increase the likelihood of the development of chronic stress and associated adverse outcomes on CG health. The progress of the dementia disease is characterized by an unpredictable and uncontrollable deterioration of various cognitive, affective and eventually physical abilities. Deepening cognitive decline as well as the patient's loss of physical capabilities lead to an overall decreased functional level associated with deficits in activities of daily living (ADL) and instrumental activities of daily living (IADL). The result is that dementia CGs must often spend more hours on caregiving compared to non-dementia CGs [9]. A number of studies have suggested that greater impairment in ADL and IADL, lower functional level and greater total care time are associated with higher levels of CG stress, subjective burden, depressiveness and lower physical health in CGs [10, 11]. Furthermore, caregiving literature has highlighted the importance of CRs' cognitive impairment, which is more common amongst dementia patients than amongst non-dementia patients [12], as a cause of worse psychological well-being and mental health as well as physical morbidity in CGs [13, 14]. Cognitive decline and changes in personality commonly present as so-called disruptive behaviors, incomprehensible, disoriented or demanding patient behaviors. These have been found to be more common in dementia than in other forms of illness and have consistently been linked to greater distress, perceived burden and depressive symptoms in CGs [6, 10–14].

To date, a large number of studies have been conducted examining psychological and physical health of CGs of dementia patients and those caring for a person with functional impairment from another type of chronic illness. Dementia caregiving status was found to be a factor associated with higher levels of stress and subjective burden, and was linked to worse overall mental health outcomes like higher psychological and psychiatric morbidity [10, 15–17]. With respect to the impact of dementia caregiving on CG's physical health results have not always been clear, but several studies revealed low levels of physical health and an increased risk of various health problems in CGs caring for dementia patients [8, 17–19]. Ory and colleagues [20] found significantly more physical strain in dementia CGs compared to those caring for elderly people with relatively unimpaired cognitive performance. However, the aforementioned studies relied to a great extent on rather small convenience samples that were recruited primarily from CG support groups or Alzheimer's associations and therefore may be susceptible to systematic recruitment biases.

More representative, unbiased samples with a greater number of participants would be essential to allow for more reliable and definite conclusions about the health-related consequences of caregiving. For this reason, the first aim of the current study was to investigate in a large, representative sample differences in health-related variables between those two subgroups of CGs.

Furthermore, a significant portion of previous research primarily focused on particular health-related aspects of informal caregiving, not taking into account the total impact of caregiving activity on the CG's overall quality of life, from now on referred to as care-related QoL. Different approaches have been made to find an appropriate definition and measure for the concept of QoL in the context of informal caregiving, but due to the multidimensional nature of this concept, no consensus has yet been reached. Some research has focused on physical and mental well-being as measures of health-related QoL (e.g. [21, 22]), but according to the WHO [23] health means not only a state of complete physical and mental well-being, but social well-being as well. Thus, not only physical and mental health, but also social and economic factors as well as familial interactions must be taken into account when discussing an individual's QoL [24, 25]. In consideration of this, Brouwer and colleagues [26] developed the CarerQoL, an instrument for the assessment of care-related QoL in informal CGs. The CarerQoL captures different aspects of the care situation affecting key domains in a person's life and at the same time allows for an evaluation of the impact of caregiving activity on the CG's overall QoL. Some attempts have been made to establish determinants of CG's QoL, finding that lower QoL levels in informal CGs seem to be associated with e.g. greater severity of the patient's behavioral problems, higher levels of CG burden and greater levels of depressiveness (e.g. [25–28]). In line with these findings, Srivastava and colleagues [29] found low levels of self-reported QoL in key CGs of dementia patients. However, this study did not involve a control group of informal CGs caring for patients with other chronic diseases. In their systematic review, Farina and colleagues [30] tried to identify factors predicting QoL in CGs of people with dementia and found that CG's better physical health, mental and emotional well-being (i.e. lower levels of depression, anxiety and perceived burden), greater CG independence, self-efficacy and coping skills were related to CG's QoL. With the exception of these findings, factors associated with QoL of CGs of dementia patients have not yet been examined to a satisfactory extent. Furthermore, no direct comparisons exist between dementia and non-dementia CGs. As previously shown, dementia CGs appear to be exposed to a greater variety of strains as well as to suffer from worse physical and mental overall health compared to non-dementia CGs. As more domains of the CG's personal life are potentially affected by dementia caregiving, it can be assumed that CGs' care-related QoL is more strongly affected in dementia CGs than in non-dementia ones. For this reason, the second aim of the current study was to examine whether caring for a person with dementia affects care-related QoL in informal CGs.

We hypothesized that

a) CGs caring for CRs with dementia would report worse physical and mental health and lower levels of care-related QoL than CGs caring for CRs with other chronic diseases
b) lower levels of the CG's care-related QoL are attributable to the CR's dementia illness

## Methods
### Research design and participants
This study is a cross-sectional study involving self-reported data. Between October 2014 and April 2015 1700 self-report questionnaires were handed out to informal CGs upon application for an initial grade or upgrade of the care level[1] of the CR at different centers of the Medical Service of Compulsory Health Insurance Funds (MDK)[2] all over Bavaria. 443 participants (26.1%) returned the questionnaires and thereby declared their consent with the utilization of their data for scientific evaluation. *Inclusion criteria* were a) providing care for someone with chronic care needs and b) CR 65 years or older. *Exclusion criteria* were a) lacking information about the presence or absence of CR's dementia and b) providing care for own children. 57 participants (13%) did not meet the conditions and thus a final total of 386 participants were included in statistical analyses.

### Measures
#### Independent variables
Demographic and background characteristics recorded were the CG's and CR's age and gender, CG's employment status and educational attainment, the relation between the relationship between the CG and CR, living situation, duration of care, total daily care time,[3] medical cause of care dependency and comorbidities (including dementia) and support received by the CG.

Physical complaints were measured using the short form of the Giessen Symptom List (GBB) [31], a reliable and valid self-assessment measure for psychosomatic health complaints. The short form consists of 24 items, all of which are measured along a five-point Likert scale (0 = 'not at all' to 4 = 'yes, absolutely'), that evaluate physical complaints on four subscales: exhaustion, gastrointestinal, musculoskeletal and cardiovascular complaints. By computing a sum score with a possible range between 0 and 96, the general impact of somatic complaints is assessed. For reasons of clarity, percentile ranks (*PR*) (median and median absolute deviation[4]) were calculated for descriptive analysis. Further analyses were carried out with the raw sum score.

To assess perceived burden, the Caregiver Strain Index (CSI) [32] was administered. The 13-item self-report questionnaire measures financial, physical, psychological, social and personal strain using a dichotomous answering format (0 = 'no', 1 = 'yes') with higher scores corresponding to higher subjective strain. Given a possible range from 0 to 13, a final score of 7 or higher reflects a considerable level of stress in the CG's life.

The Patient Health Questionnaire-9 (PHQ-9) [33] is a reliable and valid screening measure that evaluates the intensity of self-reported depressive symptoms over the last two weeks on a 4-point-scale (0 = 'not at all' to 3 = 'nearly every day'). Scores for the 9 items are summed (maximum of 27), with higher scores corresponding to greater severity of depressiveness and a total score > 9 indicating moderate or severe symptoms.

The 5-item subscale 'positive aspects' of the Berlin Inventory of Caregivers' Burden - Dementia (BIZA) [34] was used to measure positive aspects of informal caregiving, so-called benefits, on a 5-point Likert scale (0 = 'never' to 4 = 'always'). With a possible maximum sum score of 20, higher scores indicate that the CG perceived benefits to a greater extent.

#### Outcome variable
Care-related QoL in informal CGs was assessed using the *CarerQoL-7D* scale of the CarerQoL [26], a reliable and valid [35]self-report instrument measuring care-related QoL on two distinct scales. The *CarerQoL-7D* covers seven personal key domains being affected by the caregiving activity (care-related fulfillment, a mental and a physical health dimension, a social dimension and perceived support, a relational dimension, and financial security) while the *CarerQoL-VAS* allows for an evaluation of the CG's general level of happiness on a single-item visual analogue scale (VAS). Due to conceptual[5] and methodological[6] reasons, only the comprehensive set of the 7 care-related dimensions of the CarerQoL-7D was included in the survey questionnaire. Item responses are recorded on a 3-point scale (0 = 'no' to 2 = 'a lot'), resulting in a sum score with a possible range between 0 and 14. Higher scores are associated with higher care-related QoL in informal CGs; thus the CarerQoL adequately reflects care-related QoL and provides a good overview of the impact of informal care on the CG [26].

### Statistical analysis
Descriptive statistics were computed to illustrate sample characteristics in the terms of frequencies, means (*M*) and standard deviations (*SD*) of the variables.

As underlying assumptions for parametric tests were met (independence, normality and homogeneity of variance), independent t-tests and chi-squared tests were conducted to check for group differences in variables of interest between CGs caring for a dementia patient (dementia group) and those caring for relatives whose care dependency had other causes (non-dementia group).

In the next step, bivariate analyses, including Pearson's r correlations and independent t-tests, were performed to investigate the association between characteristics of the CG, CR and the care situation and CGs' self-reported QoL. Variables significant at the bivariate level were included as covariates in the initial multiple model.

The multiple analysis was conducted using a univariate covariance model (ANCOVA) with care-related QoL as the dependent variable, 'Dementia' as the fixed factor and all variables which correlated significantly with care-related QoL as covariates. Collinearity statistics were examined in advance to ensure there were no issues of multicollinearity. In an iterative approach, variables not significant at the bivariate level were added one after another to the initial model, checking whether they contributed significantly to the explained variance of QoL in the multiple model over and above the variables already included. Variables with additional explanatory power were added as further covariates into the final model.

For all analyses, a Type 1 error probability (alpha) of less than 5% was considered to constitute statistical significance. Statistical analyses were performed with SPSS v.21.

## Results

Table 1 provides the results of the descriptive analysis, including the group comparison between the two subgroups dementia vs. non-dementia in all of the variables.

Informal CGs were on average 61 years old; three quarters were female; 40% were still employed and the majority had a moderate educational level. Most of the CGs were caring either for their parents (or in-laws) or spouse, who they lived together with in 70% of the cases. During an average duration of care of 4.5 years 80% of the CGs received informal or formal support. CRs mean age was 82 years, and more than half were female. CRs in the full sample were diagnosed with three illnesses (diagnoses according to the ICD-10 [36], including dementia) on average. Dementia patients reported significantly more morbidities (two additional comorbidities apart from dementia) than those of the non-dementia group (two morbidities). The prevalence of the ten major disease groups being most frequent in the age 65–80 group in Germany as a whole [37] are also shown in Table 1, with the numbers referring to our sample.

There was no evidence for further significant differences between the two subgroups with regard to the described characteristics, with the exception of total care time: CGs in the dementia group reported a significantly higher amount of time compared to the non-dementia group.

In terms of subjective burden, CGs in both groups experienced a considerably high level of strain (CSI score > 7), with the dementia group ($n = 81$ (53%) CSI > 7) reporting significantly higher burden scores than the non-dementia group ($n = 110$ (47%) CSI > 7). Both groups reported medium levels of care-related QoL on average (CarerQoL: 8 of 14 points, range: 1–14), again with dementia CGs indicating lower levels than CGs in the non-dementia group (M = 7.4, range: 1–14 vs. M = 8.1, range: 2–14). Depressiveness scores in both groups indicated low to mild levels of depressiveness (PHQ < 9), with a tendency (though no significant difference) for the dementia group to have higher levels of depressiveness ($n = 601$ (39%) PHQ > 9 vs. non-dementia group: $n = 73$ (31%) PHQ > 9). Altogether, CGs reported psychosomatic health complaints (GBB median PR: 76) higher than in the average population (GBB median PR: 50) with no significant difference between the dementia and non-dementia group. In terms of benefits, both groups experienced positive aspects of caregiving to the same extent (BIZA: 12 of 20 points), indicating that the likelihood of experiencing benefits is higher than that of not experiencing any positive aspects of caregiving.

Bivariate correlational analyses revealed significant negative correlations between care-related QoL (CarerQoL) and depressiveness (PHQ-9), perceived burden (CSI) and physical complaints (GBB), suggesting that a greater subjective burden and physical complaints as well as lower levels of depressiveness were associated with higher levels of care-related QoL (see Table 2).

As multicollinearity analyses revealed significantly high intercorrelations ($r \geq 0.5$) between these variables, only depressiveness, which showed the strongest association with care-related QoL, was included in the final multiple model.

Furthermore, there was a significant difference in CG QoL depending on the CG's sex and employment status, indicating being male (M = 8.65, SD = 2.85 vs. female: M = 7.62, SD = 2.70) and unemployed (M = 8.25, SD = 2.91 vs. employed M = 7.29, SD = 2.44) were associated with higher levels of QoL. Hence employment status and caregiver's sex were included in the multiple model.

CR's sex, CG's and CR's age, living situation, CG's received support, relationship, educational attainment, duration of care, total care time, and benefits were not significantly associated with QoL. When entering CG's age as a covariate into the initial multiple model, an additional significant effect of age on QoL was revealed; thus, CG's age was included into the final model.

The results of a univariate covariance analysis (ANCOVA) with QoL as the independent variable, 'Dementia' as a fixed

**Table 1** Sample characteristics (N = 386)

| | Dementia (n = 153) | Non-Dementia (n = 233) | p | Total sample (N = 386) |
|---|---|---|---|---|
| Caregiver (CG) | | | | |
| Age (yrs.), M (SD) | 60.8 (13.0) | 61.6 (11.6) | 0.503 [a] | 61.3 (12.2) |
| Sex: Female, N (%) | 122 (80) | 173 (74) | 0.214 [b] | 295 (76) |
| Educational attainment (yrs.), M (SD) | 10.8 (2.7) | 10.7 (2.6) | 0.874 [b] | 10.8 (2.6) |
| Employment status: Employed, N (%) [c] | 57 (37) | 100 (43) | 0.268 [b] | 157 (41) |
| Relation: Care recipient is… N (%) | | | 0.310 [b] | |
| - mother/father (in-law) | 94 (61) | 140 (60) | | 234 (61) |
| - spouse | 50 (33) | 86 (37) | | 136 (35) |
| - other | 9 (6) | 7 (3) | | 16 (4) |
| Received support, N (%) [d] | 125 (82) | 181 (78) | 0.341 [b] | 306 (79) |
| Subjective burden (CSI), M (SD) | 7.9 (2.6) | 7.1 (2.9) | 0.004 [a] | 7.4 (2.8) |
| QoL (CarerQoL), M (SD) | 7.4 (2.8) | 8.1 (2.7) | 0.013 [a] | 7.9 (2.8) |
| Depressiveness (PHQ-9), M (SD) | 8.5 (5.0) | 7.6 (5.1) | 0.094 [a] | 8.0 (5.1) |
| Benefits (BIZA), M (SD) | 12.4 (3.9) | 12.2 (3.7) | 0.726 [a] | 12.3 (3.8) |
| Physical complaints (GBB), PR, MDN (MAD) | 80 (21.0) | 74 (23.5) | 0.132 [a] | 76 (22.7) |
| Care recipient (CR) | | | | |
| Age (yrs.), M (SD) | 82.8 (7.0) | 81.4 (7.5) | 0.063 [a] | 81.9 (7.3) |
| Sex: Female, N (%) | 101 (66) | 141 (61) | 0.275 [b] | 242 (63) |
| Number of morbidities (incl. dementia), M (SD) | 2.88 (1.68) | 2.43 (1.50) | 0.006 [a] | 2.60 (1.58) |
| Morbidities: Major disease groups (ICD-10), N (%) [e] | | | | |
| - II: Neoplasms | 6 (4) | 38 (16) | | 44 (11) |
| - IV: Endocrine, nutritional and metabolic diseases | 33 (21) [f] | 53 (23) | | 86 (22) |
| - V: Mental and behavioral disorders | 5 (3) | 7 (3) | | 12 (3) |
| - VII: Diseases of the eye and adnexa | 5 (3) | 14 (6) | | 19 (5) |
| - IX: Diseases of the circulatory system | 48 (31) | 94 (40) | | 142 (37) |
| - X: Diseases of the respiratory system | 7 (5) | 11 (5) | | 18 (5) |
| - XI: Diseases of the digestive system | 2 (1) | 5 (2) | | 7 (2) |
| - XII: Diseases of the skin and subcutaneous tissue | 1 (1) | 1 (0) | | 2 (1) |
| - XIII: Diseases of the musculoskeletal system and connective tissue | 14 (9) | 41 (18) | | 55 (14) |
| - XIV: Diseases of the genitourinary system | 3 (2) | 12 (5) | | 15 (4) |
| Care situation | | | | |
| Living situation: Together, N (%) | 108 (71) | 162 (70) | 0.824 [b] | 270 (70) |
| Duration of care (mo.), M (SD) | 52.4 (41.2) | 53.1 (57.4) | 0.892 [a] | 52.8 (51.5) |
| Total care time (hrs./day), M (SD) [g] | 11.9 (4.2) | 10.8 (4.1) | 0.010 [a] | 11.2 (4.2) |

M mean, SD standard deviation, PR Percentile Ranks, MDN Median, MAD Median absolute deviation, CSI Caregiver Strain Index (scores from 0 to 13), CarerQoL CarerQoL-7D (scores from 0 to 14), PHQ-9 Patient Health Questionnaire-9 (scores from 0 to 27), BIZA Berlin Inventory of Caregivers' Burden - Dementia (scores from 0 to 20), GBB Giessen Symptom List

[a] t-test

[b] chi-square test

[c] min. 7 yrs. (no compulsory school leaving certificate)- max. 18 yrs. (university degree)

[d] CG receives formal or/and informal support related to caregiving

[e] One or more diseases of the disease group have been reported; disease groups regarding unspecific impact factors on health (group 21) and abnormal clinical findings (group 18) are not included in the ranking

[f] not including dementia

[g] Consisting of time spent on activities of daily living (ADL), instrumental activities of daily living (IADL) and supervision of the CR (SUVI) by the CG

factor and CG's sex, age, depressiveness score and employment status as covariates are shown in Table 3.

There was a significant effect $(p = 0.034)$ of the factor 'Dementia' on QoL even after controlling for the effects of age, gender, depressiveness and employment status, suggesting that caregiving for a dementia patient was associated with lower levels of QoL in informal CGs.

## Discussion

In the present study, differences in health-related outcomes between dementia and non-dementia CGs were examined, based on a fairly large sample of CGs caring for someone legally considered to be dependent on care in Bavaria. By handing out the questionnaires directly upon the application for care level evaluation at the Medical Service of Compulsory Health Insurance Funds of Bavaria (MDK), every CG applying for an initial grade or upgrade of the care level for the CR at the Medical Service of Compulsory Health Insurance Funds of Bavaria (MDK) was addressed. In this way, systematic biases often associated with the acquisition of CGs were prevented for the recruitment of this subgroup of CGs.

Results demonstrate significant differences between the two groups of CGs regarding various health-related variables. CGs of elderly people with dementia reported a considerably high level of subjective burden, significantly higher than in the non-dementia group, which is consistent with other research on dementia caregiving

**Table 3** ANCOVA Results for QoL by 'Dementia' Controlling for the Covariates Sex CG, Age CG, Depressiveness and Employment Status $(N = 386)$

|  | SS | dF | F | p | partial $\eta^2$ |
|---|---|---|---|---|---|
| Dementia | 17.14 | 1 | 4.54 | 0.034 | .012 |
| Depressiveness (PHQ-9) | 1292.03 | 1 | 342.21 | < 0.001 | .474 |
| Sex CG | 1.82 | 1 | 0.48 | 0.489 | .001 |
| Age CG | 25.17 | 1 | 6.67 | 0.010 | .017 |
| Employment status | 30.89 | 1 | 8.18 | 0.004 | .021 |
| Error | 1434.72 | 380 | 3.78 |  |  |

*PHQ-9* Patient Health Questionnaire-9, *SS* Sum of Squares, *dF* Degrees of Freedom, *partial $\eta^2$* proportion of the total variability in *QoL* attributable to a factor or covariate (effect size measure); $R^2 = .513$ (Adj. $R^2 = .507$)

and perceived strain (e.g. [20, 38]). Along the same lines as findings suggesting more psychological morbidities in dementia CGs (e.g. [10, 39]), in our study those caring for someone with dementia tended to suffer from higher levels of depressiveness, even though the difference was not statistically significant. Despite these findings, CGs in both groups experienced positive aspects of caregiving. Contrary to our expectations based on previous literature [40] physical complaints were more or less equally pronounced in both CG groups. Furthermore, bivariate comparisons showed that dementia CGs are more involved in caregiving in terms of the hours per day that they spend on caregiving tasks (e.g. ADL and IADL), which is similar to findings by Langa and colleagues [9].

To our knowledge this study is the first to examine differences in care-related QoL between CGs of dementia patients and those caring for patients with other chronic diseases using data from a fairly large sample of CGs. Not only did bivariate comparisons show significantly lower levels of care-related QoL in dementia CGs compared to non-dementia CGs, multivariate analysis also demonstrated that these lower QoL levels appear to be due to the different experiences that dementia CGs have with caregiving rather than to CG characteristics (e.g. sex, age, employment status) or other indicators of mental health (e.g. depressiveness). Even though the effect size of dementia status as a predictor is rather small, there seems to be something unique about caring for dementia patients, over and above from sociodemographics, objective characteristics of the care situation and mental health, which leads to a poorer QoL associated with caregiving.

In addition, the results of the multiple analysis showed a strong association between higher levels of CG depressiveness and lower care-related QoL, controlling for the impact of dementia status, which corroborates previous similar findings by Santos and colleagues [25] and Farina and colleagues [30]. Further factors related to higher levels of care-related QoL seem to be an older age and being unemployed. This suggests that work might play

**Table 2** Associations of Variables of Interest with QoL (CarerQoL) $(N = 386)$

|  | Test statistic | p |
|---|---|---|
| Depressiveness (PHQ-9) | $r = -.705$ [a] | < 0.001 |
| Subjective burden (CSI) | $r = -.648$ [a] | < 0.001 |
| Physical complaints (GBB) | $r = -.668$ [a] | < 0.001 |
| Sex CG | $t = -3.146$ [b] | 0.002 |
| Employment status | $t = 3.497$ [b] | 0.001 |
| Sex CR | $t = 1.552$ [b] | 0.122 |
| Living situation | $t = -0.992$ [b] | 0.322 |
| Received support | $t = -1.121$ [b] | 0.263 |
| Relation [c] | $t = -0.299$ [b] | 0.765 |
| Educational attainment | $r = -.083$ [a] | 0.102 |
| Duration of care | $r = -.017$ [a] | 0.738 |
| Total care time | $r = -.046$ [a] | 0.365 |
| Age CG | $r = .039$ [a] | 0.449 |
| Age CR | $r = .005$ [a] | 0.918 |
| Benefits (BIZA) | $r = -.030$ [a] | 0.554 |

*CarerQoL* CarerQoL-7D, *CSI* Caregiver Strain Index, *PHQ-9* Patient Health Questionnaire-9, *GBB* Giessen Subjective Complaints List, *BIZA* Berlin Inventory of Caregivers' Burden – Dementia

[a]Pearson product moment correlation, two-tailed
[b]t-test
[c]dichotomized (spouse vs. non-spouse)

an important role in the development of stress and adverse health outcomes, either by constituting an additional stressor or as a result of a job-caregiving-conflict as explained by Pearlin (1990) in his CG stress model.

In line with previous literature, results of the current study showed that caregiving for an elderly person with dementia is associated with greater objective (e.g. total care time) and subjective strain, combined with greater depressiveness scores and a worse overall care-related QoL compared to non-dementia CGs. Although the present study provides valuable insight into the differences between dementia and non-dementia CGs, there are some limitations that must be considered when interpreting the results of this study.

### Limitations

One point of criticism of this study lays in the fact that due to high intercorrelations between subjective burden and depressiveness, only the depressiveness score was included as a covariate in the multiple prediction model for care-related QoL. Thus, the impact of dementia status on CGs' care-related QoL has not been controlled for the level of perceived burden. To rule out this putative association, future research should include perceived burden as an additional impact factor when examining the influence of dementia status on care-related QoL in multiple models.

Another limitation is that it was not possible to assess all of the variables that may have an influence on CGs' outcome variables, notably care-related QoL. With reference to Pearlin's (1990) model of CG stress, in particular secondary stressors (e.g. job-caregiving conflict) and potential moderator variables (i.e. social support) have been largely ignored. In terms of objective strain, behavioral disturbances in particular are known to typically occur as dementia progresses and have been proven to be closely correlated with CG's QoL levels [28]. Hence, these factors should be taken into consideration in future research so as to gain a more detailed and comprehensive understanding of the impact of dementia status on CGs' QoL.

As the survey questionnaires were solely handed out to CGs addressing the MDK for the care level application, our study sample is limited to a subgroup of CGs and may not represent the whole population of informal CGs, Also, with a response rate of 26.1% the study sample did not reflect the wider sample, but only the selection of CGs who were motivated to participate in the survey and able to complete the questionnaire independently. Therefore the generalizability of our findings is limited. However, another procedure would not have been feasible without a violation of the ethical principle of informed consent. Future studies of this issue should be carried out with a more comprehensive sample of CGs.

Similar to the majority of other studies in this field, our data are cross-sectional rather than longitudinal, and thus, causal conclusions need to be drawn with caution. Results from longitudinal data would be necessary to establish a more comprehensive picture of the impact of caregiving on CGs' care-related QoL when comparing dementia and non-dementia CGs. Finally, it must be noted that all data was obtained using self-report instruments, which constitutes a potential source of biases.

### Conclusions

The present study has some remarkable strengths. A large number of previous studies focusing on this issue have relied on rather small convenience samples that were recruited primarily from CG support groups or Alzheimer's associations. Data for this study were obtained from a fairly large sample that is representative for CGs applying for an initial grade or upgrade of the care level for the CR at the Medical Service of Compulsory Health Insurance Funds of Bavaria (MDK) for someone legally considered to be dependent on care in Bavaria.

The current study corroborates findings from previous research, suggesting poorer health-related outcomes like greater subjective burden, higher levels of depressiveness and lower care-related QoL levels among dementia CGs.

In addition, this study is the first to establish that lower care-related QoL levels in informal CGs are due to experiences associated with caring for dementia patients rather than CG characteristics or mental health. Still, it remains largely unclear what exactly is associated with the status of being a dementia CG that leads to such adverse effects.

### Implications for policy and practice

Nevertheless, the key take-away of this study is that it is not appropriate to generalize findings from studies examining the impact of caregiving on informal CGs caring for elderly people without dementia to dementia CGs and vice versa. Data from this study indicate that caring for a dementia patient is not only associated with greater levels of CG burden and poorer mental health, but also with lower care-related QoL compared to non-dementia CGs. In spite of these findings suggesting a greater need for support for dementia CGs, in our sample CGs in the dementia group did not receive more formal or informal support than those in the non-dementia group, despite spending a greater amount of time on caregiving. It is therefore of immediate concern to encourage dementia CGs' utilization of existing CG support services, but also to provide more specialized dementia care services, based on the specific stressors, challenges and needs associated with caregiving for elderly people with dementia. As our study revealed an association between greater depressiveness levels and decreased levels of QoL in CGs, professionals who come into contact with CGs (e.g. in CG counselling centres) should be on the lookout for CGs exhibiting depressive symptoms. In this respect, increased attention should be directed to dementia CGs once again, as they tend to show greater levels of depressiveness compared to non-dementia CGs, and therefore constitute the most vulnerable subgroup. As CG employment and a younger age seem to have adverse effects on QoL levels, a further focus should be placed on CGs facing the challenge of reconciling their job and caregiving activity, particularly when they are young.

For designing tailored intervention programs for dementia care, further research on potential causes of adverse effects of dementia caregiving as well as mediating and moderating impact factors on health itself would be valuable. Furthermore, longitudinal data would be needed to evaluate the effectiveness of potential interventions.

## Endnotes

[1]The care level describes the extent to which care is needed on a 4-level ordinal scale: 0 (no care needed), 1 (mild care needed), 2 (moderate care needed), 3 (severe care needed). It is assessed by trained experts who are independent of the insurance system. Classification is based on the need for physical care. Formal care is financed by long-term care insurance on the basis of the care level.

[2]The MDK is the official consulting and expertizing service for the statutory health and nursing care insurance (SHI). The SHI is the standard national health care insurance and covers over 85% of the German population.

[3]Total daily care time consists of the daily time required for help with ADL, IADL and supervision of the CR

[4]The median absolute deviation is a measure of statistical dispersion and is computed by averaging absolute differences between individual scores and the median of the variable. It is a more robust estimator compared to standard deviation, which is more resilient to outliers.

[5]the general experience of happiness is a broad outcome measure that does not only pertain to caregiving, but may also include aspects of well-being that are unrelated to the caregiving activity, which makes it insensitive for the assessment of *care-related* QoL

[6]two distinct scales with two scores which cannot be summed up into one comprehensive score for care-related QoL; due to the questionable benefit of a single-item VAS and to prevent potential dropouts related to CG's confusion about differing answer formats within the questionnaire (VAS vs. ordinal scale) the CarerQoL-VAS was omitted

## Abbreviations

ADL: activities of daily living; BIZA: Berlin Inventory of Caregivers' Burden - Dementia; CarerQoL: CarerQoL-7D; CG: caregiver; CR: care recipient; CSI: Caregiver Strain Index; GBB: Giessen Symptom List; IADL: instrumental activities of daily living; MDK: Medical Service of Compulsory Health Insurance Funds; PHQ-9: Patient Health Questionnaire-9; QoL: quality of life; SHI: statutory health care insurance; WHO: World Health Organisation

## Acknowledgements

We kindly thank Mrs. Graf for her support with the collection of data. We also thank all of the informal caregivers for their participation in this study. The generous provision of reference data by the BARMER GEK is also gratefully acknowledged.

## Authors' contributions

EG, OR conception, design and implementation of the study. NK, AP data analysis. EG, NK, AP data interpretation. NK, AP preparation of manuscript. EG, OR, NK, AP revision of manuscript. The present work was performed in partial fulfillment of the requirements for obtaining the degree 'Dr. rer. biol. hum.' by NK. All authors read and approved the final manuscript.

## Competing interests

The authors declare that they have no competing interests.

## Author details

[1]Department of Psychiatry and Psychotherapy, Center for Health Service Research in Medicine, Friedrich-Alexander-University Erlangen-Nuremberg, Schwabachanlage 6, D-91054 Erlangen, Germany. [2]Medical Service of Compulsory Health Insurance Funds (MDK) of Bavaria, Haidenauplatz 1, D-81667 Munich, Germany.

## References

1. Statistisches Bundesamt: Pflegestatistik 2013. Pflege im Rahmen der Pflegeversicherung. Deutschlandergebnisse; 2015.
2. Möglichkeiten und Grenzen selbstständiger Lebensführung in Privathaushalten [https://www.bundesregierung.de/Content/Infomaterial/BMFSFJ/selbststaendigkeit-im-alter_29220.html]. Accessed 20 Aug 2018.
3. Vitaliano PP, Zhang J, Scanlan JM. Is caregiving hazardous to one's physical health? A meta-analysis. Psychol Bull. 2003;129(6):946–72.
4. Pinquart M, Sörensen S. Differences between caregivers and noncaregivers in psychological health and physical health: a meta-analysis. Psychol Aging. 2003;18(2):250–67.
5. Perkins M, Howard VJ, Wadley VG, Crowe M, Safford MM, Haley WE, Howard G, Roth DL. Caregiving strain and all-cause mortality: evidence from the REGARDS study. J Gerontol Ser B Psychol Sci Soc Sci. 2013;68(4):504–12.
6. Pinquart M, Sörensen S. Associations of stressors and uplifts of caregiving with caregiver burden and depressive mood: a meta-analysis. J Gerontol Ser B Psychol Sci Soc Sci. 2003;58B(2):112–28.
7. Pinquart M, Sörensen S. Correlates of physical health of informal caregivers: a meta-analysis. J Gerontol. 2007;62b(2):126–37.
8. Brodaty H, Donkin M. Family caregivers of people with dementia. Dialogues Clin Neurosci. 2009;11(2):217–28.
9. Langa KM, Chernew ME, Kabeto MU, Herzog AR, Ofstedal MB, Willis RJ, Wallace RB, Mucha LM, Straus WL, Fendrick AM. National estimates of the quantity and cost of informal caregiving for the elderly with dementia. J Gen Intern Med. 2001;16(11):770–8.
10. Gonzalez-Salvador MT, Arango C, Lyketsos CG, Barba AC. The stress and psychological morbidity of the Alzheimer patient caregiver. Int J Geriatr Psychiatry. 1999;14(9):701–10.
11. Miyamoto Y, Tachimori H, Ito H. Formal caregiver burden in dementia: impact of behavioral and psychological symptoms of dementia and activities of daily living. Geriatr Nurs. 2010;31(4):246–53.
12. Ory MG, Yee JL, Tennstedt SL. The extent and impact of dementia care: unique challenges experienced by family caregivers. In: Schulz R, editor. Handbook on dementia caregiving: evidence-based interventions for family caregivers. New York: Springer Publishing Co.; 2000. p. 330.

13. Grau H, Graessel E, Berth H. The subjective burden of informal caregivers of persons with dementia: extended validation of the German language version of the burden scale for family caregivers (BSFC). Aging Ment Health. 2015;19(2):159–68.

14. Germain S, Adam S, Olivier C, Cash H, Ousset PJ, Andrieu S, Vellas B, Meulemans T, Reynish E, Salmon E, et al. Does cognitive impairment influence burden in caregivers of patients with Alzheimer's disease? J Alzheimers Dis. 2009;17(1):105–14.

15. McConaghy R, Caltabiano ML. Caring for a person with dementia: exploring relationships between perceived burden, depression, coping and well-being. Nurs Health Sci. 2005;7(2):81–91.

16. Laks J, Goren A, Duenas H, Novick D, Kahle-Wrobleski K. Caregiving for patients with Alzheimer's disease or dementia and its association with psychiatric and clinical comorbidities and other health outcomes in Brazil. Int J Geriatr Psychiatry. 2016;31(2):176–85.

17. Gräßel E. Häusliche Pflege dementiell und nicht dementiell Erkrankter Teil II: Gesundheit und Belastung der Pflegenden. Z Gerontol Geriatr. 1998;31(1): 57–62.

18. Fonareva I, Oken BS. Physiological and functional consequences of caregiving for relatives with dementia. Int Psychogeriatr. 2014;26(5):725–47.

19. Schulz R, Martire L. Family caregiving of persons with dementia - Prevalance, health effects, and Suppport strategies. Am J Geriatr Psychiatry. 2004;12:240–9.

20. Ory MG, Hoffman RR 3rd, Yee JL, Tennstedt S, Schulz R. Prevalence and impact of caregiving: a detailed comparison between dementia and nondementia caregivers. Gerontologist. 1999;39(2):177–85.

21. Bell CM, Araki SS, Neumann PJ. The association between caregiver burden and caregiver health-related quality of life in Alzheimer disease. Alzheimer Dis Assoc Disord. 2001;15(3):129–36.

22. The EuroQol Group. EuroQol - a new facility for the measurement of health-related quality of life. Health Policy. 1990;16:199–208.

23. World Health Organization. Preamble to the Constitution of the World Health Organization as adopted by the International Health Conference, New York, 19–22 June, 1946. New York: World Health Organization. p. 1948.

24. Glozman JM. Quality of life of caregivers. Neuropsychol Rev. 2004;14(4):183–96.

25. Santos RL, Sousa MF, Simoes-Neto JP, Nogueira ML, Belfort TT, Torres B, Rosa RD, Laks J, Dourado MC. Caregivers' quality of life in mild and moderate dementia. Arq Neuropsiquiatr. 2014;72(12):931–7.

26. Brouwer WB, van Exel NJ, van Gorp B, Redekop WK. The CarerQol instrument: a new instrument to measure care-related quality of life of informal caregivers for use in economic evaluations. Qual Life Res. 2006; 15(6):1005–21.

27. Coen RF, O'Boyle CA, Swanwick GRJ, Coakley D. Measuring the impact on relatives of caring for people with Alzheimer's disease: quality of life, burden and well-being. Psychol Health. 1999;14(2):253–61.

28. Ferrara M, Langiano E, Di Brango T, De Vito E, Di Cioccio L, Bauco C. Prevalence of stress, anxiety and depression in with Alzheimer caregivers. Health Qual Life Outcomes. 2008;6:93.

29. Srivastava G, Tripathi RK, Tiwari SC, Singh B, Tripathi SM. Caregiver burden and quality of life of key caregivers of patients with dementia. Indian J Psychol Med. 2016;38(2):133–6.

30. Farina N, Page TE, Daley S, Brown A, Bowling A, Basset T, Livingston G, Knapp M, Murray J, Banerjee S. Factors associated with the quality of life of family carers of people with dementia: a systematic review. Alzheimers Dement. 2017;13(5):572–81.

31. Brähler E, Hinz A, Scheer JW. GBB-24. Der Gießener Beschwerdebogen. Manual. Bern: Hans Huber; 2008.

32. Robinson BC. Validation of a caregiver strain index. J Gerontol. 1983;38(3):344–8.

33. Kroenke K, Spitzer RL, Williams JBW. The PHQ-9. J Gen Intern Med. 2001; 16(9):606–13.

34. Zank S, Schacke C, Leipold B. Berliner Inventar zur Angehörigenbelastung - Demenz (BIZA-D). Z Klin Psychol Psychother. 2006;35(4):296–305.

35. Lutomski JE, van Exel NJ, Kempen GI, Moll van Charante EP, den Elzen WP, Jansen AP, Krabbe PF, Steunenberg B, Steyerberg EW, Olde Rikkert MG, et al. Validation of the care-related quality of life instrument in different study settings: findings from the older persons and informal caregivers survey minimum DataSet (TOPICS-MDS). Qual Life Res. 2015;24(5):1281–93.

36. World Health Organization. The ICD-10 classification of mental and behavioural disorders: clinical descriptions and diagnostic guidelines. Geneva: World Health Organization (WHO); 1992.

37. BARMER GEK (31.10.2016). In pesonal Communication 2016.

38. Papastavrou E, Charalambous A, Tsangari H, Karayiannis G. The burdensome and depressive experience of caring: what cancer, schizophrenia, and Alzheimer's disease caregivers have in common. Cancer Nurs. 2012;35(3): 187–94.

39. Suehs BT, Shah SN, Davis CD, Alvir J, Faison WE, Patel NC, van Amerongen D, Bobula J. Household members of persons with Alzheimer's disease: health conditions, healthcare resource use, and healthcare costs. J Am Geriatr Soc. 2014;62(3):435–41.

40. Clipp EC, George LK. Dementia and cancer: a comparison of spouse caregivers. Gerontologist. 1993;33(4):534–41.

# 17

# Potentially inappropriate medication use among hypertensive older African-American adults

Mohsen Bazargan[1,2*], James L Smith[1] and Ebony O King[1,2]

## Abstract

**Background:** Inappropriate use of medications, particularly among minority older adults with co-morbidity, remains a major public health concern. The American Geriatrics Society (AGS) reports that Potentially Inappropriate Medication (PIM) continues to be prescribed for older adults, despite evidence of poor outcomes. The main objective of this study was to examine the prevalence of PIM use among underserved non-institutionalized hypertensive older African-American adults. Furthermore, this study examines potential correlations between PIM use and the number and type of chronic conditions.

**Methods:** This cross-sectional study is comprised of a convenience sample of 193 hypertensive non-institutionalized African-American adults, aged 65 years and older recruited from several senior housing units located in underserved areas of South Los Angeles. The updated 2015 AGS Beers Criteria was used to identify participants using PIMs.

**Results:** Almost one out of two participants had inappropriate medication use. While the average number of PIMs taken was 0.87 drugs, the range was from one to seven medications. Almost 23% of PIMs were due to drugs with potential drug-drug interactions. The most common PIM was the use of proton pump inhibitors (PPI) and Central Nervous System (CNS) active agents. Nearly 56% of PIMs potentially increased the risk of falls and fall-associated bone fractures. The use of PIMs was significantly higher among participants who reported a higher number of chronic conditions. Nearly 70% of participants with PIM use reported suffering from chronic pain.

**Conclusions:** The major reason for high levels of polypharmacy, PIMs, and drug interactions is that patients suffer from multiple chronic conditions. But it may not be possible or necessary to treat all chronic conditions. Therefore, the goals of care should be explicitly reviewed with the patient in order to determine which of the many chronic conditions has the greatest impact on the life goals and/or functional priorities of the patient. Those drugs that have a limited impact on the patient's functional priorities and that may cause harmful drug-drug interactions can be reduced or eliminated, while the remaining medications can focus on the most important functional priorities of the patient.

**Keywords:** Potentially inappropriate medication (PIM), Minority, Older adults, Pain, Falls

## Background

Older African-American adults have a high prevalence of many of the most potent cardiovascular disease risk factors, particularly hypertension (HTN) and diabetes mellitus [1]. The combination of HTN and diabetes is lethal and is associated with elevated all-cause and cardiovascular disease mortality among older adults [2, 3]. In 2015, more than 71% of older African American Medicare fee-for-service beneficiaries had at least two chronic conditions and 43% suffered from at least four conditions [4]. National data show that 39.8%, 45.6%, and 64.4% of older African-American Medicare adult beneficiaries have diabetes, hyperlipidemia, and HTN, respectively [5]. Effective treatment of these conditions often requires the prescribing of multiple medications. Within the last decade, prescription medication (Rx) use has increased dramatically among older adults, i.e., the median number of Rx used doubled from 2 to 4, and those

* Correspondence: mobazarg@cdrewu.edu
[1]Charles R. Drew University of Medicine and Science, 1731 East 120th Street, Los Angeles, CA 90005, USA
[2]University of California, Los Angeles, USA

taking more than 5 medications tripled from 13 to 39% [6]. This increase in medication use among older adults was driven, in part, by higher use of antidiabetics, anti-hypertensives, and statins [6]. The use of these medications has led to substantial improvements in Low-Density Lipoprotein Cholesterol, blood pressure and glycemic control. Despite these favorable outcomes, suboptimal use of medications among ethnic/racial population limits maximal health benefits [7–9]. Three major medication-related challenges that lead to suboptimal use of medications are: 1) nonadherence to prescribed drug regimens [10–16], 2) excessive and unnecessary use of medication [17, 18], and 3) inappropriate use of medications [19].

The American Geriatrics Society reports that Potentially Inappropriate Medication (PIM) continues to be prescribed for older adults, despite evidence of poor outcomes from the use of PIMs in this segment of our population [20]. Several studies documented that PIM use has been associated with an increased risk of falls and hip fractures [21]. A recent systematic review documented that PIM use was associated with a 1.6-fold increased mortality in older adults [22]. Another recent meta-analysis of PIM use in community-dwelling older American adults found the median rate of PIM to be 19.6% with a range of 4.5 to 33.3% [23].

Prevalence estimates for PIMs represent an important healthcare quality metric [24]. Specifically, given the high rate of PIM use among underserved older African-American adults, there is a need for ongoing monitoring of inappropriate medication use among this segment of our population. Additionally, it is important to continue investigating the extent and consequences of PIM use among those older African-American adults with medical conditions, such as cardiovascular disease, that place them at risk for poorer clinical outcomes. A recent study that examined PIM use among a large sample ($n = 16,588$) of non-institutionalized older adults (age $\geq 65$) from the 2006–2010 Medical Expenditure Panel Survey documented strong associations between PIM use and cardiovascular disease and other chronic conditions [24].

While several studies in the United States and other countries have examined the prevalence and correlates of PIM use among aged populations [23, 25–32], to the best of our knowledge, few studies have specifically examined the older African-American community [19]. The main objective of this study is to examine PIM use among non-institutionalized hypertensive older African-American adults, using the revised Beers' criteria (2015), to identify those individuals that may be disproportionately affected by inappropriate drug use to be targeted for appropriate interventions to reduce the use of PIMs. Furthermore, this study examines potential correlations between PIM use and the number and type of chronic conditions. In addition, we present five cases in order to gain insight into PIM use among our sample. These case studies provide a variety of actual scenarios that may help providers to reexamine PIM issues from their perspectives and then synthesize a solution in their own practice.

## Methods

This cross-sectional observational study is comprised of a convenience sample of 193 non-institutionalized African-American adults, aged 65 years and older, with a clinical diagnosis of hypertension.

### Participants and setting

Participants were recruited from several predominantly African-American senior centers and housing units located in underserved areas of South Los Angeles. This study is part of a larger effort to examine medication use among a sample of 342 African Americans aged 55 years and older. However, the current study used only participants that were 65 years of age or older (193) from the study sample to examine the use of PIMs. Only four potential subjects refused to participate in our study. No participants were selected that were residing in skilled nursing facilities. Potential participants were excluded if they were enrolled in other clinical trials. In addition, using a standard screening tool, potential participants with cognitive deficits were excluded from the study. This investigation was approved by the Charles R. Drew University of Medicine and Science Institutional Review Board. A written informed consent was collected from all participants. The study used structured, face-to-face survey interviews. Data used in the study were collected from November 2015 – February 2017.

### *Measurement*

The survey instrument was a collection of validated instruments from various sources [11, 17, 19, 33–35]. Demographic variables included age, gender, education, living arrangement, and disability status.

*Medication use* was assessed using the drug inventory method. Participants were asked to bring all over-the-counter and Rx medications that were taken within 2 weeks prior to the interviews. The interviewer transcribed from the container label the name of the medication, strength of the drug, expiration date, instructions, special warnings, providers' information, etc. The medication assessment of this study employed the methodology established by Sorensen and colleagues [36–38], which was adopted by our research team previously [11, 17, 19, 33–35].

### PIM use

The updated 2015 AGS Beers Criteria was used to identify PIM [20]. In this study PIM was defined as the number of medications that must be avoided but were prescribed for an older adult. Based on the 2015 AGS Beers Criteria, calculation of PIM should not count a prescription as a PIM in the presence of certain indications due to specific clinical conditions and criteria [Examples: use of proton-pump inhibitors (PPI) for less than 8 weeks; use of antipsychotics, first- (conventional) and second- (atypical) generation for treatment of schizophrenia, bipolar disorder, or short-term use as antiemetic during chemotherapy; use of non-cyclooxygenase-NSAIDs, oral for young-old (< 75 years) for short duration; etc.] [20]. In our study, a prescribed medication was considered appropriate (not being counted as a PIM) using the above Beers criterion in 19 PIMs (17 participants).

The AGS 2015 Updated Beers Criteria lists the drug-drug and drug-disease interactions that should be avoided in older adults. We documented the presence of these interactions by referencing this list. PIMs were counted as a total number and an adjusted number, the latter indicating a likely elimination of a medication as a PIM if a medical exception was met.

## Chronic conditions

Participants were asked to report on diagnoses only if a physician had confirmed them previously. We collected information about 13 conditions: diabetes, hypertension, thyroid disorder, cardiac disease, cancer, asthma, osteoarthritis, rheumatoid arthritis, chronic obstructive pulmonary disease, intestinal disease, depression, and hypercholesterolemia. We also used an alternative method based on the labels of medication containers to identify participants' chronic conditions. We assigned a condition to a participant if the therapeutic purpose of the medications used was clearly linked to the presence of a chronic condition. This method (examination of the medication containers) leads to an additional 25 conditions. However, a vast majority of these 25 medical conditions was not frequently diagnosed, including lupus, hepatitis, vertigo, cachexia, herpes, edema, seizures etc. Relying on self-report or administrative data alone in documenting chronic conditions underestimates the prevalence of chronic conditions, which results in biased estimates of multi-morbidity [39].

## Sample size and statistical analysis

Both descriptive and inferential statistics were used to document prevalence and correlates of PIM use among our sample. Pearson correlation coefficients, chi-squared tests, and the binary logistic regression techniques were used to examine the correlation between the PIM use and 1) number of medication use; 2) number of chronic conditions; and 3) type of chronic conditions. Examining correlation between several types of chronic conditions and

PIM, the Bonferroni correction was used to counteract the problem of inflated type I errors. All statistical analyses were performed with the Statistical Package for Social Sciences (SPSS) version 22. Based on previous studies, we expected at least 30% of study participants will be using at least one PIM [19, 23]. Therefore the sample size of 193 subjects is sufficient to determine the extent of PIM use among older African American adults.

## Results

Table 1 reports the demographic characteristics and health status of our sample. There were 193 study participants, with an age range from 65 to 96 years (M $75.2 \pm 7$). Approximately 48% of the participants were 75 years of age or older and 67% of the participants were women. The number of reported chronic illnesses ranged from one to 17, with the average being eight ($7.8 \pm 3.2$). One out of four participants had at least 10 chronic conditions. Participants were taking an average of 7.3 (SD = 3.60) prescription drugs (range: 1–24). Thirty percent of participants were using at least nine medications, whereas 27% and 43% of participants were taking five to eight and one to four prescription medications, respectively (Table 1). In addition, our data shows that nearly 21%, 36%, 60%, 65% of participants were diagnosed with depression, diabetes mellitus, hyperlipidemia, and chronic pain, respectively.

Our data indicates that inappropriate drug use occurred in 46% (99) of participants. In addition, 26% (55) 13% (25) and 8% (19) of participants were taking one, two or at least three inappropriate medications, respectively. While the average number of PIMs taken was 0.97 drugs, the range was from one to seven medications. A total of 188 PIMs were used by ninety-nine individuals. Almost 23% (43 out of 188 PIMs) were due to drugs with potential drug-drug interactions. The most common PIM was the use of proton pump inhibitors (PPI) and greater than two or more Central Nervous System (CNS) active agents, occurring at 46% and 18%, respectively. Nearly 56% (105 out of 188) of PIMs potentially increased the risk of falls and fall-associated bone fractures.

The use of PIMs was significantly higher among participants who were taking a higher number of medications ($r = 0.51$; $p < .0001$). Participants who were taking at least six medications were 3.6 times (OR = 3.6; CI: 1.91–6.7; $p < 0.001$) more likely to also be receiving inappropriate medications. Similarly, the use of PIMs was significantly higher among participants who reported a higher number of chronic conditions ($r = 0.46$; $p < 0.0001$). Participants who were diagnosed with at least six chronic conditions were 2.7 times (OR = 2.73; CI: 1.40–5.4; $p < 0.001$) more likely to be receiving inappropriate medications. In addition, three chronic medical conditions showed a statistically significant independent correlation

**Table 1** Demographic characteristics and health status of sample (N = 193)

| Demographic and health status | N (%) |
|---|---|
| Age | |
| 65–74 years | 100 (52) |
| ≥ 75 years | 93 (48) |
| Gender | |
| Male | 63 (33) |
| Female | 130 (67) |
| Education | |
| No high school diploma | 48 (25) |
| High school diploma | 68 (35) |
| Some college or more | 77 (40) |
| Living Arrangement | |
| Living alone | 150 (78) |
| Living with someone | 42 (22) |
| Disability Status | |
| Yes | 89 (44) |
| No | 104 (54) |
| Diabetes | |
| Yes | 35 (18) |
| No | 158 (82) |
| Hyperlipidemia | |
| Yes | 115 (60) |
| No | 78 (40) |
| Chronic Pain | |
| Yes | 125 (65) |
| No | 68 (35) |
| Depression | |
| Yes | 41 (21) |
| No | 152 (79) |
| Number of Prescribed Medications | |
| 0–4 | 52 (27) |
| 5–8 | 84 (43) |
| 9–24 | 57 (30) |
| Number of Chronic Conditions | |
| 1–5 | 55 (29) |
| 6–10 | 93 (48) |
| 11–17 | 45 (23) |

with PIM use. Participants who were diagnosed with chronic pain (OR = 2.4; CI: 1.3–4.5; $P < .005$), depression (OR = 2.8; CI: 1.4–5.8; $P < .005$), and gastroesophageal reflux disease (OR = 2.9; CI: 1.6–5.3; $P < .0001$) were 2.4, 2.8 and 2.9 times, respectively, more likely to use PIMs than their counterparts without these chronic conditions.

## Case studies
### Case 47
The participant is in her 70s with a medical history of osteoporosis, recent fall (12 months ago), depression, sleep disorder, and chronic pain. She has a total of 12 self-reported medical conditions and is taking a total of five potentially inappropriate medications (PIMs). At the time of the survey, the participant was taking a PPI for 12 months. PPI use longer than 8 weeks is considered a PIM as it increases the risk of developing *Clostridium difficile* infection and bone loss and fractures. She was also taking nortriptyline, a tricyclic anti-depressant with strong anti-cholinergic properties, and hydrocodone-acetaminophen. These two drugs separately and together have the potential of a > 2 CNS active agent drug-drug interaction, increasing the risk of falls and/or fractures. Lastly, the participant is taking meloxicam, a non-steroidal anti-inflammatory drug (NSAID), which in patients older than 74 years of age, poses considerable risk for peptic ulcer disease and/or development of gastrointestinal bleeding.

### Case 102
The participant is in her 70's with a medical history significant for Parkinson's disease, dependent activities of daily living (ADLs), depression and heart problems with a pacemaker. She has a total of 12 self-reported medical conditions, one-third of which are associated with PIMs that pose a significant risk of morbidity. At the time of the survey, the participant was taking a PPI for 2 weeks, although the medication had been prescribed for 12 months. She was also taking hydrocodone-acetaminophen and risperidone, which together has the potential of a > 2 CNS active agent drug-drug interaction increasing the risk of falls and/or fractures. In the case of this participant, this would hold true as the participant has both dependent ADLs and Parkinson's disease. Of particular significance is the use of the anti-psychotic risperidone in this participant with her concurrent diagnoses of Parkinson's disease. All anti-psychotics, with the exception of aripiprazole, quetiapine, and clozapine, are believed to carry the risk of the precipitation and worsening of Parkinson's symptoms.

### Case 229
The participant is in her 80s with a medical history significant for hypertension, sleep disorder and chronic pain. She has a total of eight self-reported medical conditions and a total of six PIMs including three separate drug-drug interactions. The participant is taking triamterene and lisinopril which together pose a risk for drug-drug interactions due to an increased risk of hyperkalemia. The participant is also taking temazepam, which by itself and together with nortriptyline and hydrocodone poses two separate > 2 CNS drug interactions and increases the risk of cognitive impairment, delirium, falls, fractures, and

motor-vehicle accidents. Nortriptyline by itself and to-gether with hydrocodone and temazapam has the poten-tial of two separate > 2 CNS drug-drug interactions and present a PIM with risks as described above. The partici-pant has a significant risk for morbidity for taking > 3 CNS active agents.

### Case 249

The participant is in his seventies with a medical history significant for dependent ADLs, heart problems, chronic pain and a sleep disorder. He has a total of 13 self-reported medical conditions and is taking a total of 13 medications, six of which are PIMs including three sets of drug-drug interactions. Tramadol and codeine are both opiates and are identified as PIMs as individual drugs in patients with a history or risk of falls or frac-ture, as is the case in this patient with dependent ADLs. Together these drugs also pose a > 2 CNS active drug-drug interaction. The participant is also taking a corticosteroid and NSAIDs, which together can cause a drug-drug interaction and increase the risk of peptic ulcer disease and/or gastrointestinal bleeding. Lastly, the participant is taking diphenhydramine, which by itself is a PIM in patients with a history or risks of falls and/or fractures. Diphenhydramine together with solifenacin is a risk for drug-drug interaction as both drugs are strong anticholinergics, increasing the risk of cognitive decline.

### Case 288

The participant is in her 80s with a medical history of dependent ADLs, rheumatoid arthritis, thyroid disease, and breast cancer remission. She also has a total of 16 self-reported medical conditions, is taking a total of 16 medications, seven of which are PIMs including three sets of drug-drug interactions. The participant is taking lorazepam, oxycodone, and morphine, which by them-selves are PIM in patients with a history or risk of falls and/or fracture, as is the case of this participant who has dependent ADLs. Together these CNS active agents cre-ate three different sets of > 2 CNS active agent drug-drug interactions. Lastly, the participant was taking a PPI for 7 months, which increases the risk of clostrid-ium difficile, fractures, and falls.

## Discussion

Use of medication that may cause more harm than bene-fit is considered potentially inappropriate when safer pharmacological or non-pharmacological alternatives exist [40]. Older African-American adults are a particu-larly vulnerable population as they suffer from a higher number of chronic conditions than their white counter-parts. Our data show that 41% of older hypertensive Af-rican Americans were taking at least eight medications. In addition, one out of four participants reported at least

10 chronic conditions. Yet we documented that one out of two participants are taking at least one inappropriate medication. Similar to this study, a recent study con-ducted among a sample of 400 older underserved African-American adults reported a high rate of PIM use [19]. The rate of PIM use in our study is substan-tially higher than previously reported PIM use among older adults. The 2006–2010 Medical Expenditure Panel Survey (MEPS), shows that one-third (32.8%) of older African-American adults used a PIM [24]. The higher rate of PIM use in our sample may reflect the fact that our sample has been recruited from the Service Planning Area 6 (SPA 6) of Los Angeles County, one of the most underserved minority communities in the US. We spe-cifically selected SPA 6 because nearly half of older adults living in SPA 6 are African American (49%). Home to more than one million residents, SPA 6 has disproportionately greater health disparities than the rest of Los Angeles County [41]. A good example is the age-adjusted coronary heart disease death rate which is significantly higher for SPA 6 (147.5 per 100,000 popula-tion) than the Nation (102.6) and the rest of Los Angeles County (116.7). Another example is the aged-adjusted diabetes death rate which is 37.6, 21.9, and 21.2 per 100,000 population for the SPA 6, Los Angeles County and the Nation, respectively [41].

Both quantitative analysis and the cases reported here show that chronic pain is one of the important common denominators of PIM use. Fifty-four percent of our study population who were diagnosed with chronic pain consume at least one PIM. Indeed, it is not surprising that suffering from chronic pain leads to PIM use. Previ-ous studies have also shown that inappropriate pain medications are frequently prescribed for older adults [42]. However, empirical evidence suggests that older African Americans have a higher risk for severe pain compared with non-Hispanic whites [43]. Yet severe mismanagement of pain in underserved older African Americans, particularly those with comorbidity, multiple providers, and limited access to health care has been documented [19]. A recent study shows that one in four older African American were taking NSAIDs, which can cause serious side effects in older adults with multiple chronic conditions [19]. The use of pain medication was associated with drug-drug interactions, drug duplication, and PIM use [19]. These results support the need for cli-nicians to be aware of PIM use by older adults, recognize associated medication-related adverse events, and avoid prescribing age-inappropriate medications to vulnerable older adult patients [42].

Another commonly prescribed PIM in our study was taken by participants who were diagnosed with the gas-troesophageal reflux disease (GERD). A recent study examining the PIM use among older patients with cardiovascular disease also listed the unnecessary use of PPIs common among older adults [44]. It is important that providers carefully consider the use of PPIs in older adults and monitor their continued use to prevent the drug-drug interactions and side effects, including risk of *Clostridium difficile* infection, bone loss, and fractures [45].

In addition, another common denominator for PIM use, both in our case studies and in the quantitative analysis, was diagnoses of depression among our older African-American adults. Given that several psychotropic drugs are included in Beers' list, it was not surprising to find that the presence of depressive symptoms was associated with potentially inappropriate medication use. Other studies have confirmed this association [46]. It has been empirically documented that use of anti-cholinergic medications that are listed as PIMs leads to cognitive declines and dementia among older adults [47]. Therefore, it is important that physicians avoid prescribing anti-cholinergic medication listed as PIMs, particularly for old-old adults [47]. In addition, the standard care for dementia should include careful medication review and management to avoid PIM use in this vulnerable population [48].

Another overarching theme that emerged from our case reports is the history of falls and use of PIMs that substantially increases the risk of falls among our participants. Our data shows that 56% of PIMs used by our participants potentially increased the risk of falls and fall-associated bone fractures. Several studies documented that PIM use has been associated with an increased risk of falls and hip fractures [21]. There are mixed findings in the literature in regards to the racial differences on falls among older adults. Many studies found that older non-Hispanic Whites were more likely to fall than older African Americans [49–51], yet several studies revealed no racial differences or excessive falls rates among African-American older adults compared to their White counterparts [52–55]. However, African Americans have a greater fall-risk profile when compared to non-Hispanic Whites. Older African Americans' higher fall-risk scores are attributed to their physical functioning and medication use [56] and poorer self-rated health and multiple comorbidities [57]. The 2014 Behavioral Risk Factor Surveillance System survey shows that regardless of ethnic background, the rate of fall-related injuries is significantly higher in the older adults with poor health (480 per 1000) than their counterparts with excellent health (69 per 1000) [58]. Managing at least one chronic disease increases the risk of falling by 32% [59]. The most recent report from the Center for Medicare and Medicaid Services (CMS) Chronic Condition Data Warehouse shows a higher prevalence of major chronic conditions among African-American older adults compared to their non-Hispanic White counterparts. African-American older adults experience higher rates of hypertension (68.4% vs 57.7), diabetes (39.8% vs. 24.7),

chronic kidney disease (26.7 vs. 18.2), heart failure (17.9% vs. 14.3%), Alzheimer's disease/dementia (14.2% vs. 11.3%) stroke (5.7% vs. 4.2) and cancer (10.1% vs. 9.1%). Therefore, it is imperative that providers who are prescribing medications to African-American older adults with multiple chronic conditions, be cognizant of the vulnerability of their patients and avoid prescribing the PIMs that increase the risk of falls.

### Limitations of the study

The research team did not have access to the participants' medical records to record the medications that were prescribed for participants. Medication-related information was collected directly from drug containers. Second, the study used a convenience sample, which limits the generalizability of our findings. Finally, we used a cross-sectional study design, which allowed us to collect data at only a single point in time. Nevertheless, this study provides vital information about a population (underserved African-American older adults) that has not been carefully studied to this point.

### Conclusions

The revised AGS Beers criteria provides valuable tools to guide prescribing in older adults. All clinicians who provide medical care for older adults should be familiar with this tool. However, it is important to note that reducing PIMs is only one component of improving quality of care for older adults [60]. Relying only on Beers criteria obscures the detection of important drug-related problems such as drug use without an indication, untreated conditions, or poor adherence [61]. PIM, polypharmacy, and nonadherence to medications are all interconnected, and these factors are linked to effectiveness of medications and health outcomes among older adults [11, 19, 62]. However, no intervention trials have focused on these medication-related challenges together to improve adherence to medications among African-American older adults [63]. Therefore, the first step in reducing medication-related challenges and improving the effectiveness and management of medications among older adults, particularly older African-American adults, is to conduct a comprehensive assessment of their medications [64].

The likely reason for high levels of polypharmacy, PIMs, and drug interactions is that patients suffer from multiple chronic conditions. But it may not be possible or necessary to treat all chronic conditions. Therefore, the goals of care should be explicitly reviewed with the patient (or, if the patient has limited capacity for decision making, with the patient's caretaker) in order to determine which of the many chronic conditions has the greatest impact on the life goals and/or functional priorities of the patient. Those drugs that have a limited impact on the patient's functional priorities and that may cause harmful drug-drug interactions can be reduced or eliminated, while the remaining medications can focus on the most important functional priorities of the patient.

A recent interventional study used electronic alerts at the point of computerized order-entry to reduce PIM prescribing among a large sample of older veteran adults. The study showed a modest reduction in the rate of the top 10 most common newly-prescribed PIMs (from 9.0 to 8.3%; $p = 0.016$). This intervention was only able to modify the prescribing behaviors of neurologists and detected no positive impact on prescribing of other provider specialists [65]. This is another indication that multidimensional and multicomponent interventions are needed to focus on the relationship between comorbidities and medication-related challenges among African-American older adults [66, 67].

The four case reports given above clearly show that there is additional need for multidisciplinary interventions to reduce medication-related challenges among older African-American adults with comorbidities, particularly those who suffer from pain. Safe and appropriate prescribing is a complex process, involving issues of over-prescription, under-prescription, and inappropriate prescription [68]. Without close and continuous collaboration between providers and patients with a coherent multi-pronged strategy, de-prescribing, as part of the solution to address over-prescribing and inappropriate prescribing, is almost impossible.

## Abbreviations

ADL: Activities of daily living; AGS: American Geriatrics Society; CI: Confidence intervals; CMS: Center for Medicare and Medicaid Services; CNS: Central nervous system; GERD: Gastroesophageal reflux disease; HTN: Hypertension; MEPS: Medical expenditure panel survey; NSAID: Non-steroidal anti-inflammatory drug; OR: Odds ratio; PIM: Potentially inappropriate medication; PPI: Proton pump inhibitors; Rx: Prescription medication; SPA 6: Service planning area 6; SPSS: Statistical package for social sciences

## Acknowledgements

We thank all participants who patiently participated in lengthy face-to-face interviews and allowed us to document all medications that they use. Additionally, we sincerely acknowledge the valuable suggestions and comments from Dr. Thomas Yoshikawa who carefully reviewed this manuscript.

## Funding

CMS: "1I0CMS331364–01" and NIMHD: "U54MD007598" and "R25 MD007610." The Funding agencies had no role in the design of the study and collection, analysis, interpretation of data, or in writing the manuscript.

## Authors' contributions

All authors have contributed significantly and they all are in agreement with the content of the manuscript. MB was the primary investigator, leading the study, involved in conception and design, data analysis and writing of the manuscript. JLS contributed to the acquisition of participants, data collection, and interpretation of data. EOK was involved in interpretation of data and drafting the manuscript.

## Competing interests

The authors declare that they have no competing interests.

## References

1. Howard G, Safford MM, Moy CS, et al. Racial differences in the incidence of cardiovascular risk factors in older black and white adults. J Am Geriatr Soc. 2017;65(1):83–90.
2. Oh J-Y, Allison MA, Barrett-Connor E. Different impacts of hypertension and diabetes mellitus on all-cause and cardiovascular mortality in community-dwelling older adults: the rancho Bernardo study. J Hypertens. 2017;35(1):55–62.
3. Franklin SS, Thijs L, Li Y, et al. Masked hypertension in diabetes mellitus: treatment implications for clinical practice. Hypertension. 2013;61:964–71.
4. Center for Medicare and Medicaid Services. Prevalence state level: all beneficiaries by race/ethnicity and age, 2007-2015: multiple chronic conditions prevalence state table: black or African American fee-for-service beneficiaries by age, 2015. 2016. https://www.cms.gov/Research-Statistics-Data-and-Systems/Statistics-Trends-and-Reports/Chronic-Conditions/MCC_Main.html. Accessed July 2017.
5. Center for Medicare and Medicaid Services. Chronic conditions prevalence state table: black or African American fee-for-service beneficiaries by age, 2015. 2016. https://www.cms.gov/Research-Statistics-Data-and-Systems/Statistics-Trends-and-Reports/Chronic-Conditions/MCC_Main.html. Accessed July 2017.
6. Charlesworth CJ, Smit E, Lee DS, Alramadhan F, Odden MC. Polypharmacy among adults aged 65 years and older in the United States: 1988–2010. J Gerontol A Biol Sci Med Sci. 2015;70:989–95.
7. Krousel-Wood MA, Muntner P, Islam T, Morisky DE, Webber LS. Barriers to and determinants of medication adherence in hypertension management: perspective of the cohort study of medication adherence among older adults. Med Clin North Am. 2009;93(3):753–69.
8. Young JH, Ng D, Ibe C, et al. Access to care, treatment ambivalence, medication nonadherence, and long-term mortality among severely hypertensive African Americans: a prospective cohort study. J Clin Hypertens (Greenwich). 2015;17(8):614–21.
9. Zolnierek KB, Dimatteo MR. Physician communication and patient adherence to treatment: a meta-analysis. Med Care. 2009;47(8):826–34.
10. Ayalon L, Arean PA, Alvidrez J. Adherence to antidepressant medications in black and Latino elderly patients. Am J Geriatr Psychiatr. 2005;13(7):572–80.
11. Bazargan M, Smith J, Yazdanshenas H, Movassaghi M, Martins M, Orum G. Non-adherence to medication regimens among older African-American adults. BMC Geriatr. 2017; In Print.
12. Braverman J, Dedier J. Predictors of medication adherence for African American patients diagnosed with hypertension. Ethn Dis. 2009;19(4):396–400.
13. Gerber BS, Cho YI, Arozullah AM, Lee SY. Racial differences in medication adherence: a cross-sectional study of Medicare enrollees. Am J Geriatr Pharmacother. 2010;8(2):136–45.
14. Zhang Y, Baik SH. Race/ethnicity, disability, and medication adherence among medicare beneficiaries with heart failure. J Gen Intern Med. 2014; 29(4):602–7.
15. Davis AM, Taitel MS, Jiang J, et al. A National Assessment of medication adherence to statins by the racial composition of neighborhoods. J Racial Ethn Health Disparities. 2017;4(3):462–71.
16. Lewey J, Shrank WH, Bowry AD, Kilabuk E, Brennan TA, Choudhry NK. Gender and racial disparities in adherence to statin therapy: a meta-analysis. Am Heart J. 2013;165(5):665–78 678 e661.
17. Bazargan M, Smith J, Movassaghi M, et al. Polypharmacy among underserved older African American adults. J Aging Res. 2017;2017. Article ID 6026358, 8 pages. https://doi.org/10.1155/2017/6026358.
18. Espino DV, Bazaldua OV, Palmer RF, et al. Suboptimal medication use and mortality in an older adult community based cohort: results from the Hispanic EPESE study. J Gerontol Ser A Biol Med Sci. 2006;61(2):170–5.
19. Bazargan M, Yazdanshenas H, Han S, Orum G. Inappropriate medication use among underserved elderly African Americans. J Aging Health. 2016;28(1):118–38.
20. Radcliff S, Yue J, Rocco G, et al. American Geriatrics Society 2015 updated beers criteria for potentially inappropriate medication use in older adults. J Am Geriatr Soc. 2015;63(11):2227–46.
21. Naples JG, Hanlon JT, Ruby CM, Greenspan SL. Inappropriate Medications and Risk of Falls in Older Adults. In: Huang A, Mallet L, editors. Medication-Related Falls in Older People. Adis, Cham. 2016.
22. Muhlack DC, Hoppe LK, Weberpals J, Brenner H, Schöttker B. The Association of Potentially Inappropriate Medication at older age with

cardiovascular events and overall mortality: a systematic review and meta-analysis of cohort studies. J Am Med Dir Assoc. 2017;18(3):211-20.

23. Opondo D, Eslami S, Visscher S, et al. Inappropriateness of medication prescriptions to elderly patients in the primary care setting: a systematic review. PLoS One. 2012;7(8):e43617.

24. Miller GE, Sarpong EM, Davidoff AJ, Yang EY, Brandt NJ, Fick DM. Determinants of potentially inappropriate medication use among community-dwelling older adults. Health Serv Res. 2017;52(4):1534-49.

25. Skaar DD, O'Connor HL. Use of the beers criteria to identify potentially inappropriate drug use by community-dwelling older dental patients. Oral Surg Oral Med Oral Pathol Oral Radiol. 2012;113(6):714–21.

26. Singh J. Evaluation of the appropriateness of prescribing in geriatric patients using Beers' criteria and Phadke's criteria and comparison thereof by Rima Shah and colleagues. J Pharmacol Pharmacother. 2012;3(1):81–2.

27. Vishwas HN, Harugeri A, Parthasarathi G, Ramesh M. Potentially inappropriate medication use in Indian elderly: comparison of Beers' criteria and screening tool of older Persons' potentially inappropriate prescriptions. Geriatr Gerontol Int. 2012;12(3):506–14.

28. Monroe T, Carter M, Parish A. A case study using the beers list criteria to compare prescribing by family practitioners and geriatric specialists in a rural nursing home. Geriatr Nurs. 2011;32(5):350–6.

29. Locatelli J, Lira AR, Torraga LK, Paes AT. Inappropriate medications using the beers criteria in Brazilian hospitalized elderly patients. Consult Pharm. 2010; 25(1):36–40.

30. Gallagher PF, Barry PJ, Ryan C, Hartigan I, O'Mahony D. Inappropriate prescribing in an acutely ill population of elderly patients as determined by Beers' criteria. Age Ageing. 2008;37(1):96–101.

31. Niwata S, Yamada Y, Ikegami N. Prevalence of inappropriate medication using beers criteria in Japanese long-term care facilities. BMC Geriatr. 2006;6:1.

32. van der Hooft CS, Jong GW, Dieleman JP, et al. Inappropriate drug prescribing in older adults: the updated 2002 beers criteria--a population-based cohort study. Br J Clin Pharmacol. 2005;60(2):137–44.

33. Yazdanshenas H, Bazargan M, Orum G, Loni L, Mahabadi N, Husaini B. Prescribing patterns in the treatment of hypertension among underserved African American elderly. Ethn Dis. 2014;24(4):431–7.

34. Yazdanshenas H, Bazargan M, Smith J, Martins D, Motahari H, Orum G. Pain treatment of underserved older African Americans. J Am Geriatr Soc. 2016; 64(10):2116–21.

35. Bazargan M, Yazdanshenas H, Gordon D, Orum G. Pain in community-dwelling elderly African Americans. J Aging Health. 2016;28(3):403–25.

36. Sorensen L, Stokes JA, Purdie DM, Woodward M, Roberts MS. Medication management at home: medication risk factor prevalence and inter-relationships. J Clin Pharm Ther. 2006;31(5):485–91.

37. Sorensen L, Stokes JA, Purdie DM, Woodward M, Roberts MS. Medication management at home: medication-related risk factors associated with poor health outcomes. Age Ageing. 2005;34(6):626–32.

38. Sorensen L, Stokes JA, Purdie DM, Woodward M, Elliott R, Roberts MS. Medication reviews in the community: results of a randomized, controlled effectiveness trial.[erratum appears in Br J Clin Pharmacol. 2005 mar;59(3): 376]. Br J Clin Pharmacol. 2004;58(6):648–64.

39. Fortin M, Haggerty J, Sanche S, Almirall J. Self-reported versus health administrative data: implications for assessing chronic illness burden in populations. A cross-sectional study. CMAJ Open. 2017;5(3):E729–33.

40. Tannenbaum C, Farrell B, Shaw J, et al. An ecological approach to reducing potentially inappropriate medication use: Canadian Deprescribing network—erratum. Can J Aging/La Revue canadienne du vieillissement. 2017;36(2):268–71.

41. Los Angeles County Department of Public Health, Office of Health Assessment and Epidemilogy. Key Indicators of Health by Service Planning Area. January 2017. www.publichealth.lacounty.gove/ha. Accessed 27 2018.

42. Skaar DD, O'Connor H. Using the beers criteria to identify potentially inappropriate medication use by older adult dental patients. J Am Dent Assoc. 2017;148(5):298–307.

43. Reyes-Gibby CC, Aday LA, Todd KH, Cleeland CS, Anderson KO. Pain in aging community-dwelling adults in the United States: non-Hispanic whites, non-Hispanic blacks, and Hispanics. J Pain. 2007;8(1):75–84.

44. Sheikh-Taha M, Dimassi H. Potentially inappropriate home medications among older patients with cardiovascular disease admitted to a cardiology service in USA. BMC Cardiovasc Disord. 2017;17(1):189.

45. Corleto VD, Festa S, Di Giulio E, Annibale B. Proton pump inhibitor therapy and potential long-term harm. Curr Opin Endocrinol Diabetes Obes. 2014; 21(1):3–8.

46. Lechevallier-Michel N, Gautier-Bertrand M, Alperovitch A, et al. Frequency and risk factors of potentially inappropriate medication use in a community-dwelling elderly population: results from the 3C study. Eur J Clin Pharmacol. 2005;60(11):813–9.

47. Heser K, Luck T, Rohr S, et al. Potentially inappropriate medication: association between the use of antidepressant drugs and the subsequent risk for dementia. J Affect Disord. 2018;226:28–35.

48. Wucherer D, Eichler T, Hertel J, et al. Potentially inappropriate medication in community-dwelling primary care patients who were screened positive for dementia. J Alzheimers Dis. 2017;55(2):691–701.

49. de Rekeneire N, Visser M, Peila R, et al. Is a fall just a fall: correlates of falling in healthy older persons. The health, aging and body composition study. J Am Geriatr Soc. 2003;51(6):841–6.

50. Hanlon JT, Landerman LR, Fillenbaum GG, Studenski S. Falls in African American and white community-dwelling elderly residents. J Gerontol A Biol Sci Med Sci. 2002;57(7):M473–8.

51. Karter AJ, Laiteerapong N, Chin MH, et al. Ethnic differences in geriatric conditions and diabetes complications among older, insured adults with diabetes: the diabetes and aging study. J Aging Health. 2015;27(5):894–918.

52. Faulkner KA, Cauley JA, Zmuda JM, et al. Ethnic differences in the frequency and circumstances of falling in older community-dwelling women. J Am Geriatr Soc. 2005;53(10):1774–9.

53. Means KM, O'Sullivan PS, Rodell DE. Balance, mobility, and falls among elderly African American women. Am J Phys Med Rehabil. 2000;79(1):30–9.

54. Quandt SA, Stafford JM, Bell RA, Smith SL, Snively BM, Arcury TA. Predictors of falls in a multiethnic population of older rural adults with diabetes. J Gerontol A Biol Sci Med Sci. 2006;61(4):394–8.

55. Geng Y, Lo JC, Brickner L, Gordon NP. Racial-ethnic differences in fall prevalence among older women: a cross-sectional survey study. BMC Geriatr. 2017;17(1):65.

56. Ellis R, Kosma M, Fabre JM, Moore DS, Wood RH. Proximal determinants of falls risk among independent-living older adults. Res Aging. 2012;35(4):420–36.

57. Nicklett EJ, Taylor RJ, Rostant O, Johnson KE, Evans L. Biopsychosocial predictors of fall events among older African Americans. Res Aging. 2017;39(4):501–25.

58. Bergen G, Stevens MR, Burns ER. Falls and fall injuries among adults aged >/=65 years - United States, 2014. MMWR Morb Mortal Wkly Rep. 2016; 65(37):993–8.

59. Lawlor DA, Patel R, Ebrahim S. Association between falls in elderly women and chronic diseases and drug use: cross sectional study. BMJ (Clin Res Ed). 2003;327(7417):712–7.

60. Barenholtz Levy H, Marcus E-L. Potentially inappropriate medications in older adults: why the revised criteria matter. Ann Pharmacother. 2016;50(7):599–603.

61. Verdoorn S, Kwint H-F, Faber A, Gussekloo J, Bouvy ML. Majority of drug-related problems identified during medication review are not associated with STOPP/START criteria. Eur J Clin Pharmacol. 2015;71(10):1255–62.

62. Gellad WF, Grenard JL, Marcum ZA. A systematic review of barriers to medication adherence in the elderly: looking beyond cost and regimen complexity. Am J Geriatr Pharmacother. 2011;9(1):11–23.

63. Hu D, Juarez DT, Yeboah M, Castillo TP. Interventions to increase medication adherence in African-American and Latino populations: a literature review. Hawaii J Med Public Health. 2014;73(1):11–8.

64. Bazargan M, Smith J, Yazdanshenas H, Movassaghi M, Martins D, Orum G. Non-adherence to medication regimens among older African-American adults. BMC Geriatr. 2017;17(1):163.

65. Vanderman AJ, Moss JM, Bryan WE III, Sloane R, Jackson GL, Hastings SN. Evaluating the impact of medication safety alerts on prescribing of potentially inappropriate medications for older veterans in an ambulatory care setting. J Pharm Pract. 2017;30(1):82–8.

66. Peek ME, Cargill A, Huang ES. Diabetes health disparities: a systematic review of health care interventions. Med Care Res Rev. 2007;64(5 Suppl):101S–56S.

67. Ruppar TM, Dunbar-Jacob JM, Mehr DR, Lewis L, Conn VS. Medication adherence interventions among hypertensive black adults: a systematic review and meta-analysis. J Hypertens. 2017;35(6):1145-54.

68. Spinewine A, Schmader KE, Barber N, et al. Appropriate prescribing in elderly people: how well can it be measured and optimised? Lancet. 2007; 370(9582):173–84.

# 18

# Higher levels of tumor necrosis factor β are associated with frailty in socially vulnerable community-dwelling older adults

Carla M. C. Nascimento, Marisa S. Zazzetta, Grace A. O. Gomes, Fabiana S. Orlandi, Karina Gramani-Say, Fernando A. Vasilceac, Aline C. M. Gratão, Sofia C. I. Pavarini and Marcia R. Cominetti[*] (iD)

## Abstract

**Background:** The complex physiology underpinning the frailty syndrome is responsible for the absence of robust biomarkers that can be used for screening, diagnostic and/or prognostic purposes and has made clinical implementation difficult. Considering socially vulnerable populations, who have poor health status and increased morbidity and mortality, this scenario is even more complex. However, to the best of our knowledge, there are no studies available to investigate frailty biomarkers in socially vulnerable populations. Thus, the aim of this cross-sectional study was to identify potential blood-based biomarkers of frailty in a socially vulnerable population.

**Methods:** A sample consisting of 347 community-dwelling older people living in a context of high social vulnerability was divided into non-frail (robust), pre-frail and frail groups, according to modified Fried frailty phenotype criteria. Blood samples were collected and analyzed for basic metabolic parameters and for inflammatory cytokines.

**Results:** Levels of Interleukin-1α (IL-1α) and Tumor Necrosis Factor α (TNF-α) were significantly higher in pre-frail subjects, compared to non-frail ones. Tumor Necrosis Factor β (TNF-β) levels presented higher values in the frail compared to non-frail individuals. Interleukin-6 (IL-6) levels in pre-frail and frail subjects were significantly higher compared to the levels of non-frail subjects. Using an ordinal regression analysis, we observed that socially vulnerable older people at higher risk of developing frailty were subjects above 80 years old (OR: 2.5; 95% CI: 1.1–5.6) and who presented higher levels of TNF-β (≥0.81 pg/mL, OR: 2.53; 95% CI: 1.3–4.9).

**Conclusion:** As vulnerable populations continue to age, it is imperative to have a greater understanding of the frailty condition, identifying novel potential blood-based biomarkers. The results presented here could help to implement preventive healthcare strategies by evaluating frailty and at the same time measuring a set of inflammatory biomarkers, paying special attention to TNF-β plasmatic levels.

**Keywords:** Aging, Biomarkers, Older people, Frailty, Tumor necrosis factor β

## Background

Frailty is an age-related state characterized as a syndrome in which individuals may become more vulnerable to adverse health outcomes with a higher risk for mortality when exposed to stressors [1–3]. Social vulnerability is defined as the degree to which a person's overall social situation leaves them susceptible to health problems, which include physical, mental, psychological and functional problems. Social vulnerability is particularly important for older adults as a condition related to cultural, social and economic aspects that may influence the access to goods and services. This is an important indicator to explain the high exposure of this population to the development of pathological and degenerative conditions as it increases the frailty rate [4–8].

On the other hand, knowledge regarding the cellular and molecular mechanisms related to this syndrome is limited, especially in vulnerable populations. Changes related to the immune-endocrine axis are extensively described during aging and are frequently associated to increases in morbidity and mortality [9]. These changes

* Correspondence: mcominetti@ufscar.br
Department of Gerontology, Federal University of São Carlos, Rod. Washington Luis, Km 235, Monjolinho, São Carlos, SP CEP 13565-905, Brazil

are characterized by a low-grade, controlled, asymptomatic, systemic, and chronic progressive increase in the pro-inflammatory status, also called *inflammaging* [10]. This pro-inflammatory state generated by age, sex, lifestyle, socioeconomic background, comorbidities and affective, cognitive or sensory impairments has been postulated as a potential driver of frailty pathogenesis, producing even higher levels of systemic inflammatory markers [11, 12]. Associations between frailty and endocrine and immune changes have been demonstrated, suggesting that alterations in these systems may accelerate the development of age-related diseases and consequently, frailty. [13, 14]. Considering that frailty is characterized by the loss of resilience, poor social conditions may reflect chronic stressors, which increase risk of disturbances in metabolic and immunological parameters, leading to a higher risk of developing frailty [15–17].

Previous studies have pointed out several candidates for blood-based biomarkers for frailty [18]. Those include inflammatory molecules, such as C-reactive protein (CRP) [19, 20], Interleukin-6 (IL-6) [19–22] and Tumor Necrosis Factor-α (TNF- α) [19, 21, 23], clinical parameters such as hemoglobin [19, 24] and serum albumin [25], hormones, such as dehydroepiandrosterone sulfate (DHEA-S) [26], testosterone [27], Insulin-like Growth Factor-1 (IGF-1) [28] and vitamin D [29], among others. To the best of our knowledge, however, no study has described the differences of clinical parameters and pro-inflammatory cytokines so far among different frailty statuses of older adults living in socially vulnerable populations.

As a result, we performed a cross-sectional study to investigate potential blood-based biomarkers for frailty under a social vulnerability context, considering demographic, psychological and clinical characteristics. The results of this study could contribute to a greater understanding of frailty syndrome in socially vulnerable populations, as well as to the biology of frailty with regards to the panel of expressed inflammatory cytokines. Moreover, identifying potential blood-based biomarkers will enable the development of interventions and specific policies for this public.

## Methods
### Sample
A total of 852 older adults fulfilled the eligibly criteria and were registered in the database. Based on this, the adequate sample size was calculated according to the multinomial statistics analysis. Thus, 347 representative participants were stratified according to sex and age sample. This sample size provided a power of 95%, considering a medium effect size (50%; $p = 0.50$). Participants who accepted to take part in the study and signed the consent term were asked to collect blood samples. Immediately after drawing blood, the clinical assessment for frailty status was scheduled.

### Study protocol
The study protocol (860.653/2014) and informed consent form received ethics approval from the Federal University of São Carlos Ethics Committee on Human Experimentation. Written informed consent concerning the conduct of the survey was obtained from each participant, and complete anonymity of participants was assured as described earlier [30].

Brazil has a Unified Health System (*Sistema Único de Saúde - SUS*), and it is estimated that more than 75% of the Brazilian population rely exclusively on it for their health care. The Family Health Program is a part of the unified health system created to provide mainly primary care health [31]. Since we consider that these units are located mainly in vulnerable areas, most people living in these zones are users and are registered on the *SUS* database. All people that use the health care service must be registered and accompanied by a team of health professionals. For this study, older adults (60 years and over) were selected, who were registered in the *SUS* database in a region with a high rate of social vulnerability and poverty in São Carlos, São Paulo, Brazil, called "*Cidade Aracy*", which is a region with a high rate of poverty that unifies five public clinical practice units. Social vulnerability was determined using the Paulista Social Vulnerability Index (PSVI) that measures social exclusion in different cities in São Paulo state, Brazil [32]. SVI allows the classification of a determined population into seven groups: 1 - extremely low; 2 - very low; 3 - low; 4 - medium; 5 - high; 6 - very high vulnerability and 7 - rural areas of high vulnerability (Additional file 1). Based on these criteria, the study population was classified as level 5 of vulnerability, which represents populations living in urban areas with high vulnerability. This instrument was used with the unique intention to determine the social vulnerability of the studied population, not for comparison purposes.

Subjects were classified according to diagnostic criteria based on the classification proposed by Fried and co-workers [1] and validated in Brazil by Nunes and colleagues [33], as described in the study protocol. According to these criteria, the subjects were classified into three groups: frail (scores 3–5), pre-frail (scores 1, 2), and non-frail (score 0). For the diagnosis of frailty, five items were considered: 1) non intentional weight loss was evaluated by means of self-report considering losses of more than 4.5 kg during the last year; 2) fatigue was assessed considering the answers given to two items from the Center of Epidemiological Study Center Scale (CES-D): "*Have you felt that you had to make an effort to do your customary tasks?*" and "*Were you unable to proceed when doing your things?*" [34]; 3) Handgrip strength was measured using a manual dynamometer and was considered the measure of the highest force possible produced for the dominant upper limb in three attempts. These values were adjusted considering gender and body mass index (BMI) for the final criteria; 4) physical inactivity was evaluated by applying the International Physical Activity Questionnaire (IPAQ) [35], which assesses the amount of physical activity performed by the individual and the estimated caloric expenditure. Individuals with a caloric expenditure in the first quintile were considered positive for this item; 5) low-gait speed was measured using a 4.6-m-long circuit and the time spent to go through the circuit. The individuals in the first quintile, after adjusting their respective heights and genders, were considered positive for this item.

Sociodemographic and clinical data were also assessed: age, sex, education, ethnicity, cognitive function measured by the Mini Mental State Examination [36], depressive symptoms measured by the Geriatric Depression Scale, GDS-15, Brazilian version [37], leisure-time of physical activity measured by the self-report specific part of the International Physical Activity Questionnaire [35], medications, Body Mass Index (BMI), marital status and per capita income. In an effort to avoid potential sources of bias, all the interviews were conducted by trained gerontologists and data was included using the software Epidata® software.

### Analysis of biomarkers

Fasting blood samples were collected on a visit closest to the frailty assessment. Samples were collected using EDTA tubes, mixed by inversion and centrifuged (3000 rpm, 5 min) to separate plasma. Plasma samples were stored at − 80 °C until they were analyzed. One plasma aliquot was used to perform measures of glucose, insulin, total cholesterol, triglycerides, urea, creatinine, dehydroepiandrosterone (DHEA), dehydroepiandrosterone sulfate (S-DHEA), human growth hormone (GH), insulin-like growth factor 1 (IGF-1) and glycated hemoglobin in a specialized clinical laboratory.

Another aliquot was used to measure the level of inflammatory cytokines. For that, 25 μL of samples were added to each well of a 96-well plate provided with the kit (HCYTOMAG, MILLIPLEX® MAP Kit EMD Millipore Corp., MA, USA). Plates were incubated under agitation on a shaker for 2 h at room temperature (20–25 °C). Next, after washing according to the instructions provided in the kit, 25 μL of premixed beads containing the primary antibodies to detect the specific cytokines evaluated (Interleukin-1α; Interleukin-1β; Interleukin-6; Tumor Necrosis Factor α and Tumor Necrosis Factor β) were inserted in each well. The plate was sealed and incubated for 2 h at room temperature (20–25 °C). Afterwards, the plates were washed twice with the washing solution provided and 25 μL of streptavidin-phycoerythrin solution was added to each well and plates were incubated with

agitation on a shaker for 30 min at room temperature. A standard curve was prepared with the reagents provided in the kit and luminescence readings were performed on a plate reader (Luminex xMAP®).

### Statistical analysis

To describe the profile samples for all variables, data were presented in frequency tables for categorical data and descriptive statistics were applied for numerical data with means and standard deviation. In order to compare categorical data, the chi-square and the Fisher exact tests were used. When comparisons involved three levels of frailty (non-frail, pre-frail and frail individuals), the *Kruskal-Wallis* test was used due to the non-normal distribution of the data. To compare numerical variables according to frailty status adjusted for sex and age, an analysis of covariance (ANCOVA) was applied. Univariate analysis was performed to assess the association between factors and outcome measures. Variables considered with a significance of at least 20% ($p < =0.20$) in the univariate analysis were all included in the multivariable ordinal logistic regression. In this model, variables were considered significant at $p \leq 0.05$. All statistical analyses were performed using the SAS System for Windows (Statistical Analysis System), version 9.2 (SAS Institute Inc., 2002–2008, Cary, NC, USA).

### Results

The mean age of the study cohort was $70.1 \pm 7.7$ years, mostly female (56.2%) with a low education level ($3.8 \pm 2.3$ years) (data not shown). In this sample, 34 subjects (9.8%) were non-frail, 197 (56.8%) were classified as pre-frail and 116 (33.4%) subjects fulfilled the criteria for physical frailty. Considering age, as expected, frail individuals were significantly older than their non-frail counterparts (Table 1).

Results showed significant differences between groups concerning the sex, indicating that women were more frequent in the non-frail group, while men were most frequent in pre-frail and frail categories. Regarding age, as expected, older people (> 80 years) were frailer compared to those in the age groups of 60–69 and 70–79 years. The Geriatric Depression Scale (GDS) indicated that prevalence of depressive symptoms was also higher in pre-frail and frail, compared to non-frail individuals. Frail individuals also presented insufficient levels of physical activity evaluated by the International Physical Activity Questionnaire (IPAQ) (Table 1), which is consistent to the frailty condition.

Considering the results of metabolic parameters and biomarker evaluation, we observed that urea and TNF-β were significantly higher in frail participants compared to non-frail individuals. Levels of creatinine and IL-6 were higher among pre-frail and frail individuals, compared to

**Table 1** Sociodemographic characteristics and clinical parameters of participants distributed according to the Fried frailty scale, $n = 347$

| | Non-frail | Pre-frail | Frail | p-value |
|---|---|---|---|---|
| | $n = 34$ (9.8%) | $n = 197$ (56.8%) | $n = 116$ (33.4%) | |
| Age (%) | | | | **0.003** |
|   60–69 years | 52.9 | 59.4* | 43.1 | |
|   70–79 years | 47.1* | 28.4 | 37.1 | |
|   > 80 years | 0.0 | 12.2 | 19.8* | |
| Sex (Men/women, %) | 20.6/79.4* | 43.1*/56.9 | 51.7*/48.3 | **0.005** |
| Schooling (%) | | | | 0.161 |
|   0 years | 0.0 | 1.5 | 4.3 | |
|   1–4 years | 76.9 | 72.8 | 82.6 | |
|   > 5 years | 23.1 | 25.7 | 13.1 | |
| Ethnicity (White/non-white, %) | 44.1/55.9 | 39.5/50.5 | 43.9/56.1 | 0.700 |
| Global Cognitive State-MMSE (%) | | | | 0.132 |
|   Without cognitive impairment | 58.8 | 60.7 | 49.1 | |
|   With cognitive impairment | 41.2 | 39.3 | 50.9 | |
| Depressive Symptoms-GSD (%) | 11.8 | 31.1* | 40.5* | **0.006** |
| Physically Active Enough-IPAQ score (%) | 73.5 | 61.9 | 29.3* | **< 0.001** |
| Medications (%) | | | | 0.388 |
|   0–5 medications | 75.0 | 67.8 | 62.3 | |
|   > 6 medications | 25.0 | 32.2 | 37.7 | |
| Body Mass Index | 29.5 ± 6.5 | 28.6 ± 5.9 | 28.2 ± 6.1 | 0.906 |
| Marital status (With/without partner, %) | 64.7/35.3 | 59.7/40.3 | 52.6/47.4 | 0.325 |
| Per capita income | 280.4 ± 151.3 | 239.2 ± 127.7 | 220.3 ± 126.5 | 0.169 |

*Notes:* Data are expressed as mean ± SD or percentage of total sample; Body Mass Index was calculated as weight in kilograms divided by height in square meters. GDS: Geriatric Depression Scale; MMSE: Mini-Mental State Examination. Per capita incomes are in US dollars, according to the quotation made on October/ 2017. Chi-square test ($\chi w^2$) was used for categorical variables and Kruskal-Wallis test for numerical variables. *Values with statistical significance ($p < 0.05$) All other bold entries represent the $p$ values of significant results

non-frail ones. Cytokines IL-1α and TNF-α levels were higher in pre-frail, compared to non-frail, but no statistically significant differences for these cytokines were found comparing non-frail with frail individuals (Table 2).

We performed a univariate regression analysis to track the main variables that seem to contribute to the frailty phenotype considering the three groups (frail vs pre-frail vs non-frail) evaluated. Variables were considered to be part of the ordinal model when they presented a statistical significance above 20% ($p < 0.20$). Thus, we considered the following variables for our model: sex, age, HDL and VLDL cholesterols, urea, creatinine, triglycerides IL-1β, IL-6 and TNF-β (Table 3).

Given these results, an ordinal regression model was conducted in order to predict which variables were significantly associated with frailty. Results showed that age and TNF-β levels were significantly associated with frail phenotype. Older people with increased risk to becoming frail were those older than 80 years (OR: 2.5; 95% CI: 1.09–5.61) and who presented higher levels of TNF-β (OR: 2.5; 95% CI: 1.30–4.9) (Table 4).

## Discussion

Frailty is a geriatric syndrome associated with disability and mortality outcomes in older people. In a recent multicenter, a population-based cross-sectional study showed a prevalence around 38% of frailty in Brazilian community-dwelling older people [38]. We identified in our sample, in which all individuals were living in a high social vulnerability context, that 33.4% of aged subjects investigated fulfilled criteria for physical frailty. A possible explanation for these differences may be related to the fact that in our study, most of the participants were in the 60 to 69 year old age group (53.3%; data not shown) and few participants were above 80 years old (13.5%; data not shown), while in a study carried out by Pereira et al. [38] the age group ranging from 60 to 69 years old represented only 36.4% of the sample. More importantly, in the study by Pereira et al. [38], the authors did not evaluate frailty using Fried's score, but instead used the frailty index (FI), which probably contributed to the difference found in both studies, regarding frailty prevalence. Accordingly, Collard et al.

**Table 2** Peripheral biomarkers of participants distributed according to the Fried frailty scale, $n = 347$

| | Non-frail<br>$n = 34$<br>(11.2%) | Pre-frail<br>$n = 197$<br>(58.2%) | Frail<br>$n = 116$<br>(30.6%) | p-value |
|---|---|---|---|---|
| Glucose (mg/dL) | 95.5 ± 27.5 | 98.7 ± 44.5 | 106.4 ± 52.2 | 0.640 |
| Glycated hemoglobin (%) | 5.8 ± 1.7 | 5.7 ± 2.4 | 5.7 ± 2.8 | 0.874 |
| Insulin (μmol/L) | 8.4 ± 5.5 | 8.6 ± 7.8 | 8.7 ± 8.1 | 0.663 |
| Total cholesterol (mg/dL) | 200.2 ± 40.4 | 195.2 ± 43.1 | 193.3 ± 45.7 | 0.435 |
| HDL cholesterol (mg/dL) | 49.4 ± 11.2 | 48.3 ± 13.5 | 47.2 ± 11.6 | 0.497 |
| LDL cholesterol (mg/dL) | 119.8 ± 37.8 | 119.6 ± 34.2 | 115.2 ± 34.2 | 0.441 |
| VLDL cholesterol (mg/dL) | 32.3 ± 23.0 | 28.4 ± 13.6 | 30.2 ± 16.3 | 0.818 |
| Triglycerides (mg/dL) | 146.2 ± 61.2 | 148.5 ± 82.7 | 151.4 ± 89.7 | 0.939 |
| Urea (mg/dL) | 34.5 ± 10.1 | 35.5 ± 11.6 | 40.1 ± 14.9 | **0.013***[a] |
| Creatinine (mg/dL) | 0.8 ± 0.2 | 0.96 ± 0.3 | 1.1 ± 0.5 | **0.004***[a,b] |
| DHEA (ng/mL) | 4.1 ± 4.5 | 4.4 ± 4.3 | 4.3 ± 4.5 | 0.407 |
| S-DHEA (μg/dL) | 55.8 ± 40.3 | 67.2 ± 48.4 | 67.2 ± 53.3 | 0.423 |
| IGF-1 (ng/mL) | 113.2 ± 42.4 | 119.7 ± 47.5 | 117.2 ± 43.2 | 0.776 |
| Hydroxyvitamin D (ng/mL) | 22.1 ± 5.6 | 23.2 ± 8.6 | 22.2 ± 7.8 | 0.693 |
| Inflammatory markers (pg/mL) | | | | |
| Interleukin-1α | 3.0 ± 5.2 | 6.8 ± 12.5 | 9.2 ± 21.8 | **0.027***[b] |
| Interleukin-1β | 1.9 ± 2.8 | 3.1 ± 4.2 | 3.4 ± 4.4 | 0.056 |
| Interleukin-6 | 1.9 ± 1.6 | 2.1 ± 4.2 | 4.2 ± 7.6 | **0.012***[a,b] |
| Interleukin-10 | 1.3 ± 2.0 | 1.7 ± 3.2 | 3.6 ± 12.4 | 0.571 |
| Tumor Necrosis Factor-α | 2.0 ± 2.0 | 3.6 ± 5.8 | 4.7 ± 10.2 | **0.035***[b] |
| Tumor Necrosis Factor-β | 0.5 ± 0.5 | 3.0 ± 11.5 | 3.0 ± 10.1 | **0.033***[a] |

*Notes:* DHEA: Dehydroepiandrosterone; S-DHEA: Dehydroepiandrosterone sulfate; GH: Growth Hormone; IGF-1: Insulin-like growth factor 1. Kruskal-Wallis test.
*Values with statistical significance ($p < 0.05$). [a]Non-frail vs frail; [b]non-frail vs pre-frail
All other bold entries represent the $p$ values of significant results

[39], in a systematic review of 21 studies ($n = 61,500$), described that the prevalence of frailty in a community-dwelling population has a high variability, ranging from 4 to 59.1%. Moreover, in another study, Moreira and Lourenço [40] found a prevalence of 9.1% of frailty when a different scale was applied to track this phenotype, while Sousa et al. [41] found a prevalence of 17.1% for Brazilian older people using Fried's phenotype scale. These variations may be highlighted by the different operationalization of frailty status used in the studies, resulting in widely different frailty prevalences.

The frail condition in our sample was also more frequent in men, which is different from previously published epidemiological data that showed higher rates of frailty in women [42, 43]. It has been demonstrated that men frequently have more acute illnesses, while women have more comorbidities and disabilities [44, 45]. This may consequently lead to men becoming more vulnerable to frailty in advanced ages. Additionally, it is important to consider that Brazilian population social inequalities in health behavior are very relevant to explain the particularity of some results found for our sample. It has already been demonstrated

that in low-income, less schooled people and those without private health insurance, Brazilian men were found to have more risk behavior, including smoking, sedentary lifestyles and bad quality of food, with a low intake of fruit and vegetables [46]. Furthermore, another investigation found that around 1.1% among men and 0.3% among women in this social condition have never visited a physician and 35% and 52% of men and women respectively, had not visited a physician in the last year [47]. These findings help to elucidate the underutilization of health care services among individuals of the lowest economic class, but especially among men, which may characterize them as a more vulnerable group for frailty. On the other hand, our data is in accordance with other research, indicating that frailty increases with age and low levels of physical activity [39].

The aging process frequently results in a decline of the immune function, known as immunosenescense, which was related to the role of inflammation in frailty [48]. These alterations are characterized by around 2-fold increased levels of cytokine production when compared to young individuals' levels. Increases in adipose tissue, low levels of physical activity and the senescent cellular

**Table 3** Results of the univariate ordinal logistic regression analysis among groups (frail vs pre-frail vs non-frail)

| Variable | Category | Univariate Regression | | *p*-value |
| | | O.R. | 95% CI | |
|---|---|---|---|---|
| Sex | Women (ref.) | 1.00 | --- | --- |
| | Men | 1.85 | 1.21–2.82 | **0.004*** |
| Age (years) | 60–69 years (ref.) | 1.00 | – | – |
| | 70–79 years | 1.29 | 0.81–2.05 | 0.278 |
| | ≥80 years | 2.65 | 1.41–5.00 | **0.003*** |
| Glucose (mg/dL) (tertile) | ≤83 (ref.) | 1.00 | – | – |
| | 84–96 | 0.99 | 0.59–1.67 | 0.979 |
| | ≥97 | 1.06 | 0.64–1.77 | 0.816 |
| HDL cholesterol (mg/dL) (tertile) | ≥51 (ref.) | 1.00 | – | – |
| | 42–50 | 1.18 | 0.70–1.97 | 0.538 |
| | ≤41 | 1.42 | 0.85–2.40 | **0.184*** |
| LDL cholesterol (mg/dL) (tertile) | ≤99 (ref.) | 1.00 | – | – |
| | 100–129 | 1.18 | 0.70–1.98 | 0.531 |
| | ≥130 | 0.83 | 0.49–1.41 | 0.493 |
| VLDL cholesterol (mg/dL) (tertile) | ≤20 (ref.) | 1.00 | – | – |
| | 21–31 | 0.59 | 0.35–1.01 | **0.051*** |
| | ≥32 | 1.00 | 0.59–1.69 | 1.000 |
| Urea (mg/dL) (tertile) | ≤30 (ref.) | 1.00 | – | – |
| | 31–39 | 1.21 | 0.71–2.08 | 0.480 |
| | ≥40 | 2.01 | 1.19–3.41 | **0.010*** |
| Creatinine (mg/dL) (tertile) | ≤0.7 (ref.) | 1.00 | – | – |
| | 0.8–1.0 | 0.85 | 0.48–1.50 | 0.569 |
| | ≥1.1 | 1.96 | 1.05–3.66 | **0.034*** |
| DHEA (ng/mL) (tertile) | ≤2.31 (ref.) | 1.00 | – | – |
| | 2.32–4.28 | 0.90 | 0.54–1.52 | 0.699 |
| | ≥4.29 | 0.98 | 0.58–1.63 | 0.922 |
| Hydroxyvitamin D (ng/mL) (tertile) | ≥25 (ref.) | 1.00 | – | – |
| | 19–24 | 0.96 | 0.58–1.59 | 0.880 |
| | ≤18 | 1.10 | 0.66–1.84 | 0.720 |
| Insulin (µmol/L) (tertile) | ≥9 (ref.) | 1.00 | – | – |
| | 5–8 | 1.31 | 0.79–2.16 | 0.298 |
| | ≤4 | 0.93 | 0.55–1.55 | 0.769 |
| Triglycerides (mg/dL) (em tertile) | ≤103 (ref.) | 1.00 | – | – |
| | 104–158 | 0.53 | 0.32–0.90 | **0.019*** |
| | ≥159 | 0.88 | 0.53–1.47 | 0.627 |
| Total cholesterol (mg/dL) (tertile) | ≤174 (ref.) | 1.00 | – | – |
| | 175–211 | 1.16 | 0.69–1.94 | 0.577 |
| | ≥212 | 0.72 | 0.43–1.21 | 0.211 |
| S-DHEA (µg/dL) (tertile) | ≤36 (ref.) | 1.00 | – | – |
| | 37–73 | 1.17 | 0.69–1.97 | 0.556 |
| | ≥74 | 1.37 | 0.81–2.30 | 0.243 |
| IGF-1 (ng/mL) (tertile) | ≤91.5 (ref.) | 1.00 | – | – |
| | 91.6–134.3 | 0.98 | 0.58–1.64 | 0.932 |
| | ≥134.4 | 1.14 | 0.68–1.91 | 0.621 |

**Table 3** Results of the univariate ordinal logistic regression analysis among groups (frail vs pre-frail vs non-frail) *(Continued)*

| Variable | Category | Univariate Regression | | |
|---|---|---|---|---|
| | | O.R. | 95% CI | *p*-value |
| Glycated hemoglobin (%) (tertile) | ≤5.5 (ref.) | 1.00 | – | – |
| | 5.6–6.3 | 0.70 | 0.41–1.17 | 0.173 |
| | ≥6.4 | 0.90 | 0.54–1.51 | 0.694 |
| IL-10 (pg/dL) (tertile) | ≤0.39 (ref.) | 1.00 | – | – |
| | 0.40–1.05 | 1.11 | 0.63–1.96 | 0.720 |
| | ≥1.06 | 1.31 | 0.74–2.32 | 0.362 |
| IL-1α (pg/dL) (tertile) | ≤0.60 (ref.) | 1.00 | – | – |
| | 0.70–3.35 | 1.30 | 0.74–2.28 | 0.355 |
| | ≥3.36 | 1.22 | 0.69–2.13 | 0.498 |
| IL-1β (tertile) | ≤0.86 (ref.) | 1.00 | – | – |
| | 0.87–2.30 | 1.21 | 0.69–2.12 | 0.507 |
| | ≥2.31 | 1.47 | 0.83–2.59 | **0.183\*** |
| IL-6 (tertile) | ≤1.50 (ref.) | 1.00 | – | – |
| | 1.51–2.60 | 1.62 | 0.96–2.72 | **0.071\*** |
| | ≥2.61 | 1.67 | 0.99–2.81 | **0.052\*** |
| TNF-α (tertile) | ≤0.96 (ref.) | 1.00 | – | – |
| | 0.97–2.89 | 0.92 | 0.53–1.61 | 0.776 |
| | ≥2.90 | 0.99 | 0.57–1.76 | 0.993 |
| TNF-β (tertile) | ≤0.29 (ref.) | 1.00 | – | – |
| | 0.30–0.80 | 1.24 | 0.70–2.20 | 0.459 |
| | ≥0.81 | 2.39 | 1.33–4.28 | **0.003\*** |

Variables with P < 0.20 were entered in the multivariable logistic regression model, *n* = 347. *Notes:* OR: Odds ratio shows the increase in odds for frailty. 95% CI = 95% of confidence interval for odds ratio; ref. = category chosen as reference. \*Values with statistical significance (*p* < 0.2)
All other bold entries represent the *p* values of significant results

process itself were suggested as mainly factors to drive this phenomenon that results in a low-grade chronic inflammatory state [49]. However, it is difficult to establish the relationship between inflammation and frailty, considering that both conditions linearly increase with advancing age, thus avoiding a clear answer to determine whether inflammation is a cause or a consequence of the frailty phenotype. Nevertheless, in a recent meta-analysis involving 32 cross-sectional studies and 23,910 older people, it was demonstrated that frail and pre-frail conditions are related to increased levels of serum cytokines, when compared to the levels of non-frail participants [50]. Our results corroborate the literature, demonstrating that an increased pro-inflammatory state is also present in frail older adults living in a context of social vulnerability.

Using an ordinal regression model, we found that TNF-β was significantly associated to the frail phenotype. Abnormalities in TNF-α or TNF-β expression have been implicated in several diseases [51–53]. A TNF-β signaling pathway seems to be involved in the support of efficient immune responses against pathogens, which is a key point in the immunosenescense [54]. An important link between the lack of adaptability of immunological

function during aging and increased risk for frailty in the vulnerable oldest old individuals was found in our study and may indicate that imbalances in immune functions seem to trigger physical frailty in this population. Similarly, in a systematic and meta-analysis review, Soysal and co-workers [50] demonstrated that three large prospective studies failed to find any association between higher inflammatory levels and frailty. The authors attribute this result to the paucity of data, to an over-adjustment of the analyses and/or to the fact that frail people were prone to diseases that might have increased the levels of inflammatory cytokines during the follow-up period and the lack of an adjustment for inherent changes to these markers in their analyses.

As an important limitation of this work, we can point out that this is a cross-sectional study, which does not follow individuals over time. A follow-up study using the same approaches to investigate frailty in this population is currently underway in our group. On the other hand, the statistical power of our sample size allows the expansion of our findings to other already recognized socially vulnerable populations. Notwithstanding, the knowledge of the characteristics related to socioeconomic and biological conditions configures an important tool to raise

**Table 4** Results of multivariable ordinal logistic regression for frailty (*n* = 257)

| Variable | Category | O.R. | 95% CI | *p*-value |
|---|---|---|---|---|
| Sex | Female (ref.) | 1.00 | – | – |
| | Male | 1.61 | 0.89–2.92 | 0.116 |
| Age | 60–69 years (ref.) | 1.00 | – | – |
| | 70–79 years | 1.26 | 0.72–2.21 | 0.422 |
| | ≥80 years | 2.47 | 1.09–5.61 | **0.031*** |
| HDL (mg/dL, tertile) | ≥51 (ref.) | 1.00 | – | – |
| | 42–50 | 1.02 | 0.55–1.89 | 0.942 |
| | ≤41 | 1.03 | 0.53–2.02 | 0.931 |
| VLDL (mg/dL, tertile) | ≤20 (ref.) | 1.00 | – | – |
| | 21–31 | 1.49 | 0.21–10.51 | 0.687 |
| | ≥32 | 1.38 | 0.09–21.22 | 0.818 |
| Urea (mg/dL, tertile) | ≤30 (ref.) | 1.00 | – | – |
| | 31–39 | 1.28 | 0.66–2.46 | 0.469 |
| | ≥40 | 1.73 | 0.86–3.45 | 0.123 |
| Creatinine (mg/dL, tertile) | ≤0.7 (ref.) | 1.00 | – | – |
| | 0.8–1.0 | 0.67 | 0.33–1.34 | 0.256 |
| | ≥1.1 | 1.21 | 0.51–2.91 | 0.668 |
| Triglycerides (mg/dL, tertile) | ≤103 (ref.) | 1.00 | – | – |
| | 104–158 | 0.39 | 0.06–2.78 | 0.350 |
| | ≥159 | 0.72 | 0.05–10.92 | 0.810 |
| IL-1β (pg/mL, tertile) | ≤0.86 (ref.) | 1.00 | – | – |
| | 0.87–2.30 | 1.05 | 0.54–2.05 | 0.890 |
| | ≥2.31 | 0.88 | 0.44–1.74 | 0.707 |
| IL-6 (pg/mL, tertile) | ≤1.50 (ref.) | 1.00 | – | – |
| | 1.51–2.60 | 1.80 | 0.92–3.54 | 0.088 |
| | ≥2.61 | 1.84 | 0.93–3.64 | 0.078 |
| TNF-β (pg/mL, tertile) | ≤0.29 (ref.) | 1.00 | – | – |
| | 0.30–0.80 | 1.14 | 0.59–2.18 | 0.698 |
| | ≥0.81 | 2.53 | 1.30–4.90 | **0.006*** |

*Notes:* OR (*Odds Ratio*) = risk of frailty. 95% CI = 95% Confidence interval for odds ratio. *Values with statistical significance (*p* < 0.05)
Score Test for the Proportional Odds Assumption: X2 = 17.59; DF = 19; *P* = 0.550; *n* = 29 non-frail, *n* = 143 pre-frail and *n* = 85 frail
All other bold entries represent the *p* values of significant results

preventive strategies to decrease frailty risk in the most vulnerable populations.

## Conclusions

Taken together, the results presented here could help to implement preventive healthcare strategies by evaluating frailty and at the same time measuring a set of inflammatory biomarkers, paying special attention to TNF-β plasmatic levels. This could enable health teams to plan and improve care actions for this population, especially in the community and in primary health services.

## Abbreviations

BMI: Body Mass Index; DHEA: Dehydroepiandrosterone; DHEA-S: Dehydroepiandrosterone sulfate; GDS: Geriatric Depression Scale; GH: Human Growth Hormone; IGF-1: Insulin-like Growth Factor-1; IL-1α: Interleukin-1α; IL-1β: Interleukin-1β; IL-6: Interleukin-6; IPAQ: International Physical Activity Questionnaire; SVI: Social Vulnerability Index; TNFα: Tumor Necrosis Factor α; TNFβ: Tumor Necrosis Factor β

## Acknowledgments

The authors are grateful to the team of gerontologists and nurses who performed the data collection and biological material and to all the family members and older adults who participated in this study.

## Funding

This work was supported by the Research Program for SUS-PPSUS/Ministry of Health and São Paulo Research Foundation (FAPESP) grant #2014/50104-0, the National Council for Scientific and Technological Development (CNPq) and the Coordination of Improvement of Higher Education Personnel - Brazil (CAPES) - Grant #001. CMCN has a postdoc fellowship from FAPESP, grant #2014/21066-2.

## Authors' contributions

CMCN collected and analyzed the data; GAOG, FSO, KG-S, FAV, ACMG, MSZ, SCIP, MRC participated in the conception and design of the study; CMCN and MRC prepared the manuscript. All authors revised the final version of the manuscript. The sponsors of this study were not involved in the design, methods, subject recruitment, data collections, analysis, or preparation of paper. All authors read and approved the final manuscript.

## Competing interests

The authors declare that they have no competing interests.

## References

1. Fried LP, Tangen CM, Walston J, Newman AB, Hirsch C, Gottdiener J, Seeman T, Tracy R, Kop WJ, Burke G, et al. Frailty in older adults: evidence for a phenotype. J Gerontol A Biol Sci Med Sci. 2001;56(3):M146–56.
2. Kulmala J, Nykanen I, Hartikainen S. Frailty as a predictor of all-cause mortality in older men and women. Geriatr Gerontol Int. 2014;14(4):899–905.
3. Mitnitski AB, Rutenberg AD, Farrell S, Rockwood K. Aging, frailty and complex networks. Biogerontology. 2017;18(4):433–46.
4. Andrew MK, Keefe JM. Social vulnerability from a social ecology perspective: a cohort study of older adults from the National Population Health Survey of Canada. BMC Geriatr. 2014;14:90.
5. Andrew MK, Mitnitski AB, Rockwood K. Social vulnerability, frailty and mortality in elderly people. PLoS One. 2008;3(5):e2232.
6. Andrew MK. Frailty and social vulnerability. Interdiscip Top Gerontol Geriatr. 2015;41:186–95.
7. Andrew MK, Rockwood K. Social vulnerability predicts cognitive decline in a prospective cohort of older Canadians. Alzheimers Dement. 2010;6(4):319–25 e311.
8. Curcio CL, Henao GM, Gomez F. Frailty among rural elderly adults. BMC Geriatr. 2014;14:2.
9. De Martinis M, Franceschi C, Monti D, Ginaldi L. Inflammation markers predicting frailty and mortality in the elderly. Exp Mol Pathol. 2006;80(3):219–27.
10. Franceschi C, Bonafe M, Valensin S, Olivieri F, De Luca M, Ottaviani E, De Benedictis G. Inflamm-aging. An evolutionary perspective on immunosenescence. Ann N Y Acad Sci. 2000;908:244–54.
11. Chang SS, Weiss CO, Xue QL, Fried LP. Association between inflammatory-related disease burden and frailty: results from the Women's health and aging studies (WHAS) I and II. Arch Gerontol Geriatr. 2012;54(1):9–15.
12. Mocchegiani E, Corsonello A, Lattanzio F. Frailty, ageing and inflammation: reality and perspectives. Biogerontology. 2010;11(5):523–5.
13. Baylis D, Bartlett DB, Syddall HE, Ntani G, Gale CR, Cooper C, Lord JM, Sayer

AA. Immune-endocrine biomarkers as predictors of frailty and mortality: a 10-year longitudinal study in community-dwelling older people. Age. 2013; 35(3):963–71.

14. Hubbard RE, Woodhouse KW. Frailty, inflammation and the elderly. Biogerontology. 2010;11(5):635–41.

15. Darvin K, Randolph A, Ovalles S, Halade D, Breeding L, Richardson A, Espinoza SE. Plasma protein biomarkers of the geriatric syndrome of frailty. J Gerontol A Biol Sci Med Sci. 2014;69(2):182–6.

16. Kanapuru B, Ershler WB. Inflammation, coagulation, and the pathway to frailty. Am J Med. 2009;122(7):605–13.

17. Puts MTE, Visser M, Twisk JWR, Deeg DJH, Lips P. Endocrine and inflammatory markers as predictors of frailty. Clin Endocrinol. 2005;63(4):403–11.

18. Calvani R, Marini F, Cesari M, Tosato M, Anker SD, von Haehling S, Miller RR, Bernabei R, Landi F, Marzetti E, et al. Biomarkers for physical frailty and sarcopenia: state of the science and future developments. J Cachexia Sarcopenia Muscle. 2015;6(4):278–86.

19. Cesari M, Penninx BW, Pahor M, Lauretani F, Corsi AM, Rhys Williams G, Guralnik JM, Ferrucci L. Inflammatory markers and physical performance in older persons: the InCHIANTI study. J Gerontol A Biol Sci Med Sci. 2004;59(3):242–8.

20. Tiainen K, Hurme M, Hervonen A, Luukkaala T, Jylha M. Inflammatory markers and physical performance among nonagenarians. A Biol Sci Med Sci. 2010;65(6):658–63.

21. Visser M, Pahor M, Taaffe DR, Goodpaster BH, Simonsick EM, Newman AB, Nevitt M, Harris TB. Relationship of interleukin-6 and tumor necrosis factor-alpha with muscle mass and muscle strength in elderly men and women: the health ABC study. J Gerontol A Biol Sci Med Sci. 2002;57(5):M326–32.

22. Verghese J, Holtzer R, Oh-Park M, Derby CA, Lipton RB, Wang C. Inflammatory markers and gait speed decline in older adults. J Gerontol A Biol Sci Med Sci. 2011;66(10):1083–9.

23. Penninx BW, Kritchevsky SB, Newman AB, Nicklas BJ, Simonsick EM, Rubin S, Nevitt M, Visser M, Harris T, Pahor M. Inflammatory markers and incident mobility limitation in the elderly. J Am Geriatr Soc. 2004;52(7):1105–13.

24. Penninx BWJH, Pahor M, Cesari M, Corsi AM, Woodman RC, Bandinelli S, Guralnik JM, Ferrucci L. Anemia is associated with disability and decreased physical performance and muscle strength in the elderly. J Am Geriatr Soc. 2004;52(5):719–24.

25. Visser M, Kritchevsky SB, Newman AB, Goodpaster BH, Tylavsky FA, Nevitt MC, Harris TB, Composition HAB. Lower serum albumin concentration and change in muscle mass: the health, Aging and Body Composition Study. Am J Clin Nutr. 2005;82(3):531–7.

26. Voznesensky M, Walsh S, Dauser D, Brindisi J, Kenny AM. The association between dehydroepiandosterone and frailty in older men and women. Age Ageing. 2009;38(4):401–6.

27. Araujo AB, Travison TG, Bhasin S, Esche GR, Williams RE, Clark RV, McKinlay JB: Association between testosterone and estradiol and age-related decline in physical function in a diverse sample of men. J Am Geriatr Soc 2008, 56(11):2000–2008.

28. Onder G, Liperoti R, Russo A, Soldato M, Capoluongo E, Volpato S, Cesari M, Ameglio F, Bernabei R, Landi F. Body mass index, free insulin-like growth factor I, and physical function among older adults: results from the ilSIRENTE study. Am J Phys Endocrinol Metab. 2006;291(4):E829–34.

29. Mastaglia SR, Seijo M, Muzio D, Somoza J, Nunez M, Oliveri B. Effect of vitamin D nutritional status on muscle function and strength in healthy women aged over sixty-five years. J Nutr Health Aging. 2011;15(5):349–54.

30. Zazzetta MS, Gomes GA, Orlandi FS, Gratao AC, Vasilceac FA, Gramani-Say K, Ponti MA, Castro PC, Pavarini SC, Menezes AL, et al. Identifying frailty levels and associated factors in a population living in the context of poverty and social vulnerability. J Frailty Aging. 2017;6(1):29–32.

31. Pessoa VM, Rigotto RM, Carneiro FF, Teixeira AC. Meanings and methods of territorialization in primary health care. Cien Saude Colet. 2013;18(8):2253–62.

32. Dados S-FSEdAd. Índice Paulista de Vulnerabilidade Social, vol. 17. São Paulo: Fundação SEADE; 2013.

33. Nunes DP, Duarte YA, Santos JL, Lebrao ML. Screening for frailty in older adults using a self-reported instrument. Revista de saude publica. 2015;49:2.

34. Batistoni SST, Neri AL, Cupertino APFB. Validity of the center for epidemiological studies depression scale among brazilian elderly. Revista de saude publica. 2007;41(4):598–605.

35. Hagstromer M, Oja P, Sjostrom M. The international physical activity questionnaire (IPAQ): a study of concurrent and construct validity. Public Health Nutr. 2006;9(6):755–62.

36. Brucki SM, Nitrini R, Caramelli P, Bertolucci PH, Okamoto IH. Suggestions for utilization of the mini-mental state examination in Brazil. Arq Neuropsiquiatr. 2003;61(3B):777–81.

37. Almeida OP, Almeida SA. Reliability of the Brazilian version of the + +abbreviated form of geriatric depression scale (GDS) short form. Arq Neuropsiquiatr. 1999;57(2B):421–6.

38. Pereira AA, Borim FSA, Neri AL. Absence of association between frailty index and survival in elderly Brazilians: the FIBRA study. Cad Saude Publica. 2017; 33(5):e00194115.

39. Collard RM, Boter H, Schoevers RA, Oude Voshaar RC. Prevalence of frailty in community-dwelling older persons: a systematic review. J Am Geriatr Soc. 2012;60(8):1487–92.

40. Moreira VG, Lourenco RA. Prevalence and factors associated with frailty in an older population from the city of Rio de Janeiro, Brazil: the FIBRA-RJ study. Clinics. 2013;68(7):979–85.

41. Sousa AC, Dias RC, Maciel AC, Guerra RO. Frailty syndrome and associated factors in community-dwelling elderly in Northeast Brazil. Arch Gerontol Geriatr. 2012;54(2):e95–e101.

42. Buckinx F, Rolland Y, Reginster JY, Ricour C, Petermans J, Bruyere O. Burden of frailty in the elderly population: perspectives for a public health challenge. Arch Public Health. 2015;73(1):19.

43. Gordon EH, Peel NM, Samanta M, Theou O, Howlett SE, Hubbard RE. Sex differences in frailty: a systematic review and meta-analysis. Exp Gerontol. 2017;89:30–40.

44. Theou O, Rockwood MR, Mitnitski A, Rockwood K. Disability and co-morbidity in relation to frailty: how much do they overlap? Arch Gerontol Geriatr. 2012;55(2):e1–8.

45. Banks J, Muriel A, Smith JP. Disease prevalence, disease incidence, and mortality in the United States and in England. Demography. 2010; 47(Suppl):S211–31.

46. de Azevedo Barros MB, Lima MG, LdPB M, Szwarcwald CL, Malta DC. Social inequalities in health behaviors among Brazilian adults: National Health Survey, 2013. Int J Equity Health. 2016;15(1):148.

47. Boccolini CS, de Souza Junior PR. Inequities in healthcare utilization: results of the Brazilian National Health Survey, 2013. Int J Equity Health. 2016;15(1):150.

48. Goronzy JJ, Weyand CM. Understanding immunosenescence to improve responses to vaccines. Nat Immunol. 2013;14(5):428–36.

49. Wilson D, Jackson T, Sapey E, Lord JM. Frailty and sarcopenia: the potential role of an aged immune system. Ageing Res Rev. 2017;36:1–10.

50. Soysal P, Stubbs B, Lucato P, Luchini C, Solmi M, Peluso R, Sergi G, Isik AT, Manzato E, Maggi S, et al. Inflammation and frailty in the elderly: a systematic review and meta-analysis. Ageing Res Rev. 2016;31:1–8.

51. Komaki Y, Yamada A, Komaki F, Kudaravalli P, Micic D, Ido A, Sakuraba A. Efficacy, safety and pharmacokinetics of biosimilars of anti-tumor necrosis factor-alpha agents in rheumatic diseases; a systematic review and meta-analysis. J Autoimmun. 2017;79:4–16.

52. Willrich MA, Murray DL, Snyder MR. Tumor necrosis factor inhibitors: clinical utility in autoimmune diseases. Transl Res. 2015;165(2):270–82.

53. Speeckaert MM, Speeckaert R, Laute M, Vanholder R, Delanghe JR. Tumor necrosis factor receptors: biology and therapeutic potential in kidney diseases. Am J Nephrol. 2012;36(3):261–70.

54. Tumanov AV, Christiansen PA, Fu YX. The role of lymphotoxin receptor signaling in diseases. Curr Mol Med. 2007;7(6):567–78.

# 19

# Prevalence of frailty, cognitive impairment, and sarcopenia in outpatients with cardiometabolic disease in a frailty clinic

Yoshiaki Tamura[1*], Joji Ishikawa[2], Yoshinori Fujiwara[3], Masashi Tanaka[4], Nobuo Kanazawa[5], Yuko Chiba[1], Ai Iizuka[3], Sho Kaito[3], Jun Tanaka[2], Masamitsu Sugie[2], Takashi Nishimura[6], Akiko Kanemaru[7], Keigo Shimoji[8], Hirohiko Hirano[9], Ko Furuta[10], Akihiko Kitamura[3], Satoshi Seino[3], Shoji Shinkai[3], Kazumasa Harada[2], Shunei Kyo[6], Hideki Ito[1] and Atsushi Araki[1]

## Abstract

**Background:** Although frailty and cognitive impairment are critical risk factors for disability and mortality in the general population of older inhabitants, the prevalence and incidence of these factors in individuals treated in the specialty outpatient clinics are unknown.

**Methods:** We recently established a frailty clinic for comprehensive assessments of conditions such as frailty, sarcopenia, and cognition, and planned 3-year prospective observational study to identify the risk factors for progression of these aging-related statuses. To date, we recruited 323 patients who revealed symptoms suggestive of frailty mainly from a specialty outpatient clinic of cardiology and diabetes. Frailty status was diagnosed by the modified Cardiovascular Health Study (mCHS) criteria and some other scales. Cognitive function was assessed by Mini-Mental State Examination (MMSE), Japanese version of the Montreal Cognitive Assessment (MoCA-J), and some other modalities. Sarcopenia was defined by the criteria of the Asian Working Group for Sarcopenia (AWGS). In this report, we outlined our frailty clinic and analyzed the background characteristics of the subjects.

**Results:** Most patients reported hypertension (78%), diabetes mellitus (57%), or dyslipidemia (63%), and cardiovascular disease and probable heart failure also had a higher prevalence. The prevalence of frailty diagnosed according to the mCHS criteria, cognitive impairment defined by MMSE ($\leq$27) and MoCA-J ($\leq$25), and of AWGS-defined sarcopenia were 24, 41, and 84, and 31%, respectively. The prevalence of frailty and cognitive impairment increased with aging, whereas the increase in sarcopenia prevalence plateaued after the age of 80 years. No significant differences were observed in the prevalence of frailty, cognitive impairment, and sarcopenia between the groups with and without diabetes mellitus, hypertension, or dyslipidemia with a few exceptions, presumably due to the high-risk subjects who had multiple cardiovascular comorbidities. A majority of the frail and sarcopenic patients revealed cognitive impairment, whereas the frequency of suspected dementia among these patients were both approximately 20%.

**Conclusions:** We found a high prevalence of frailty, cognitive impairment, and sarcopenia in patients with cardiometabolic disease in our frailty clinic. Comprehensive assessment of the high-risk patients could be useful to identify the risk factors for progression of frailty and cognitive decline.

**Keywords:** Frailty, Frailty clinic, Modified CHS criteria, Cognitive impairment, Sarcopenia, Cardiometabolic diseases

* Correspondence: tamurayo@tmghig.jp
[1]Department of Diabetes, Metabolism, and Endocrinology, Tokyo Metropolitan Geriatric Hospital, Tokyo, Japan
Full list of author information is available at the end of the article

## Background

Recently, although life expectancies in the developed countries, including Japan, have been increasing, the number of older people with functional disabilities who need assistance from others is also on rise. Extending healthy life expectancy is an urgent task for the gerontologists.

Frailty is a state in which an older person becomes vulnerable to the external stresses due to declining age-related physiological reserve and can lead to disabilities, falls, fractures, and death [1, 2]. Frailty is a reversible condition because physical and nutritional intervention can improve a person's physical condition. The concept of multidimensional frailty based on a comprehensive geriatric assessment has been proposed because cognitive and social frailties, as well as physical frailty, have a major effect on disability and mortality. Thus, it is essential to screen for frailty and cognitive deficits in the older people to prevent deterioration of their functional ability.

The prevalence of frailty has been reported to be approximately10% in the general population of older inhabitants. Although cardiometabolic diseases [diabetes mellitus (DM), hypertension (HT), dyslipidemia (DL), and heart failure] have been associated with the prevalence of frailty in epidemiological studies, this prevalence in the individuals treated in the cardiology and diabetes specialty outpatient clinics remains unknown.

However, it is difficult to complete the multidimensional assessment of frailty during the routine visits in the outpatient clinics. Therefore, we recently established a frailty clinic and identified a cohort group of patients in the clinic for inclusion in a 3-year prospective longitudinal study.

The aim of this prospective study was to answer the following questions: first, what is the prevalence and incidence of frailty in the specialized frailty clinic? what are the associations, if any, between frailty status and clinical outcomes of fall, cardiovascular disease, dementia, hospitalization, functional disability, and death? and what are the most useful indices for predicting these outcomes in evaluating frailty status?

In this article, we describe our frailty clinic and the baseline characteristics of the patients in a cohort for the prospective longitudinal study.

## Methods

### Frailty clinic

Our frailty clinic was opened to comprehensively assess frailty, sarcopenia, cognition, psychological condition, nutrition, medications, and social status of patients in October 2015. At present, doctors from the departments of endocrinology and cardiology examine the patients in the frailty clinic in a rotational system. One to two clinical psychologists are present in the clinic every day to interview the patients.

### Subjects

Three hundred twenty-five patients were recruited mainly from the outpatient clinics of cardiology and diabetes departments of our hospital who gave their consent to be assessed for frailty. When the subjects initially visited the frailty clinic, informed consent was obtained for inclusion in a planned 3-year observational study. After a short interview to gather information on their medical history, family history, and life history, a brief systematic physical examination was performed by a physician to identify any underlying disease. Patients who revealed a history of advanced cancer, acute severe diseases or conditions requiring hospitalization, and severely impaired activities of daily living (ADL) and/or cognitive function, were excluded. Only one patient was excluded by these criteria, because of severe heart failure. Patients who were free of these diseases were subjected to questionnaires, physical function tests, and a body composition assessment, as described below. All patients underwent the same assessments. The flow chart of the method is shown in Fig. 1. Six hospitalized patients with DM and HT, who were

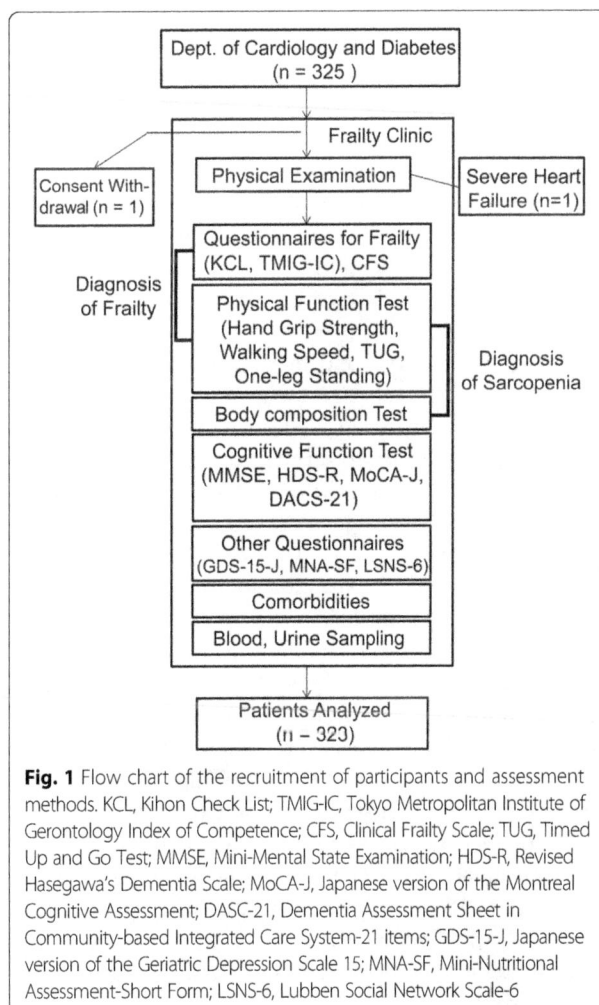

**Fig. 1** Flow chart of the recruitment of participants and assessment methods. KCL, Kihon Check List; TMIG-IC, Tokyo Metropolitan Institute of Gerontology Index of Competence; CFS, Clinical Frailty Scale; TUG, Timed Up and Go Test; MMSE, Mini-Mental State Examination; HDS-R, Revised Hasegawa's Dementia Scale; MoCA-J, Japanese version of the Montreal Cognitive Assessment; DASC-21, Dementia Assessment Sheet in Community-based Integrated Care System-21 items; GDS-15-J, Japanese version of the Geriatric Depression Scale 15; MNA-SF, Mini-Nutritional Assessment-Short Form; LSNS-6, Lubben Social Network Scale-6

generally stable, were also included. One subject withdrew the consent. Finally, a total of 323 patients were enrolled for the analysis in this study.

In this report, the subjects were registered as the first cohort between June 22, 2015 and Mar 10, 2017; however, as this is an ongoing study, the number of subjects will increase to up to 800 as the final cohort.

### Frailty status

Frailty status was evaluated according to the following four criteria: I) The modified version of the Cardiovascular Health Study (CHS) criteria (mCHS). CHS criteria were originally proposed by Fried et al. [1] and comprised five indices of frailty: weight loss, exhaustion, weakness, inactivity, and low walking speed. We modified the CHS based on the report by Makizono et al. [3] in which their criteria were adapted to a Japanese population. For assessing weakness, hand grip strength < 26 kg (males) and < 18 kg (females) were set as the cutoff points regardless of the body mass index (BMI). To evaluate the slow gait speed, 4-m walk tests were administered, and a walk speed < 1.0 m/s, regardless of sex or body height, was set as a cutoff. We further modified the CHS criteria by using certain questions in the Kihon Check List (KCL) [4]. For evaluating the body weight loss and exhaustion, the KCL questions, "Did you experience >2–3 kg of body weight loss in the last 6 months?" and "In the last 2 weeks, have you felt tired without a reason?" were asked. For the question of low physical activity, those who answered either "No" for the question "Do you go out at least once a week?" or "Yes" for the question "Do you go out less frequently than you did last year?" were defined as positive. Subjects who were positive in three of the five indices were diagnosed as frail, and those positive in one or two indices were diagnosed as prefrail.

II) Clinical Frailty Scale (CFS); patients were classified into nine categories based on their dependence on others [5]. We defined subjects whose CFS scores were ≥ 4 as frail, although in the original report, the term "frail" was used for scores ≥5.

III) KCL; the KCL was created by the Ministry of Health, Labor, and Welfare of the Japanese government for screening the older frail group and comprised 25 items that evaluate not only ADL and physical function but also nutrition, oral health, social withdrawal, cognition, and depression. Subjects whose scores were ≥ 8 were diagnosed as frail [4]. IV) The Tokyo Metropolitan Institute of Gerontology Index of Competence (TMIG-IC); the TMIG-IC was originally created by our institute to evaluate the higher-level functional capacity [6]. It comprises 13 items, evaluating the instrumental ADL (5 items), intellectual activity (4 items), and social role (4 items). Subjects whose scores were ≤ 9 were diagnosed as frail.

### Cognitive function assessment

The Mini-Mental State Examination (MMSE) and Hasegawa's Dementia Scale-Revised (HDS-R) were used for the functional assessments. We also performed the Japanese version of the Montreal Cognitive Assessment (MoCA-J) [7]. We further performed the Dementia Assessment Sheet in Community-based Integrated Care System-21 items (DASC-21), a questionnaire set used to easily evaluate the impaired cognitive function and basic ADL at the same time [8]. Cognitive impairment was defined as an MMSE score ≤ 27 or an MoCA-J ≤ 25 [7, 9], and suspected dementia was defined as an MMSE score ≤ 23, HDS-$R$ ≤ 20, or DASC-21 ≥ 31.

### Depressive mood, nutritional status, and social support network

The Japanese version of the Geriatric Depression Scale 15 (GDS-15-J) was used to evaluate depressive mood [10]. Subjects whose scores were ≥ 5 were suspected to have a depressive tendency. To evaluate the subjects' nutritional status, the Mini-Nutritional Assessment-Short Form (MNA-SF) was used [11], which comprised 6 items, with a highest score of 14; subjects with scores from 8 to 11 were suspected to be at risk of malnutrition, whereas subjects with scores of ≤7 were suspected as being malnourished. The status of the subjects' social support was evaluated by using the Japanese version of the Lubben Social Network Scale-6 (LSNS-6) [12]. Scores ranged from 0 to 30, and lower scores indicate a lack of social support.

### Physical performance tests

Hand grip, usual walking speed, timed up and go test (TUG), and one-leg standing were performed. Hand grip strength was measured by using a dynamometer (Takei Scientific Instruments Co., Ltd., Niigata, Japan) for both hands, and the best results were recorded. To measure usual walking speed, patients were instructed to walk for 6 m at their ordinary speed. The time spent for walking the middle 4 m was measured, and the walking speed was calculated. Hand grip and walking speed were measured twice, and the best result was recorded. Details of TUG have been described elsewhere [13]. Briefly, the time spent for the following series of movement was measured: standing up, walking (at a maximum speed) to a mark 3 m ahead, turning, walking (at a maximum speed) back to a seat, and sitting down. For one-leg standing, patients were instructed to stand on either of their legs for maximum duration, and the time was recorded. The TUG and one-leg standing test were administered twice, and the average value was recorded; however, for the one-leg standing test, if the better value was more than twice the other, the better value was recorded, and if a subject could stand for > 60 s for either of the two trials, the time was recorded as 60 s. If a subject could not complete the 4-m walking test or TUG, their data were omitted, whereas the time of those who could not stand on either leg was recorded as 0 s.

### Body composition test and diagnosis of sarcopenia

Body composition was evaluated by bioimpedance analysis using an InBody 770® (InBody Japan Inc., Tokyo, Japan). Skeletal muscle mass index (SMI) was calculated by dividing the appendicular muscle mass (kg) by the square of body height (m). Sarcopenia was diagnosed according to the criteria of the Asian Working Group for Sarcopenia (AWGS) [14]. Those who also exhibited low SMI in conjunction with either low grip strength or slow walking speed were diagnosed as having sarcopenia.

### Comorbidities

The concurrent diseases were diagnosed by descriptions in the clinical records. History of coronary artery disease (CAD) was defined as a history of either angina pectoris or myocardial infarction or both. History of stroke was defined as a history of either cerebral infarction or cerebral bleeding or both. Probable heart failure was diagnosed either by the clinical record or as brain natriuretic peptide (BNP) values ≥100 pg/mL.

### Blood sampling

Blood was collected ad libitum. Blood cell count, blood biochemistry tests, and measurement of glycohemoglobin (HbA1c) and plasma BNP were performed as normally done in the clinic. Serum was preserved at − 20 °C for further investigation.

### Other evaluation tests

Self-measured blood pressure at home, ambulatory blood pressure monitoring, central arterial pressure, ankle brachial pressure index, pulse wave velocity, carotid Doppler ultrasonography, echocardiography, brain magnetic resonance imaging, lower extremity motor function analysis to measure power, speed, and balance during a standing-up motion (zaRitz®; Tanita Corp., Tokyo, Japan) and an autonomic nervous function test (Kiritsu-Meijin®; Crosswell Co., Ltd., Kanagawa, Japan) were performed in some patients when necessary. To assess the quality of life of health status, the Japanese version of the questionnaire EQ-5D-5 L was used [15]. To evaluate physical activity, the International Physical Activity Questionnaire was used [16]. To assess the frequency of going outdoors and social participation, questionnaires adopted in the previous reports were used [17, 18]. In addition, the subjects were asked if they had a certified level of support or care needs or if they had received any long-term care services from the health insurance system in Japan.

### Outcomes of the longitudinal study

During the 3-year longitudinal observational study, the following outcomes were evaluated annually using questionnaires and medical charts: (1) incidence of fall and fracture; (2) incidence or progression of frailty status; (3) dementia; (4) cardiovascular disease (myocardial infarction, stroke, cardiovascular interventions); (5) hospitalization; (6) certified level of support or long-term care needs from the insurance system; and (7) death.

### Statistical analysis

To test the difference in the frequencies between groups of categorical data, we used the chi-square test. To compare the continuous valuables between the two groups, we used the Mann–Whitney test. All statistical analyses were performed by using the SPSS Statistics 20 software package (IBM, Armonk, NY, USA). In all comparisons, the significance level was set at $P < 0.05$.

## Results

### Background of the subjects

The study participants included 323 patients who visited the frailty clinic. The characteristics of the subjects are summarized in Table 1. These patients were aged between

**Table 1** Background characteristics of subjects ($n = 323$)

| | |
|---|---|
| Age (y) | 78 (75–82) |
| Male (%) | 37.8 |
| BMI (kg/m²) | 23.0 (21.3–25.5) |
| Systolic BP (mmHg) ($n = 320$) | 130 (120–140) |
| Diastolic BP (mmHg) ($n = 320$) | 74 (65–82) |
| HbA1c (%) ($n = 321$) | 6.4 (5.9–7.1) |
| TC (mg/dl) ($n = 321$) | 191 (168–215) |
| TG (mg/dl) ($n = 321$) | 119 (84–164) |
| HDL-cholesterol (mg/dl) ($n = 321$) | 55 (47–66) |
| eGFR (mL/min/1.73m²) ($n = 321$) | 58 (47–68) |
| BNP (pg/mL) ($n = 287$) | 35 (21–70) |
| Hypertension (%) ($n = 320$) | 78.0 |
| Diabetes Mellitus (%) | 57.3 |
| Dyslipidemia (%) | 62.5 |
| CAD (%) | 18.0 |
| Stroke (%) ($n = 312$) | 10.9 |
| Probable Heart Failure (%) ($n = 288$) | 22.2 |
| GDS-15-J ($n = 322$) | 4 (2–7) |
| MNA-SF ($n = 322$) | 12 (10–13) |
| LSNS-6 ($n = 309$) | 12 (8–16) |

*Abbreviations: BMI* body mass index, *BP* blood pressure, *HbA1c* glycohemoglobin, *TC* total cholesterol, *TG* triglyceride, *HDL* high-density lipoprotein, *eGFR* estimated glomerular filtration rate, *CAD* coronary artery disease, *GDS-15-J* Japanese version of the Geriatric Depression Scale 15, *MNA-SF* Mini-Nutritional Assessment-Short Form, *LSNS-6* Lubben Social Network Scale-6
For continuous variables, values indicate median (25–75th percentile)

50 and 95 years, but 97% were ≥ 65 years, with a median age of 78 years. Reflecting the background of the subjects recruited from the endocrinology and cardiology departments, the major comorbidities of the subjects were the metabolic and cardiac diseases, including HT (78%), DM (57%), dyslipidemia (DL, 63%), CAD (18%), stroke (11%), and probable heart failure (22%). Scores of GDS-15-J, MNA-SF, and the Japanese version of LSNS-6 are also summarized in Table 1. Forty-eight percent of the patients scored ≥5 points in the GDS-15-J. Nutritional statuses were fairly good in this population.

### Prevalence of frailty, cognitive impairment, and sarcopenia

The prevalence of frailty and cognitive impairment is summarized in Table 2. The prevalence of subjects who were robust, prefrail, and frail diagnosed by the mCHS were 26, 50, and 24%, respectively. According to the CFS, KCL, and TMIG-IC criteria, 32, 34, and 27%, respectively, of the subjects were diagnosed as being frail.

The median MMSE, HDS-R, MoCA-J, and DASC-21 scores were 28, 27, 22, and 24, respectively. The prevalence of cognitive impairment was higher than that for suspected dementia but was significantly different between the evaluation methods; the assessment by an MMSE score ≤ 27 revealed prevalence of 41%, while the prevalence according to

**Table 2** Background characteristics of frailty and cognitive function

| Frailty status | |
|---|---|
| mCHS status (n = 303) | |
| Robust (%) | 26.1 |
| Prefrailty (%) | 49.8 |
| Frailty (%) | 24.1 |
| Frailty (%) by CFS (n = 315) | 31.7 |
| Frailty (%) by KCL (n = 311) | 33.8 |
| Frailty (%) by TMIG-IC (n = 320) | 26.6 |
| Cognitive function | |
| MMSE (n = 320) | 28 (26–29) |
| HDS-R (n = 320) | 27 (24–29) |
| MoCA-J (n = 320) | 22 (19–25) |
| DASC-21 (n = 264) | 24 (23–27) |
| Cognitive impairment | |
| MMSE ≤27 (%)(n = 320) | 40.9 |
| MoCA -J ≤ 25 (%)(n = 320) | 84.1 |
| Suspected dementia | |
| MMSE ≤23 (%)(n = 320) | 12.8 |
| HDS-R ≤ 20 (%)(n = 320) | 11.6 |
| DASC-21 ≥ 31 (%)(n = 264) | 14.8 |

Abbreviations: SMI Skeletal Muscle Mass Index, TUG Timed up and go test For continuous variables, values indicate median (25–75th percentile)

the criteria of MoCA-J ≤ 25 was 84%. The prevalence of suspected dementia was comparable between the evaluation methods; assessment by an MMSE score ≤ 23, HDS-R ≤ 20, and DASC-21 ≥ 31 revealed prevalence of 13, 12, and 15%, respectively.

The results of body composition, physical performance tests and sarcopenia are summarized in Table 3. The prevalence of sarcopenia in males and females were 33 and 30%, respectively. For the diagnostic elements, approximately half of the patients matched the criteria of low SMI and low hand grip in both sexes. In contrast, the number of patients with low gait speed was significantly small.

### Prevalence of frailty, cognitive impairment, and sarcopenia stratified by age

Figure 2 presents the prevalence of frailty, suspected dementia, cognitive impairment, and sarcopenia stratified by age categories of 65–74, 75–79, 80–84, and ≥ 85 years. The percentage of robust subjects diagnosed according to the mCHS criteria decreased significantly with the increasing age, whereas the percentages of subjects who were frail and had suspected dementia, cognitive impairment, and sarcopenia, were all significantly increased with the increasing age. Almost half of the subjects who were ≥ 85 years old were frail, and the prevalence of cognitive impairment (defined by the MoCA-J ≤ 25) and sarcopenia in subjects ≥80 years were approximately 90 and 50%, respectively. The increase in sarcopenia prevalence plateaued after the age of 80 years.

### Prevalence of patients with frailty, sarcopenia, and cognitive impairment among the DM, HT, and DL subjects

Tables 4 and 5 summarizes the prevalence of patients with frailty (Table 4), suspected dementia, cognitive impairment and sarcopenia (Table 5) compared between those with and without DM, with and without HT, and with and without DL stratified by age. There were no significant differences, except for the significantly higher and lower prevalence of sarcopenia in the ≤74 years age group of DM and the 80–84 years age group of HT, respectively.

### Overlap of frailty, sarcopenia, and cognitive impairment/ suspected dementia

The overlap of frailty, sarcopenia, and suspected dementia (MMSE ≤23)/cognitive impairment (MoCA-J ≤ 25) are presented in Fig. 3a and b. Approximately, 60% of the frail subjects were also sarcopenic and 40% of those with sarcopenia were also frail. Of interest, patterns of the diagrams are significantly different in relation to the cognitive function. Approximately, 20% each of the subjects with frailty or with sarcopenia were also diagnosed as having suspected dementia, whereas almost all of the

**Table 3** Background characteristics of body composition, physical function, and sarcopenia

|  | Total | Male | Female |
|---|---|---|---|
| SMI (kg/m$^2$) | 6.3 (5.6–7.0) (n = 312) | 7.0 (6.6–7.7) (n = 119) | 5.8 (5.3–6.4) (n = 193) |
| Hand Grip (kg) | 20.3 (16.1–25.5) (n = 313) | 27.0 (22.3–32.3) (n = 118) | 17.5 (14.5–20.9) (n = 195) |
| Walk Speed (m/s) | 1.11 (0.91–1.29) (n = 312) | 1.11 (0.90–1.28) (n = 119) | 1.11 (0.91–1.30) (n = 193) |
| Low SMI (%) | 45.2 (n = 312) | 48.7 (n = 119) | 43.0 (n = 193) |
| Low Hand Grip (%) | 49.5 (n = 313) | 44.9 (n = 118) | 52.3 (n = 195) |
| Slow Walk Speed (%) | 15.4 (n = 312) | 13.4 (n = 119) | 16.6 (n = 193) |
| Sarcopenia (%) | 31.4 (n = 309) | 33.1 (n = 118) | 30.4 (n = 191) |
| TUG (s) | 7.7 (6.6–9.6) (n = 301) | 7.3 (6.2–9.3) (n = 116) | 7.9 (6.7–9.8) (n = 185) |
| One Leg Standing (s) | 7.1 (2.3–24.4) (n = 312) | 6.9 (2.5–25.2) (n = 119) | 7.1 (2.1–23.6) (n = 193) |

*Abbreviations*: *mCHS* modified Cardiovascular Health Study, *CFS* Clinical Frailty Scale, *KCL* Kihon Check List, *TMIG-IC* Tokyo Metropolitan Institute of Gerontology Index of Competence, *MMSE* Mini-Mental State Examination, *HDS-R* Hasegawa's Dementia Scale for Revised, *MoCA-J* Japanese version of the Montreal Cognitive Assessment, *DASC-21* Dementia Assessment Sheet in Community-based Integrated Care System-21 itemsFor continuous variables, values indicate median (25–75$^{th}$ percentile)

frail (97%) and sarcopenic (90%) subjects were diagnosed as having cognitive impairment.

## Discussion

In this study, we described our recently established frailty clinic, which mainly treats patients with cardiometabolic diseases. At present, there is an urgent need to assess frailty and cognition in older individuals with cardiometabolic disease because diabetes and cardiovascular disease are associated with the aging process and with frailty and cognitive impairment [19]. We performed a comprehensive geriatric assessment for these patients to evaluate frailty, suspected dementia, cognitive impairment, and sarcopenia and found that the prevalence of all of these conditions increased with increasing age (Fig. 2).

The prevalence of frailty diagnosed according to the mCHS criteria in our study population was about twice as high as that of the recently reported community-dwelling older persons, and in most of those, the prevalence was approximately 10% [20–22]. One reason for the discrepancy was the difference in the diagnostic criteria. We

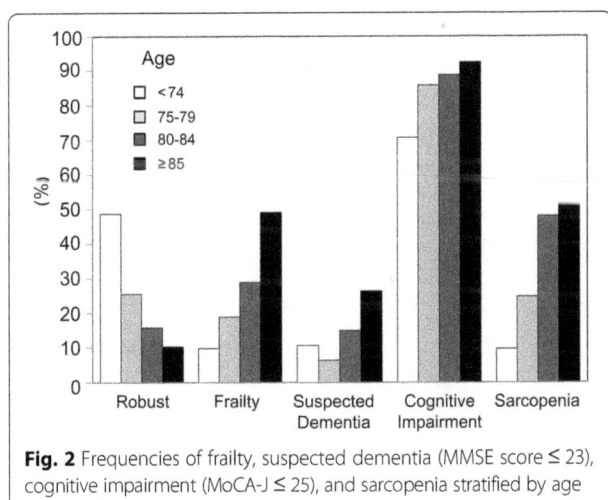

**Fig. 2** Frequencies of frailty, suspected dementia (MMSE score ≤ 23), cognitive impairment (MoCA-J ≤ 25), and sarcopenia stratified by age

modified the cutoff points for SMI, grip strength, and walking speed, and we substituted some questions from the KCL for the original ones since they were easier to obtain answers from the subjects; however, the major reasons for the discrepancy was that our study populations included higher rate of patients aged over 80 and that they comprised outpatients, especially those who had cardiometabolic diseases, since most of them were recruited from the departments of cardiology or diabetes.

In this report, we attempted to evaluate frailty status using several different scales, but the prevalence of frailty varied from 24 to 34% depending on the scale. The highest prevalence was observed in the KCL criteria, which was 10% higher than that in the mCHS criteria, perhaps because the KCL questionnaire assesses multidimensional aspects of frailty, including physical, cognitive, and social frailty; malnutrition; poor oral health; and depression. The high prevalence of cardiometabolic diseases could explain this discrepancy, particularly with DM, which is frequently associated with physical frailty as well as mental disorders, as is the case with the TMIG-IC criteria, which includes questionnaires regarding intellectual activity and social roles. The CFS criterion showed a high prevalence of frailty when we defined it using a cutoff value of ≥4 instead of the original cutoff value of > 5 (the prevalence rate was reduced to 8.6% when we diagnosed frailty using the ≥5 cutoff). In a prospective study, we believe that all of these results will be useful in clarifying the most appropriate diagnostic criteria for predicting functional disability or mortality in patients with cardiovascular risk factors.

Although a few patients were suspected of having dementia, there were a substantial number of patients with mildly impaired cognitive function, and the frequency of the MoCA-J ≤ 25 was revealed to be ≥80%. It has been reported that mild cognitive impairment (MCI) could

**Table 4** Frequency of frailty diagnosed by mCHS criteria among DM, HT, and DL patients [values indicate number (%)]

| Age | Frailty Status | DM (−) | DM (+) | P value | HT (−) | HT (+) | P value | DL (−) | DL (+) | P value |
|---|---|---|---|---|---|---|---|---|---|---|
| 50–74 | Robust | 18 (60) | 17 (41) | 0.147 | 10 (50) | 25 (48) | 0.577 | 13 (59) | 22 (44) | 0.480 |
| | Prerail | 11 (37) | 19 (45) | | 7 (35) | 23 (44) | | 7 (32) | 23 (46) | |
| | frail | 1 (3) | 6 (14) | | 3 (15) | 4 (8) | | 2 (9) | 5 (10) | |
| 75–79 | Robust | 12 (30) | 15 (23) | 0.706 | 5 (26) | 22 (25) | 0.950 | 7 (20) | 20 (28) | 0.381 |
| | Prerail | 21 (53) | 38 (58) | | 10 (53) | 49 (56) | | 19 (54) | 40 (56) | |
| | frail | 7 (18) | 13 (20) | | 4 (21) | 16 (18) | | 9 (26) | 11 (16) | |
| 80–84 | Robust | 4 (11) | 8 (20) | 0.327 | 1 (6) | 11 (19) | 0.393 | 5 (17) | 7 (15) | 0.740 |
| | Prerail | 19 (53) | 23 (58) | | 11 (61) | 31 (53) | | 15 (50) | 27 (59) | |
| | frail | 13 (36) | 9 (23) | | 6 (33) | 16 (27) | | 10 (33) | 12 (26) | |
| ≥85 | Robust | 4 (14) | 1 (5) | 0.113 | 2 (17) | 3 (8) | 0.412 | 2 (7) | 3 (14) | 0.755 |
| | Prerail | 8 (29) | 12 (57) | | 6 (50) | 14 (38) | | 11 (41) | 9 (41) | |
| | frail | 16 (57) | 8 (38) | | 4 (33) | 20 (54) | | 14 (52) | 10 (55) | |

*Abbreviations: DM* diabetes mellitus, *HT* hypertension, *DL* dyslipidemia

already be a significant risk for progression of disabilities in older persons [23], and screening these patients is vital. Similar to frailty, the prevalence of cognitive impairment was significantly different among diagnostic criteria. It is known that MoCA is more sensitive than the MMSE for detecting MCI because it assesses cognitive domain impairment, including executive functioning, attention and concentration, visuospatial skills, and memory. In a report by Trzepacz et al., a score of 25 for MoCA was equivalent to a score of 29 for the MMSE and a score of 26–30 for MoCA was equivalent to a score of 30 for the MMSE [24]. Thus, MoCA may be more sensitive than the MMSE in detecting cognitive impairment. In fact, reports have shown the superiority of MoCA over the MMSE in screening for MCI in patients with DM [25] and heart failure [26].

The prevalence of sarcopenia in our population was considerably higher than that of community-dwelling people in the Asian countries (males, 7.1%; females, 19.8%) [14]. This is natural because most of our subjects were affected by various chronic diseases. Indeed, both DM and heart failure are known to be risk factors for skeletal muscle mass reduction [27, 28]. Similar to our study, Han et al. have reported that the prevalence of sarcopenia in China increased with the accumulation of cardiovascular risk factors, DM, HT, and DL using the

**Table 5** Frequency of suspected dementia, cognitive impairment, and sarcopenia among DM, HT, and DL patients [values indicate number (%)]

| Age | DM (-) | DM (+) | P value | HT (-) | HT (+) | P value | DL (-) | DL (+) | P value |
|---|---|---|---|---|---|---|---|---|---|
| Frequency of suspected dementia | | | | | | | | | |
| 50–74 | 3 (10) | 5 (11) | 1.000 | 2 (10) | 6 (11) | 1.000 | 4 (17) | 4 (8) | 0.259 |
| 75–79 | 4 (10) | 3 (4) | 0.257 | 2 (10) | 5 (5) | 0.606 | 0 (0) | 7 (9) | 0.094 |
| 80–84 | 5 (14) | 7 (16) | 1.000 | 3 (16) | 9 (15) | 1.000 | 5 (16) | 7 (14) | 1.000 |
| ≥85 | 8 (27) | 6 (26) | 1.000 | 2 (15) | 12 (30) | 0.473 | 8 (28) | 6 (25) | 1.000 |
| Frequency of cognitive impairment | | | | | | | | | |
| 50–74 | 19 (61) | 34 (77) | 0.198 | 13 (65) | 40 (73) | 0.572 | 17 (71) | 36 (71) | 1.000 |
| 75–79 | 34 (83) | 62 (87) | 0.580 | 15 (75) | 81 (88) | 0.159 | 31 (86) | 65 (86) | 1.000 |
| 80–84 | 31 (86) | 40 (91) | 0.724 | 16 (84) | 55 (90) | 0.437 | 29 (94) | 42 (86) | 0.470 |
| ≥85 | 29 (97) | 20 (87) | 0.305 | 11 (85) | 38 (95) | 0.249 | 28 (97) | 21 (88) | 0.318 |
| Frequency of sarcopenia | | | | | | | | | |
| 50–74 | 0 (0) | 7 (17) | 0.017* | 3 (15) | 4 (8) | 0.388 | 2 (9) | 5 (10) | 1.000 |
| 75–79 | 7 (18) | 20 (29) | 0.250 | 6 (32) | 21 (23) | 0.559 | 11 (32) | 16 (21) | 0.238 |
| 80–84 | 17 (50) | 20 (47) | 0.821 | 14 (78) | 23 (39) | 0.006** | 13 (45) | 24 (50) | 0.814 |
| ≥85 | 16 (53) | 10 (48) | 0.779 | 7 (58) | 19 (49) | 0.743 | 16 (55) | 10 (46) | 0.577 |

*Abbreviations: DM* diabetes mellitus, *HT* hypertension, *DL* dyslipidemia
*p < 0.05. **p < 0.01

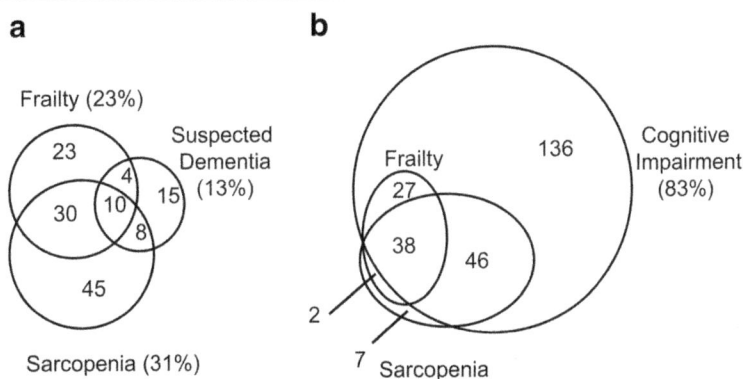

**Fig. 3** Overlap of frailty, sarcopenia, and suspected dementia (MMSE score ≤ 23) (**a**) and overlap of frailty, sarcopenia, and cognitive impairment (MoCA-J ≤ 25) (**b**). Numbers indicates the number of patients included in the area

AWGS criteria [29]. However, the prevalence of sarcopenia in individuals with these diseases was 11.1–22.2%, which was low compared with that in our subjects [29]; this could be explained by the difference in age of the study subjects as well as the exclusion criteria regarding patients with previous cardiovascular diseases. Notably, among the diagnostic items of sarcopenia, the majority of patients met the criterion of low muscle mass and muscle weakness, whereas almost all did not meet that of walking speed (Table 3). In the AWGS criteria, the cutoff points for SMI and grip strength were slightly lower than those of the European Working Group on Sarcopenia in Older People [30]; however, the cutoff point for walking speed remained unchanged. It is suspected that SMI of the Japanese is considerably smaller than that of the European people reflecting their small body size, whereas in contrast, walking speed in the Japanese older people is comparatively faster [31]. Considering these specific characteristics of Japanese, it might be necessary to produce a more appropriate diagnostic criterion for sarcopenia in the Japanese older persons. In addition to the items needed for the diagnosis of sarcopenia, we performed the one-leg standing and TUG tests. It has been reported that both indices are associated with instrumental ADL status [13, 32] and falls [33, 34].

In this study, we also evaluated the depressive mood, nutritional status, and social support network since several reports have revealed that depressive mood and malnutrition could be risks for frailty [35, 36], and a recent report revealed that the older persons living alone are susceptible to becoming frail [37], which indicates that the lack of social support also could be a crucial risk factor for frailty.

We found that the prevalence of frailty, cognitive impairment, and sarcopenia increased with advancing age; however, the prevalence of sarcopenia plateaued in the subjects > 80 years of age. Few studies have investigated sarcopenia in very old subjects (≥85 years). Our ceiling effect could be accounted for by selection bias. Because our

study was held mainly in an outpatient clinic, those who registered and were > 85 years old were relatively healthy and did not represent the general population of the same age. In the Newcastle 85+ study, the authors mentioned that low BMI (≤18.5) was a significant risk factor for the prevalence and incidence of sarcopenia in this age group [38]. In our patients ≥85 years; however, the median BMI was 21.6, and most of the patients had normal nutrition.

It has been reported that DM are associated with high prevalence and incidence of frailty [39, 40], and that HT is also related to prevalent frailty [41, 42], our results stratified by age revealed almost no significant difference in the prevalence of frailty by DM or HT. It is also known that DM is associated with cognitive dysfunction [43] and sarcopenia [44], but no difference was observed except for the prevalence of sarcopenia in the youngest group. This result may also be due to a selection bias in the specialty clinic. Although these subjects became stable, they might have been referred from general practitioners because they had poor control of glucose or blood pressure and multi-morbidities, such as CAD, stroke, or heart failure. These backgrounds of the subjects could have diluted the effects of each single disease, especially in those in the older age groups. For example, it has been reported that chronic heart failure was associated with frailty [45] and cognitive impairment [46]. However, even when considering the bias above, the prevalence of frailty, sarcopenia, and cognitive impairment in the youngest DM group appears to be high, suggesting the importance of taking all possible measures to prevent frailty from occurring at an earlier stage in DM patients.

The prevalence of frailty in the oldest DM group (aged ≥85 years) showed a trend of reduction compared to that in the non-DM group; however, this was not the case for HT, and the reason for this discrepancy remains unclear. Perhaps, some selection or survivorship bias might have influenced these results. Nevertheless, it is unclear why the prevalence of sarcopenia was low in HT subjects aged 80–84 years.

It has been reported in the Japanese population that frailty is associated with both sarcopenia and cognitive decline [47]; however, our results provide valuable new information about how these conditions related to aging overlap with each other. Although the prevalence of cognitive impairment was high, it is noteworthy that almost all of the frail and sarcopenic subjects were cognitively impaired. Alternatively, the prevalence of suspected dementia among the frail and sarcopenic subjects were relatively small. The factors that determine the coincidence of progression of physical function and cognitive decline should further be elucidated by observing this cohort longitudinally.

The strength of our study was that this is the first study to describe the establishment of a frailty clinic with the unique unprecedented backgrounds of our clinic's patients. Several studies have evaluated frailty status in their own frailty clinics; however, their patients' backgrounds were quite different from ours. Tavasson et al. reported that the prevalence of frailty in those who visited their original frailty clinic was 54.5%, which was considerably higher than ours [48]. Their registration criterion was "those considered as frail by their physician" so that they could include several patients with functional disabilities; this was evidenced by the low mean gait speed of their participants of 0.78 m/s. The prevalence of frailty in other studies assessed in "geriatric outpatient clinics" were approximately 35% [49, 50], which were close to the prevalence in our study; however, the sample numbers were small ($n < 200$), the studies were conducted in the US or Canada, and although the prevalence of hypertension was higher in one of the studies, there appeared to be few patients with metabolic diseases. Our study appears to be the first that was conducted in Japanese patients with mainly cardiometabolic diseases who were self-supported but at high risk of becoming frail.

Another strength of our study is that we evaluated frailty and cognitive status by using multiple test modalities, including the CHS, CFS, KCL, and TMIG-IC for frailty and the MMSE, HDS-R, MoCA-J, and DASC-21 for cognitive impairment. This study characteristic is also unprecedented. Using these precise datasets, we could determine the index for frailty and cognitive function that is most associated with and most appropriate to predict a specific outcome. The comprehensive assessment using patients with cardiometabolic disease at baseline will help us to explore risk factors for the progression of frailty and cognitive decline in an ongoing 3-year longitudinal prospective observational study concerning frailty in patients with diabetes or heart diseases.

Our study had some limitations. First, the study was conducted with a relatively small sample size to detect a difference in the age- and disease-stratified analyses.

Nevertheless, our results have clarified for the first time the prevalence of frailty, sarcopenia, and cognitive impairment in patients with a wide range of age who presented with cardiometabolic diseases. Second, this study was performed only in one Japanese institution. Our results should be confirmed in large multicenter and multiracial studies. In addition, the heterogeneity of our subjects' backgrounds may make it difficult to apply the results to the general population. We plan to expand the subject samples to include a wide variety of diseases. Third, as this analysis was performed in a cross-sectional study design, the causal associations between cardiometabolic diseases and frailty, sarcopenia, or cognitive impairment remain unknown. To clarify the exact associations, further longitudinal studies are warranted.

## Conclusion

We established a frailty clinic in our institution and selected a cohort to be analyzed in the follow-up studies. The subjects' statuses of frailty, cognitive function, and sarcopenia were assessed. By using this group of patients, we hope to discover useful information concerning frailty, cognitive impairment, sarcopenia, and other aging-related disabilities in older adults.

**Abbreviations**

ADL: Activity of daily living; AWGS: Asian Working Group for Sarcopenia; CAD: Coronary artery disease; CFS: Clinical Frailty Scale; DASC-21: Dementia Assessment Sheet in Community-based Integrated Care System-21 items; DL: Dyslipidemia; DM: Diabetes mellitus; GDS-15-J: Japanese version of the Geriatric Depression Scale 15; HbA1c, glycohemoglobin; HDS-R: Hasegawa's Dementia Scale for Revised; HT: Hypertension; KCL: Kihon Check List; LSNS-6: Lubben Social Network Scale-6; mCHS: Modified Cardiovascular Health Study; MCI: Mild cognitive impairment; MMSE: Mini-Mental State Examination; MNA-SF: Mini-Nutritional Assessment-Short Form; MoCA-J: Japanese version of the Montreal Cognitive Assessment; SMI: Skeletal Muscle Mass Index; TMIG-IC: Tokyo Metropolitan Institute of Gerontology Index of Competence; TUG: Timed up and go test

**Acknowledgments**

The authors thank Dr. Tsuyoshi Maruyama for blood and urine sample management; clinical psychologists Mr. Masahiro Cho, Ms. Kanako Ito, Ms. Manami Ogawa, Ms. Tomomi Kobayashi, and Ms. Aiko Cho for interviewing and performing physical function tests; and Ms. Kazuko Minowa and Ms. Minako Yabuki for data management.

**Funding**

This study was supported by a grant from the Research Funding for Longevity Sciences (28–30) from the National Center for Geriatrics and Gerontology.

**Authors' contributions**

YT, JI, and AA designed the study, analyzed the data, and wrote the draft of the manuscript. YC, AI, SKa, JT, MS, and TM contributed to data collection, analysis, and interpretation of the data. YF, MT, NK, TN, Aka, KS, HH, KF, Aki, SSe, SSh, KH, SKy, and HI contributed to data interpretation and critically reviewed the manuscript. All authors read and approved the final manuscript.

## Competing interests

Araki A has received speaker honoraria from pharmaceutical companies, Merck Sharp & Dohme, Dainippon Sumitomo Parma Co. Ltd., Kyowa Hakko Kirin Co. Ltd., Astellas Pharma Inc., AstraZeneca, Astellas Pharma Inc., Tanabe Mitsubishi Pharma Corporation, Eli Lilly Japan Co. Ltd., Ono Pharmaceutical Co. Ltd., Taisho Toyama Pharmaceutical Co. Ltd., Novo Nordisk Pharma Ltd., Takeda Pharmaceutical Co. Ltd., Boehringer Ingelheim GmbH, and Novartis Pharma Co. Ltd.

zaRitz® was provided free of charge by Tanita Corp.

## Author details

[1]Department of Diabetes, Metabolism, and Endocrinology, Tokyo Metropolitan Geriatric Hospital, Tokyo, Japan. [2]Department of Cardiology, Tokyo Metropolitan Geriatric Hospital, Tokyo, Japan. [3]Research Team for Social Participation and Community Health, Tokyo Metropolitan Institute of Gerontology, Tokyo, Japan. [4]Department of Clinical Laboratory, Tokyo Metropolitan Geriatric Hospital, Tokyo, Japan. [5]Department of Surgery, Tokyo Metropolitan Geriatric Hospital, Tokyo, Japan. [6]Department of Cardiac Surgery, Tokyo Metropolitan Geriatric Hospital, Tokyo, Japan. [7]Department of Rehabilitation, Tokyo Metropolitan Geriatric Hospital, Tokyo, Japan. [8]Department of Diagnostic Radiology, Tokyo Metropolitan Geriatric Hospital, Tokyo, Japan. [9]Department of Dentistry and Oral Surgery, Tokyo Metropolitan Geriatric Hospital, Tokyo, Japan. [10]Department of Psychiatry, Tokyo Metropolitan Geriatric Hospital, Tokyo, Japan.

## References

1. Fried LP, Tangen CM, Walston J, Newman AB, Hirsch C, Gottdiener J, et al. Frailty in older adults: evidence for a phenotype. J Gerontol A Biol Sci Med Sci. 2001;56:M146–56.
2. Ensrud KE, Ewing SK, Taylor BC, Fink HA, Cawthon PM, Stone KL, et al. Comparison of 2 frailty indexes for prediction of falls, disability, fractures, and death in older women. Arch Intern Med. 2008;168:382–9.
3. Makizako H, Shimada H, Doi T, Tsutsumimoto K, Suzuki T. Impact of physical frailty on disability in community-dwelling older adults: a prospective cohort study. BMJ Open. 2015;5:e008462.
4. Sewo Sampaio PY, Sampaio RA, Yamada M, Arai H. Systematic review of the Kihon checklist: is it a reliable assessment of frailty? Geriatr Gerontol Int. 2016; 16:893–902.
5. Rockwood K, Song X, MacKnight C, Bergman H, Hogan DB, McDowell I, et al. A global clinical measure of fitness and frailty in elderly people. CMAJ. 2005;173:489–95.
6. Koyano W, Shibata H, Nakazato K, Haga H, Suyama Y. Measurement of competence: reliability and validity of the TMIG index of competence. Arch Gerontol Geriatr. 1991;13:103–16.
7. Fujiwara Y, Suzuki H, Yasunaga M, Sugiyama M, Ijuin M, Sakuma N, et al. Brief screening tool for mild cognitive impairment in older Japanese: validation of the Japanese version of the Montreal cognitive assessment. Geriatr Gerontol Int. 2010;10:225–32.
8. Awata S, Sugiyama M, Ito K, Ura C, Miyamae F, Sakuma N, et al. Development of the dementia assessment sheet for community-based integrated care system. Geriatr Gerontol Int. 2016;16(Suppl 1):123–31.
9. Saxton J, Morrow L, Eschman A, Archer G, Luther J, Zuccolotto A. Computer assessment of mild cognitive impairment. Postgrad Med. 2009;121:177–85.
10. Sugishita K, Sugishita M, Hemmi I, Asada T, Tanigawa T. A Validity and Reliability study of the Japanese version of the geriatric depression scale 15 (GDS-15-J). Clin Gerontol. 2017;40:233–40
11. Rubenstein LZ, Harker JO, Salvà A, Guigoz Y, Vellas B. Screening for undernutrition in geriatric practice: developing the short-form mini-nutritional assessment (MNA-SF). J Gerontol A Biol Sci Med Sci. 2001;56:M366–72.
12. Kurimoto A, Awata S, Ohkubo T, Tsubota-Utsugi M, Asayama K, Takahashi K, et al. Reliability and validity of the Japanese version of the abbreviated Lubben social network scale. Nihon Ronen Igakkai Zasshi. 2011;48:149–57.
13. Podsiadlo D, Richardson S. The timed "up & go": a test of basic functional mobility for frail elderly persons. J Am Geriatr Soc. 1991;39:142–8.
14. Chen LK, Liu LK, Woo J, Assantachai P, Auyeung TW, Bahyah KS, et al. Sarcopenia in Asia: consensus report of the Asian working Group for Sarcopenia. J Am Med Dir Assoc. 2014;15:95–101.
15. Herdman M, Gudex C, Lloyd A, Janssen M, Kind P, Parkin D, et al. Development and preliminary testing of the new five-level version of EQ-5D (EQ-5D-5L). Qual Life Res. 2011;20:1727–36.
16. Craig CL, Marshall AL, Sjöström M, Bauman AE, Booth ML, Ainsworth BE, et al. International physical activity questionnaire: 12-country reliability and validity. Med Sci Sports Exerc. 2003;35:1381–95.
17. Fujita K, Fujiwara Y, Chaves PH, Motohashi Y, Shinkai S. Frequency of going outdoors as a good predictors for incident disability of physical function as well as disability recovery in community-dwelling older adults in rural Japan. J Epidemiol. 2006;16:261–70.
18. Kanamori S, Kai Y, Aida J, Kondo K, Kawachi I, Hirai H, et al. Social participation and the prevention of functional disability in older Japanese: the JAGES cohort study. PLoS One. 2014;9:e99638.
19. Lee JS, Auyeung TW, Leung J, Kwok T, Leung PC, Woo J. Physical frailty in older adults is associated with metabolic and atherosclerotic risk factors and cognitive impairment independent of muscle mass. J Nutr Health Aging. 2011;15:857–62.
20. Kojima G, Iliffe S, Taniguchi Y, Shimada H, Rakugi H, Walters K. Prevalence of frailty in Japan: a systematic review and meta-analysis. J Epidemiol. 2017;27:347–53.
21. Collard RM, Boter H, Schoevers RA, Oude Voshaar RC. Prevalence of frailty in community-dwelling older persons: a systematic review. J Am Geriatr Soc. 2012;60:1487–92.
22. Choi J, Ahn A, Kim S, Won CW. Global prevalence of physical frailty by Fried's criteria in community-dwelling elderly with National Population-Based Surveys. J Am Med Dir Assoc. 2015;16:548–50.
23. Doi T, Shimada H, Makizako H, Tsutsumimoto K, Hotta R, Nakakubo S, et al. Mild cognitive impairment, slow gait, and risk of disability: a prospective study. J Am Med Dir Assoc. 2015;16:1082–6.
24. Trzepacz PT, Hochstetler H, Wang S, Walker B, Saykin AJ. Alzheimer's Disease Neuroimaging Initiative. Relationship between the Montreal cognitive assessment and mini-mental state examination for assessment of mild cognitive impairment in older adults. BMC Geriatr. 2015;15:107.
25. Alagiakrishnan K, Zhao N, Mereu L, Senior P, Senthilselvan A. Montreal cognitive assessment is superior to standardized mini-mental status exam in detecting mild cognitive impairment in the middle-aged and elderly patients with type 2 diabetes mellitus. Biomed Res Int. 2013;2013:186106.
26. Alagiakrishnan K, Mah D, Dyck JR, Senthilselvan A, Ezekowitz J. Comparison of two commonly used clinical cognitive screening tests to diagnose mild cognitive impairment in heart failure with the golden standard European consortium criteria. Int J Cardiol. 2017;228:558–62.
27. Park SW, Goodpaster BH, Lee JS, Kuller LH, Boudreau R, de Rekeneire N, et al. Excessive loss of skeletal muscle mass in older adults with type 2 diabetes. Diabetes Care. 2009;32:1993–7.
28. Fülster S, Tacke M, Sandek A, Ebner N, Tschöpe C, Doehner W, et al. Muscle wasting in patients with chronic heart failure: results from the studies investigating co-morbidities aggravating heart failure (SICA-HF). Eur Heart J. 2013;34:512–9.
29. Han P, Yu H, Ma Y, Kang L, Fu L, Jia L, et al. The increased risk of sarcopenia in patients with cardiovascular risk factors in suburb-dwelling older Chinese using the AWGS definition. Sci Rep. 2017;7:9592.
30. Cruz-Jentoft AJ, Baeyens JP, Bauer JM, Boirie Y, Cederholm T, Landi F, et al. Sarcopenia: European consensus on definition and diagnosis: report of the European working group on sarcopenia in older people. Age Ageing. 2010; 39:412–23.
31. Seino S, Shinkai S, Fujiwara Y, Obuchi S, Yoshida H, Hirano H, et al. Reference values and age and sex differences in physical performance measures for community-dwelling older Japanese: a pooled analysis of six cohort studies. PLoS One. 2014;9:e99487.
32. Vellas BJ, Rubenstein LZ, Ousset PJ, Faisant C, Kostek V, Nourhashemi F, et al. One-leg standing balance and functional status in a population of 512 community-living elderly persons. Aging (Milano). 1997;9:95–8.
33. Vellas BJ, Wayne SJ, Romero L, Baumgartner RN, Rubenstein LZ, Garry PJ. One-leg balance is an important predictor of injurious falls in older persons. J Am Geriatr Soc. 1997;45:735–8.
34. Kojima G, Masud T, Kendrick D, Morris R, Gawler S, Treml J, et al. Does the timed up and go test predict future falls among British community-dwelling older people? Prospective cohort study nested within a randomised controlled trial. BMC Geriatr. 2015;15:38.
35. Lakey SL, LaCroix AZ, Gray SL, Borson S, Williams CD, Calhoun D, et al. Antidepressant use, depressive symptoms, and incident frailty in women

aged 65 and older from the Women's Health Initiative observational study. J Am Geriatr Soc. 2012;60:854–61.

36. Kaiser M, Bandinelli S, Lunenfeld B. Frailty and the role of nutrition in older people. A review of the current literature. Acta Biomed. 2010;81(Suppl 1):37–45.

37. Yamanashi H, Shimizu Y, Nelson M, Koyamatsu J, Nagayoshi M, Kadota K, et al. The association between living alone and frailty in a rural Japanese population: the Nagasaki Islands study. J Prim Health Care. 2015;7:269–73.

38. Dodds RM, Granic A, Davies K, Kirkwood TB, Jagger C, Sayer AA, et al. Prevalence and incidence of sarcopenia in the very old: findings from the Newcastle 85+ study. J Cachexia Sarcopenia Muscle. 2017;8:229–37.

39. Castrejón-Pérez RC, Gutiérrez-Robledo LM, Cesari M, Pérez-Zepeda MU. Diabetes mellitus, hypertension and frailty: a population-based, cross-sectional study of Mexican older adults. Geriatr Gerontol Int. 2017;17:925–30.

40. Espinoza SE, Jung I, Hazuda H. Frailty transitions in the San Antonio longitudinal study of aging. J Am Geriatr Soc. 2012;60:652–60.

41. Aprahamian I, Sassaki E, Dos Santos MF, Izbicki R, Pulgrossi RC, Biella MM, et al. Hypertension and frailty in older adults. J Clin Hypertens (Greenwich). 2018;20:186–92.

42. Ramsay SE, Arianayagam DS, Whincup PH, Lennon LT, Cryer J, Papacosta AO, et al. Cardiovascular risk profile and frailty in a population-based study of older British men. Heart. 2015;101:616–22.

43. Biessels GJ, Staekenborg S, Brunner E, Brayne C, Scheltens P. Risk of dementia in diabetes mellitus: a systematic review. Lancet Neurol. 2006;5: 64–74.

44. Trierweiler H, Kisielewicz G, Hoffmann Jonasson T, Rasmussen Petterle R, Aguiar Moreira C. Zeghbi Cochenski Borba V. sarcopenia: a chronic complication of type 2 diabetes mellitus. Diabetol Metab Syndr. 2018;10:25.

45. Denfeld QE, Winters-Stone K, Mudd JO, Gelow JM, Kurdi S, Lee CS. The prevalence of frailty in heart failure: a systematic review and meta-analysis. Int J Cardiol. 2017;236:283–9.

46. Cannon JA, Moffitt P, Perez-Moreno AC, Walters MR, Broomfield NM, McMurray JJV, et al. Cognitive impairment and heart failure: systematic review and meta-analysis. J Card Fail. 2017;23:464–75.

47. Nishiguchi S, Yamada M, Fukutani N, Adachi D, Tashiro Y, Hotta T, et al. Differential association of frailty with cognitive decline and sarcopenia in community-dwelling older adults. J Am Med Dir Assoc. 2015;16:120–4.

48. Tavassoli N, Guyonnet S, Abellan Van Kan G, Sourdet S, Krams T, Soto ME, et al. Description of 1,108 older patients referred by their physician to the "geriatric frailty clinic (G.F.C) for assessment of frailty and prevention of disability" at the gerontopole. J Nutr Health Aging. 2014;18:457–64.

49. Kim H, Higgins PA, Canaday DH, Burant CJ, Hornick TR. Frailty assessment in the geriatric outpatient clinic. Geriatr Gerontol Int. 2014;14:78–83.

50. Pritchard JM, Kennedy CC, Karampatos S, Ioannidis G, Misiaszek B, Marr S, et al. Measuring frailty in clinical practice: a comparison of physical frailty assessment methods in a geriatric out-patient clinic. BMC Geriatr. 2017;17:264.

# 20

# The effect of body mass index, lower extremity performance, and use of a private car on incident life-space restriction: a two-year follow-up study

Taishi Tsuji[1]* ⓘ, Merja Rantakokko[2], Erja Portegijs[2], Anne Viljanen[2] and Taina Rantanen[2]

## Abstract

**Background:** The purpose of the study was to explore the single and combined contributions of body mass index (BMI) and lower extremity performance as modifiable physical factors, and the influence of use of a private car as an environmental factor on prevalent and incident life-space restriction in community-dwelling older people.

**Methods:** Community-dwelling people aged 75–90 years ($n = 823$) participated in the Life-Space Mobility in Old Age (LISPE) two-year follow-up study. Participants who reported that the largest life-space area they had attained, without aid from any device or another person, was the neighborhood or less were considered to have life-space restriction. Incident life-space restriction was the endpoint of Cox's proportional hazard model. BMI, lower extremity performance (Short Physical Performance Battery, SPPB), and use of a private car were predictors.

**Results:** At baseline, people who had both obesity (BMI ≥30.0) and impaired lower extremity performance (SPPB 0–9) had a higher prevalence of life-space restriction (prevalence ratio 3.6, 95% confidence interval, CI, 2.0–6.3) compared to those with normal weight (BMI 23.0–24.9) and intact physical performance (SPPB 10–12). The 581 people without life-space restriction at the baseline contributed 1033 person-years during the two-year follow-up. Incident life-space restrictions were reported by 28.3% participants. A higher hazard ratio (HR) for incident life-space restriction was observed in subjects having both obesity and impaired lower extremity performance (HR 3.6, 95% CI, 1.7–7.4), impaired lower extremity performance only (HR 1.9, 95% CI 0.9–4.1), and obesity only (HR 1.8, 95% CI, 0.9–3.5) compared to those with normal weight and intact performance. Private car passengers (HR 2.0, 95% CI, 1.3–3.0) compared to car drivers had a higher risk of life-space restriction. All models were adjusted for age, sex, chronic diseases, and education.

**Conclusions:** Older people with impaired lower extremity performance have an increased risk of incident life-space restriction especially if combined with obesity. Also, not driving a car renders older people vulnerable to life-space restriction.

**Keywords:** Mobility limitation, Obesity, Physical performance, Aging

* Correspondence: tsuji.t@chiba-u.jp
[1]Center for Preventive Medical Sciences, Chiba University, 1-8-1 Inohana, Chuo Ward, Chiba City, Chiba 260-8670, Japan
Full list of author information is available at the end of the article

## Background

The maintenance of good mobility is vital to attaining active aging, being closely linked to physical and psychological health status and quality of life [1, 2]. Life-space mobility refers to the spatial extent of the actual mobility performance, which depends on the balance between older adults' internal physiologic capacity and the external challenges and resources encountered in their daily environment [3]. Previous cross-sectional studies have revealed that life-space mobility is positively associated with physical [4–6] and psychological health [4] and quality of life [7, 8]. Furthermore, low life-space mobility predicts future falls [9], incident activities of daily living (ADL) disability [10], a rapid decline in cognitive function [11], health care utilization [12], and premature death [13]. Few reports have investigated the factors that may induce the incidence of life-space restriction. To date, hearing difficulties [14], low executive function [15], and frailty [16] have been reported as factors causing life-space restriction.

Life-space mobility considers the size of the spatial area (bedroom, home, yard outside home, neighborhood, town, distant locations) a person purposely moves through in daily life and the frequency of travel within a specific time and needs for assistance for that travel [4]. Movement through smaller life-space areas is more likely to occur using active forms of transportation, such as walking. In turn, traveling longer distances is more dependent on using a car or other modes of passive transportation [17]. Several cross-sectional studies have suggested that driving a car is associated with a larger life-space [18–20]. Consequently, the absence of a private car, which can be driven at will, may be a crucial environmental factor that negatively affects life-space.

Body mass index (BMI) and lower extremity performance are modifiable physical characteristics. Earlier studies have indicated that low life-space mobility is more widespread among very obese (BMI ≥35.0 kg/m$^2$) community-dwelling older individuals [5, 21]. The lower extremity performance of older individuals contributes substantially to the variability in life-space mobility [4–6]. Portegijs et al. [6] reported that poor balance, walking speed, and chair standing test performance were associated with reduced life-space mobility. Obesity and poor lower extremity performance may cause life-space restriction, which in turn, may result in a vicious cycle of increasing body weight and decreasing performance.

The present study aimed to explore the single and combined contributions of BMI and lower extremity performance and the use of a private car on incident life-space restriction in community-dwelling older people.

## Methods

### Study design and participants

The Life-Space Mobility in Old Age (LISPE) project, a two-year prospective cohort study, included 848 community-dwelling individuals aged 75–90 years residing in the municipalities of Jyväskylä and Muurame, Finland. The participants were recruited from a random sample drawn from the national population register. The inclusion criteria were a willingness to participate, community-dwelling in the study area, and ability to communicate. Participants were interviewed in their homes during spring 2012 and followed up by telephone one (mean 362 ± 9 days) and 2 years (mean 721 ± 8 days) after the baseline assessment. The recruitment and study methods, including nonrespondents, have been previously published [3].

Figure 1 shows the procedure for sample selection in our study. Of the baseline participants, those with missing data pertaining to BMI or lower extremity performance ($n = 25$) were excluded from the cross-sectional analyses leaving 823 participants. After excluding participants with life-space restriction ($n = 226$), 597 participants (262 male and 335 female) were included in the present longitudinal analyses.

### Measurements

#### Life-space mobility

Life-space mobility was assessed with the 15-item University of Alabama at Birmingham Study of Aging Life-Space Assessment [4] in a face-to-face interview at the baseline and telephone interviews at the 1st and 2nd follow-ups. Participants reported how many days a week they had attained each life-space level (0, bedroom; 1, other rooms; 2, outside home; 3, neighborhood; 4, town; 5, beyond town) during the preceding 4 weeks and whether they needed help from another person or assistive devices. When the largest life-space area attained without assistance from any device or another person was the neighborhood or less (i.e., maximal independent life-space score ≤ 3), subjects were considered to have life-space restriction. Subjects admitted to institutional care were also assigned incident life-space restriction.

#### Body mass index

Self-reported body height and weight were obtained at the baseline. BMI was calculated as weight (kg) divided by height squared (m$^2$). We classified participants as obese (≥30.0 kg/m$^2$) and overweight (25.0–29.9 kg/m$^2$) based on World Health Organization (WHO) guidelines [22]. We categorized those participants as normal weight (23.0–24.9 kg/m$^2$) and low weight (< 23.0 kg/m$^2$) based on the Mini Nutritional Assessment [23]. As only seven of the participants met the WHO criteria for underweight (< 18.5 kg/m$^2$) in the longitudinal analyses.

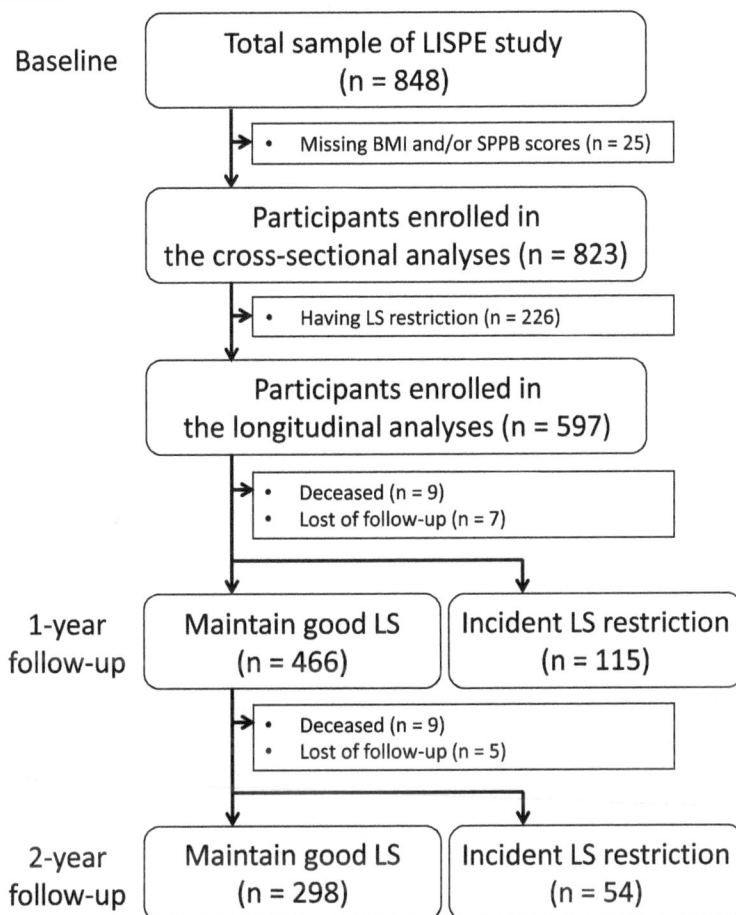

**Fig. 1** Flow of participants in the study from the Life-space mobility in old age (LISPE) project 2012–2014. LISPE: the Life-space mobility in old age study, BMI: body mass index, LS: life-space

*Lower extremity performance*

We objectively evaluated lower extremity performance using the Short Physical Performance Battery (SPPB) [24] at baseline. SPPB comprises three tests assessing standing balance, walking speed over 2.44 m, and five timed chair rises. Each task was scored 0–4 points according to established age- and sex-specific cutoff points [25]. A sum score was calculated (range, 0–12). When at least two tests were completed the result was included in the analyses and being scaled to represent the range. Higher scores indicated better performance. We categorized the participants as having intact (10–12) or impaired (0–9) physical performance.

*Use of a private car*

At the baseline, participants were asked how often they drive a car or travel by car as a passenger. The response options were daily or almost daily, a few times a week, a few times a month, a few times a year, less than once a year, and never. To be categorized as a car driver, or a private car passenger, participants needed to report

using a private car at least on a monthly basis. In case they reported both drivers and being a passenger, the more frequent role was selected for the categorization. If the frequency of driving and traveling as a passenger were equal, the participant was categorized as a car driver. If the participant reported using a private car less than monthly, the person was categorized as not using a private car.

*Covariates*

Information regarding age and sex was derived from the national population register. Years of education was self-reported. The number of chronic diseases was calculated from a list of 22 self-reported, physician-diagnosed chronic diseases (asthma, chronic obstructive pulmonary disease, chronic bronchitis, myocardial infarction, coronary heart disease, heart failure, hypertension, stroke, thrombosis, rheumatic arthritis, osteoarthritis, chronic back pain or problems, chronic neck pain or problems, cataract (not surgically repaired), glaucoma, macular degeneration, hearing disorders, diabetes mellitus, malignant cancer, Parkinson's disease, Alzheimer's disease or dementia, depression or other psychiatric disorder) and an additional open-ended question concerning any other physician-diagnosed chronic conditions [6].

## Statistical analyses

Group differences in baseline characteristics were investigated using ANOVA, chi-square, Kruskal-Wallis, and Mann-Whitney $U$ tests. The main outcome of this study was incident life-space restriction. A multivariate Poisson regression analysis was conducted to confirm the cross-sectional association of each BMI and SPPB category and the use of a private car with the prevalence of life-space restriction. The results were presented as prevalence ratios (PRs) with 95% confidence intervals (CIs). Because the percentages of individuals with life-space restriction (27.5%) were > 10%, the adjusted odds ratio derived from logistic regression could no longer approximate the PR [26]. Cox's proportional hazards models were used to test the longitudinal association of each BMI and SPPB category and the use of a private car with incident life-space restriction. Ties were handled using the Breslow method. The results were presented as hazard ratios (HRs) with 95% CIs. The follow-up period for each participant was defined from the baseline examination to the time point of the first incidence of life-space restriction, the time point of death, or the last study contact, whichever came first (i.e., 1st or 2nd follow-up) to calculate person-years. Five models were constructed in both the cross-sectional and longitudinal analyses. Model 1 and 2 independently included BMI (with normal weight as reference) and SPPB categories (with intact physical performance as reference), respectively. BMI and SPPB categories were jointly included in model 3 and covariates were added. After creating eight dummy variables by combining 4 BMI × 2 SPPB categories, these and all covariates were included in model 4 with normal weight and intact physical performance as a reference, and use of a private car was added in model 5 with car driver as a reference. SPSS Statistics 22 (IBM, Armonk, NY, USA) was used for all statistical analyses. The statistical significance was set at $P < 0.05$.

## Results

Table 1 shows participants' characteristics according to both BMI and SPPB categories. Participants with a BMI ≥30.0 kg/m² were more often women and younger than subjects with a lower BMI. The most prevalent use of a private car in participants with normal weight was driving; whereas in those with low weight, obesity, or who were overweight, being a passenger was most common. Those with impaired lower

extremity performance were older and had a higher BMI, more chronic diseases, less education, and more restricted life-space area than those with intact lower extremity performance.

Table 2 shows the results of multivariate Poisson regression analyses having life-space restriction at the baseline. Among those with impaired performance, all BMI groups had a significantly higher risk of restricted life-space than the group with normal weight and intact physical performance in the fully adjusted model (PR varies between 2.71 and 3.31).

The flow of participants is indicated in Fig. 1. The 581 older people without life-space restriction at baseline contributed 1033 person-years during the two-year follow-up. During follow-up, incident life-space restrictions were reported by 28.3% participants (event rate 164 per 1000 person-years). Figure 2 shows the incidence rates of life-space restriction at each follow-up according to the combined BMI and SPPB categories. The incidence rate was 21.8% (18.1%–28.4% among BMI categories) among those with intact lower extremity performance and 47.4% (42.3–65.0% among BMI categories) among those with an impaired performance from baseline to two-year follow-up.

Table 3 shows the results of multiple Cox's proportional hazard regression analyses. Subjects with a BMI ≥30.0 kg/m² were 1.73 (95% CI, 1.05–2.86) times more likely to develop life-space restriction compared with people with a BMI 23.0–24.9 kg/m². The corresponding figure was 2.44 (95% CI, 1.80–3.32) among people with impaired lower extremity performance vs. those with intact performance. In the model including both BMI and SPPB categories and covariates, SPPB remained significant (HR 2.39, 95% CI 1.75–3.27) but the effect of BMI was attenuated (BMI ≥30.0 kg/m²: HR 1.65, 95% CI 0.99–2.75). The model examining the combined effect of BMI and SPPB catergories revealed that subjects with both obesity and impaired lower extremity performance had the highest hazard for incident life-space restriction (HR 3.79, 95% CI 1.84–7.83), followed by those with impaired lower extremity performance only (HR 2.50, 95% CI 1.18–5.29), and those with obesity only (HR 1.70, 95% CI, 0.88–3.29), after adjusting for age, sex, number of chronic diseases, and year of education. In the full model including combined BMI × SPPB categories, use of a private car, and covariates, those overweight and obese subjects with impaired lower extremity performance remained significant (HR 2.77 and 3.57, respectively), and private car passengers had a significantly higher hazard for incident life-space restriction than car drivers (HR 1.96, 95% CI, 1.27–3.01). Age, numbers of chronic diseases, and years of education were statistically significant as potential confounding factors; however, sex was not.

**Table 1** Descriptive baseline data of participants according to BMI and lower extremity performance

| Variables | Low weight (BMI < 23.0) | Normal weight (BMI 23.0–24.9) | Overweight (BMI 25.0–29.9) | Obese (BMI ≥30.0) | P | Intact LEP (SPPB 10–12) | Impaired LEP (SPPB 0–9) | P |
|---|---|---|---|---|---|---|---|---|
| | n = 156 | n = 166 | n = 375 | n = 126 | | n = 523 | n = 300 | |
| **Characteristics** | | | | | | | | |
| Age (year), M ± SD | 81.2 ± 4.3 | 79.9 ± 4.2 | 80.0 ± 4.3 | 79.4 ± 4.1 | .003 [a] | 79.7 ± 4.2 | 80.8 ± 4.3 | <.001 [a] |
| Women, n (%) | 100 (64.1%) | 88 (53.0%) | 226 (60.3%) | 97 (77.0%) | <.001 [b] | 318 (60.8%) | 193 (64.3%) | .315 [b] |
| Height (cm), M ± SD | 163.8 ± 9.0 | 166.7 ± 9.0 | 164.9 ± 9.0 | 162.4 ± 7.7 | <.001 [a] | 165.0 ± 8.4 | 164.0 ± 9.7 | .104 [a] |
| Body weight (kg), M ± SD | 56.8 ± 8.3 | 66.9 ± 7.4 | 73.7 ± 8.4 | 86.9 ± 11.0 | <.001 [a] | 70.8 ± 11.8 | 71.7 ± 13.8 | .317 [a] |
| BMI (kg/m2), M ± SD | 21.1 ± 1.6 | 24.0 ± 0.5 | 27.0 ± 1.4 | 32.9 ± 2.9 | <.001 [a] | 26.0 ± 3.8 | 26.6 ± 4.3 | .029 [a] |
| Chronic diseases (n), Med (IQR) | 4 (4) | 4 (3) | 4 (3) | 4 (3) | .007 [c] | 4 (3) | 5 (4) | <.001 [d] |
| Education (year), Med (IQR) | 9 (5) | 9 (5) | 8 (5) | 8 (5) | .060 [c] | 9 (5) | 8 (4) | <.001 [d] |
| **Life-space** | | | | | | | | |
| Maximal independent LS (score), Med (IQR) | 4 (2) | 5 (1) | 4 (2) | 4 (4) | .019 [c] | 5 (1) | 4 (4) | <.001 [d] |
| **Short Physical Performance Battery** | | | | | | | | |
| Total (score), Med (IQR) | 11.0 (3.0) | 11.0 (3.0) | 10.0 (3.0) | 10.0 (3.0) | .006 [c] | 11.0 (1.0) | 8.0 .0) | <.001 [d] |
| Impaired (SPPB 0–9), n (%) | 56 (35.9%) | 48 (28.9%) | 144 (38.4%) | 52 (41.3%) | .113 [b] | – | – | |
| **Use of a private car, n (%)** | | | | | | | | |
| Car driver | 51 (32.7%) | 78 (47.0%) | 160 (42.7%) | 37 (29.4%) | .006 [b] | 246 (47.0%) | 80 (26.7%) | <.001 [b] |
| Private car passenger | 77 (49.4%) | 66 (39.8%) | 165 (44.0%) | 75 (59.5%) | | 216 (41.3%) | 167 (55.7%) | |
| No use of a private car | 28 (17.9%) | 22 (13.3%) | 50 (13.3%) | 14 (11.1%) | | 61 (11.7%) | 53 (17.7%) | |

n = 823

M mean, SD standard deviation, Med median, IQR interquartile range, BMI body mass index, LEP lower extremity performance, SPPB short physical performance battery, LS life-space

[a] one-way analysis of variance; [b] chi-square test; [c] Kruskal-Wallis test; [d] Mann-Whitney U test

## Discussion

This two-year prospective study reveals that community-dwelling older people who are overweight or obese and also have impaired lower extremity performance exhibit a higher risk of both current and future life-space restriction than those who are not overweight or obese, with or without impaired lower extremity performance. Furthermore, not driving a car also renders older people vulnerable to having a restricted life-space. These results suggest that we should approach the subject of life-space mobility in older people from the aspects of both physical characteristics and transportation options.

We found that impaired lower extremity performance was a crucial contributing factor to incident life-space restriction. Previous cross-sectional studies have established that a good lower extremity performance in older adults is an important factor underlying better life-space mobility [4–6]. Lower extremity performance also contributes to incident mobility disability and limitations in ADL [27–29]. Most previous longitudinal studies have assessed the self-reported ability to perform specific tasks (e.g., walking a half mile, climbing stairs, using toilets, or bathing) with or without difficulties or help. A life-space assessment has the advantage of revealing how

far participants move, which is determined by their internal physiologic capacity and their immediate environmental challenges [3]. The results of the present study suggest that lower extremity performance may correspond to the internal physiological capacity contributing to individuals' life-space, and it may also play an important role when addressing environmental challenges.

Our results support previous cross-sectional study findings that highly obese older people (BMI ≥35.0 kg/m²) were significantly more likely to attain low life-space mobility scores [5]. Furthermore, systematic reviews and meta-analyses of longitudinal studies have revealed that obesity was a strong predictor of long-term risk for mobility disability and limitations in ADL [30, 31]. Excess body weight in older individuals may cause a mechanical burden potentially leading to altered walking patterns with lower energetic efficiency [32] and overall strain experienced when in motion. Additionally, increasing body weight triggers lower extremity pain (especially in the knee and ankle), which may contribute to mobility disability in older people. [30]. The joint pain may induce fear of movement and avoidance of weight-bearing tasks that trigger pain [33]. These negative consequences associated with obesity may correspond to a poor internal physiological capacity, making it difficult to tackle

**Table 2** Association of BMI and lower extremity performance with life-space restriction (cross-sectional analysis)

| | Model 1 | | Model 2 | | Model 3[a] | | Model 4[a] | | Model 5[a] | |
|---|---|---|---|---|---|---|---|---|---|---|
| | PR | 95% CI | PR | 95% CI | PR | 95% CI | PR | 95% CI | PR | 95% CI |
| Single association | | | | | | | | | | |
| BMI | | | | | | | | | | |
| < 23 | 1.36 | (0.93, 1.98) | | | 1.03 | (0.74, 1.44) | | | | |
| 23–25 | 1.00 | | | | 1.00 | | | | | |
| 25–30 | 1.21 | (0.86, 1.69) | | | 1.01 | (0.75, 1.36) | | | | |
| ≥ 30 | 1.68 | (1.16, 2.44) | | | 1.24 | (0.89, 1.73) | | | | |
| Lower extremity performance | | | | | | | | | | |
| Intact (SPPB 10–12) | | | 1.00 | | 1.00 | | | | | |
| Impaired (SPPB 0–9) | | | 3.31 | (2.62, 4.18) | 2.58 | (2.05, 3.25) | | | | |
| Combined association | | | | | | | | | | |
| Intact LEP with BMI | | | | | | | | | | |
| < 23 | | | | | | | 1.15 | (0.60, 2.23) | 1.09 | (0.56, 2.11) |
| 23–25 | | | | | | | 1.00 | | 1.00 | |
| 25–30 | | | | | | | 1.18 | (0.66, 2.11) | 1.19 | (0.67, 2.12) |
| ≥ 30 | | | | | | | 1.48 | (0.77, 2.82) | 1.43 | (0.76, 2.71) |
| Impaired LEP with BMI | | | | | | | | | | |
| < 23 | | | | | | | 3.03 | (1.73, 5.31) | 2.71 | (1.55, 4.74) |
| 23–25 | | | | | | | 3.14 | (1.74, 5.67) | 2.73 | (1.53, 4.89) |
| 25–30 | | | | | | | 2.89 | (1.68, 4.97) | 2.66 | (1.56, 4.53) |
| ≥ 30 | | | | | | | 3.55 | (2.02, 6.27) | 3.31 | (1.89, 5.81) |
| Use of a private car | | | | | | | | | | |
| Car driver | | | | | | | | | 1.00 | |
| Private car passenger | | | | | | | | | 2.07 | (1.39, 3.07) |
| No use a private car | | | | | | | | | 2.15 | (1.41, 3.28) |

n = 823

PR prevalence ratio, CI confidence interval, BMI body mass index, LEP lower extremity performance, SPPB short physical performance battery

[a]Adjusting for sex, age, chronic diseases, and education

environmental challenges. Therefore, life-space in obese people is more likely to be restricted. After adjusting for lower extremity performance and covariates, however, the statistical significance of obesity was lost in the current study. As indicated above, BMI considerably impacts lower extremity performance and chronic diseases and may be a confounding factor itself [34].

The principal finding of the present study was that impaired lower extremity performance combined with overweight or obesity increased the risk of incident life-space restriction more than either one alone. Recently, dynapenic obesity, a condition of coexisting low muscle strength and obesity, received attention as a relative or contributing factor for falls [35], a decline in physical function [36, 37], and limitations in mobility and ADL [36]. Stenholm et al. [36] showed that obese older persons with low knee extensor muscle strength experienced significantly greater declines in walking speed and mobility than persons with either condition

alone over a six-year follow-up. People with poor lower extremity muscular function may not have enough physical capacity to carry their body mass, and, consequently, their life-space mobility declines even further than those with only obesity or impaired lower extremity performance. Among people with impaired lower extremity performance, its negative impact was compensated by the use of a private car in those with low or normal weight but not in those who were overweight or obese. These results suggest that improving alternative transportation options may aid those people with low or normal weight to maintain their life-space even if their lower extremity performance is impaired. However, for obese people improvements in transportation options alone may not be sufficient to prevent life-space restriction.

The present study revealed that driving one's private car was important for maintaining life-space in community-dwelling older people. This result is in line with previous findings showing an association between

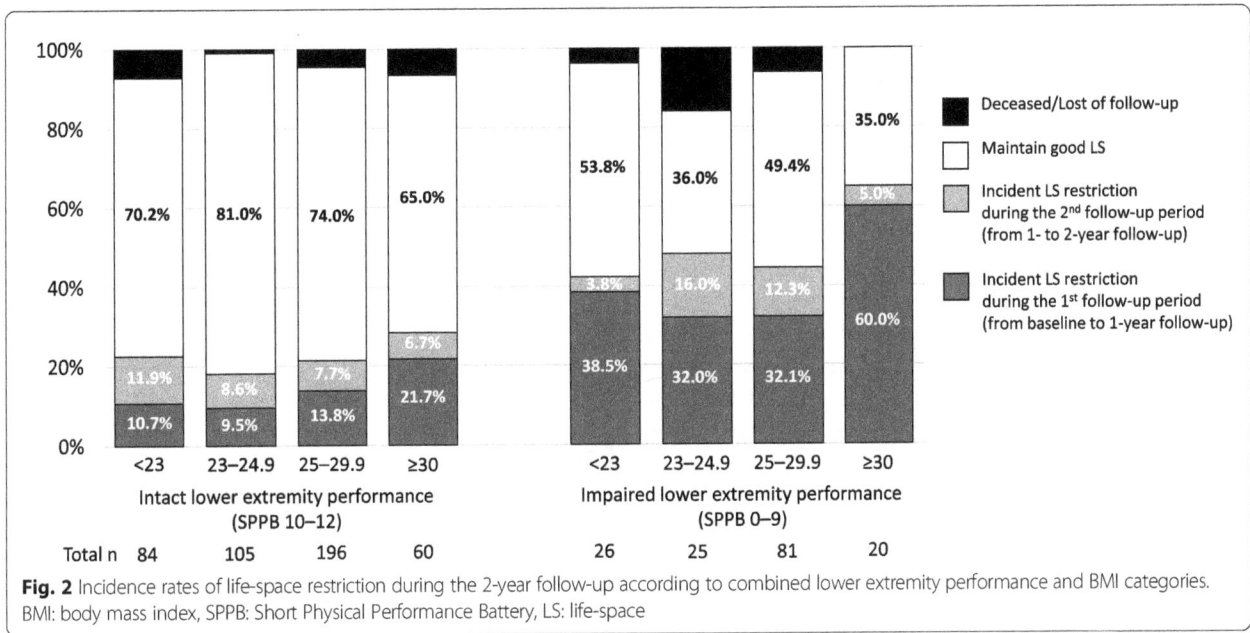

**Fig. 2** Incidence rates of life-space restriction during the 2-year follow-up according to combined lower extremity performance and BMI categories. BMI: body mass index, SPPB: Short Physical Performance Battery, LS: life-space

**Table 3** Effect of BMI and lower extremity performance on incident life-space restriction (longitudinal analysis)

| | Model 1 | | Model 2 | | Model 3[a] | | Model 4[a] | | Model 5[a] | |
|---|---|---|---|---|---|---|---|---|---|---|
| | HR | 95% CI | HR | 95% CI | HR | 95% CI | HR | 95% CI | HR | 95% CI |
| Single effect | | | | | | | | | | |
| BMI | | | | | | | | | | |
| < 23 | 1.19 | (0.72, 1.97) | | | 1.03 | (0.62, 1.70) | | | | |
| 23–25 | 1.00 | | | | 1.00 | | | | | |
| 25–30 | 1.21 | (0.80, 1.84) | | | 1.07 | (0.70, 1.62) | | | | |
| ≥ 30 | 1.73 | (1.05, 2.86) | | | 1.65 | (0.99, 2.75) | | | | |
| Lower extremity performance | | | | | | | | | | |
| Intact (SPPB 10–12) | | | 1.00 | | 1.00 | | | | | |
| Impaired (SPPB 0–9) | | | 2.44 | (1.80, 3.32) | 2.39 | (1.75, 3.27) | | | | |
| Combined effect | | | | | | | | | | |
| Intact LEP with BMI | | | | | | | | | | |
| < 23 | | | | | | | 1.02 | (0.54, 1.93) | 1.00 | (0.53, 1.89) |
| 23–25 | | | | | | | 1.00 | | 1.00 | |
| 25–30 | | | | | | | 1.06 | (0.61, 1.84) | 1.06 | (0.61, 1.83) |
| ≥ 30 | | | | | | | 1.70 | (0.88, 3.29) | 1.78 | (0.92, 3.47) |
| Impaired LEP with BMI | | | | | | | | | | |
| < 23 | | | | | | | 2.40 | (1.16, 4.97) | 2.03 | (0.98, 4.22) |
| 23–25 | | | | | | | 2.50 | (1.18, 5.29) | 1.91 | (0.90, 4.08) |
| 25–30 | | | | | | | 2.57 | (1.46, 4.52) | 2.77 | (1.57, 4.87) |
| ≥ 30 | | | | | | | 3.79 | (1.84, 7.83) | 3.57 | (1.72, 7.38) |
| Use of a private car | | | | | | | | | | |
| Car driver | | | | | | | | | 1.00 | |
| Private car passenger | | | | | | | | | 1.96 | (1.27, 3.01) |
| No use a private car | | | | | | | | | 1.51 | (0.87, 2.62) |

581 people without life-space restriction at the baseline contributed 1033 person-years during two-year follow-up
HR hazard ratio, CI confidence interval, BMI body mass index, LEP lower extremity performance, SPPB short physical performance battery
[a]Adjusting for sex, age, chronic diseases, and education

driving a car and a larger life-space [18, 19]. Shah et al. [19] reported that people who were licensed to drive were less likely to be restricted in their life-space over the average four-year follow-up compared to people without a driver's license. The results of this study have also revealed that use of a private car, not as a driver but as a passenger, was associated with life-space restriction independently from individuals' physical characteristics, which is consistent with a previous cross-sectional study [20]. However, the risk of incident life-space restriction was increased without statistical significance in people who did not use a private car in the present study. Even among those people, some may have frequently used public transportation modes, which are also associated with life-space [38, 39]. According to a previous cross-sectional study, the risk of life-space restriction in public transportation users did not differ significantly from private car drivers among older people without walking difficulties [20]. Further studies taking into consideration the use of public transportation modes are warranted.

The strengths of the present study were the use of high-quality longitudinal data with an excellent follow-up rate for a large population-based sample and exploring the contributing factors of life-space restriction, which is a topical issue, by focusing on both modifiable physical factors and an environmental factor. However, several study limitations warrant further consideration. Firstly, BMI was calculated from self-reported height and weight, not from objective measurements. Secondly, because of the bias of the participants' BMI distribution, we classified those with $BMI < 23.0$ $kg/m^2$ as low weight. However, this classification does not conform to the WHO guidelines [22] which state that a $BMI < 18.5$ $kg/m^2$ should be classified as underweight. This change may have resulted in an underestimation of the contribution of low weight on incident life-space restriction. Thirdly, we did not collect BMI and SPPB data at the follow-ups. Therefore, we could not address whether a change in BMI or lower extremity performance in older age contributes to incident life-space restriction.

## Conclusions

Community-dwelling older adults with impaired lower extremity performance have an increased risk of both current and future life-space restriction, especially when overweight or obese. Furthermore, not driving a private car renders older people vulnerable to life-space restriction. Programs to improve lower extremity performance and to prevent excess body weight may have the potential to maintain life-space and even prevent social isolation, a potential consequence of restricted life-space mobility. Improvements in alternative transportation options, especially for older people who do not drive a car, is also essential.

## Abbreviations
ADL: Activities of daily living; BMI: Body mass index; CI: Confidence interval; HR: Hazard ratio; LISPE: Life-Space Mobility in Old Age; PR: Prevalence ratio; SPPB: Short Physical Performance Battery

## Acknowledgements
We would like to thank the study participants. The Gerontology Research Center (GEREC) is a joint effort between University of Jyväskylä and University of Tampere, Finland.

## Funding
This work was supported by Grant-in-Aid for JSPS Fellows (grant number 13 J00010), Grant-in-Aid for Scientific Research (KAKENHI) from the Japanese Society for the Promotion of Science (grant number 16 K16595), Academy of Finland (future of living and housing program ASU-LIVE, grant number 255403), and Finnish Ministry of Education and Culture. The funders had no role in study design, data collection and analysis, decision to publish, or preparation of the manuscript.

## Authors' contributions
TT: conception, design, analysis and interpretation of the data, and writing the article; MR, EP, and AV: conception, design, data collection and critical revision of the article; TR: conception, design, data collection, critical revision of the article, and principal investigator for the LISPE project. All authors approved the final draft submitted.

## Competing interests
The authors declare that they have no competing interest.

## Author details
$^1$Center for Preventive Medical Sciences, Chiba University, 1-8-1 Inohana, Chuo Ward, Chiba City, Chiba 260-8670, Japan. $^2$Gerontology Research Center, Faculty of Sport and Health Sciences, University of Jyvaskyla, PO Box 35, FI-40014 Jyväskylä, Finland.

## References
1. Brown CJ, Flood KL. Mobility limitation in the older patient: a clinical review. JAMA. 2013;310:1168–77.
2. La Grow S, Yeung P, Towers A, Alpass F, Stephens C. The impact of mobility on quality of life among older persons. J Aging Health. 2013;25:723–36.
3. Rantanen T, Portegijs E, Viljanen A, Eronen J, Saajanaho M, Tsai LT, et al. Individual and environmental factors underlying life space of older people - study protocol and design of a cohort study on life-space mobility in old age (LISPE). BMC Public Health. 2012;12:1018.
4. Baker PS, Bodner EV, Allman RM. Measuring life-space mobility in community-dwelling older adults. J Am Geriatr Soc. 2003;51:1610–4.
5. Al Snih S, Peek KM, Sawyer P, Markides KS, Allman RM, Ottenbacher KJ. Life-space mobility in Mexican Americans aged 75 and older. J Am Geriatr Soc. 2012;60:532–7.
6. Portegijs E, Rantakokko M, Mikkola TM, Viljanen A, Rantanen T. Association between physical performance and sense of autonomy in outdoor activities and life-space mobility in community-dwelling older people. J Am Geriatr Soc. 2014;62:615–21.
7. Rantakokko M, Portegijs E, Viljanen A, Iwarsson S, Rantanen T. Life-space mobility and quality of life in community-dwelling older people. J Am Geriatr Soc. 2013;61:1830–2.
8. Bentley JP, Brown CJ, McGwin G Jr, Sawyer P, Allman RM, Roth DL.

Functional status, life-space mobility, and quality of life: a longitudinal mediation analysis. Qual Life Res. 2013;22:1621–32.

9. Lo AX, Rundle AG, Buys D, Kennedy RE, Sawyer P, Allman RM, et al. Neighborhood disadvantage and life-space mobility are associated with incident falls in community-dwelling older adults. J Am Geriatr Soc. 2016;64: 2218–25.

10. Portegijs E, Rantakokko M, Viljanen A, Sipila S, Rantanen T. Identification of older people at risk of ADL disability using the life-space assessment: a longitudinal cohort study. J Am Med Dir Assoc. 2016;17:410–4.

11. Silberschmidt S, Kumar A, Raji MM, Markides K, Ottenbacher KJ, Al SS. Life-space mobility and cognitive decline among Mexican Americans aged 75 years and older. J Am Geriatr Soc. 2017;65:1514–20.

12. Kennedy RE, Williams CP, Sawyer P, Lo AX, Connelly K, Nassel A, et al. Life-space predicts health care utilization in community-dwelling older adults. J Aging Health. 2017. https://doi.org/10.1177/0898264317730487.

13. Kennedy RE, Sawyer P, Williams CP, Lo AX, Ritchie CS, Roth DL, et al. Life-space mobility change predicts 6-month mortality. J Am Geriatr Soc. 2017; 65:833–8.

14. Polku H, Mikkola TM, Rantakokko M, Portegijs E, Tormakangas T, Rantanen T, et al. Self-reported hearing difficulties and changes in life-space mobility among community-dwelling older adults: a two-year follow-up study. BMC Geriatr. 2015;15:121.

15. Poranen-Clark T, von Bonsdorff MB, Rantakokko M, Portegijs E, Eronen J, Pynnonen K, et al. The temporal association between executive function and life-space mobility in old age. J Gerontol A Biol Sci Med Sci. 2018;73: 835–9.

16. Portegijs E, Rantakokko M, Viljanen A, Sipila S, Rantanen T. Is frailty associated with life-space mobility and perceived autonomy in participation outdoors? A longitudinal study. Age Ageing. 2016;45:550–3.

17. Collia DV, Sharp J, Giesbrecht L. The 2001 National Household Travel Survey: a look into the travel patterns of older Americans. J Saf Res. 2003;34:461–70.

18. Stalvey BT, Owsley C, Sloane ME, Ball K. The life space questionnaire: a measure of the extent of mobility of older adults. J Appl Gerontol. 1999;18: 460–78.

19. Shah RC, Maitra K, Barnes LL, James BD, Leurgans S, Bennett DA. Relation of driving status to incident life space constriction in community-dwelling older persons: a prospective cohort study. J Gerontol A Biol Sci Med Sci. 2012;67:984–9.

20. Viljanen A, Mikkola TM, Rantakokko M, Portegijs E, Rantanen T. The association between transportation and life-space mobility in community-dwelling older people with or without walking difficulties. J Aging Health. 2016;28:1038–54.

21. Ritchie CS, Locher JL, Roth DL, McVie T, Sawyer P, Allman R. Unintentional weight loss predicts decline in activities of daily living function and life-space mobility over 4 years among community-dwelling older adults. J Gerontol A Biol Sci Med Sci. 2008;63:67–75.

22. Obesity: preventing and managing the global epidemic. Report of a WHO consultation. World Health Organ Tech Rep Ser. 2000;894:i-xii, 1–253.

23. Vellas B, Villars H, Abellan G, Soto ME, Rolland Y, Guigoz Y, et al. Overview of the MNA--its history and challenges. J Nutr Health Aging. 2006;10:456–63 discussion 63-5.

24. Guralnik JM, Simonsick EM, Ferrucci L, Glynn RJ, Berkman LF, Blazer DG, et al. A short physical performance battery assessing lower extremity function: association with self-reported disability and prediction of mortality and nursing home admission. J Gerontol. 1994;49:M85–94.

25. Mänty M, Sihvonen S, Hulkko T, Lounamaa A. Iäkkäiden Henkilöiden Kaatumistapaturmat. Opas Kkaatumisten ja Murtumien Ehkäisyyn, 2nd Ed. Kansanterveyslaitoksen julkaisuja· Helsinki; 2007.

26. Zhang J, Yu KF. What's the relative risk? A method of correcting the odds ratio in cohort studies of common outcomes. JAMA. 1998;280:1690–1.

27. Guralnik JM, Ferrucci L, Simonsick EM, Salive ME, Wallace RB. Lower-extremity function in persons over the age of 70 years as a predictor of subsequent disability. N Engl J Med. 1995;332:556–61.

28. Deshpande N, Metter EJ, Guralnik J, Bandinelli S, Ferrucci L. Predicting 3-year incident mobility disability in middle-aged and older adults using physical performance tests. Arch Phys Med Rehabil. 2013;94:994–7.

29. den Ouden ME, Schuurmans MJ, Arts IE, van der Schouw YT. Physical performance characteristics related to disability in older persons: a systematic review. Maturitas. 2011;69:208–19.

30. Vincent HK, Vincent KR, Lamb KM. Obesity and mobility disability in the older adult. Obes Rev. 2010;11:568–79.

31. Backholer K, Wong E, Freak-Poli R, Walls HL, Peeters A. Increasing body weight and risk of limitations in activities of daily living: a systematic review and meta-analysis. Obes Rev. 2012;13:456–68.

32. Ko S, Stenholm S, Ferrucci L. Characteristic gait patterns in older adults with obesity--results from the Baltimore longitudinal study of aging. J Biomech. 2010;43:1104–10.

33. Gooberman-Hill R, Woolhead G, Mackichan F, Ayis S, Williams S, Dieppe P. Assessing chronic joint pain: lessons from a focus group study. Arthritis Rheum. 2007;57:666–71.

34. Sharts-Hopko NC, Sullivan MP. Obesity as a confounding health factor among women with mobility impairment. J Am Acad Nurse Pract. 2003;15: 438–43.

35. Scott D, Sanders KM, Aitken D, Hayes A, Ebeling PR, Jones G. Sarcopenic obesity and dynapenic obesity: 5-year associations with falls risk in middle-aged and older adults. Obesity (Silver Spring). 2014;22:1568–74.

36. Stenholm S, Alley D, Bandinelli S, Griswold ME, Koskinen S, Rantanen T, et al. The effect of obesity combined with low muscle strength on decline in mobility in older persons: results from the InCHIANTI study. Int J Obes. 2009; 33:635–44.

37. Bouchard DR, Janssen I. Dynapenic-obesity and physical function in older adults. J Gerontol A Biol Sci Med Sci. 2010;65:71–7.

38. Murata C, Kondo T, Tamakoshi K, Yatsuya H, Toyoshima H. Factors associated with life space among community-living rural elders in Japan. Public Health Nurs. 2006;23:324–31.

39. Wilkie R, Peat G, Thomas E, Croft P. Factors associated with restricted mobility outside the home in community-dwelling adults ages fifty years and older with knee pain: an example of use of the international classification of functioning to investigate participation restriction. Arthritis Rheum. 2007;57:1381–9.

# 21

# A need to improve the assessment of environmental hazards for falls on stairs and in bathrooms: results of a scoping review

Rosanne Blanchet[1]* ⓘ and Nancy Edwards[2]

## Abstract

**Background:** Falls occurring on stairs or in bathrooms are associated with a high risk of injuries among older adults. Home environmental assessments are frequently used to guide fall-prevention interventions. The aims of this review were to describe how, where, by whom, and for whom environmental hazard checklists are used, and to examine the characteristics of environmental hazard assessment checklists with specific attention to features of bathrooms and stairs/steps assessed in them.

**Methods:** Studies published before January 5, 2018, were identified using several databases. Publications reporting the use and/or evaluation of environmental hazard checklists were eligible if they assessed bathrooms or stairs/steps in homes of older adults (≥65 years). Content analysis was conducted on publications that provided a complete list of specific environmental hazards assessed. Checklist items related to bathrooms and stairs/steps were extracted and categorized as structural or non-structural and as objective or subjective.

**Results:** 1119 studies were appraised. A pool of 136 published articles and 4 checklists from the grey literature were included in this scoping review. Content analysis was conducted on 42 unique checklists. There was no widely used checklist and no obvious consensus definition of either environmental hazards overall or of single hazards listed in checklists. Checklists varied greatly with respect to what rooms were assessed, whether or not outdoor stair/steps hazards were assessed, and how responses were coded. Few checklists examined person-environment fit. The majority of checklists were not oriented towards structural hazards in bathrooms. Although the majority of checklists assessing stair/steps hazards evaluated structural hazards, most features assessed were not related to the construction geometry of stairs/steps. Objective features of bathrooms and stairs/steps that would deem them safe were rarely specified. Rather, adequacy of their characteristics was mostly subjectively determined by the evaluator with little or no guidance or training.

**Conclusion:** The lack of standard definitions and objective criteria for assessing environmental hazards for falls is limiting meaningful cross-study comparisons and slowing advances in this field. To inform population health interventions aimed at preventing falls, such as building code regulations or municipal housing by-laws, it is essential to include objectively-assessed structural hazards in environmental checklists.

**Keywords:** Environmental hazards, Falls, Seniors, Built environment, Scoping review, Bathroom, Stairs

* Correspondence: rblan035@uottawa.ca
[1]School of Nursing, University of Ottawa, 1 Stewart Street, Room 212, Ottawa, ON K1H 8M5, Canada
Full list of author information is available at the end of the article

# Background

Falls among older adults are considered a major public health concern [1]. Falls can lead to loss of autonomy, greater isolation and depression, reduced mobility, and increased morbidity and mortality [2]. In Canada, the direct and indirect costs of falls among older adults are estimated at over $3 billion annually [3]. Aging-in-place policies highlight the importance of mitigating fall risks in the home [4]; safer homes may enable independent rather than dependent living arrangements for older persons.

Although causes of falls are considered multi-factorial, it is well-established that environmental hazards are implicated in as many as one third of all falls among older adults [5–9]. Research on falls indicates that two areas in the home are particularly hazardous for injurious falls; bathrooms, and indoor or outdoor stairs or steps [10–12]. In the most recently available National Electronic Injury Surveillance data for 2017, for example, the product category stairs, ramps, landings and floors is the top-ranked location of injuries in the United States for those 65 years and older, while bathtub and shower structures rank fourth for this age group [13]. Furthermore, when time spent on stairs or in bathrooms (risk exposure time) is taken into account, these locations account for a significantly higher incidence of falls than other room locations (Jake Pauls, personal communications, June 12, 2018). Stairs and bathrooms are problematic because they involve navigating transitions and transfers, and structural features of these locations (such as poor stair geometry or the lack of transfer assists) may challenge an individual's capacity to respond to the pressure exerted by these environmental features, thereby exceeding optimal person-environment fit parameters [14–23].

Both primary studies and systematic reviews have documented the effectiveness of efforts to address environmental hazards generally, or more specifically in bathrooms and stairs [4, 6, 24–30]. Still, studies that assessed the influence of home environmental hazards, or of removing such hazards, on the occurrence of falls have frequently shown no significant associations [5, 31–39] or conflicting results [7] even if this relationship makes intuitive sense. It is our contention that these discrepant findings are influenced by how and which hazards are assessed or removed. Indeed, systematic reviews of fall prevention initiatives show that a variety of checklists have been used to assess environmental hazards and that information about their strengths and weaknesses is sparse [4, 6, 40]. Therefore, a review of what environmental hazard checklists have been developed and used is needed to more effectively prevent falls and to assess the potential for data on environmental hazards to inform policies such as building code legislation and regulated universal design.

The purpose of this scoping review was three-fold: a) to summarise how environmental hazards are defined by those developing or using environmental hazard checklists; b) to describe how, where, by whom, and for whom environmental hazard checklists are used; and, c) to examine the characteristics of environmental hazard checklists, with specific attention to features of bathrooms, and stairs/steps assessed in same. This review complements those that have focused on the relationships between falls and environmental hazards [4, 6, 40, 41] and provides a detailed examination of the assessment criteria used for two important locations in homes for injurious falls involving environmental hazards, namely bathrooms and stairs/steps.

# Methods

This scoping review was conducted in a systemic manner according to the steps outlined by Arksey and O'Malley [42], and Levac et al. [43]. Reporting follows the PRISMA (Preferred Reporting Items for Systematic Reviews and Meta-Analyses) statement guidelines, as appropriate. Ethics approval was not required.

### Identification of relevant articles

Papers were identified using various databases, namely: Medline, Embase, Web of Science, Scopus, CINAHL, AgeLine, HAPI, and PsychTESTS. No restrictions were set regarding the publication year. The search covered articles published up to January 5, 2018. A combination of descriptors (e.g. MESH terms) and key words was used. The authors reviewed the search syntax and strategy and provided additional search terms. The search strategy was finalized after consultation with a professional librarian and tailored for each database (Additional file 1). As an example, the following strategy was used for the search in Medline:

- (Fall OR accident OR accidental fall)
- AND (home adj3 hazard* OR environment* adj3 hazard*)
- AND (housing OR public housing OR Housing for the elderly OR home OR dwelling)

Backward searching from reference lists of reviewed articles was also done.

### Inclusion and exclusion criteria

We applied inclusion and exclusion criteria in two stages. The first stage yielded a more complete set of articles, all with at least some information about environmental hazard checklists. For the first stage, the inclusion criteria were:

- Assess environmental hazards for falls in one or more of the following settings: personal homes or apartments, public housing, and housing for older persons including retirement residences, even if the checklist was not entirely described.
- Include an assessment of environmental hazards in bathrooms and/or on stairs/steps by lay and/or

professional raters (e.g. nurses providing home healthcare services).

- Involve a population aged 65 years of age or older.
- Primary research study or research protocols for primary studies.

Exclusion criteria used for this first stage were:

- Focus exclusively on hospital or long-term care settings.
- Focus exclusively on a population aged less than 65 years of age (e.g. children).
- Not written in English or French.
- Conference and poster abstracts; letters, commentaries, editorials, reviews (e.g. narrative reviews, systematic reviews, meta-analysis studies), and practice guideline papers.

The second stage identified a subset of publications included in stage one that either included the checklists or provided a list of all specific environmental hazards assessed.

### Study selection

Figure 1 summarizes the two-stage process used to identify and select papers included in this review. The initial database searches yielded a total of 1114 articles. The search in HAPI and PsychTESTS yielded five additional articles, for a total of 1119 articles. All articles were entered in Zotero. Duplicates were removed, leaving 470 articles. First stage inclusion and exclusion criteria were pilot-tested and refined on a subset of 10 random titles and abstracts by the two authors. Titles and abstracts were then reviewed for stage one eligibility by two independent raters (first author and a research associate)

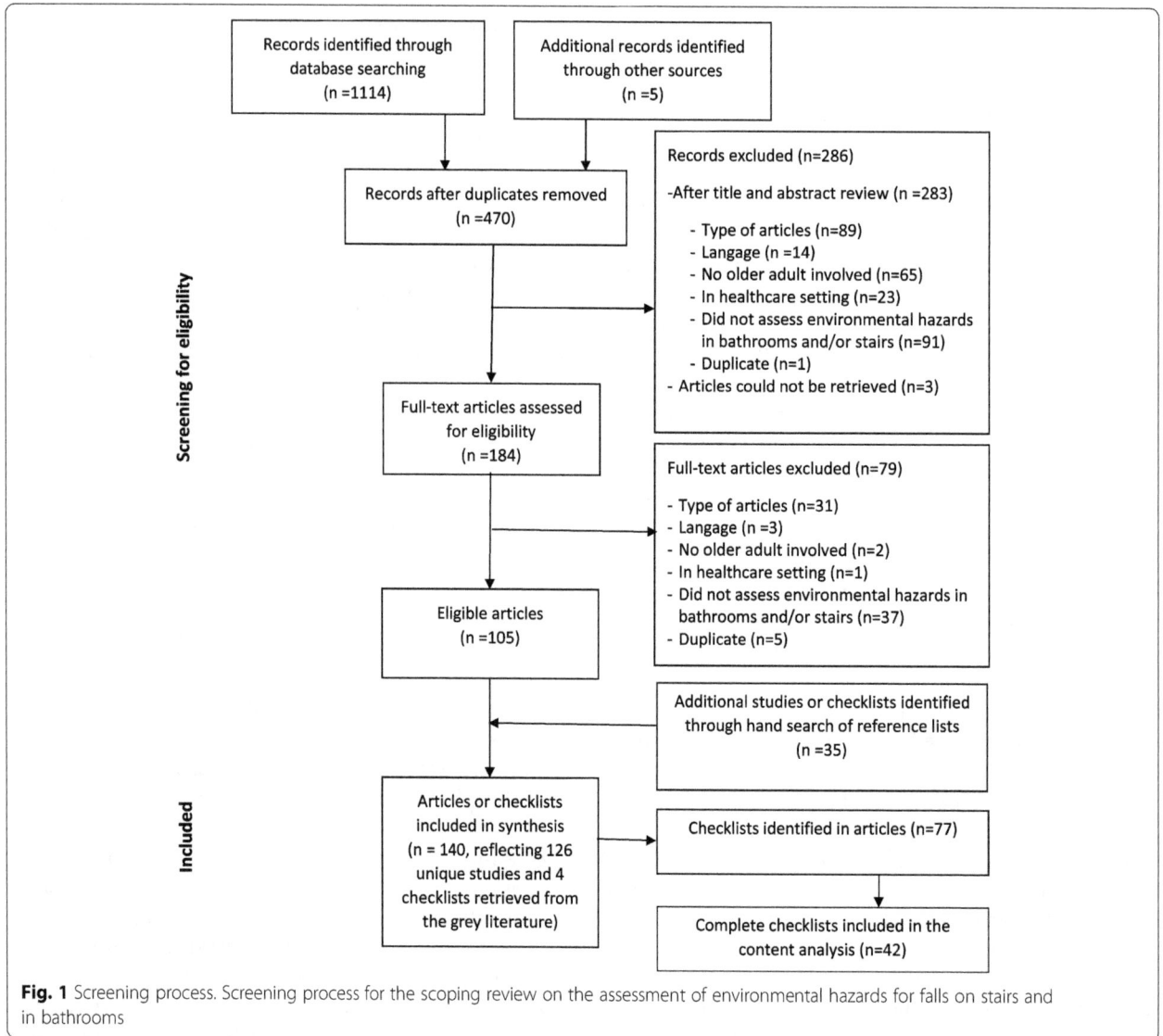

**Fig. 1** Screening process. Screening process for the scoping review on the assessment of environmental hazards for falls on stairs and in bathrooms

and classified as eligible ($n = 36$), ineligible ($n = 284$) or unclear ($n = 150$). Any discrepancies in eligibility were discussed until a consensus was reached. Articles classified as eligible or unclear underwent full-text review by the first author. After full-text review, 105 articles were deemed eligible. An additional 35 eligible articles or checklists were identified through the hand search of reference lists.

A pool of 136 published articles [1, 5, 7, 8, 14–39, 44–64, 65–147] and 4 checklists from the grey literature [148–151] were included in the first stage of this scoping review. The 136 published articles represented 126 unique studies—nine studies had multiple citations.

From these documents, 42 unique checklists were identified and included in the second stage of this review [8, 15–17, 20–23, 34, 44, 49, 51, 53, 58, 66, 69, 72, 79, 82, 86, 87, 98, 102, 108, 110–112, 115, 121, 124, 126, 132, 135, 137, 139, 140, 144, 148–152].

### Data extraction

Each of the 140 articles or checklists identified during stage one was read thoroughly and all pertinent information extracted in Excel by the first author. Extraction was overseen by the second author. The key data fields extracted are detailed in Table 1. During stage two, the first author extracted details about which and how hazards were assessed in bathrooms or on stairs/steps (indoor and outdoor). Data extracted about studies described in multiple articles were combined. When checklists were described in multiple articles, data for the checklists were combined from all sources.

An asterisk was inserted in database cells when information was not reported or not applicable. Questions that arose during the process about what data to extract were discussed until consensus was reached. The database is available upon request from the corresponding author.

### Data coding and analysis
#### Stage 1
We grouped studies or checklists into four main categories based on their objectives: 1- developed a checklist and/or tested its validity or reliability; 2- used a checklist to assess environmental hazards or the impact of environmental hazards on falls; 3- used a checklist in an intervention study and/or reported home modifications; 4- not applicable, checklist only. We dichotomized checklists according to reports of psychometric testing (those with versus those without reports of validity and/or reliability testing in current or previous studies) and assessor training (authors did or did not report training of assessors). Checklists were categorized according to whether they assessed solely fall-related hazards or whether they included non-fall-related environmental hazards. The former items were defined as "aspects of the physical environment, including objects, space and the elements in and about the house that pose a risk or danger of causing the person to fall" [56] (p. 171). Items

**Table 1** Key data extraction fields for stage one and stage two publications

| Stage and Fields | Description (and response options where applicable) |
| --- | --- |
| Stage 1 | |
| Definition of environmental hazards | The definition of environmental hazards |
| Definition of falls | The definition of falls |
| Study objective | The objective of the study |
| Year | Year of the article publication; if more than one article originating from the same study, the year of the first article was selected |
| Country(ies) | Country(ies) where the study was conducted |
| Population | Specific characteristics of the study population |
| Assessors | Who assessed environmental hazards (occupational therapist; physiotherapist, nurse; researcher or research assistant; other professional; participants or family members) |
| Training or experience | Whether assessors were trained to use the checklist or experienced with home assessment (yes or no) |
| Quality of the training | Details about the training provided to assessors |
| Checklist name | The name of the specific checklist used |
| Psychometric properties | Validity or reliability of the checklist reported for the current study or another study using the same checklist. |
| Stage 2 | |
| Environmental hazards analyzed/reported | All information provided about what and how hazards were evaluated in bathrooms and on stairs/steps (indoor and/or outdoor), and if and how the person-environment fit was assessed |
| Number of items | How many fall-related items were in the checklist (in total; in bathrooms; on indoor stairs/steps; and on outdoor stairs/steps) |

considered unrelated to falls included fire hazards, medication misuse, and wandering.

Descriptive analyses were conducted in IBM SPSS Statistics for Windows (version 24.0, Armonk, NY). We examined whether or not reports of training assessors were associated with reports of developing checklist or testing its validity or reliability (yes/no) using a Pearson chi-square test. We tested the association between time (by 1-year and 5-year period) and the proportion of studies using checklists with prior psychometric testing using Spearman correlations. $P$ values $< 0.05$ were considered significant.

### Stage 2

Detailed information was extracted about how hazards were evaluated in bathrooms and on stairs/steps (indoor and/or outdoor), and if and how person-environment fit was assessed. This data was then content analyzed [43, 153] using two sets of categorical descriptors. First, we rated hazards as structural or non-structural. We defined structural hazards as environmental features that were anchored in walls or on floors (e.g., grab bars affixed to wall, handrails on stairs) or were features of building construction (e.g. stair geometry). We defined non-structural hazards as environmental features that were not anchored in walls or on floors (e.g., presence of bathmats, cluttered stairs). Second, we rated assessment criteria as objective or subjective. We defined objective criteria as defined physical properties not involving personal judgment (e.g. presence of handrail, tread length, lumens of light on stairs). We defined subjective criteria as undefined descriptors requiring the individual judgement of the assessor (e.g., steep or narrow stairs/steps, sturdy handrails or grab bars, slippery surface). Using these definitions, all items for the three locations of hazards (bathrooms, indoor stairs/steps and outdoor stairs/steps) were independently rated by the authors using the two sets of categories for increased internal reliability. Any discrepancies in ratings were discussed until a consensus was reached.

## Results
### Stage 1
#### Definitions of environmental hazards

Only 22 studies (17%) provided a definition for the term environmental hazards, and there was considerable variation in these definitions across studies. Most authors who defined hazards, described them by giving examples such as, "features of the home environment such as loose rugs, floor clutter, and poor lighting" [19] (p. 2) or "environmental features such as poor lighting, lack of handrails on staircases, objects in pathways, and slippery rugs" [25] (p. 16). The most comprehensive definition provided was "home fall hazards are aspects of the

physical environment, including objects, space and the elements in and about the house that pose a risk or danger of causing the person to fall and, therefore, risk injury" [56] (p. 171).

### Geographic location and objectives of studies

The 126 eligible studies and 4 checklists assessed hazards in 25 countries (Additional file 2: Table S1), with the leading sites being USA ($n = 43$, 33%), Australia ($n = 17$, 13%) and Canada ($n = 13$, 10%). Most studies had been undertaken in higher-income countries ($n = 112$, 86%).

Forty-one per cent ($n = 52$, 41%) of publications described used a checklist to assess environmental hazards and/or their impact on falls. Another 36% ($n = 45$, 36%) of publications presented intervention studies that aimed to prevent falls by reducing home environmental hazards. One quarter of studies ($n = 32$, 25%) reported the development of a checklist or tested its validity or reliability. Six studies were classified simultaneously in two of the above categories ($n = 6$, 5%), and six additional entries were categorized as solely the environmental hazard checklist (n = 6, 5%).

### Checklist used

Seventy-seven different checklists were reported, with just one fourth ($n = 19$, 25%) used in two or more studies (see Table 2). Five checklists (6%) were used in at least five studies (Additional file 3: Table S2), the Westmead Home Safety Assessment (WeHSA, $n = 10$) [24, 48, 55–58, 61, 68, 136, 145], Minimum Data Set–Home Care instrument (MDS-HC; $n = 7$) [52, 54, 74, 99, 106, 112, 147], Tideiksaar et al. checklist (n = 7) [5, 14, 70, 94, 100, 129, 140], Home Falls and Accidents Screening Tool (HOME FAST; $n = 6$) [27, 101–103, 110, 122], and Housing Enabler Instrument ($n = 5$) [80, 83, 84, 118, 154]. A majority of studies ($n = 57$, 74%) used "in house" questionnaires. Only three checklists, the MDS-HC, Housing Enabler and Housing Enabler-screening tool had been used in cross-country studies [49, 80, 83, 84, 112].

### Psychometric properties of checklists

Most studies summed up hazardous items into an overall safety score. There was little discussion of the clinical appropriateness of this approach. Studies varied markedly in terms of the psychometric data presented. Some authors reported criterion validity [49, 62, 110, 112, 120, 124], others reported content validity [56, 81, 82, 91, 97, 103] or predictive validity [27]. Only two authors reported sensitivity and specificity of checklists items [62, 103]. Thirty studies reported inter-rater reliability [8, 14, 15, 19, 23, 51, 54, 57–59, 72, 77, 80, 81, 84, 85, 98, 103, 106, 110–112, 115, 120–123, 133, 135, 152]; fewer reported test-retest reliability [36, 81, 98, 122] or internal consistency [53, 81, 86, 97]. The inter-rater reliability of checklists, when used

**Table 2** Environmental hazard checklists included in the content analysis

| Checklist | Author | Year | Countries where checklists have been used | Total #of fall-related items in checklist | Psychometric data reported (Y/N) | Bathrooms | | | | Indoor stairs/steps | | | | Outdoor stairs/steps | | | |
|---|---|---|---|---|---|---|---|---|---|---|---|---|---|---|---|---|---|
| | | | | | | #of fall-related items in bathrooms | >50% of items are subjective (Y/N) | >50 of items are non-structural hazards (Y/N) | Assessed grab bars (Y/N) | #of fall-related items on indoor stairs/steps | >50% of items are subjective (Y/N) | >50 of items are non-structural hazards (Y/N) | Assessed handrails (Y/N) | #of fall-related items on outdoor stairs/steps | >50% of items are subjective (Y/N) | >50 of items are non-structural hazards (Y/N) | Assessed handrails (Y/N) |
| Carter et al. | Carter et al. [51] | 1997 | Australia | 99 | Y | 24 | N | Y | Y | 16 | Y | N | Y | 2 | Y | Y | N |
| CDC Home checklist | CDC [148] | 2005 | USA, Singapore | 25 | N | 6 | Y | Y | N | 7 | N | N | Y | 7 | N | N | Y |
| Cougar[1] | Fisher et al. [71] | 2006 | USA | 56 | Y | 5 | Y | Y | Y | 5 | Y | N | Y | 1 | Y | Y | N |
| Edwards & Jones | Edwards & Jones [66] | 1998 | South Wales | 14 | N | 5 | N | Y | Y | 1 | N | N | Y | 0 | a | a | a |
| Environmental Safety Checklist | Huang et al. [16] | 2005 | China | 31 | Y | 5 | Y | Y | Y | 4 | Y | Y | Y | 1 | a | a | a |
| Evci et al. | Evci et al. [69] | 2006 | Turkey | 15 | N | 6 | N | N | Y | 5 | N | N | Y | 0 | a | a | a |
| Greene et al. | Greene et al. [79] | 2009 | USA | 15 | N | 2 | N | N | Y | 4 | N | N | Y | 4 | N | N | N |
| Healthy housing index | Keall et al. [90] | 2008 | New Zealand | 26 | N | 3 | Y | N | | 12 | Y | Y | | 9 | Y | Y | |
| HEAP | Gitlin et al. [15] | 2002 | USA | 69 | Y | 10 | N | Y | Y | 6 | Y | Y | Y | 6 | Y | N | Y |
| HEAVI | Yonge et al. [22] | 2017 | USA | 127 | Y | 15 | N | Y | Y | 17 | N | N | Y | 19 | N | N | Y |
| HEROS Environmental Safety Check | Sadasivam et al. [124] | 2014 | USA | 5 | Y | 6 | Y | Y | Y | 0 | a | a | a | 0 | a | a | a |
| Home Environment Survey | Rodriguez et al. [121] | 1995 | USA | 17 | Y | 4 | N | N | Y | Can't tell | a | a | a | Can't tell | a | a | a |
| HOME FAST | Mackenzie et al. [102] | 2000 | Australia, Scotland, Malaysia, England | 25 | Y | 6 | Y | Y | Y | 4 | Y | Y | N | 1 | Y | N | Y |
| HOME FAST – Self-Report Assessment | Mehraban et al. [110] | 2011 | Australia | 87 | Y | 7 | Y | Y | Y | 11 | Y | N | Y | 3 | Y | N | Y |
| Home fall hazard assessment | You et al. (2004) [23] | 2004 | China | 60 | Y | 16 | Y | Y | Y | 10 | Y | Y | | 0 | a | a | |
| Home-screen safe | Johnson et al. [86] | 2001 | Australia | 10 | N | 2 | Y | Y | N | Can't tell | a | a | a | Can't tell | a | a | a |
| Housing Enabler[2] | Iwarsson & Björn [149] | 2010 | Sweden | 188 | Y | 13 | N | N | Y | 11 | N | N | Y | 11 | N | N | Y |
| Housing Enabler screening tool | Carlsson et al. [49] | 2009 | Sweden, Germany, Latvia, Hungary, Denmark, Finland, Iceland, England | 61 | Y | 10 | Y | Y | Y | 6 | Y | N | Y | 6 | Y | N | Y |
| Isbener et al. | Isbener et al. [82] | 1998 | USA | 21 | N | 0 | a | a | a | 10 | Y | N | Y | 2 | N | N | N |
| Kamei et al. | Kamei et al. [87] | 2015 | USA | 33 | N | 7 | Y | Y | Y | Can't tell | Y | N | Y | Can't tell | a | a | a |

**Table 2** Environmental hazard checklists included in the content analysis (*Continued*)

| Checklist | Author | Year | Countries where checklists have been used | Total #of fall-related items in checklist | Psychometric data reported (Y/N) | Bathrooms #of fall-related items in bathrooms | Bathrooms >50% of items are subjective (Y/N) | Bathrooms >50 of items are non-structural hazards (Y/N) | Assessed grab bars (Y/N) | Indoor stairs/steps #of fall-related items on indoor stairs/steps | Indoor >50% of items are subjective (Y/N) | Indoor >50 of items are non-structural hazards (Y/N) | Assessed handrails (Y/N) | Outdoor stairs/steps #of fall-related items on outdoor stairs/steps | Outdoor >50% of items are subjective (Y/N) | Outdoor >50 of items are non-structural hazards (Y/N) | Assessed handrails (Y/N) |
|---|---|---|---|---|---|---|---|---|---|---|---|---|---|---|---|---|---|
| Kellogg international work group | Kellogg international work group [139] | 1987 | Canada, USA | 40 | N | 4 | Y | Y | Y | 6 | Y | N | Y | 0 | a | a | a |
| Lan et al. | Lan et al. [17] | 2009 | | 6 | N | 3 | Y | Y | Y | 0 | a | a | a | 1 | Y | N | Y |
| Lim & Sung | Lim & Sung [126] | 2012 | Korea | 3 | N | 1 | N | Y | N | 0 | a | a | a | 0 | a | a | a |
| MAHC-10 Fall Checklist | Bamgbade & Dearmon [44] | 2016 | USA | 1 | N | <1 | a | a | N | Can't tell | a | a | a | Can't tell | a | a | a |
| Marshall et al. | Marshall et al. [108] | 2005 | USA | 10 | N | 2 | N | N | Y | 1.5 | N | N | Y | 1.5 | N | N | Y |
| McLean & Lord | McLean & Lord [34] | 1996 | Australia | 15 | N | 4 | N | Y | Y | 0 | a | a | a | 2 | N | N | Y |
| MDS-HC | Morris et al. [112] | 1997 | Canada, Hong Kong, USA, Korea, Italy, Australia, Czech Republic, Japan | 8 | Y | 1 | Y | Y | Y | 1 | Y | N | N | 1 | Y | Y | N |
| Morgan et al. | Morgan et al. [111] | 2005 | | 73 | Y | 13 | Y | Y | Y | 2 | Y | N | Y | 4 | N | N | Y |
| Nevit et al. | Nevit et al. [7] reported in Northridge et al. [115] | 1898 | USA | 22 | Y | 8 | Y | Y | Y | 0 | a | a | a | 0 | a | a | a |
| Safe living guide | Public Health Agency of Canada [151] | 2015 | Canada | 34 | Y | 9 | Y | Y | Y | 6 | Y | Y | Y | 2 | Y | N | Y |
| SAFER-HOME | Chiu & Oliver [53] | 2006 | Canada, USA | 17 | Y | 7 | Y | Y | Y | 2 | Y | N | Y | 0 | a | a | N |
| SAFER Tool | Letts et al. [98] | 1998 | Canada | 17 | Y | 5 | Y | Y | Y | 2 | Y | N | Y | 0 | a | a | N |
| Sattin et al. | Sattin et al. [8] | 1998 | USA | 10 | Y | 3 | N | Y | Y | 0 | a | a | a | 0 | a | a | a |
| Sophonratanapokin et al. | Sophonratanapokin et al. [132] | 2012 | Thailand | 9 | N | 4 | N | N | Y | 2 | N | N | Y | 1 | N | N | N |
| Stalenhoef et al. | Stalenhoef et al. [135] | 1998 | Netherlands | 116 | Y | 17 | Y | Y | Y | 11 | Y | N | Y | 0 | a | a | a |
| Stevens et al. | Stevens et al. [137] | 2001 | Australia | 14 | N | 8 | Y | Y | N | 2 | N | N | N | 0 | a | a | a |
| Tanner | Tanner [20] | 2003 | USA | 20 | N | 2 | N | N | Y | Can't tell | Y | N | Y | Can't tell | a | a | a |
| Tideiksaar et al. | Tideiksaar et al. [140] | 1987 | Canada, England, USA | 37 | Y | 6 | Y | N | Y | 4 | Y | N | Y | 5 | Y | N | Y |
| Vladutiu et al. | Vladutiu et al. [144] | 2012 | USA | 6 | N | 2 | N | N | Y | 3 | N | N | Y | 1 | N | N | N |

**Table 2** Environmental hazard checklists included in the content analysis (*Continued*)

| Checklist | Author | Year | Countries where checklists have been used | Total #of fall-related items in checklist | Psychometric data reported (Y/N) | Bathrooms | | | | Indoor stairs/steps | | | | Outdoor stairs/steps | | | |
|---|---|---|---|---|---|---|---|---|---|---|---|---|---|---|---|---|---|
| | | | | | | #of fall-related items in bathrooms | >50% of items are subjective (Y/N) | >50 of items are non-structural hazards (Y/N) | Assessed grab bars (Y/N) | #of fall-related items on indoor stairs/steps | >50% of items are subjective (Y/N) | >50 of items are non-structural hazards (Y/N) | Assessed handrails (Y/N) | #of fall-related items on outdoor stairs/steps | >50% of items are subjective (Y/N) | >50 of items are non-structural hazards (Y/N) | Assessed handrails (Y/N) |
| WeSHA | Clemson et al. [58] | 1992 | Australia, England, New Zealand, USA | 72 | Y | 10 | Y | Y | Y | 7 | Y | N | Y | 5 | Y | N | Y |
| Wyman et al. | Wyman et al. [21] | 2007 | USA | 37 | Y | 12 | Y | Y | Y | 7 | Y | N | Y | 0 | a | a | a |
| Zhang et al. | Zhang et al. [152] | 2016 | China | 30 | Y | 8 | Y | Y | Y | 6 | Y | N | Y | 1 | Y | N | N |

Y=Yes, N=No
CDC: Center for disease control
HEAP: Home Environmental Assessment Protocol
HEAVI: Home Environment Assessment for the Visually Impaired
HOME FAST: Home Falls and Accidents Screening Tool
MAHC-10: Missouri Alliance for Home Care-10
MDS-HC: Minimum Data Set-Home Care
SAFER-HOME: Safety Assessment of Function and the Environment for Rehabilitation–Health Outcome Measurement and Evaluation
SAFER Tool: Safety Assessment of Function and the Environment for Rehabilitation
WeHSA: Westmead Home Safety Assessment
aLocation not assessed
[1] Version 1.0 and 2.0;
[2] Original, revised and Nordic

by professional and lay older adult pairs, was reported in four studies; three showed that professionals identified more hazards than lay older adults [23, 111, 133] and one showed that lay older adults reported more of some hazards, while professionals reported more of other hazards [110]. Further, the reliability of items on a checklist was often reported as excellent for some but poor for others [8, 19, 58, 80, 103, 110, 111, 115, 121]. Two authors noted that objective items had a higher reliability coefficient than subjective items [19, 80]. Interestingly, no time trend was observed in the proportion of studies using checklists with prior psychometric testing versus checklists without this prior testing (see Fig. 2).

### Study populations

About half of the studies ($n = 73$, 57%) drew their sample from the general population. The remainder targeted populations at a higher risk of falls such as individuals who had fallen in the previous year; frail individuals; or individuals with mental or visual impairments.

Almost no studies adapted the type of specific home hazards assessed to the specific needs of participants. There were two exceptions. The HEAVI was developed for visually impaired individuals and focusses on related environmental features such as lighting and visual cues [19]. The HEAP was developed for individuals with dementia and includes an assessment of pressure gates at the top and bottom of stairways [15, 78].

### Who completed the assessment

Among the studies that assessed environmental hazards ($n = 122$), evaluations were conducted by occupational therapists ($n = 45$, 37%), nurses ($n = 28$, 23%), researchers or research assistants ($n = 20$, 16%), the participant or a family member ($n = 18$, 15%), other professionals ($n = 16$, 13%; e.g.; physicians, home inspectors, house retailers),

or physiotherapists ($n = 7$, 6%). In 17 studies (14%), two or more types of assessors conducted assessments. Assessors were not described in 7 studies (6%). Forty-nine (40%) studies specified that assessors had been trained or had experience in home assessment, and two studies (2%) mentioned that the checklist used does not require prior training in home evaluation or modification [18, 21]. The rest of the studies ($n = 69$, 57%) provided no details about training. The assessments in 22 (32%) of these latter studies were conducted by occupational therapists. When described, training approaches varied in duration (one-hour to one-week workshop) and format (theoretical lectures, video of home assessment or practical sessions using the checklist in real/mock homes). Studies that described training assessors were more likely to report developing a checklist or testing its validity or reliability ($X^2 = 15.840$, df = 1, $p < 0.0001$, Table 3).

### Stage 2

Most checklists assessed solely fall-related environmental hazards; a quarter of them ($n = 10$) were imbedded in a checklist designed to also capture non-fall related hazards. As shown in Tables 2 and 4, checklists varied greatly in their length and in the number of bathroom and stair items assessed. Checklists differed with respect to what rooms were assessed (e.g. all bathrooms or bathroom most often used), whether or not outdoor hazards were assessed, and how responses were coded. Some hazards were assessed using dichotomous response categories (e.g.; present/absent); others were coded as continuous variables (e.g.; number of stairs/steps).

### Person-environment fit

Most checklists did not assess person-environment fit. There were a few exceptions [15, 34, 53, 58, 69, 83, 87,

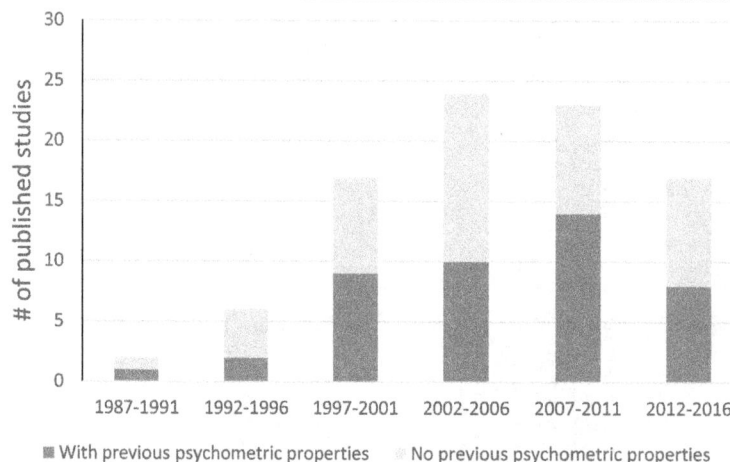

**Fig. 2** Number of articles published according to whether the checklist used had prior psychometric testing ($n = 96$)

**Table 3** Association between training assessors and developing a checklist or testing its validity or reliability

| | Report developing a checklist or testing its validity or reliability | | |
|---|---|---|---|
| Report training assessors | Yes (n = 67) | No (n = 53) | p* |
| Yes | 56.7% | 20.8% | < 0.0001 |
| No | 43.3% | 79.2% | |

*Chi-square analysis

98, 102, 110, 140]. Examples of items that assessed person-environment fit included either participants' self-reports or assessors' observations of difficulties (or lack or thereof) walking from room to room, over different floor surfaces; climbing and descending stairs/steps; transferring from beds, chairs, and toilets; and getting in and out of bathtubs or showers. Notably, the Housing Enabler Instrument [83] assesses the environment and older adults' functional limitations separately. Uniquely, these authors provide an analytic matrix and a software program to examine the gap between the environment and the person's limitations.

### Summary of key findings related to bathrooms
Thirty-nine checklists assessed bathrooms. Few checklists indicated which bathroom to assess when there were more than one in the home. As shown in Table 5, a majority of checklists (n = 25, 63%) used mostly subjective items to assess hazards in bathrooms. For instance, they assessed an "awkward toilet seat", or "slippery floor". Similarly, over three quarters of checklists (n = 30, 77%) assessed primarily non-structural hazards such as non-skid mats, abrasive strips in the bath or shower, or objects on the bathroom floor. The most frequently assessed structural hazard was the absence of grab bars.

**Grab bars** Although most checklists assessed grab bars in bathrooms, there was a lot of variation as to where (in the bathtub, shower and/or next to the toilet) and how they were assessed. For instance, in some checklists, grab bars were assessed with a single item and a bathroom would need to have grab bars in three locations (toilet, bath, shower) not to be hazardous, while in others, grab bars were also assessed with a single item but the presence of only one grab bar was enough to code the item as having the grab bar present. In other

studies, each location was assessed separately and one, two or three items were listed in the checklist accordingly. Two checklists coded the lack of grab bars as a hazard only if the person needed them [23, 115], one coded using a grab bar as a hazard [20], and another described grab bars as assistive devices and did not consider their absence to be an environmental hazard [108].

None of the checklists distinguished between diagonal, horizontal or vertical grab bars in the tub/shower; or documented where they were situated (e.g. side wall and/or back wall). Four checklists assessed grab bar placement; one had objective height measures [149], whereas others relied on subjective criteria such as "properly installed" [71], "properly placed" [151], or "can be reached without leaning enough to lose balance" [102]. Four checklists assessed if grab bars were sturdy or well anchored to walls [16, 139, 140, 151]. Illustrations of grab bars in another checklist included two types that were not fixed to a wall [111]. Only three checklists provided a definition of grab bars or specified that towel racks are not grab bars [102, 111, 121].

### Summary of key findings related to stairs/steps
Thirty-nine checklists included items on stairs and/or steps. Most (n = 22, 63%) assessed both indoor and outdoor stairs/steps, while eleven (31%) assessed only indoor stairs/steps and two assessed only outdoor stairs/steps. The location of stairs/steps (whether indoors or outdoors) was not differentiated in four of the checklists (10%). Very few checklists assessed the number of stairs/steps or staircases in the home.

**Indoor stairs/steps** Among the 33 checklists that assessed indoor stairs/steps, twenty-six (79%) assessed features of stairs/steps not related to handrails (see Table 6). Most checklists (n = 23, 70%) used a majority of subjective items (e.g. stairs/steps in need of repair,

**Table 4** Bathroom and stair locations included in checklists and range and average number of items evaluated (n = 42 checklists)

| Location of assessment items | Checklists including ≥1 items n (%) | Range for number of items | Average (SD) number of items |
|---|---|---|---|
| Bathrooms | 39 (92.9%) | 1–24 | 7.2 (5.1) |
| Indoor stairs/steps | 33 (78.5%) | 1–17 | 6.0 (4.2) |
| Outdoor stairs/steps | 23 (54.7%) | 1–19 | 4.2 (4.2) |
| All locations | 42 (100%) | 1–188 | 38.1 (38.8) |

Range and average are shown only for tools including 1 or more assessment item in location

**Table 5** Summary of findings on how environmental hazards are assessed in bathrooms (*n* = 39 checklists)

| Characteristics of items assessed on checklists | n (%) |
|---|---|
| Overall | |
| > 50% of items are subjective | 25 (63%) |
| > 50% of items are non-structural hazards | 30 (77%) |
| Frequently assessed hazards | |
| Assessed the presence of throw rugs and/or if they were well anchored to the floor (non-structural hazards) | 20 (51%) |
| Assessed the lack of a non-skid mat or strips in the tub and/or shower (non-structural hazards) | 22 (56%) |
| Assessed the absence of grab bars (structural hazards) | 35 (90%) |

sloping or broken steps, stairs too steep) and most (*n* = 30, 91%) included a majority of structural items. Yet, most structural features assessed were not related to the construction geometry of stairs/steps (e.g., height of riser, tread width).

**Indoor handrails** Handrails were the most commonly assessed structural features of stairs/steps (n = 30, 91%). Eight checklists (27%) solely assessed if handrails were present; the others assessed specific features of handrails: sturdiness (*n* = 18, 60%); height, length and/or if they were continuous (*n* = 13, 43%); and diameter or ease of grip (*n* = 7, 23%). There was also variability in the number of handrails that needed to be present to code stairs/steps as not hazardous. For the majority (*n* = 24, 80%) the presence of only one handrail resulted in this categorization, while for six checklists (*n* = 6, 20%), two handrails had to be present for this categorization.

**Outdoor stairs/steps** There were fewer items and fewer features assessed for outdoor than indoor stairs/steps. Of the 23 checklists that assessed outdoor stairs/steps, eight (35%) assessed some features of stairs/steps other than handrails. Assessment criteria were predominantly subjective in most of these checklists (*n* = 13, 57%). Most checklists assessed structural hazards (*n* = 20, 87%). Yet, similarly to indoor stairs/steps, the features assessed were not related to their construction geometry.

**Table 6** Summary of findings on how environmental hazards are assessed in stairs/steps

| Characteristics of items assessed on checklists | n (%) |
|---|---|
| Indoor stairs/steps (*n* = 33 checklists) | |
| > 50% of items are subjective | 23 (70%) |
| > 50% of items are non-structural hazards | 3 (9%) |
| Assessed handrails absence or features (structural hazard) | 30 (91%) |
| Outdoor stairs/steps (n = 23 checklists) | |
| > 50% of items are subjective | 13 (57%) |
| > 50% of items are non-structural hazards | 3 (13%) |
| Assessed handrails absence or features (structural hazard) | 15 (65%) |

**Outdoor handrails** Handrails were assessed in 15 (65%) checklists. Almost all of these checklists assessed at least one specific feature of handrails (n = 13, 87%): sturdiness (*n* = 7, 50%); height, length and/or if they were continuous (*n* = 5, 31%); and diameter or ease of grip (n = 2, 13%). Similarly to the assessment of indoor handrails, 87% (n = 13) of checklists required the presence of only one handrail to code outdoor stairs/steps as not hazardous.

## Discussion

This is the first scoping review to examine the characteristics of environmental hazards checklists. Given the pervasive presence of environmental hazards in homes and their causal relationship with falls and independent functional mobility among the older adults, examining the status and quality of such checklists is imperative.

Despite over three decades of research in this field, there are still no widely used environmental assessment checklists. There is a lot of variability among checklists in terms of the number of items, which parts of the home were assessed, and among those assessing bathrooms and stairs/steps whether checklists emphasized structural or non-structural features or used primarily objective or subjective criteria for assessments. The lack of standardized assessment items in checklists severely limits cross-study comparisons [58]. In 2003, Gitlin concluded that there was a "lack of psychometrically sound measures" to assess home environments and that most assessment methods used were study-specific with unknown reliability and validity [155]. Our review indicates that this conclusion still largely holds. Developing "gold standard" environmental hazards checklists with known psychometric properties is critical to advance the field and inform fall-related prevention practices. This requires the development of a consensus definition of environmental hazards [58], and the identification of priority structural and non-structural attributes of safe bathrooms and safe stairs/steps. There is substantial data available from ergonomic studies to support this prioritization. Furthermore, statistical modeling of the relationship between checklist items and falls would help establish the predictive validity of checklist items, determine if it is clinically appropriate to sum all items into an overall hazard score, and identify priority objective measures for inclusion in abbreviated checklists.

We found limited descriptions of training approaches used and a lack of information on whether or not assessors were trained to use checklists. We recognize that training is costly, but agree with authors who have suggested that training is essential to achieve consistent assessments among raters [57]. For instance, interviewers have been shown to incorrectly identify towel racks as grab bars [8], highlighting the need to train them and to provide definitions of hazards. We also think that scaling-up the use of robust environmental hazard assessment checklists is important; their reach could be extended by training lay people to conduct assessments, and reducing the number of items on hazard checklists.

Given the disproportionately high rate of injurious falls that occur on stairs/steps and in bathrooms [10–12], it was surprising to us that checklists did not always include an assessment of these locations and that outdoor stairs/steps were so infrequently included. Outdoor stairs/steps often comprise part of older adults' walking paths (Edwards & Dulai, under review); affect the visitability of a home; and may be more prone to hazardous characteristics since they may not be covered by building code legislation. In our view, comprehensive environmental hazard checklists need to assess both indoor and outdoor home environments.

Most of the authors describing environmental hazard checklists seemed to conceptualize the environment as an independent static entity, ignoring how older adults interact with their environment or the degree of their exposure [155, 156]. Ideally, checklists that assess person-environment fit and/or dynamic variability of the environment would be used alongside standard checklists, providing more insights on how older adults navigate their home environment in ways that either reduce or increase their risk of falls [157]. For example, checklists should assess whether older adults use stair handrails to compensate for poor balance or use a toilet or bathtub grab bar to aid transfers. Checklists should also contain items and directions pertaining to assessing the dynamic and variable nature of some environmental hazards (e.g. outdoor stairs/steps that were dry versus covered in ice or snow, friction coefficient of wet versus dry bathroom floor, combinations of natural and artificial lighting on stairs/steps that changed at different times of the day) [56].

There has been a tendency to define the problem of environmental risk modification as an individual behaviour change problem rather than as an environmental issue that requires a multi-level and inter-sectoral approach such as building code legislation and regulated universal design [158]. This behavioural emphasis may in part, explain the emphasis on subjective and non-structural items that was evident in checklists that assessed bathrooms and stairs/steps. In the longer-term, policy interventions, are likely to be more effective than behavioural interventions in facilitating some environmental modifications, such as safer stair geometry and universal access to grab bars for toilets, showers and bathtubs [159, 160]. It is imperative that we identify those constellations of hazards that are priorities and best tackled through policy change. This requires cumulative knowledge about the prevalence of structural environmental hazards and their relationship to falls. The inclusion of consistent, objectively-assessed, structural items in environmental hazard checklists could help address this knowledge gap.

## Limitations

This review has several limitations. First, we focussed on hazards related to bathrooms and stairs/steps. This may have resulted in the exclusion of a few checklists assessing solely other parts of homes. Second, we did not attempt to access unpublished training manuals for checklists, which may include descriptions of items that would have led us to categorize them as objective rather than subjective. However, most studies did not mention training their assessors or having a training manual, so it seems unlikely that this would have substantially shifted our results. Third, it was sometimes hard to categorize items as structural or non-structural, or as objective or subjective due to the limited descriptors of hazards contained in many checklists. For instance, "dim lightning" could be caused by a lack of proper ceiling light fixtures (structural) or by a burned-out light bulb (non-structural). To improve reliability, both authors independently rated the environmental hazard items on checklists and discussed discrepant results until a consensus emerged. However, it might have been more rigorous to involve an independent rater in this process. Lastly, we did not judge the appropriateness of objective criteria used to evaluate hazards. We did observe that objective criteria were inconsistent across checklists. In the future, an assessment of objective criteria should include a quality assessment against standards such as those suggested in ergonomic studies or those used in existing building code legislation.

## Conclusion

The lack of standard definitions and consistent objective criteria for assessing environmental hazards for falls is limiting meaningful cross-study comparisons and slowing advances in this field. This gap may partly explain conflicting results regarding the effectiveness of interventions targeting home environmental hazards (in particular those involving bathrooms and stairs/steps) to prevent falls among older adults. This field of research would be improved with standardized environmental hazard checklists containing objective criteria to assess structural hazards. To inform population health interventions aimed at preventing falls, such as building code regulations or municipal housing by-laws, it is essential to include objectively-assessed, structural hazards in environmental checklists.

## Abbreviations
CDC: Center for Disease Control; CINAHL: Cumulative Index to Nursing and Allied Health Literature; HAPI: Health and Psychosocial Instruments; HEAP: Home Environmental Assessment Protocol; HEAVI: Home Environment Assessment for the Visually Impaired; HOME FAST: Home Falls and Accidents Screening Tool; MAHC-10: Missouri Alliance for Home Care-10; MDS-HC: Minimum Data Set-Home Care; MeSH: Medical Subject Headings; PRISMA: Preferred Reporting Items for Systematic Reviews and Meta-Analyses; WeHSA: Westmead Home Safety Assessment

## Acknowledgements
The authors would like to thank Yeonjung Yoo for her help screening potential articles.

## Funding
This research was carried out with funding support from the Canadian Institutes of Health Research, grant number #122510.

## Authors' contributions
RB: Contributed to the study design, acquired and extracted data for analysis, performed statistical analyses, interpreted the data and drafted the manuscript. NE: Designed the study, oversaw data extraction, interpreted the data, drafted some sections of the manuscript and edited the overall manuscript for critical content. Both authors have read and approved the final manuscript.

## Competing interests
The authors declare that they have no competing interests.

## Author details
[1]School of Nursing, University of Ottawa, 1 Stewart Street, Room 212, Ottawa, ON K1H 8M5, Canada. [2]School of Nursing, University of Ottawa, 1 Stewart Street, Room 205, Ottawa, ON K1H 8M5, Canada.

## References
1. Tinetti ME, Speechley M, Ginter SF. Risk factors for falls among elderly persons living in the community. N Engl J Med. 1988;319:1701–7.
2. Public Health Agency of Canada. Seniors' falls in Canada: Second report. 2014. https://www.canada.ca/en/public-health/services/health-promotion/aging-seniors/publications/publications-general-public/seniors-falls-canada-second-report.html. Accessed 29 Sep 2017.
3. Parachute. The cost of injury in Canada. Toronto: Parachute; 2015.
4. Clemson L, Mackenzie L, Ballinger C, Close JCT, Cumming RG. Environmental interventions to prevent falls in community-dwelling older people: a meta-analysis of randomized trials. J Aging Health. 2008;20:954–71.
5. Gill TM, Williams CS, Tinetti ME. Environmental hazards and the risk of nonsyncopal falls in the homes of community-living older persons. Med Care. 2000;38:1174–83.
6. Gillespie L, Robertson M, Gillespie W, Sherrington C, Gates S, Clemson L, et al. Interventions for preventing falls in older people living in the community. Cochrane Database Syst Rev. 2012;9:CD007146. https://doi.org/10.1002/14651858.CD007146.pub3.
7. Nevitt MC, Cummings SR, Kidd S, Black D. Risk factors for recurrent nonsyncopal falls. A prospective study. JAMA. 1989;261:2663–8.
8. Sattin RW, Rodriguez JG, DeVito CA, Wingo PA. Home environmental hazards and the risk of fall injury events among community-dwelling older persons. Study to assess falls among the elderly (SAFE) group. J Am Geriatr Soc. 1998;46:669–76.
9. Speechley M, Tinetti M. Falls and injuries in frail and vigorous community elderly persons. J Am Geriatr Soc. 1991;39:46–52.
10. Blazewick DH, Chounthirath T, Hodges NL, Collins CL, Smith GA. Stair-related injuries treated in United States emergency departments. Am J Emerg Med. 2017. https://doi.org/10.1016/j.ajem.2017.09.034.
11. Stevens JA, Haas EN, Haileyesus T. Nonfatal bathroom injuries among persons aged ≥15 years--United States, 2008. J Saf Res. 2011;42:311–5.
12. Hanba C, Gupta A, Svider PF, Folbe AJ, Eloy JA, Zuliani GF, et al. Forgetful but not forgotten: bathroom-related craniofacial trauma among the elderly. Laryngoscope. 2017;127:820–7.
13. Consumer Product Safety Commission. 2017 NEISS data highlights: top 20 injury estimates by age. Maryland: Consumer Product Safety Commission; 2018. https://www.cpsc.gov/s3fs-public/2017-NEISS-data-highlights-age.pdf?pKuMH.4NqENxSLlyA9fVd1U0g0F5MGV
14. Gill TM, Williams CS, Robison JT, Tinetti ME. A population-based study of environmental hazards in the homes of older persons. Am J Public Health. 1999;89:553–6.
15. Gitlin LN, Schinfeld S, Winter L, Corcoran M, Boyce AA, Hauck W. Evaluating home environments of persons with dementia: interrater reliability and validity of the home environmental assessment protocol (HEAP). Disabil Rehabil. 2002;24:59–71.
16. Huang TT. Home environmental hazards among community-dwelling elderly persons in Taiwan. J Nurs Res JNR. 2005;13:49–57.
17. Lan TY, Wu SC, Chang WC, Chen CY. Home environmental problems and physical function in Taiwanese older adults. Arch Gerontol Geriatr. 2009;49:335–8.
18. Leclerc BS, Bégin C, Cadieux E, Goulet L, Allaire J-F, Meloche J, et al. Relationship between home hazards and falling among community-dwelling seniors using home-care services. Rev Epidemiol Sante Publique. 2010;58:3–11.
19. Swenor BK, Yonge AV, Goldhammer V, Miller R, Gitlin LN, Ramulu P. Evaluation of the home environment assessment for the visually impaired (HEAVI): an instrument designed to quantify fall-related hazards in the visually impaired. BMC Geriatr. 2016;16:214. https://doi.org/10.1186/s12877-016-0391-2.
20. Tanner EK. Assessing home safety in homebound older adults. Geriatr Nurs N Y N. 2003;24:250–4 256.
21. Wyman JF, Croghan CF, Nachreiner NM, Gross CR, Stock HH, Talley K, et al. Effectiveness of education and individualized counseling in reducing environmental hazards in the homes of community-dwelling older women: education and individualized counseling to reduce environmental hazards. J Am Geriatr Soc. 2007;55:1548–56.
22. Yonge AV, Swenor BK, Miller R, Goldhammer V, West SK, Friedman DS, et al. Quantifying fall-related hazards in the homes of persons with glaucoma. Ophthalmology. 2017;124:562–71.
23. You L, Deans C, Liu K, Zhang MF, Zhang J. Raising awareness of fall risk among Chinese older adults. Use of the home fall hazards assessment tool. J Gerontol Nurs. 2004;30:35–42.

24. Cumming RG, Thomas M, Szonyi G, Salkeld G, O'Neill E, Westbury C, et al. Home visits by an occupational therapist for assessment and modification of environmental hazards: a randomized trial of falls prevention. J Am Geriatr Soc. 1999;47:1397–402.

25. Hornbrook MC, Stevens VJ, Wingfield DJ, Hollis JF, Greenlick MR. Preventing falls among community-dwelling older persons: results from a randomized trial. Gerontologist. 1994;34:16–23.

26. La Grow SJ, Robertson MC, Campbell AJ, Clarke GA, Kerse NM. Reducing hazard related falls in people 75 years and older with significant visual impairment: how did a successful program work? Inj Prev J Int Soc Child Adolesc Inj Prev. 2006;12:296–301.

27. Mackenzie L, Byles J, D'Este C. Longitudinal study of the home falls and accidents screening tool in identifying older people at increased risk of falls. Australas J Ageing. 2009;28:64–9.

28. Palvanen M, Kannus P, Piirtola M, Niemi S, Parkkari J, Jarvinen M. Effectiveness of the Chaos falls clinic in preventing falls and injuries of home-dwelling older adults: a randomised controlled trial. Injury. 2014;45:265–71.

29. Steinberg M, Cartwright C, Peel N, Williams G. A sustainable programme to prevent falls and near falls in community dwelling older people: results of a randomised trial. J Epidemiol Community Health. 2000;54:227–32.

30. Sze P-C, Cheung WH, Lam PS, Lo HS, Leung KS, Chan T. The efficacy of a multidisciplinary falls prevention clinic with an extended step-down community program. Arch Phys Med Rehabil. 2008;89:1329–34.

31. Elley CR, Robertson MC, Garrett S, Kerse NM, McKinlay E, Lawton B, et al. Effectiveness of a falls-and-fracture nurse coordinator to reduce falls: a randomized, controlled trial of at-risk older adults. J Am Geriatr Soc. 2008;56: 1383–9.

32. Hendriks MR, Bleijlevens MH, van Haastregt JC, Crebolder HF, Diederiks JP, Evers SM, et al. Lack of effectiveness of a multidisciplinary fall-prevention program in elderly people at risk: a randomized, controlled trial. J Am Geriatr Soc. 2008;56:1390–7.

33. Keskinoglu P, Picakciefe M, Bilgic N, Giray H, Karakus N, Ucku R. Home accidents in the community-dwelling elderly in Izmir, Turkey: how do prevalence and risk factors differ between high and low socioeconomic districts? J Aging Health. 2008;20:824–36.

34. McLean D, Lord S. Falling in older people at home: transfer limitations and environmental risk factors. Aust Occup Ther J. 2010;43:13–8.

35. Pardessus V, Puisieux F, Di Pompeo C, Gaudefroy C, Thevenon A, Dewailly P. Benefits of home visits for falls and autonomy in the elderly: a randomized trial study. Am J Phys Med Rehabil. 2002;81:247–52.

36. Pattaramongkolrit S, Sindhu S, Thosigha O, Somboontanot W. Fall-related factors among older, visually-impaired Thais. Pac Rim Int J Nurs Res. 2013;17: 181–96.

37. Peel N, Steinberg M, Williams G. Home safety assessment in the prevention of falls among older people. Aust N Z J Public Health. 2000;24:536–9.

38. Salminen MJ, Vahlberg TJ, Salonoja MT, Aarnio PTT, Kivelä SL. Effect of a risk-based multifactorial fall prevention program on the incidence of falls: fall prevention and incidence of falls. J Am Geriatr Soc. 2009;57:612–9.

39. van Bemmel T, Vandenbroucke JP, Westendorp RG, Gussekloo J. In an observational study elderly patients had an increased risk of falling due to home hazards. J Clin Epidemiol. 2005;58:63–7.

40. Karlsson MK, Vonschewelov T, Karlsson C, CÅster M, Rosengen BE. Prevention of falls in the elderly: a review. Scand J Public Health. 2013;41:442–54.

41. Chase CA, Mann K, Wasek S, Arbesman M. Systematic review of the effect of home modification and fall prevention programs on falls and the performance of community-dwelling older adults. Am J Occup Ther. 2012;66:284–91.

42. Arksey H, O'Malley L. Scoping studies: towards a methodological framework. Int J Soc Res Methodol. 2005;8:19–32.

43. Levac D, Colquhoun H, O'Brien KK. Scoping studies: advancing the methodology. Implement Sci. 2010;5:69. https://doi.org/10.1186/1748-5908-5-69.

44. Bamgbade S, Dearmon V. Fall prevention for older adults receiving home healthcare. Home Healthc Now. 2016;34:68–75.

45. Bleijlevens MH, Hendriks MR, Van Haastregt JC, Crebolder HF, Van Eijk JT. Lessons learned from a multidisciplinary fall-prevention programme: the occupational-therapy element. Scand J Occup Ther. 2010;17:319–25.

46. Brotherton SS, Krause JS, Nietert PJ. Falls in individuals with incomplete spinal cord injury. Spinal Cord. 2007;45:37–40.

47. Camilloni L, Farchi S, Rossi PG, Chini F, Di Giorgio M, Molino N, et al. A case-control study on risk factors of domestic accidents in an elderly population. Int J Inj Control Saf Promot. 2011;18:269–76.

48. Campbell AJ. Randomised controlled trial of prevention of falls in people aged >=75 with severe visual impairment: the VIP trial. BMJ. 2005;331:817 https://doi.org/10.1136/bmj.38601.447731.55.

49. Carlsson G, Schilling O, Slaug B, Fänge A, Ståhl A, Nygren C, et al. Toward a screening tool for housing accessibility problems: a reduced version of the housing enabler. J Appl Gerontol. 2009;28:59–80.

50. Carter SE, Campbell EM, Sanson-Fisher RW, Gillespie WJ. Accidents in older people living at home: a community-based study assessing prevalence, type, location and injuries. Aust N Z J Public Health. 2000;24:633–6.

51. Carter SE, Campbell EM, Sanson-Fisher RW, Redman S, Gillespie WJ. Environmental hazards in the homes of older people. Age Ageing. 1997;26:195–202.

52. Cesari M, Landi F, Torre S, Onder G, Lattanzio F, Bernabei R. Prevalence and risk factors for falls in an older community-dwelling population. J Gerontol A Biol Sci Med Sci. 2002;57:M722–6.

53. Chiu T, Oliver R. Factor analysis and construct validity of the SAFER-HOME. OTJR Occup Particip Health. 2006;26:132–42.

54. Chou KL, Chi I. The temporal relationship between falls and fear-of-falling among Chinese older primary-care patients in Hong Kong. Ageing Soc. 2007;27:181–93.

55. Clemson L, Cumming RG, Roland M. Case-control study of hazards in the home and risk of falls and hip fractures. Age Ageing. 1996;25:97–101.

56. Clemson L, Fitzgerald MH, Heard R. Content validity of an assessment tool to identify home fall hazards: the Westmead home safety assessment. Br J Occup Ther. 1999;62:171–9.

57. Clemson L, Fitzgerald MH, Heard R, Cumming RG. Inter-rater reliability of a home fall hazards assessment tool. Occup Ther J Res. 1999;19:83–100.

58. Clemson L, Roland M, Cumming R. Occupational therapy assessment of potential hazards in the homes of elderly people: an inter-rater reliability study. Aust Occup Ther J. 1992;39:23–6.

59. Clemson L, Roland M, Cumming RG. Types of hazards in the homes of elderly people. Occup Ther J Res. 1997;17:200–13.

60. Close J, Ellis M, Hooper R, Glucksman E, Jackson S, Swift C. Prevention of falls in the elderly trial (PROFET): a randomised controlled trial. Lancet Lond Engl. 1999;353:93–7.

61. Close JC, Wesson J, Sherrington C, Hill KD, Kurrle S, Lord SR, et al. Can a tailored exercise and home hazard reduction program reduce the rate of falls in community dwelling older people with cognitive impairment: protocol paper for the i-FOCIS randomised controlled trial. BMC Geriatr. 2014;14:89. https://doi.org/10.1186/1471-2318-14-89.

62. Daniel N, Oesch P, Stuck A, Born S, Bachmann S, Schoenenberger A. Evaluation of a novel photography-based home assessment protocol for identification of environmental risk factors for falls in elderly persons. Swiss Med Wkly. 2013. https://doi.org/10.4414/smw.2013.13884.

63. Edwards N, Birkett N, Nair R, Murphy M, Roberge G, Lockett D. Access to bathtub grab bars: evidence of a policy gap. Can J Aging/Rev Can Vieil. 2006;25:295–304.

64. Diener DD, Mitchell JM. Impact of a multifactorial fall prevention program upon falls of older frail adults attending an adult health day care center. Top Geriatr Rehabil. 2005;21:247–57.

65. Edwards N, Lockett D, Aminzadeh F, Nair RC. Predictors of bath grab-bar use among community-living older adults. Can J Aging/Rev Can Vieil. 2003; 22:217–27.

66. Edwards NI, Jones DA. Ownership and use of assistive devices amongst older people in the community. Age Ageing. 1998;27:463–8.

67. El-Faizy M, Reinsch S. Home safety intervention for the prevention of falls. Phys Occup Ther Geriatr. 1994;12:33–49.

68. Elley CR, Robertson MC, Kerse NM, Garrett S, McKinlay E, Lawton B, et al. Falls assessment clinical trial (FACT): design, interventions, recruitment strategies and participant characteristics. BMC Public Health. 2007;7. https://doi.org/10.1186/1471-2458-7-185.

69. Evci ED, Ergin F, Beser E. Home accidents in the elderly in Turkey. Tohoku J Exp Med. 2006;209:291–301.

70. Faul AC, Yankeelov PA, Rowan NL, Gillette P, Nicholas LD, Borders KW, et al. Impact of geriatric assessment and self-management support on community-dwelling older adults with chronic illnesses. J Gerontol Soc Work. 2009;52:230–49.

71. Fisher GS, Baker A, Koval D, Lishok C, Maisto E. A field test of the cougar home safety assessment (version 2.0) in the homes of older persons living alone. Aust Occup Ther J. 2007;54:124–30.

72. Fisher GS, Coolbaugh K, Rhodes C. A field-test of the cougar home safety assessment for older persons: version 1.0. Californian J Health Promot. 2006;4:181–96.

73. Fitzharris MP, Day L, Lord SR, Gordon I, Fildes B. The Whitehorse NoFalls trial: effects on fall rates and injurious fall rates. Age Ageing. 2010;39:728–33.

74. Fletcher PC, Hirdes JP. Risk factors for falling among community-based seniors using home care services. J Gerontol A Biol Sci Med Sci. 2002;57:M504–10.

75. Gershon RR, Dailey M, Magda LA, Riley HE, Conolly J, Silver A. Safety in the home healthcare sector: development of a new household safety checklist. J Patient Saf. 2012;8:51–9.

76. Gill TM, Robison JT, Williams CS, Tinetti ME. Mismatches between the home environment and physical capabilities among community-living older persons. J Am Geriatr Soc. 1999;47:88–92.

77. Gitlin LN, Winter L, Dennis MP, Corcoran M, Schinfeld S, Hauck WW. A randomized trial of a multicomponent home intervention to reduce functional difficulties in older adults. J Am Geriatr Soc. 2006;54:809–16.

78. Gitlin LN, Hodgson N, Piersol CV, Hess E, Hauck WW. Correlates of quality of life for individuals with dementia living at home: the role of home environment, caregiver, and patient-related characteristics. Am J Geriatr Psychiatry. 2014;22:587–97.

79. Greene D, Sample P, Fruhauf C. Fall-prevention pilot: Hazard survey and responses to recommendations. Occup Ther Health Care. 2009;23:24–39.

80. Helle T, Nygren C, Slaug B, Brandt A, Pikkarainen A, Hansen A-G, et al. The Nordic housing enabler: inter-rater reliability in cross-Nordic occupational therapy practice. Scand J Occup Ther. 2010;17:258–66.

81. Huang TT, Acton GJ. Effectiveness of home visit falls prevention strategy for Taiwanese community-dwelling elders: randomized trial. Public Health Nurs Boston Mass. 2004;21:247–56.

82. Isberner F, Ritzel D, Sarvela P, Brown K, Hu P, Newbolds D. Falls of elderly rural home health clients. Home Health Care Serv Q. 1998;17:41–51.

83. Iwarsson S, Horstmann V, Carlsson G, Oswald F, Wahl H-W. Person—environment fit predicts falls in older adults better than the consideration of environmental hazards only. Clin Rehabil. 2009;23:558–67.

84. Iwarsson S, Nygren C, Slaug B. Cross-national and multi-professional inter-rater reliability of the housing enabler. Scand J Occup Ther. 2005;12:29–39.

85. Iwarsson S, Slaug B, Fänge AM. The housing enabler screening tool: feasibility and interrater agreement in a real estate company practice context. J Appl Gerontol. 2012;31:641–60.

86. Johnson M, Cusick A, Chang S. Home-screen: a short scale to measure fall risk in the home. Public Health Nurs Boston Mass. 2001;18:169–77.

87. Kamei T, Kajii F, Yamamoto Y, Irie Y, Kozakai R, Sugimoto T, et al. Effectiveness of a home hazard modification program for reducing falls in urban community-dwelling older adults: a randomized controlled trial. Jpn J Nurs Sci. 2015;12:184–97.

88. Kampe K, Kohler M, Albrecht D, Becker C, Hautzinger M, Lindemann U, et al. Hip and pelvic fracture patients with fear of falling: development and description of the "step by step" treatment protocol. Clin Rehabil. 2017;31:571–81.

89. Keall MD, Howden-Chapman P, Baker MG, Kamalesh V, Cunningham M, Cunningham C, et al. Formulating a programme of repairs to structural home injury hazards in New Zealand. Accid Anal Prev. 2013 Aug;57:124–30.

90. Keall MD, Baker M, Howden-Chapman P, Cunningham M. Association between the number of home injury hazards and home injury. Accid Anal Prev. 2008;40:887–93.

91. Kittipimpanon K, Amnatsatsue K, Kerdmongkol P, Maruo SJ, Nityasuddhi D. Development and evaluation of a community-based fall prevention program for elderly Thais. Pac Rim Int J Nurs Res. 2012;16:222–35.

92. Lamontagne I, Lévesque B, Gingras S, Maurice P, Verreault R. Dangers environmentaux de chute dans des habitations à loyer modique pour personnes âgées [Environmental hazards for falls in elders in low income housing]. Rev Epidemiol Sante Publique. 2004;52:19–27.

93. Larsen ER, Mosekilde L, Foldspang A. Correlates of falling during 24 h among elderly Danish community residents. Prev Med. 2004;39:389–98.

94. Leclerc BS, Begin C, Cadieux E, Goulet L, Leduc N, Kergoat MJ, et al. Risk factors for falling among community-dwelling seniors using home-care services: an extended hazards model with time-dependent covariates and multiple events. Chronic Dis Can. 2008;28:111–20.

95. Leclerc BS, Bégin C, Cadieux E, Goulet L, Allaire J-F, Meloche J, et al. A classification and regression tree for predicting recurrent falling among community-dwelling seniors using home-care services. Can J Public Health Rev Can Sante Publique. 2009;100:263–7.

96. Lee HC, Chang KC, Tsauo JY, Hung JW, Huang YC, Lin SI, et al. Effects of a multifactorial fall prevention program on fall incidence and physical function in community-dwelling older adults with risk of falls. Arch Phys Med Rehabil. 2013;94:606–15.

97. Letts L, Marshall L. Evaluating the validity and consistency of the SAFER tool. Phys Occup Ther Geriatr. 1996;13:49–66.

98. Letts L, Scott S, Burtney J, Marshall L, McKean M. The reliability and validity of the safety assessment of function and the environment for rehabilitation (SAFER tool). Br J Occup Ther. 1998;61:127–32.

99. Leung A, Chi I, Lou VWQ, Chan KS. Psychosocial risk factors associated with falls among Chinese community-dwelling older adults in Hong Kong. Health Soc Care Community. 2010;18:272–81.

100. Lowery K, Buri H, Ballard C. What is the prevalence of environmental hazards in the homes of dementia sufferers and are they associated with falls. Int J Geriatr Psychiatry. 2000;15:883–6.

101. Lawton K, Laybourne AH, Whiting DG, Martin FC. Can fire and rescue services and the National Health Service work together to improve the safety and wellbeing of vulnerable older people? Design of a proof of concept study BMC Health Serv Res. 2010;10:327. https://doi.org/10.1186/1472-6963-10-327.

102. Mackenzie L, Byles J, Higginbotham N. Designing the home falls and accidents screening tool (HOME FAST): selecting the items. Br J Occup Ther. 2000;63:260–9.

103. Mackenzie L, Byles J, Higginbotham N. Reliability of the home falls and accidents screening tool (HOME FAST) for identifying older people at increased risk of falls. Disabil Rehabil. 2002;24:266–74.

104. Mahoney JE, Shea TA, Przybelski R, Jaros L, Gangnon R, Cech S, et al. Kenosha county falls prevention study: a randomized, controlled trial of an intermediate-intensity, community-based multifactorial falls intervention: multifactorial falls intervention. J Am Geriatr Soc. 2007;55:489–98.

105. Mann WC, Hurren D, Tomita M, Bengali M, Steinfeld E. Environmental problems in homes of elders with disabilities. Occup Ther J Res. 1994;14:191–211.

106. Markle-Reid M, Browne G, Gafni A, Roberts J, Weir R, Thabane L, et al. A cross-sectional study of the prevalence, correlates, and costs of falls in older home care clients "at risk" for falling. Can J Aging Rev Can Vieil. 2010;29:119–37.

107. Marquardt G, Johnston D, Black BS, Morrison A, Rosenblatt A, Lyketsos CG, et al. A descriptive study of home modifications for people with dementia and barriers to implementation. J Hous Elder. 2011;25:258–73.

108. Marshall SW, Runyan CW, Yang J, Coyne-Beasley T, Waller AE, Johnson RM, et al. Prevalence of selected risk and protective factors for falls in the home. Am J Prev Med. 2005;28:95–101.

109. Matchar DB, Duncan PW, Lien CT, Ong MEH, Lee M, Gao F, et al. Randomized controlled trial of screening, risk modification, and physical therapy to prevent falls among the elderly recently discharged from the emergency department to the community: the steps to avoid falls in the elderly study. Arch Phys Med Rehabil. 2017;98:1086–96.

110. Mehraban AH, Mackenzie LA, Byles JE. A self-report home environment screening tool identified older women at risk of falls. J Clin Epidemiol. 2011;64:191–9.

111. Morgan R, Devito C, Stevens J, Branche C, Virnig B, Wingo P, et al. A self-assessment tool was reliable in identifying hazards in the homes of elders. J Clin Epidemiol. 2005;58(12):1252–9.

112. Morris JN, Fries BE, Steel K, Ikegami N, Bernabei R, Carpenter GI, et al. Comprehensive clinical assessment in community setting: applicability of the MDS-HC. J Am Geriatr Soc. 1997;45:1017–24.

113. Nikolaus T, Bach M. Preventing falls in community-dwelling frail older people using a home intervention team (HIT): results from the randomized falls-HIT trial. J Am Geriatr Soc. 2003;51:300–5. https://doi.org/10.1046/j.1532-5415.2003.51102.x.

114. Northridge ME, Nevitt MC, Kelsey JL. Non-syncopal falls in the elderly in relation to home environments. Osteoporos Int. 1996;6:249–55.

115. Northridge ME, Nevitt MC, Kelsey JL, Link B. Home hazards and falls in the elderly: the role of health and functional status. Am J Public Health. 1995;85:509–15.

116. Oliver R, Blathwayt J, Brackley C, Tamaki T. Development of the safety assessment of function and the environment for rehabilitation (SAFER) tool. Can J Occup Ther Rev Can Ergother. 1993;60:78–82.

117. Pereira CL, Baptista F, Infante P. Role of physical activity in the occurrence of falls and fall-related injuries in community-dwelling adults over 50 years old. Disabil Rehabil. 2014;36:117–24.

118. Rantakokko M, Törmäkangas T, Rantanen T, Haak M, Iwarsson S. Environmental barriers, person-environment fit and mortality among community-dwelling very old people. BMC Public Health. 2013;13. https://doi.org/10.1186/1471-2458-13-783.

119. Renfro MO, Fehrer S. Multifactorial screening for fall risk in community-dwelling older adults in the primary care office: development of the fall risk assessment & screening tool. J Geriatr Phys Ther. 2011;34:174–83.

120. Ritchey KC, Meyer D, Ice GH. Non-therapist identification of falling hazards in older adult homes using digital photography. Prev Med Rep. 2015;2:794–7.

121. Rodriguez JG, Baughman AL, Sattin RW, de Vito CA, Ragland DL, Bacchelli S, et al. A standardized instrument to assess hazards for falls in the home of older persons. Accid Anal Prev. 1995;27:625–31.

122. Romli MH, Mackenzie L, Lovarini M, Tan MP, Clemson L. The interrater and test-retest reliability of the home falls and accidents screening tool (HOME FAST) in Malaysia: using raters with a range of professional backgrounds. J Eval Clin Pract. 2017;23:662–9.

123. Russell MA, Hill KD, Blackberry I, Day LL, Dharmage SC. Falls risk and functional decline in older fallers discharged directly from emergency departments. J Gerontol A Biol Sci Med Sci. 2006;61:1090–5.

124. Sadasivam RS, Luger TM, Coley HL, Taylor BB, Padir T, Ritchie CS, et al. Robot-assisted home hazard assessment for fall prevention: a feasibility study. J Telemed Telecare. 2014;20:3–10.

125. Salkeld G, Cumming RG, O'Neill E, Thomas M, Szonyi G, Westbury C. Cost effectiveness of a home hazard reduction program to reduce falls among older persons. Aust N Z J Public Health. 2000;24:265–71.

126. Lim YM, Sung MH. Home environmental and health-related factors among home fallers and recurrent fallers in community dwelling older Korean women: falls in Korean older women. Int J Nurs Pract. 2012;18:481–8.

127. Scharlach AE, Graham CL, Berridge C. An integrated model of co-ordinated community-based care. Gerontologist. 2015;55:677–87.

128. Schwarz DF, Grisso JA, Miles C, Holmes JH, Sutton RL. An injury prevention program in an urban African-American community. Am J Public Health. 1993;83:675–80.

129. Shaw FE, Bond J, Richardson DA, Dawson P, Steen IN, McKeith IG, et al. Multifactorial intervention after a fall in older people with cognitive impairment and dementia presenting to the accident and emergency department: randomised controlled trial. BMJ. 2003;326:73 https://doi.org/10.1136/bmj.326.7380.73.

130. Sheffield C, Smith CA, Becker M. Evaluation of an agency-based occupational therapy intervention to facilitate aging in place. Gerontologist Gerontologist. 2013;53:907–18.

131. Sjosten NM, Salonoja M, Piirtola M, Vahlberg T, Isoaho R, Hyttinen H, et al. A multifactorial fall prevention programme in home-dwelling elderly people: a randomized-controlled trial. Public Health. 2007;121:308–18.

132. Sophonratanapokin B, Sawangdee Y, Soonthorndhada K. Effect of the living environment on falls among the elderly in Thailand. Southeast Asian J Trop Med Public Health. 2012;43:1537–47.

133. Sorcinelli A, Shaw L, Freeman A, Cooper K. Evaluating the safe living guide: a home hazard checklist for seniors. Can J Aging/Rev Can Vieil. 2007;26:127–37.

134. Staeger P, Burnand B, Santos-Eggimann B, Klay M, Siffert C, Livio JJ, et al. Prevention of recurrent hip fracture. Aging Clin Exp Res. 2000;12:13–21.

135. Stalenhoef P, Diederiks J, Knottnerus A, Witte LD, Crebolder H. How predictive is a home-safety checklist for indoor fall risk for the elderly living in the community? Eur J Gen Pract. 1998;4:114–20.

136. Stark S, Somerville E, Keglovits M, Conte J, Li M, Hu YL, et al. Protocol for the home hazards removal program (HARP) study: a pragmatic, randomized clinical trial and implementation study. BMC Geriatr. 2017;17:90. https://doi.org/10.1186/s12877-017-0478-4.

137. Stevens M, Holman CD, Bennett N. Preventing falls in older people: impact of an intervention to reduce environmental hazards in the home. J Am Geriatr Soc. 2001;49:1442–7.

138. Stevens M, Holman CD, Bennett N, de Klerk N. Preventing falls in older people: outcome evaluation of a randomized controlled trial. J Am Geriatr Soc. 2001;49:1448–55.

139. The prevention of falls in later life. A report of the Kellogg International Work Group on the Prevention of Falls by the Elderly. Dan Med Bull. 1987; 34(Suppl 4):1–24.

140. Tideiksaar R. Fall prevention in the home. Top Geriatr Rehabil. 1987;3:57–64.

141. Trader SE, Newton RA, Cromwell RL. Balance abilities of homebound older adults classified as fallers and nonfallers. J Geriatr Phys Ther. 2003;26:3–8.

142. Tynan C, Cardea JM. Home health hazard assessment. J Gerontol Nurs. 1987; 13:25–8.

143. van Haastregt JCM, van Rossum E, Diederiks JPM, Voorhoeve PM, de Witte LP, Crebolder HFJM. Preventing falls and mobility problems in community-dwelling elders: the process of creating a new intervention. Geriatr Nur. 2000;21:309–14.

144. Vladutiu CJ, Casteel C, Marshall SW, McGee KS, Runyan CW, Coyne-Beasley T. Disability and home hazards and safety practices in US households. Disabil Health J. 2012;5:49–54.

145. Wesson J, Clemson L, Brodaty H, Lord S, Taylor M, Gitlin L, et al. A feasibility study and pilot randomised trial of a tailored prevention program to reduce falls in older people with mild dementia. BMC Geriatr. 2013;13:89.

146. Yates SM, Dunnagan TA. Evaluating the effectiveness of a home-based fall risk reduction program for rural community-dwelling older adults. J Gerontol A Biol Sci Med Sci. 2001;56:M226–30.

147. Yoo IY. Recurrent falls among community-dwelling older Koreans: prevalence and multivariate risk factors. J Gerontol Nurs. 2011;37:28–40.

148. Centers for Disease Control and Prevention. Check for safety: A home fall prevention checklist for older adults. 2005 https://www.cdc.gov/steadi/pdf/check_for_safety_brochure-a.pdf .

149. Iwarsson S, Björn S. Environmental component, the complete housing enabler instrument. 2010. http://www.enabler.nu/Environmental_component.pdf. Accessed 14 Nov 2017.

150. Keall M, Baker M, Howden-Chapman P, Cunningham M, Cunningham C. Healthy housing index pilot study. Final report.2007. Wellington, New Zeland: He Kainga Oranga / Housing and Health Research Programme, Department of Public Health, University of Otago; 2006.

151. Public Health Agency of Canada. The Safe Living Guide—A guide to home safety for seniors. Ottawa: Public Health Agency of Canada; 2015.

152. Zhang L, Yan T, You L, Li K, Gao Y. Social isolation and physical barriers in the houses of stroke survivors in rural China. Arch Phys Med Rehabil. 2016;97:2054–60.

153. Hsieh H-F, Shannon SE. Three approaches to qualitative content analysis. Qual Health Res. 2005;15:1277–88.

154. Iwarsson S. The housing enabler: an objective tool for assessing accessibility. Br J Occup Ther. 1999;62:491–7.

155. Gitlin LN. Conducting research on home environments: lessons learned and new directions. Gerontologist. 2003;43:628–37.

156. Wahl HW, Fange A, Oswald F, Gitlin LN, Iwarsson S. The home environment and disability-related outcomes in aging individuals: what is the empirical evidence? Gerontologist. 2009;49:355–67.

157. Nygren C, Oswald F, Iwarsson S, Fänge A, Sixsmith J, Schilling O, et al. Relationships between objective and perceived housing in very old age. Gerontologist. 2007;47:85–95.

158. Edwards NC. Preventing falls among seniors: the way forward. J Saf Res. 2011;42:537–41.

159. Edwards N. Chapter 15: knowledge translation for intersectoral action: the case of Canada's building codes. In: Bourgeault IL, Labonte R, Packer C, Runnels V, editors. Population health in Canada: issues, research, and action. Toronto: Canada Scholars Press; 2017. p. 156–60.

160. Monson AZ, Pauls J, Leverett M. Applying the regulatory powers of public health. J Law Med Ethics. 2003;31(4 Suppl):68–9.

# 22

# Home and community-based services coordination for homebound older adults in home-based primary care

Gregory J. Norman*, Amy J. Wade, Andrea M. Morris and Jill C. Slaboda

## Abstract

**Background:** Medically complex vulnerable older adults often face social challenges that affect compliance with their medical care plans, and thus require home and community-based services (HCBS). This study describes how non-medical social needs of homebound older adults are assessed and addressed within home-based primary care (HBPC) practices, and to identify barriers to coordinating HCBS for patients.

**Methods:** An online survey of members of the American Academy of Home Care Medicine (AAHCM) was conducted between March through November 2016 in the United States. A 56-item survey was developed to assess HBPC practice characteristics and how practices identify social needs and coordinate and evaluate HCBS. Data from 101 of the 150 surveys received were included in the analyses. Forty-four percent of respondents were physicians, 24% were nurse practitioners, and 32% were administrators or other HBPC team members.

**Results:** Nearly all practices (98%) assessed patient social needs, with 78% conducting an assessment during the intake visit, and 88% providing ongoing periodic assessments. Seventy-four percent indicated 'most' or 'all' of their patients needed HCBS in the past 12 months. The most common needs were personal care (84%) and medication adherence (40%), and caregiver support (38%). Of the 86% of practices reporting they coordinate HCBS, 91% followed-up with patients, 84% assisted with applications, and 83% made service referrals. Fifty-seven percent reported that coordination was 'difficult.' The most common barriers to coordinating HCBS included cost to patient (65%), and eligibility requirements (63%). Four of the five most frequently reported barriers were associated with practices reporting it was 'difficult' or 'very difficult' to coordinate HCBS (OR from 2.49 to 3.94, p-values < .05).

**Conclusions:** Despite the barriers to addressing non-medical social needs, most HBPC practices provided some level of coordination of HCBS for their high-need, high-cost homebound patients. More efforts are needed to implement and scale care model partnerships between medical and non-medical service providers within HBPC practices.

**Keywords:** Home-based primary care, Community-based services, Care coordination, Homebound

## Background

Approximately two million older adults aged 65 and older in the United States meet the criteria for being homebound [1, 2]. Homebound older adults have great difficulty living in their home independently, have high-levels of frailty and physical disability, and often have cognitive, behavioral, and psychiatric impairments [3, 4]. Without regular access to primary preventative care, they resort to high emergency department and

hospital use as a way of coping with fluctuations in their physical health [5, 6]. Homebound older adults respond well to routine medical care provided in their home, known as home-based primary care (HBPC), because it is effective at keeping patients medically stable, preventing hospitalization, and reducing medical spending [5–9].

HBPC is a multidisciplinary team-based approach to providing longitudinal in-home medical care to high-need high-cost patients with limited mobility. It has been shown to be a care model that reduces costs per patient while maintaining quality of care as well as patient and provider satisfaction compared to usual care [10–12]. A

* Correspondence: gjnorman@westhealth.org
West Health Institute, 10350 North Torrey Pines Road, La Jolla, CA 92037, USA

major advantage of long-term care provided in the home is that it enables the physician to evaluate the patient's home environment, and be responsive to changes in health status, patient goals, and family caregiving capacity [13]. Unfortunately, of the 2 to 4 million people in the U.S. who are homebound only about one quarter receives medical care at home [2].

Many HBPC practices in the U.S. are provider-led by a physician or nurse practitioner. The practice may also include a registered nurse, and medical assistants who support providers by triaging patients, assisting with patient intakes, and handling medication refills [11, 14]. Larger practices may employ administrative coordinators who provide scheduling, billing, procurement of supplies, and other administrative tasks; social workers who focus on the patient's home environment and link patients to community supports and services; medical coders and billers; and transition nurses who facilitate the patient transfer from the hospital to the HBPC practice [3].

In addition to being medically complex, homebound older adults often have a variety of non-medical health-related social needs (also referred to as social determinants of health) that include: housing, transportation, nutrition, social support, and assistance with activities of daily living. There is evidence to suggest that unmet social needs significantly impact health outcomes, increase healthcare utilization and costs [15–18]. As a result, comprehensive HBPC must consider the full spectrum of patient needs, both medical and non-medical, to better support this complex population and enable homebound older adults to age in place [19–21]. Non-medical home and community-based services (HCBS) can allow older adults to remain in their homes and avoid long-term care facilities, a goal that is shared with HBPC providers and their patients [22]. Assessing and addressing these non-medical social needs requires coordination between medical providers and HCBS providers. However, there is a gap in understanding how HBPC practices coordinate with HCBS providers to meet patients' unmet social needs. Specifically, more information is needed about how nonmedical services are requested, to what extent there is ongoing coordination with HCBS providers, and what factors are assessed related to patient eligibility for services.

Care management models have been developed that include coordination of medical and non-medical patient needs [5, 15, 19, 20, 23], but these models have not been widely adopted by primary care in the U.S [21]. These models typically include staff resources to conduct assessments, identify community resources/partners, and define communication pathways that can include electronic or verbal [15]. For example, a health plan and a local Area Agency on Aging (AAA) in Arizona partnered to assess for social determinants of health with

high-risk, dually-enrolled Medicaid/Medicare patients living in their home and provided connections to the appropriate community services under AAA contract, conducted ongoing assessments, and shared information between AAA and the health plan [19].

Several barriers exist to connecting high-risk older adults with the HCBS services they need, many of which apply to HBPC practices. An estimated 70% of older adults in the U.S. will need HCBS at some point [24]. While many older adults want to learn about HCBS, they often lack knowledge of the available services in their area, how to secure them, or how to pay for them [24, 25]. Similarly, medical providers may not know or understand how to refer and coordinate HCBS services [25, 26]. Demand for HCBS services may be greater than the availability of services within the community [27]. Finally, a recognized significant barrier is paying for HCBS [5, 27]. In the U.S. HCBS are covered by state government Medicaid, however not all older adults who need services will meet Medicaid's eligibility requirements, forcing individuals to pay from their personal funds [28]. Often, older adults must spend down their savings before they are eligible for Medicaid coverage [27].

Based on models such as the Chronic Care Model [29], which postulates effective care for patients with multiple chronic conditions requires systems of coordinated medical and social services, we aimed to better understand non-medical care coordination for HCBS within HBPC practices. We surveyed HBPC practices in the U.S. to learn the extent social needs of patients are assessed and coordinated, and to determine the most salient barriers HBPC providers encounter in the coordination process, and if those barriers impact the frequency of coordination for the practices. While this is mainly a descriptive study, we hypothesized barriers to non-medical care coordination would be positively associated with difficulty and frequency of coordination among HBPC providers.

## Methods

Development of the survey instrument was informed by reviewing the relevant literature and by a previous survey of members of the American Academy of Home Care Medicine (AAHCM) [3]. Additional questions were developed collaboratively through an iterative process with project team members. The final version of the survey contained 56 questions and was divided into four sections: 1.) Identifying and Assessing Non-Medical Social Needs (14 questions); 2.) Coordinating and Evaluating Home and Community-based Services (10 questions); 3.) Oral Health Care Needs (11 questions); and 4.) Practice Characteristics (21 questions). Oral health questions were not included in this analysis. Non-medical social needs were defined to include: transportation, home-delivered meals, food preparation, personal care (e.g., bathing, toileting, etc.), housekeeping, housing assistance, home modifications and/or repairs, caregiver supports and/or training, financial advice, legal advice, case management, and medication adherence.

A link to the online survey was posted in the AAHCM electronic newsletter and was available to all AAHCM members over an eight-month period (March to November 2016). The survey was administered using Survey-Gizmo software (www.surveygizmo.com). Two reminders were sent to AAHCM members to encourage participation. Western Institutional Review Board reviewed and approved exemption status for this study.

## Analysis

The unit of analysis was the individual HBPC practice site. For multi-site house calls practices, respondents were asked to provide information about the specific practice site where they provided services. For cases where more than one response was received from a multi-site practice, responses were cross-checked by IP address and responder role within the practice to ensure that the response was not a duplication.

Data were analyzed using SAS Studio Release: 3.6 (SAS Institute Inc., Cary, NC, USA). Descriptive statistics were assessed for HBPC practice characteristics, including practice size and location, number of practice sites and settings, funding structure, and profit status. Descriptive statistics were also used to describe how HBPC practices addressed social needs, including whether HBPC providers assessed patients for social needs, and the extent they coordinated social needs as part of their HBPC practice model.

Using univariate logistic regression models, we analyzed associations between the five most common barriers to coordinating HCBS (availability of local service providers; eligibility requirements; insurance coverage; cost to patient; time delays) and three dependent variables: 'Does your practice coordinate HCBS?'; 'How difficult is it to coordinate HCBS?'; and of the practices that coordinate HCBS, 'How often does the practice coordinate HCBS?' (often/always vs. never, rarely, sometimes). A logistic regression model was also used to regress the three dependent variables on the number of barriers (0 to 5) to coordination reported.

## Results
### Survey respondents

A total of 150 responses to the survey were submitted online. Of the 150, eight surveys were not eligible for inclusion (respondents were not part of a HBPC practice). An additional 41 surveys were excluded due to insufficient data for analyses. The final analytic sample consisted of 101 surveys. All respondents were part of a HBPC practice located in the United States. Forty-four

percent of respondents were physicians, 24% were nurse practitioners, and 32% were administrators or other HBPC team members.

### Practice characteristics

Nearly all practices (86%) reported that 75–100% of their patients were ages 65 and older, and 26 practices (26%) indicated their entire patient population was 65 or older. Table 1 presents characteristics of the HBPC. A majority of practices (58%) were in the Northeast or the Midwest regions of the U.S. and most practices operated in urban and suburban settings. Only 13% of practices operated in rural areas. This geographical distribution of practices is comparable to a previous survey of AAHCM members [3]. Practices tended (56%) to operate independently. Most practices (63%) reported a patient census of more than 500 and consisted of a single site (74%). Group practices (68%) predominated over solo practices (32%).

Most practices (77%) reported receiving funding for HCBS through insurance reimbursement (Medicaid, Medicare Advantage); 22% reported self-pay patients; and 19% received subsidized funding from philanthropy or through a hospital or health system. Seventy-four percent of practices indicated that their dually enrolled (Medicare and Medicaid covered) patients constituted less than 50% of their practice. The most common methods of payment for HCBS was through Medicaid (40%) and self-payment from the patient (20%). Most of practices were for-profit (61%), and most practices (78%) provided services for patients with primary Medicare Managed Care.

### Assessing and addressing social needs

Table 2 presents practice operations around assessing patients' non-medical social needs. Nearly all HBPC practices (98%) assessed patient needs for HCBS. Seventy-eight percent provide an assessment during the intake visit, 88% provide ongoing periodic assessments, and 88% document this in the patient care plan. Referrals for HCBS were typically initiated by the healthcare provider (64%) and caregivers (12%). Seventy-four percent of providers noted that 'most' or 'all' of their patients needed HCBS in the past 12 months. The most common service needs were personal care (84%) and medication adherence (40%).

Table 3 describes current practices for coordinating and evaluating HCBS. Eighty-six percent of practices reported they coordinate HCBS for their patients, and of those who do, 85% do so 'often' or 'always.' Of these practices, the most common coordination activities were following up with patients (91%), assisting with applications (84%), and service referrals (83%). Forty-eight percent of practices had nurse practitioners provide HCBS coordination. Nearly all practices that coordinate HCBS

**Table 1** Characteristics of Home-based Primary Care Practices

| Survey Question | N | N% |
|---|---|---|
| What region of the United States is your practice located? | | |
| Northeast | 27 | 30% |
| Midwest | 25 | 28% |
| Southwest | 14 | 16% |
| Southeast | 13 | 15% |
| West | 12 | 14% |
| Primary sponsor/ owner of the practice? | | |
| Independent Provider (MD, NP, PA) / Provider Group | 50 | 56% |
| Hospital or Health System | 22 | 24% |
| Other | 7 | 8% |
| Home Health Care Company | 4 | 4% |
| Government Organization | 4 | 4% |
| Independent Investor Group | 3 | 3% |
| Total practice census | | |
| < 500 Patients | 56 | 63% |
| ≥ 500 Patients | 33 | 37% |
| Number of sites that your practice operates | | |
| 1 | 74 | 74% |
| 2+ | 26 | 26% |
| Predominant practice setting | | |
| Urban | 44 | 44% |
| Suburban/Rural | 41 | 41% |
| ≥ 2 Settings | 16 | 16% |
| Practice Type | | |
| Group or Other | 61 | 68% |
| Solo | 29 | 32% |
| Practice funding structure/revenue model *(Select all that apply)* | | |
| Insurance Reimbursement (Medicare, Medicaid, private insurers) | 78 | 77% |
| Self-pay | 22 | 22% |
| Subsidized (hospital, health system, or philanthropy) | 19 | 19% |
| Percentage of patients dually enrolled in both Medicare and Medicaid | | |
| < 50% | 61 | 74% |
| ≥ 50% | 21 | 26% |
| How are HCBS for your patients typically paid for? | | |
| Medicaid | 40 | 40% |
| Self-pay | 20 | 20% |
| Profit status of HBPC your practice | | |
| For profit | 54 | 61% |
| Not-for-profit | 34 | 39% |
| Does HBPC practice provide services for patients with primary Medicare Managed Care? | | |
| Yes | 69 | 78% |
| No | 20 | 22% |

**Table 2** Practice Operations: Identifying and Assessing Social Needs

| Survey Question | N | N% |
|---|---|---|
| Does your practice assess patient needs for HCBS? | | |
| Yes | 98 | 98% |
| No | 1 | 1% |
| Unknown | 1 | 1% |
| How are patient needs for HCBS assessed? *(Select all that apply)* | | |
| Periodic ongoing reassessments | 86 | 88% |
| Initial intake assessment | 76 | 78% |
| Other | 12 | 12% |
| Are HCBS needs documented in the care plan? | | |
| Yes | 86 | 88% |
| No | 9 | 9% |
| Unknown | 3 | 3% |
| What typically initiates a referral for HCBS? | | |
| Healthcare provider recommendation / observation | 63 | 64% |
| Caregiver request | 12 | 12% |
| Social worker recommendation / observation | 8 | 8% |
| Patient request | 6 | 6% |
| Other | 9 | 9% |
| How many of your patients or caregivers had HCBS needs (past 12 months) | | |
| Most/All | 73 | 74% |
| None/Few/Some | 25 | 26% |
| What were the most common service needs? *(Select all that apply)* (Top 5 listed) | | |
| Personal care (e.g., bathing, toileting, etc.) | 82 | 84% |
| Medication adherence | 39 | 40% |
| Caregiver supports / training | 37 | 38% |
| Case management | 35 | 36% |
| Transportation | 31 | 32% |

connect with multiple service providers or agencies (92%). HCBS agencies were usually characterized as local community service agencies (72%), and individual HCBS providers (70%). Word of mouth from patients (44%) was the most common way of determining the quality of an HBCS provider. Only 8% assessed quality through other agencies such as AAAs, and only 1% used the internet.

Table 4 shows across all practices, 57% reported that coordination was 'difficult' or 'very difficult.' The most common barriers to coordinating HCBS included cost to patient (65%), and eligibility requirements (63%). When asked what would make coordination of services easier, no clear answer emerged. The top two answers included a point person in the practice to coordinate services for every patient (27%), and a local service that could handle

**Table 3** Practice Operations: Coordinating and Evaluating HCBS

| Survey Question | N | N% |
|---|---|---|
| Does your practice coordinate HCBS for your patients? | | |
| Yes | 87 | 86% |
| No | 14 | 14% |
| How often does the practice coordinate HCBS?[a] | | |
| Often/Always | 73 | 85% |
| Rarely/Sometimes | 13 | 15% |
| What level of coordination is provided? *(Select all that apply)*[a] | | |
| Follow up with patients and caregivers | 79 | 91% |
| Assistance completing applications | 73 | 84% |
| Make service referrals | 72 | 83% |
| Determine eligibility for services | 61 | 70% |
| Follow up with community service providers | 55 | 63% |
| Identify services | 46 | 53% |
| Assess service needs on an ongoing basis | 34 | 39% |
| Who in the practice is responsible for coordinating HCBS needs for patients (or caregivers)? *(Select all that apply)*[a] | | |
| Nurse Practitioner | 41 | 48% |
| Physician | 33 | 38% |
| Social Worker | 25 | 29% |
| Case Manager | 21 | 24% |
| Does the practice coordinate patient HCBS with one or more community service providers/agencies?[a] | | |
| Yes, with more than one | 79 | 92% |
| Yes, with one community service provider/agency | 6 | 7% |
| No | 1 | 2% |
| What types of organizations do you coordinate services with? *(Select all that apply)*[a] | | |
| Local community service agencies (e.g., AAA, ADRC) | 62 | 72% |
| Individual HCBS providers | 60 | 70% |
| Hospital systems | 45 | 52% |
| Senior centers | 44 | 51% |
| When making a referral, how do you primarily determine the quality of HCBS providers/agencies?[a] | | |
| Word of mouth from patient | 38 | 44% |
| Other | 18 | 21% |
| Report from service provider | 16 | 19% |
| AAA, ADRC | 7 | 8% |
| Internet | 1 | 1% |

Note. [a] Question asked only of respondents who replied, "Yes" to "Does your practice coordinate home and community-based services?"

**Table 4** Barriers and Potential Solutions to Coordinating HCBS

| Survey Question | N | N% |
|---|---|---|
| How difficult is it to coordinate HCBS for your patients? | | |
| Difficult/Very Difficult | 56 | 57% |
| Neutral/Easy/Very Easy | 42 | 43% |
| Top barriers to coordinating HCBS for patients/caregivers *(Select all that apply)* | | |
| Cost to patient | 66 | 65% |
| Eligibility requirements | 64 | 63% |
| Insurance coverage | 61 | 60% |
| Availability of local service providers | 40 | 40% |
| Time delays | 40 | 40% |
| What do you think would make the coordination of HCBS easier? *(Select all that apply)* | | |
| A point person in the practice to coordinate services for every patient | 27 | 27% |
| A local service that could handle everything | 24 | 24% |
| Other | 16 | 16% |
| More knowledge of local available services | 13 | 13% |
| Defined quality measures for long-term services and supports (LTSS) | 12 | 12% |
| Unknown | 9 | 9% |
| Is your practice EMR interoperable with other HCBS providers or agencies? | | |
| No | 66 | 81% |
| Yes | 15 | 19% |

eligibility requirements; insurance coverage; availability of local service providers; and time delays) and whether practices coordinated HCBS; how difficult it was to coordinate services; and how often practices coordinate services (Table 5). Cost to patients was the barrier most strongly associated with practices reporting they conduct care coordination (OR = 2.96, 95% CI = 0.94–9.38, $p$ = .06). Four of the five barriers were significantly associated with HBPC practices reporting it was 'difficult' or 'very difficult' to coordinate HCBS compared to those who reported it was 'neutral,' 'easy,' or 'very easy' (OR ranging from 2.49 to 3.94, all $p$ values < .05). Number of reported barriers was also associated with an increased difficulty with HCBS coordination (OR = 1.77, 95%CI = 1.32–2.37; $p$ = .0001). Frequently providing HCBS coordination was defined as those practices providing coordination 'always' or 'often' versus 'sometimes,' 'rarely,' or 'never.' Among practices indicating they currently coordinate HCBS services, patient eligibility (OR 5.96, 95% CI: 1.65, 21.55; $p$ = 0.007) and time delays (OR 9.90 95% CI: 1.22, 80.11, $p$ = 0.032) were associated with practices providing frequent coordination. When assessing the number of reported barriers, each additional barrier

everything (24%). Only 19% of practices reported having an EMR interoperable with HCBS providers.

**Barriers associated with HCBS coordination**

We tested associations between the five most common barriers to coordinating HCBS (i.e., cost to patient;

**Table 5** Associations Between Barriers to Coordination of HCBS and Coordination Difficulty and Frequency

| Barriers | Does your practice coordinate HCBS? OR, p-value | How difficult is it to coordinate HCBS? OR, p-value | Of the practices that coordinate ($N = 87$), how often does the practice coordinate HCBS? OR, p-value |
|---|---|---|---|
| Provider availability | 1.21, $p = 0.75$<br>For Yes:<br>Barrier (87.5%)<br>Not Barrier (85.3%) | 3.94, $p = 0.003$<br>For Difficult:<br>Barrier (76.3%)<br>Not Barrier (45.0%) | 4.29, $p = 0.07$<br>For Often/Always:<br>Barrier (94.1%)<br>Not Barrier (78.6%) |
| Eligibility requirements | 2.67, $p = 0.09$<br>Barrier (90.6%)<br>Not Barrier (78.4%) | 2.49, $p = 0.04$<br>Barrier (65.1%)<br>Not Barrier (42.9%) | 5.96, $p = 0.007$<br>Barrier (93.0%)<br>Not Barrier (69.0%) |
| Insurance | 2.29, $p = 0.16$<br>Barrier (90%)<br>Not Barrier (80%) | 2.52, $p = 0.03$<br>Barrier (66.1%)<br>Not Barrier (43.6%) | 1.07, $p = 0.92$<br>Barrier (85.0%)<br>Not Barrier (84.0%) |
| Cost to patient | 2.96, $p = 0.06$<br>Barrier (90.9%)<br>Not Barrier (77.1%) | 3.01, $p = 0.01$<br>Barrier (66.2%)<br>Not Barrier (39.4%) | 1.45, $p = 0.55$<br>Barrier (86.0%)<br>Not Barrier (81.5%) |
| Time delay | 1.21, $p = 0.75$<br>Barrier (87.5%)<br>Not Barrier (85.3%) | 2.33, $p = 0.05$<br>Barrier (69.2%)<br>Not Barrier (49.1%) | 9.9, $p = 0.03$<br>Barrier (97.1%)<br>Not Barrier (76.9%) |
| Number of barriers | 1.28, $p = 0.15$ | 1.77, $p = 0.0001$ | 1.89, $p = 0.008$ |

increased the odds that practices were frequently, rather than infrequently, providing coordination (OR = 1.88, 95% CI: 1.18, 2.99, $p = 0.008$).

## Discussion

This study revealed that in the majority of HBPC practices, most or all their patients had nonmedical social needs within the past 12 months, and nearly all practices assessed these needs both initially and periodically on an ongoing basis. HBPC providers reported being actively engaged in assessing, documenting, and coordinating HCBS for their patients. Respondents indicated cost to the patient, eligibility requirements, and insurance coverage were the top barriers to coordinating HCBS.

The high patient need for HCBS reflects the patient population characterized as frail, medically complex homebound older adults, which is consistent with other reports on HBPC [14, 30]. Most of these patients are in the last years of life and their goal is often to remain at home and out of the hospital and long-term care facilities [22]. To meet this goal requires meeting the non-medical, social service needs of homebound patients. Medical care for these patients is mostly centered on keeping their chronic conditions stable and reconciling multiple medications.

Unfortunately, more than half of the providers indicated HCBS coordination was difficult or very difficult. While barriers did not differentiate if a practice coordinated HCBS, all the top five barriers were associated with HBPC practices indicating HCBS coordination was difficult. Eligibility requirements and time delays were the two barriers associated with frequency of HCBS

coordination. This suggests that these two barriers may add to HBPC providers work load around HCBS coordination. The barriers HBPC providers most frequently reported their patients encountered were financial in nature, including the cost to the patient, eligibility requirements, and insurance coverage. This is consistent with other studies stating that in the U.S. Medicare coverage for HCBS is negligible, and those who need them often fall into a gap where they lack the financial means to pay for HCBS but do not meet Medicaid's eligibility requirements to receive coverage [5, 27, 28]. Interestingly, while over three quarters of HBPC practices reported they provide medical services for Medicare Advantage (MA) patients, only about 12% of patients received HCBS through MA.

In the U.S., MA plans and other capitated payment models, as well as alternative payment models with shared risk or shared savings incentives, create opportunities to finance integrated medical and non-medical care for homebound frail older adults [15]. These models align Medicare payment incentives with conducting high-quality care to avoid high-cost medical care such as emergency department visits and hospitalizations [31]. For example, the Comprehensive Primary Care Plus Model (CPC+), an advanced primary care medical home model, is a proactive, team-based approach to care that focuses on a patient-centered care plan provided through home-visits, e-visits, and telephone [32]. The CPC+ model has several payment components including a care management fee, a performance-based incentive payment, and a fee-for-service payment. The model is specifically designed to address the longitudinal chronic care needs of medically complex older adults.

The other two top barriers to patients receiving HCBS services identified in the survey were availability of service providers and time delays. HCBS provider availability may reflect both lack of service options, and HBPC practitioners' lack of awareness of the HCBS services available within their community [25]. Time delays and service availability both likely reflect scarce and stretched HCBS providers that may vary in quality of service delivery. Survey responses indicated there was no consistent method for HBPC practices to learn about and determine the quality of potential HCBS options. Patient word-of-mouth reports were cited as the top option providers relied upon to assess quality. A recent literature review concluded there is a need for quality measures to address the non-medical, health-related social needs of older adults [33]. Lynn [28] reaffirmed these needs, stating that most communities lack a centralized system for evaluating and determining the quality and parity of services, and reforms have failed to address these needs at a local level. Interestingly, 48 U.S. states do conduct quality assessments of HCBS in Medicaid as part of 1915(c) waivers, which allows states to shift care from institutional to community based settings [34]. However, these measures tend to be process-oriented and not focused on the quality of care beneficiaries receive. A quality measurement framework has been recently developed by the National Quality Forum to address gaps in performance measurement of HCBS in eleven domains (e.g., person-centered planning and coordination, community inclusion, and workforce) [35].

Practices endorsed several viable options to ease the burden of HCBS coordination. About a third of practices indicated a good option would be to designate a point person in the practice to manage this process. To address the implementation of possible HCBS coordination solutions, HBPC practices can look to existing innovative models of care that are partnerships between health care and community-based organizations that have been developed and evaluated [15, 36, 37]. Evidence supports the efficacy of nutritional assistance, case management and community outreach programs for high-need, low income older adults [38]. For example, the Geriatric Resources for Assessment and Care of Elders (GRACE) model was designed for low-income community dwelling older adults most of whom have multiple chronic conditions. The model includes in-home assessments and an individualized care plan developed by a nurse practitioner and social worker team in conjunction with the primary care physician. In a controlled trial over a two-year intervention period, GRACE reduced hospital costs for high-risk patients [23]. Unfortunately, only 10% of GRACE program costs are covered under traditional FFS Medicare, but the program would be feasible through Medicare managed care capitated payment [21].

While this program along with several other successful programs designed for high-risk older adults have common components such as comprehensive need assessments, patient-centered care planning, caregiver engagement, and care coordination, there has not been wide-spread adoption in practice [15, 36].

Study limitations include a low response rate to the survey and reliance on self-report measures, both of which may limit the generalizability of these findings. Of the approximately 1000 members of AAHCM, we received 101 complete responses. There may be a self-selection bias where HBPC providers who are already offering HCBS assessment and coordination in their practice were more likely to complete the survey. The proportion of HBPC practices that assess, refer, and coordinate HCBS may be lower in the overall population.

The study findings are from self-report survey responses, and there was no method to validate the responses. However, we have no reason to believe respondents had a 'social desirability' bias to exaggerate the extent of their care coordination efforts for patients. Other study methods, such as structured interviews, might result in information about barriers that did not surface through our survey. Future studies could use mixed-methods and include other stakeholders such as patients and family members to corroborate and expand on these findings. Study strengths include a comprehensive survey of non-medical care coordination completed by a diverse sample of HBPC practices in the US.

## Conclusions

Despite the barriers to coordinating HCBS, most HBPC practices in the U.S. provided some level of coordination of non-medical services for their high-need, high-cost homebound patients. More efforts are needed to implement and scale care model partnerships between medical and non-medical service providers for this vulnerable population of older adults, but adequate payment methods and quality measurements must be in place to ensure high quality care is delivered at a reasonable cost relative to other treatment options such as long-term institutional care and frequent inpatient care. Since 'days spent at home,' verses in health care facilities, has been recognized as the preference of most patients toward end-of-life [22], it makes sense to recognize 'days spent at home' as a patient-centered outcome that can be achieved through integrated care of HBPC and HCBS.

**Abbreviations**

AAA: Area Agency on Aging; AAHCM: American Academy of Home Care Medicine; CI: Confidence interval; CPC +: Comprehensive Primary Care Plus Model.; FFS: Fee-for-service; GRACE: Geriatric Resources for Assessment and Care of Elders; HBPC: Home-based primary care; HCBS: Home and community-based services; MA: Medicare Advantage; OR: Odds ratio

## Acknowledgments

We thank Dr. Bruce Leff for sharing his survey instrument previously used to assess home-based primary care practice characteristics. Portions of this work were presented at the 2016 Annual Meeting of The American Geriatrics Society.

## Funding

There was no extramural support for this research. GN, AW, AM, JS are employees of the West Health Institute. They have no potential competing interests to disclose.

## Authors' contributions

GN participated in the acquisition of the data, conducted data analyses, interpreted the data and prepared the manuscript for publication. AW conducted data analyses, interpreted the data, and prepared the manuscript for publication. AM and JS participated in the data collection, interpretation of the data and manuscript preparation. All authors approved the final version of the manuscript for publication.

## Competing interests

The authors declare that they have no competing interests.

## References

1. Ornstein KA, Leff B, Covinsky KE, et al. Epidemiology of the homebound population in the United States. JAMA Intern Med. 2015;175(7):1180–6.
2. Leff B, Carlson CM, Saliba D, Ritchie C. The invisible homebound: setting quality-of-care standards for home-based primary and palliative care. Health Aff (Millwood). 2015;34(1):21–9.
3. Leff B, Weston CM, Garrigues S, Patel K, Ritchie C. Home-based primary care practices in the United States: current state and quality improvement approaches. J Am Geriatr Soc. 2015;63(5):963–9.
4. Qiu WQ, Dean M, Liu T, et al. Physical and mental health of homebound older adults: an overlooked population. J Am Geriatr Soc. 2010;58(12):2423–8.
5. Feinglass J, Norman G, Golden RL, Muramatsu N, Gelder M, Cornwell T. Integrating social services and home-based primary Care for High-Risk Patients. In: Popul health Manag; 2017.
6. Cornwell T. Home-Based Primary Care's Perfect Storm. Home centered care institute: home centered care institute; March 2, 2015.
7. Totten AM, White-Chu EF, Wasson N, et al. Home-based primary care interventions. Agency for Healthcare Research and Quality;2016.
8. Edes T, Kinosian B, Vuckovic NH, Nichols LO, Becker MM, Hossain M. Better access, quality, and cost for clinically complex veterans with home-based primary care. J Am Geriatr Soc. 2014;62(10):1954–61.
9. DeCherrie LV, Soriano T, Hayashi J. Home-based primary care: A needed primary-care model for vlnerable populations. Mt Sinai J Med. 2012;79: 425–32.
10. De Jonge KE, Jamshed N, Gilden D, Kubisiak J, Bruce SR, Taler G. Effects of home-based primary care on Medicare costs in high-risk elders. J Am Geriatr Soc. 2014;62(10):1825–31.
11. Reckrey JM, Soriano TA, Hernandez CR, et al. The team approach to home-based primary care: restructuring care to meet individual, program, and system needs. J Am Geriatr Soc. 2015;63(2):358–64.
12. Rotenberg J, Kinosian B, Boling P, Taler G. Independence at home learning collaborative writing G. home-based primary care: beyond extension of the Independence at home demonstration. J Am Geriatr Soc. 2018;66(1):812–7.
13. Boling PA, Chandekar RV, Hungate B, Purvis M, Selby-Penczak R, Abbey LJ. Improving outcomes and lowering costs by applying advanced models of in-home care. Cleve Clin J Med. 2013;80 Electronic Suppl 1:eS7–14.
14. Melnick GA, Green L, Rich J. House calls: California program for homebound patients reduces monthly spending, delivers meaningful care. Health Aff (Millwood). 2016;35(1):28–35.
15. Shier G, Ginsburg M, Howell J, Volland P, Golden R. Strong social support services, such as transportation and help for caregivers, can lead to lower health care use and costs. Health Aff (Millwood). 2013;32(3):544–51.
16. Remington PL, Catlin BB, Gennuso KP. The county health rankings: rationale and methods. Popul Health Metrics. 2015;13(11):1–12.
17. Bradley EH, Canavan M, Rogan E, et al. Variation in health outcomes: the role of spending on social services, public health, and health care, 2000-09. Health Aff (Millwood). 2016;35(5):760–8.
18. Arbaje AI, Wolff JL, Yu Q, Powe NR, Anderson GF, Boult C. Postdischarge environmental and socioeconomic factors and the likelihood of early hospital readmission among community-dwelling Medicare beneficiaries. The Gerontologist. 2008;48(4):495–504.
19. Meiners MR, Mokler PM, Kasunic ML, et al. Insights from a pilot program to integrate medical and social services. Home Health Care Serv Q. 2014;33(3):121–36.
20. Fraze T, Lewis VA, Rodriguez HP, Fisher ES. Housing, transportation, and food: how ACOs seek to improve population health by addressing nonmedical needs of patients. Health Aff (Millwood). 2016;35(11):2109–15.
21. Bielaszka-DuVernay C. The 'GRACE' model: in-home assessments lead to better care for dual eligibles. Health Aff (Millwood). 2011;30(3):431–4.
22. Groff AC, Colla CH, Lee TH. Days spent at home - a patient-centered goal and outcome. N Engl J Med. 2016;375(17):1610–2.
23. Counsell SR, Callahan CM, Clark DO, et al. Geriatric care management for low-income seniors: a randomized controlled trial. JAMA. 2007;298(22):2623–33.
24. Henning-Smith CE, Shippee TP. Expectations about future use of long-term services and supports vary by current living arrangement. Health Aff (Millwood). 2015;34(1):39–47.
25. Siegler EL, Lama SD, Knight MG, Laureano E, Reid MC. Community-based supports and Services for Older Adults: a primer for clinicians. J Geriatr. 2015;2015:1–6.
26. Buckley DI, McGinnis P, Fagnan LJ, Mardon R, Johnson M, Dymek C. Clinical Community Relationships Evaluation Roadmap. Rockville, MD: Agency for Healthcare Research and Quality; July 2013 2013.
27. Weaver RH, Roberto KA. Home and community-based service use by vulnerable older adults. Gerontologist. 2017;57(3):540–51.
28. Lynn J. Reliable and sustainable comprehensive care for frail elderly people. JAMA. 2013;310(18):1935–6.
29. Wagner EH, Austin BT, Davis C, Hindmarsh M, Schaefer J, Bonomi A. Improving chronic illness care: translating evidence into action. Health Aff. 2001;20(6):64–78.
30. Hayes SL, Salzberg CA, McCarthy D, et al. High-need, high-cost patients: who are they and how do they use health care? A population-based comparison of demographics, health care use, and expenditures the Commonwealth Fund; August 2016. 1897.
31. Ling SM, McGann P. Changing healthcare service delivery to improve health outcomes for older adults: opportunities not to be missed. J Am Geriatr Soc. 2018;66(2):235–8.
32. Meltzer DO, Ruhnke GW. Redesigning care for patients at increased hospitalization risk: the comprehensive care physician model. Health Aff (Millwood). 2014;33(5):770–7.
33. MacLeod S, Schwebke K, Hawkins K, Ruiz J, Hoo E, Yeh CS. The need for comprehensive health care quality meausures for older adults. In: Popul health Manag; 2017.
34. Hartman L, Lukanen E. Quality measurement for home and community based services (HCBS) and behavioral health in Medicaid. State Health Access Data Assistance Center; December 2016.
35. Forum NQ. Quality in Home and Community-Based Services to Support Community Living: Addressing Gaps in Performance Measurement. Washington, DC: National Quality Forum; September 2016 2016. Final Report.
36. McCarthy D, Ryan J, Klein S. Models of care for high-need, high-cost patients: An evidence synthesis. The Commonwealth Fund. 2015.
37. Szanton SL, Leff B, Wolff JL, Roberts L, Gitlin LN. Home-based care program reduces disability and promotes aging in place. Health Aff (Millwood). 2016; 35(9):1558–63.
38. Taylor LA, Coyle CE, Ndumele C, et al. Leveraging the social determinants of health: what works? June 2015.

# 23

# Environmental factors and risk of delirium in geriatric patients: an observational study

Sigurd Evensen[1,2*] ⓘ, Ingvild Saltvedt[1,2], Stian Lydersen[3], Torgeir Bruun Wyller[4,5], Kristin Taraldsen[2] and Olav Sletvold[1,2]

## Abstract

**Background:** Patients with delirium have increased risk of death, dementia and institutionalization, and prognosis differs between delirium motor subtypes. A few studies have identified associations between environmental factors like room-transfers and time spent in the emergency department (ED) and delirium, but no studies have investigated if environmental factors may influence delirium motor subtypes. We wanted to explore if potentially stressful events like ward-transfers, arriving ED at nighttime, time spent in ED and nigthttime investigations were associated with development of delirium (incident delirium) and delirium motor subtypes.

**Methods:** We used the DSM-5 criteria to diagnose delirium and the Delirium Motor Subtype Scale for motor subtyping. We defined hyperactive and mixed delirium as delirium with hyperactive symptoms, and hypoactive and no-subtype delirium as delirium without hyperactive symptoms. We registered ward-transfers, time of arrival in ED, time spent in ED and nighttime investigations (8 p.m. to 8 a.m.), and calculated Global Deterioration Scale (GDS) and Cumulative Illness Rating Scale (CIRS) to adjust for cognitive impairment and comorbidity. We used logistic regression analyses with incident delirium and delirium with hyperactive symptoms as outcome variables, and ward-transfers, arriving ED at nighttime, time spent in ED and nighttime investigations as exposure variables, adjusting for age, GDS and CIRS in the analyses for incident delirium.

**Results:** We included 254 patients, mean age 86.1 years (SD 5.2), 49 (19.3%) had incident delirium, 22 with and 27 without hyperactive symptoms. There was a significant association between nighttime investigations and incident delirium in both the unadjusted (odds ratio (OR) 2.22, 95% confidence interval (CI) 1.17 to 4.22, $p = 0.015$) and the multiadjusted model (OR 2.61, CI 1.26 to 5.40, $p = 0.010$). There were no associations between any other exposure variables and incident delirium. No exposure variables were associated with delirium motor subtypes.

**Conclusions:** Nighttime investigations were associated with incident delirium, even after adjusting for age, cognitive impairment and comorbidity. We cannot out rule that the medical condition leading to nighttime investigations is the true delirium-trigger, so geriatric patients must still receive emergency investigations at nighttime. Hospital environment in broad sense may be a target for delirium prevention.

**Keywords:** Delirium, Risk factors, Geriatric patients, Hospital, Environmental

---

\* Correspondence: sigurd.evensen@ntnu.no
[1]Department of Geriatrics, St. Olavs hospital, Trondheim University Hospital, Trondheim, Norway
[2]Department of Neuromedicine and Movement Science, Faculty of Medicine and Health Sciences, Norwegian University of Science and Technology (NTNU), N-7491 Trondheim, Norway
Full list of author information is available at the end of the article

# Background

Delirium is an acute disturbance of attention, awareness and cognition, affecting one third of older medical inpatients [1]. High age, cognitive impairment and comorbidity are the most important risk factors [2]. Patients suffering from delirium have increased risk of death, cognitive impairment and institutionalization [3], and delirium has substantial medical, societal and economical implications on the entire health care system [4]. Four different motor subtypes of delirium have been described; hyperactive delirium, hypoactive delirium, mixed delirium with both hyperactive and hypoactive features and no-subtype delirium without motor disturbances [5]. Most studies find that hypoactive delirium has worst prognosis [5–9]. It is unclear whether risk factors and etiology differ between motor subtypes [8, 10, 11].

The Diagnostic and Statistical Manual of Mental Disorders (DSM-5) criteria [12] are physiologically oriented and state that delirium is caused by medical conditions, substance intoxication or withdrawal, exposure to a toxin, or is due to multiple etiologies. On the other hand, non-pharmacological intervention programs focusing on activity, orientation and sleep hygiene are effective to prevent delirium [13, 14], indicating that environmental factors may have a role in development of delirium. There are previous reports on both sensory deprivation [15] and sensory overload [16] as contributors to delirium, and three studies have identified associations between specific environmental factors in the hospital care pathway and delirium. Goldberg et al. and Bo et al. found associations between room-transfers and time spent in the emergency department (ED) and development of delirium, respectively [17, 18], and McCusker et al. found that increasing number of room-transfers increased the severity of delirium [15]. These associations seem plausible since both room-transfers and long time spent in ED can be stressfull events that might be able to induce aberrant stress responses eventually contributing to delirium [19]. To our knowledge, no studies have investigated the association between environmental factors and motor subtypes of delirium, which is of interest since the motor subtypes have different prognosis.

Due to the substantial impact of delirium and the increasing number of delirium-prone older patients in strained and crowded hospitals [20], there is a need to further explore the associations between potentially stressful environmental factors in the hospital care patway and delirium. The aim of this study is to specifically investigate if ward-transfers, arriving ED at nighttime, time spent in ED and visits from other specialists and radiological procedures at nighttime (nighttime investigations) are associated with development of delirium (incident delirium) and delirium motor subtypes in patients acutely admitted to a geriatric ward.

# Methods

## Design, settings and participants

This is a prospective observational study conducted at the medical geriatric ward at St. Olavs hospital, Trondheim University Hospital, Norway, between May 6 2015 and January 31 2017. The ward has 15 single-bed rooms, and the patients receive comprehensive geriatric assessment and care [21] by an interdisciplinary geriatric team consisting of physicians, nurses, occupational therapists and physiotherapists. Ninety per cent of the patients are acutely admitted with conditions like infections, injuries after falls, cardiopulmonary conditions and dehydration [22]. Acutely admitted patients arrive via the ED which has ten regular rooms, three acute-rooms and eight beds in a triage room. Nurses collect blood-samples in the ED. Physicians examine the patients in the ED before the patients as soon as possible are transferred to a relevant ward. The patients frequently receive radiological procedures during transfer between ED and the ward. As in other hospitals [20], the ED is frequently chaotic and over-crowded.

The inclusion criteria were age $\geq 75$ years and acute admittance. Patients transferred from other wards were eligible for inclusion if they met the inclusion criteria. We excluded patients previously taking part in the study and patients with delirium on admittance. Nurses, physiotherapists or a physician (SE) included all patients within 24 h after arriving the ward.

## Diagnosis of delirium and delirium motor subtypes

We diagnosed delirium according to the DSM-5 criteria, judging consciousness, awareness and arousal clinically, testing attention using the digit span forwards and backwards [23] and cognitive impairment using the ten orientation items and the three word short time memory test from the Mini Mental Status Excamination [24]. In this population of elderly patients we particularily stressed that the present symptoms could not be better explained by preexisting dementia and that the delirium episode had to be a consequence of physiological disturbances. We based the final diagnosis on all available information, i.e. first day visits to all patients, interviews with nurses and proxies and careful chart review as described by Inouye [25], since this combined approach increases the number of patients correctly diagnosed with delirium [26]. When in doubt concerning the diagnosis, and if the staff noticed changes in mental status, we visited the patient several times.

After diagnosing delirium, we did motor subtyping using the Delirium Motor Subtype Scale (DMSS) [27]. The DMSS lists four hyperactive and seven hypoactive features. To fulfill the criteria for a certain motor subtype, the patient must have at least two of these features. Patients having both hyperactive and hypoactive features get the diagnosis of mixed delirium, and patients with one or less motor feature get the diagnosis of no-subtype delirium. Due to a small number of observations, we combined the patients with hyperactive and mixed delirium to create the category "delirium with hyperactive symptoms" and the patients with hypoactive and no-subtype delirium to create the category "delirium without hyperactive symptoms." In patients not visited due to logistical reasons, we based the diagnosis of delirium and motor subtype on careful chart review. We were not able to secure that the delirium assessors were completely blinded to exposure status of environmental factors.

## Data collection

We registered time of arrival at the ED and total time in the ED retrospectively using the hospital's ED database. We defined nighttime between 8 p.m. and 8 a.m. We registered cerebral MRI-scans, other radiological investigations (CT-scans, ultrasound and x-rays) and visits from other specialties at nighttime retrospectively reviewing the hospital records. Due to small numbers of cerebral MRI-scans and visits from other specialties we combined these with other radiological investigations and created the category investigations at nighttime, despite that MRI-scans might be a stronger contributor to incident delirium due to noise and narrowness. Nurses registered ward-transfers consecutively (yes/no).

To be able to adjust for cognitive impairment, we scored the Global Deterioration Scale (GDS) [28]. The GDS ranges from one to seven, one indicates no cognitive symptoms, seven indicates end-stage dementia. We defined dementia as a GDS-score more than four. To be able to adjust for comorbidity, we calculated the Cumulative Illness Rating Scale (CIRS) retrospectively reviewing the hospital records [29]. CIRS ranges from 0 to 56; higher score indicates increasing comorbidity.

We used the Barthel Index (BI, 0 to 20, 20 best score) as a baseline measure of personal Activities of Daily Living [30] prior to hospitalization and the Short Physical Performance Battery (SPPB, 0 to 12, 12 best score) as a baseline measure of general health and frailty [31]. We used a modified APACHE II-score (0 to 71, increasing score indicates more severe illness) as a baseline measure of acute illness [32]. We collected demographic data from the hospital records.

## Ethics

The Regional Committee for Medical and Health Research Ethics of Mid-Norway approved the study (REC Central 2015/474). Since there were no elements of invasive or uncomfortable procedures, the patients could consent for participation even if they had signs of cognitive impairment. If the patient was unable to give consent, a proxy could sign the consent form. Independent of cognitive status, we never included patients who expressed concerns about participation.

## Statistical analysis

We present descriptive data for continuous variables as means and standard deviations (SD), and for dichotomous and categorical variables as percentages. To investigate if the exposure variables ward-transfers, arrival at nighttime, time spent in ED and nighttime investigations were associated with incident delirium, we used logistic regression analyses, unadjusted and multiadjusted, with incident delirium as outcome variable. To adjust for important risk factors for delirium we also included the covariates age, GDS (cognitive function) and CIRS (comorbidity) in the analyses. We used the same strategy to study the relation between the exposure variables and motor subtypes, using incident delirium with hyperactive symptoms as outcome variable. Due to a small numbers of observations, we did not include the covariates age, GDS and CIRS in the latter analysis. This study is part of a project where the main aim was to detect differences in one-year mortality between patients with hypoactive and hyperactive delirium, and we based power calculation on an assumption of 50% mortality among 60 patients with hypoactive delirium and 20% mortality among 40 patients with hyperactive delirium, giving a power of 87.9% with $\alpha = 0.05$. We report odds ratios (OR) with 95% confidence intervals (CI) from the logistic regression analyses and judge two-sided $p$-values $< 0.05$ as statistically significant. We completed all analyses using SPSS version 25.

## Results

In total, 311 patients took part in the study. After reviewing the medical notes from the ED and other wards, we excluded 54 patients with delirium on admittance. As illustrated in Fig. 1 we excluded one patient who died the night of inclusion and two patients who were discharged the next day. This article thus reports analyses of 254 patients. As shown in Table 1, mean age was 86.1 years (SD 5.2), 151 (58.4%) were female and 133 (52.4%) had dementia.

Fourty-nine patients had incident delirium, of which we diagnosed 41 through direct assessment by the first author and the remaining eight through chart review. Eleven had hyperactive delirium, 11 mixed delirium, 18 hypoactive delirium and nine had no-subtype delirium. Thus, 22 patients had delirium with hyperactive symptoms and 27 had delirium without hyperactive symptoms. Regarding exposure variables, 42 out of 254 patients (16.5%) were transferred from other wards, 44 (17.3%) arrived at nighttime and 77 (30.3%) received

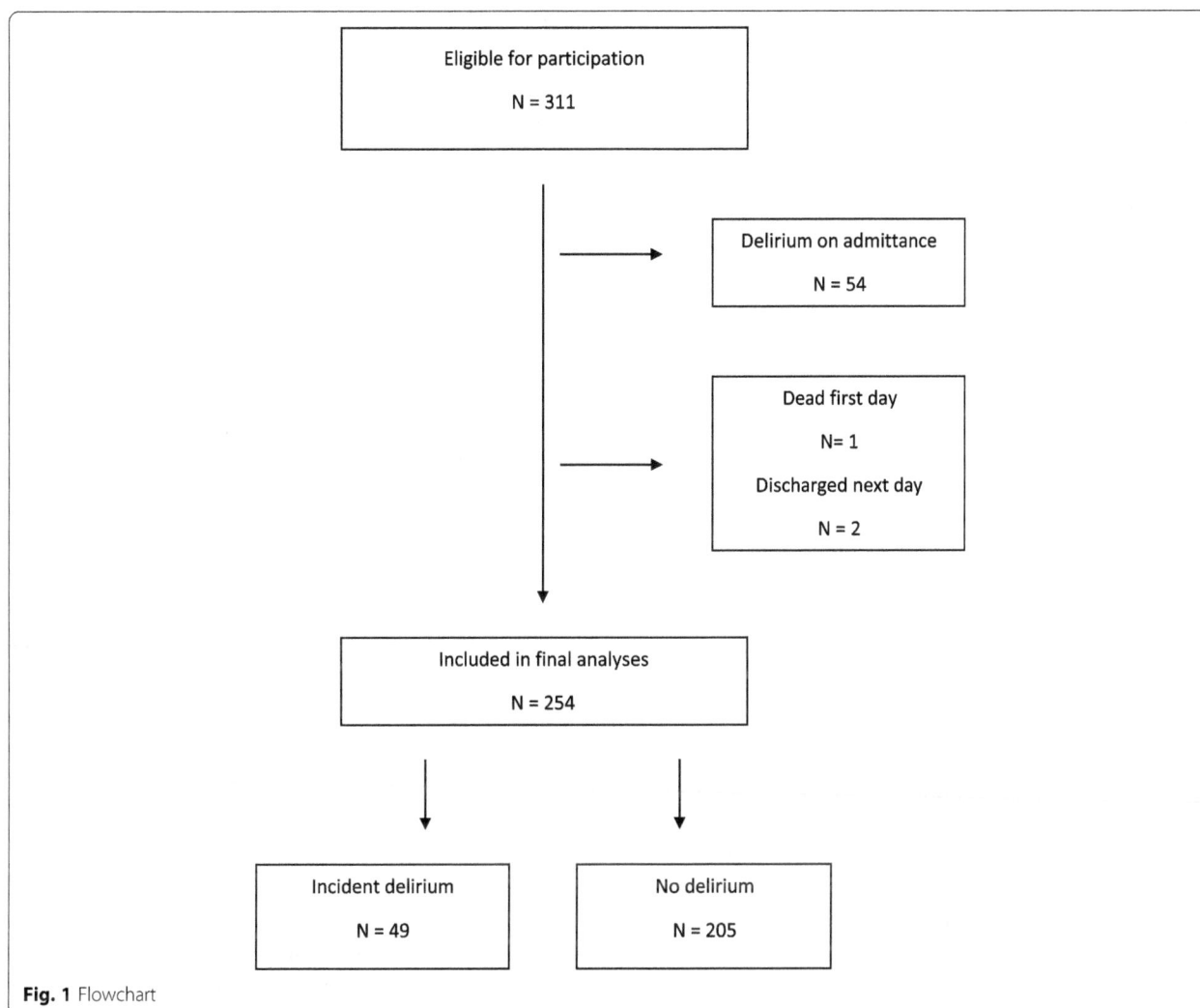

**Fig. 1** Flowchart

**Table 1** Baseline characteristics for all patients, patients with incident delirium and patients remaining free of delirium

| | All (254) Mean; SD | Incident delirium (n = 49) Mean; SD | No delirium (n = 205) Mean; SD | p-values[a] |
|---|---|---|---|---|
| Age (years) | 86.1; 5.2 | 86.9; 5.0 | 85.8; 5.2 | 0.20 |
| Body Mass Index | 24.2; 4.3 | 23.4; 3.6 | 24.4; 4.4 | 0.12 |
| GDS[b] (1–7) | 3.4; 1.7 | 4.3; 1.3 | 3.2; 1.7 | < 0.001 |
| CIRS[c] (0–56) | 12.9; 4.4 | 14.3; 4.6 | 12.6; 4.3 | 0.020 |
| APACHE (0–71) | 8.9; 2.7 | 9.3; 2.7 | 8.8; 2.7 | 0.30 |
| Barthel Index (0–20) | 16.3; 3.6 | 14.9; 4.0 | 16.7; 3.4 | 0.002 |
| SPPB[d] (0–12) | 4.0; 3.0 | 2.5; 2.6 | 4.3; 3.1 | < 0.001 |
| Female | 151 (59.4%) | 23 (46.9%) | 128 (62.4%) | 0.049 |
| Home-dwelling | 246 (96.9%) | 46 (93.9%) | 200 (97.6%) | 0.19 |
| Dementia (GDS > 4) | 133 (52.4%) | 38 (77.6%) | 95 (46.3%) | < 0.001 |

Baseline characteristics for all patients, patients with incident delirium and patients remaining free of delirium
[b]Global Deterioration Scale
[c]Cumulative Illness Rating Scale
[d]Short Physical Performance Battery

nighttime investigations of which three had cerebral MRI-scans, 65 other radiological investigations and nine received visits from other specialities. Those arriving at nighttime received 25 (32.5%) of the nighttime investigations. The mean time spent in ED was 4.1 h (SD 0.9).

Table 2 and Table 3 show results of the logistic regression analyses. In the unadjusted model, nighttime investigations were significantly associated with incident delirium (OR 2.22, CI 1.17 to 4.22, $p = 0.015$), indicating a more than doubled risk of incident delirium if the patient was exposed to nighttime investigations. In the multiadjusted model, nighttime investigations remained significantly associated with incident delirium (OR 2.61, CI 1.26 to 5.40, $p = 0.010$). Figure 2 illustrates the associations between ward-transfers, arriving at nighttime, nighttime investigations, time spent in ED and incident delirium. There were no significant associations between any of the exposure variables and the two groups of delirium motor subtypes.

## Discussion

In this observational study in acutely admitted geriatric patients, there was a significantly increased risk of incident delirium associated with exposure to nighttime investigations, even after adjusting for age, cognitive impairment and comorbidity, all well-known risk factors for delirium. There were no significant associations between ward-transfers, arrival at nighttime, time spent in ED and incident delirium. There were no associations between any of the exposure variables and delirium motor subtypes.

Previous studies have identified associations between room-transfers [15, 17] and time spent in ED [18] and delirium. These previous findings as well as our result seem biologically plausible since both room-transfers, long time spent in ED and nighttime investigations are potentially stressfull events that could induce aberrant stress responses which is a widely held hypothesis [19]

regarding the pathophysiology of delirium. On the other hand, the association between nighttime investigations and incident delirium might be a spurious finding since the medical condition leading to nighttime investigations might be the true trigger of delirium, and not the investigation itself. The uncertainty about what is the true delirium trigger could have been reduced if we had reliable admission diagnoses, but in our opinion diagnoses on admission forms, at least in our hospital, are too unreliable to be used for this purpose. Like all observational studies, our study is unable to establish firm causality, and our findings must not be overinterpreted. In our opinion, clinicians must still refer geriatric patients to medically indicated nighttime investigations, but hospital organizers should secure that non-emergency investigations are done in a predictable way at daytime.

These associations between environmental factors and delirium are supported by studies showing that non-pharmacological, mainly environmental intervention programs are effective in preventing delirium [13, 14, 33]. Since delirium is common [1], has poor prognosis [3] and substantial economical impact [2], there seems to be a large potential for both health-related and economical benefits through focus on hospital environment and implementation of non-pharmacological delirium intervention programs. Such interventions also seem to have benefits beyond delirium prevention. In addition to a 44% reduction in delirium incidence, a meta-analysis from 2015 reports a 64% reduction in fall rates and a trend towards reduced length of stay and institutionalization rates in the intervention groups [13].

We found no association between ward-transfers and incident delirium. A possible explanation is that all ward-transfers are done in a predictable way at daytime. Another explanation may be that the geriatric ward provides a multicomponent intervention program against delirium that may out-weigh the potentially negative effect of ward-transfers. If so, this effect could also have influenced

**Table 2** Logistic regression analyses with incident delirium ($n = 49$) as outcome variable, unadjusted and multiadjusted, for all the listed covariates, for all 254 patients

|  | Unadjusted | | | Multiadjusted | | |
|---|---|---|---|---|---|---|
|  | OR | 95% CI | $p$-value | OR | 95% CI | $p$-value |
| Ward-transfers | 0.98 | 0.42 to 2.28 | 0.97 | 0.70 | 0.28 to 1.72 | 0.43 |
| Arrive late[a] | 0.76 | 0.32 to 1.82 | 0.53 | 0.56 | 0.20 to 1.55 | 0.26 |
| Time spent in ED (hours) | 0.89 | 0.75 to 1.06 | 0.20 | 0.85 | 0.69 to 1.04 | 0.12 |
| Investigations at nighttime[a] | 2.22 | 1.17 to 4.22 | 0.015 | 2.61 | 1.26 to 5.40 | 0.010 |
| Age (years) | 1.04 | 0.98 to 1.11 | 0.20 | 1.03 | 0.97 to 1.10 | 0.37 |
| GDS[b] | 1.54 | 1.24 to 1.91 | < 0.001 | 1.59 | 1.26 to 1.99 | < 0.001 |
| CIRS[c] | 1.09 | 1.01 to 1.17 | 0.020 | 1.08 | 1.00 to 1.18 | 0.049 |

[a]Between 8 p.m. and 8 a.m
[b]Global Deterioration Scale
[c]Cumulative Illness Rating Scale

**Table 3** Logistic regression analyses with delirium with hyperactive symptoms (*n*=22) as outcome variable, unadjusted and multiadjusted, for all the listed covariates, for all 254 patients

| | Unadjusted | | | Multiadjusted | | |
|---|---|---|---|---|---|---|
| | OR | 95% CI | *p*-value | OR | 95% CI | *p*-value |
| Ward-transfers | 1.14 | 0.36 to 3.54 | 0.83 | 1.11 | 0.35 to 3.49 | 0.86 |
| Arrive late[a] | 0.74 | 0.21 to 2.60 | 0.63 | 0.41 | 0.10 to 1.62 | 0.20 |
| Time spent in ED (hours) | 0.80 | 0.60 to 1.05 | 0.11 | 0.75 | 0.56 to 1.02 | 0.065 |
| Investigations at nighttime[a] | 1.67 | 0.68 to 4.09 | 0.26 | 2.00 | 0.77 to 5.16 | 0.15 |

[a]Between 8 p.m. and 8 a.m

the associations between the other exposure variables and incident delirium. The lack of association between time spent in the ED and incident delirium might reflect that the ED in our hospital emphasises initial examination and short stay before transfer to a relevant ward, thereby providing less insult to vulnerable patients than the ED as described by Bo et al. [18]. Another explanation may be that physicians identify the patients prone to develop delirium as more vulnerable and examine these patients rapidly.

The lack of significant associations between any of the variables and delirium motor subtypes must be interpreted carefully due to a small number of observations. There is a trend towards less delirium with hyperactive symptoms with increasing time spent in the ED, which is plausible since the staff in ED might register signs of hyperactivity and therefore transfer these patients fast. An alternative hypothesis is that too quick transfers could be stressful and thereby inducing delirium. It remains uncertain if this trend would have reached statistical significance if the study was designed for this purpose. The results of previous studies addressing the relation between motor subtypes and etiology are diverging.

A recent cross-sectional study found a negative association between use of atypical antipsychotics and hypoactive delirium and a positive association between intravenous lines and mixed delirium [11], possibly indicating differences in etiology between the subtypes. On the other hand, two reports from a longitudinal study designed to investigate the relationship between motor subtypes and other factors found no associations between motor subtypes and etiology [8], age and preexisting dementia [10]. Our results complies with the two latter reports.

### Strengths and limitations

The major strength of this study is that we have diagnosed delirium using the DSM-5 criteria directly and based the diagnoses on a combination of interviews with patients, nurses and proxies and a validated chart review method. The completeness of all variables of interest is another strength. The major limitation is the small number of patients with incident delirium. The limited sample size is particularly important when it comes to the analyses of environmental factors and delirium motor

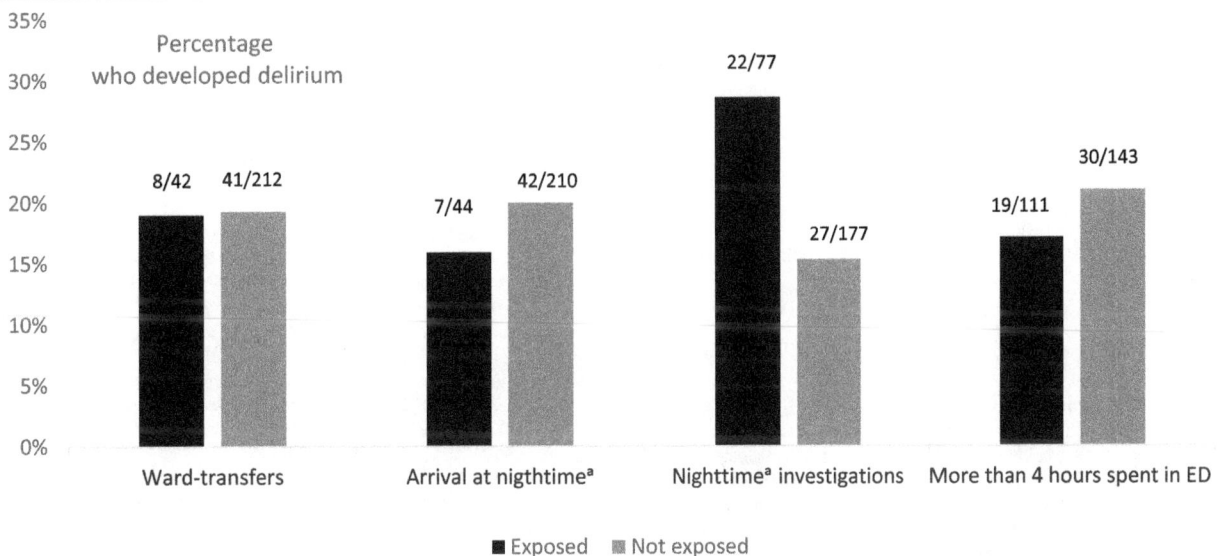

**Fig. 2** Percentages of patients who developed delirium among those who were exposed (black bars) and unexposed (grey bars) to the environmental factors. [a]Between 8 p.m. and 8 a.m

subtypes. Uncertainty about what is triggering delirium could have been reduced if we had reliable diagnoses for admissions to both hospital and nighttime investigations, and lack of such information is a limitation. A further limitation is that we were not strictly blinded to the exposure of environmental factors when diagnosing delirium, but we believe this has minor implications since we were focusing the presence of physiological disturbance resulting in delirium. Finally, our findings are not necessarily generalizable to non-geriatric wards and younger patients, or to EDs organized in a different way than in our hospital.

## Conclusions

In this observational study on 254 acutely admitted geriatric patients we found an association between nighttime investigations and incident delirium, but no associations between any of the exposure variables and delirium motor subtypes. In general, investigations should therefore be done in a predictable way at daytime, althoug patients should have emergency investigations at nighttime when indicated. Hospital environment in broad sense may be a target for delirium prevention along with non-pharmacological delirium intervention programs. There is a need for larger studies with both accurate registrations of environmental factors and a precise diagnostic work-up of delirium.

### Abbreviations
APACHE: Acute Physiology And Chronic Health Evaluation; BI: Barthel Index; CI: Confidence Interval; CIRS: Cumulative Illness Rating Scale; DMSS: Delirium Motor Subtype Scale; DSM: Diagnostic and Statistical Manual of Mental Disorders; ED: Emergency Department; GDS: Global Deterioration Scale; OR: Odds Ratio; SD: Standard Deviations; SPPB: Short Physical Performance Battery

### Acknowledgements
Warm thanks to the staff at the geriatric ward for help with inclusion of patients and data collection.

### Funding
The Liaison Committee for education, research and innovation in Central Norway funded the project. We confirm that the funder had no role in designing the study, in the collection, analyses or interpretation of data or in writing/ submitting the manuscript.

### Authors' contributions
SE did the initial drafting of the article, had the main responsibility for data collection and for diagnosing and subtyping delirium. IS participated in designing and planning the study with particular responsibility in data collection at the geriatric ward. SL had the main responsibility for the statistical analyses. TBW participated in designing and planning the study with particular responsibility in the diagnostic work-up of delirium and subtyping. KT participated in designing and planning the study. OS is the project manager and designed the study. He also participated in diagnosing and subtyping of delirium. All authors have critically read and approved the final manuscript.

### Competing interests
The authors declare that they have no competing interests.

### Author details
[1]Department of Geriatrics, St. Olavs hospital, Trondheim University Hospital, Trondheim, Norway. [2]Department of Neuromedicine and Movement Science, Faculty of Medicine and Health Sciences, Norwegian University of Science and Technology (NTNU), N-7491 Trondheim, Norway. [3]Regional Centre for Child and Youth Mental Health and Child Welfare, NTNU, Norwegian University of Science and Technology, Trondheim, Norway. [4]Oslo Delirium Research Group, Department of Geriatric Medicine, Oslo University Hospital, Oslo, Norway. [5]Institute of Clinical Medicine, University of Oslo, Oslo, Norway.

### References
1.  Marcantonio ER. Delirium in hospitalized older adults. N Engl J Med. 2017; 377(15):1456–66.
2.  Inouye SK, Westendorp RG, Saczynski JS. Delirium in elderly people. Lancet. 2014;383(9920):911–22.
3.  Witlox J, Eurelings LS, de Jonghe JF, Kalisvaart KJ, Eikelenboom P, van Gool WA. Delirium in elderly patients and the risk of postdischarge mortality, institutionalization, and dementia: a meta-analysis. JAMA. 2010;304(4): 443–51.
4.  Oh ES, Fong TG, Hshieh TT, Inouye SK. Delirium in older persons: advances in diagnosis and treatment. JAMA. 2017;318(12):1161–74.
5.  Liptzin B, Levkoff SE. An empirical study of delirium subtypes. Br J Psychiatry. 1992;161:843–5.
6.  Bellelli G, Speciale S, Barisione E, Trabucchi M. Delirium subtypes and 1-year mortality among elderly patients discharged from a post-acute rehabilitation facility. J Gerontol A Biol Sci Med Sci. 2007;62(10):1182–3.
7.  Kiely DK, Jones RN, Bergmann MA, Marcantonio ER. Association between psychomotor activity delirium subtypes and mortality among newly admitted post-acute facility patients. J Gerontol A Biol Sci Med Sci. 2007; 62(2):174–9.
8.  Meagher DJ, Leonard M, Donnelly S, Conroy M, Adamis D, Trzepacz PT. A longitudinal study of motor subtypes in delirium: relationship with other phenomenology, etiology, medication exposure and prognosis. J Psychosom Res. 2011;71(6):395–403.
9.  Yang FM, Marcantonio ER, Inouye SK, Kiely DK, Rudolph JL, Fearing MA, Jones RN. Phenomenological subtypes of delirium in older persons: patterns, prevalence, and prognosis. Psychosomatics. 2009;50(3):248–54.
10. Meagher DJ, Leonard M, Donnelly S, Conroy M, Adamis D, Trzepacz PT. A longitudinal study of motor subtypes in delirium: frequency and stability during episodes. J Psychosom Res. 2012;72(3):236–41.
11. Morandi A, Di Santo SG, Cherubini A, Mossello E, Meagher D, Mazzone A, Bianchetti A, Ferrara N, Ferrari A, Musicco M, et al. Clinical features associated with delirium motor subtypes in older inpatients: results of a multicenter study. Am J Geriatr Psychiatry. 2017;25(10):1064–71.
12. Association AP. DSM-5 classification. Washington: American Psychiatric Publishing; 2013.
13. Hshieh TT, Yue J, Oh E, Puelle M, Dowal S, Travison T, Inouye SK. Effectiveness of multicomponent nonpharmacological delirium interventions: a meta-analysis. JAMA Intern Med. 2015;175(4):512–20.
14. Inouye SK, Bogardus ST Jr, Charpentier PA, Leo-Summers L, Acampora D, Holford TR, Cooney LM Jr. A multicomponent intervention to prevent delirium in hospitalized older patients. N Engl J Med. 1999;340(9):669–76.
15. McCusker J, Cole M, Abrahamowicz M, Han L, Podoba JE, Ramman-Haddad L. Environmental risk factors for delirium in hospitalized older people. J Am Geriatr Soc. 2001;49(10):1327–34.
16. Beresin EV. Delirium in the elderly. J Geriatr Psychiatry Neurol. 1988;1(3):127–43.
17. Goldberg A, Straus SE, Hamid JS, Wong CL. Room transfers and the risk of delirium incidence amongst hospitalized elderly medical patients: a case-control study. BMC Geriatr. 2015;15:69.
18. Bo M, Bonetto M, Bottignole G, Porrino P, Coppo E, Tibaldi M, Ceci G, Raspo S, Cappa G, Bellelli G. Length of stay in the emergency department and occurrence of delirium in older medical patients. J Am Geriatr Soc. 2016; 64(5):1114–9.
19. Maclullich AM, Ferguson KJ, Miller T, de Rooij SE, Cunningham C. Unravelling the pathophysiology of delirium: a focus on the role of aberrant stress responses. J Psychosom Res. 2008;65(3):229–38.

20. Carpenter CR, Bromley M, Caterino JM, Chun A, Gerson LW, Greenspan J, Hwang U, John DP, Lyons WL, Platts-Mills TF, et al. Optimal older adult emergency care: introducing multidisciplinary geriatric emergency department guidelines from the American College of Emergency Physicians, American Geriatrics Society, emergency nurses association, and Society for Academic Emergency Medicine. J Am Geriatr Soc. 2014;62(7):1360–3.

21. Ellis G, Gardner M, Tsiachristas A, Langhorne P, Burke O, Harwood RH, Conroy SP, Kircher T, Somme D, Saltvedt I, et al. Comprehensive geriatric assessment for older adults admitted to hospital. Cochrane Database Syst Rev. 2017;9:CD006211.

22. Evensen S, Sletvold O, Lydersen S, Taraldsen K. Physical activity among hospitalized older adults - an observational study. BMC Geriatr. 2017;17(1):110.

23. Hall RJ, Meagher DJ, MacLullich AM. Delirium detection and monitoring outside the ICU. Best Pract Res Clin Anaesthesiol. 2012;26(3):367–83.

24. Folstein MF, Folstein SE, McHugh PR. "Mini-mental state". A practical method for grading the cognitive state of patients for the clinician. J Psychiatr Res. 1975;12(3):189–98.

25. Inouye SK, Leo-Summers L, Zhang Y, Bogardus ST Jr, Leslie DL, Agostini JV. A chart-based method for identification of delirium: validation compared with interviewer ratings using the confusion assessment method. J Am Geriatr Soc. 2005;53(2):312–8.

26. Saczynski JS, Kosar CM, Xu G, Puelle MR, Schmitt E, Jones RN, Marcantonio ER, Wong B, Isaza I, Inouye SK. A tale of two methods: chart and interview methods for identifying delirium. J Am Geriatr Soc. 2014;62(3):518–24.

27. Meagher D, Moran M, Raju B, Leonard M, Donnelly S, Saunders J, Trzepacz P. A new data-based motor subtype schema for delirium. J Neuropsychiatry Clin Neurosci. 2008;20(2):185–93.

28. Reisberg B, Ferris SH, de Leon MJ, Crook T. The global deterioration scale for assessment of primary degenerative dementia. Am J Psychiatry. 1982; 139(9):1136–9.

29. Salvi F, Miller MD, Grilli A, Giorgi R, Towers AL, Morichi V, Spazzafumo L, Mancinelli L, Espinosa E, Rappelli A, et al. A manual of guidelines to score the modified cumulative illness rating scale and its validation in acute hospitalized elderly patients. J Am Geriatr Soc. 2008;56(10):1926–31.

30. Mahoney FI, Barthel DW. Functional evaluation: the Barthel index. Md State Med J. 1965;14:61–5.

31. Guralnik JM, Simonsick EM, Ferrucci L, Glynn RJ, Berkman LF, Blazer DG, Scherr PA, Wallace RB. A short physical performance battery assessing lower extremity function: association with self-reported disability and prediction of mortality and nursing home admission. J Gerontol. 1994;49(2):M85–94.

32. Knaus WA, Draper EA, Wagner DP, Zimmerman JE. APACHE II: a severity of disease classification system. Crit Care Med. 1985;13(10):818–29.

33. Siddiqi N, Harrison JK, Clegg A, Teale EA, Young J, Taylor J, Simpkins SA. Interventions for preventing delirium in hospitalised non-ICU patients. Cochrane Database Syst Rev. 2016;3:CD005563.

# 24

# Serum cystatin C, impaired kidney function, and geriatric depressive symptoms among older people living in a rural area: a population-based study

Ling Wu[1,2], Zhongrui Yan[2]* (iD), Hui Jiang[3], Huaimei Xing[1,2], Haohao Li[1,2] and Chengxuan Qiu[4,5]*

## Abstract

**Background:** The relationship between kidney function and depressive symptoms among elderly people has been rarely investigated in settings of the general population. The aim of our study was to examine the association of serum cystatin C (cysC) and impaired kidney function with geriatric depressive symptoms among older people living in a rural community in China.

**Methods:** This population-based cohort study included 1440 individuals (age $\geq$ 60 years) who were recruited for the Confucius Hometown Aging Project in 2010–2011; of the 1124 persons who were free of depressive symptoms, 669 (59.5%) were re-examined in 2014–2016. At baseline, data on demographics, lifestyle factors, health conditions, and medical history were collected through interviews, clinical examinations, and laboratory tests. We defined impaired kidney function as the cystatin C-based estimated glomerular filtration rate ($eGFR_{cysC}$) < 60 ml/min/1. 73 $m^2$, and depressive symptoms as a score $\geq$ 5 on the 15-item Geriatric Depression Scale. Data were analyzed using multiple logistic and Cox proportional-hazards models.

**Results:** Of the 1440 participants, 316 (21.9%) were defined to have geriatric depressive symptoms at baseline. Serum cysC levels of 1.01–1.25 and > 1.25 mg/L (vs. $\leq$1.00 mg/L) were associated with a multiple-adjusted odds ratio (OR) of 1.41 (95% CI 1.01–1.97) and 3.20 (2.32–4.41), respectively, for having geriatric depressive symptoms ($P_{trend}$ < 0.001). Of the 669 people who were free of depressive symptoms at baseline, 157 had incident depressive symptoms at the follow-up examination. The multiple-adjusted hazard ratio (HR) for incident depressive symptoms were 2.16 (95% CI 1.43–3.27) for serum cysC > 1.25 mg/L (vs. < 1.00 mg/L). Impaired kidney function was cross-sectionally (multiple-adjusted OR = 2.95; 95% CI 2.22–3.92) and longitudinally (multiple-adjusted HR 1.54; 95% CI 1. 03–2.30) associated with an increased risk of geriatric depressive symptoms.

**Conclusion:** Elevated serum cysC levels and impaired kidney function are associated with an increased risk of geriatric depressive symptoms among Chinese older people living in a rural community.

**Keywords:** Aging, Cystatin C, Kidney function, Depressive symptoms, Cohort study, China

* Correspondence: zhongruiy@163.com; chengxuan.qiu@ki.se
[2]Department of Neurology, Jining No. 1 People's Hospital, Jiankang Road 6, Jining 272111, Shandong, China
[4]Department of Neurology, Shandong Provincial Hospital, Jinan, Shandong, China
Full list of author information is available at the end of the article

# Background

As population ages, geriatric depression has become a public health concern. Depression in older people is related not only to poor health-related quality of life [1], but also to morbidity, mortality, and even suicide [2]. The Global Burden of Disease 2010 study identified that depressive disorder was a leading cause of years lived with disability (YLDs), and that major depressive disorder accounted for 8.2% of global YLDs [3]. In China, the meta-analyses showed that the prevalence of depression ranges from ~ 20% to ~ 30% among older adults living in communities, with the pooled prevalence being ~ 23% [4, 5]. However, depression has been both underdiagnosed and undertreated in primary care settings owing to common co-occurrence with other geriatric conditions in older adults [6]. Therefore, it is particularly important to identify risk factors related to geriatric depression for possible intervention.

Chronic kidney disease or decreased renal function is increasingly common as people age [7]. In US, chronic kidney disease, defined as an estimated glomerular filtration rate (eGFR) $< 60$ mL/min/1.73 m$^2$, affected nearly one-third of community-dwelling adults aged over 70 years [8]. However, only a few population-based studies have so far examined the relationship between kidney function and depression in older adults, with mixed results. For instance, a cross-sectional study of Chinese older people aged 70–84 years indicated that eGFR $< 60$ mL/min/1.73 m$^2$ was associated with depressive symptoms [9], whereas the Singapore Longitudinal Aging Study found no association between the serum creatinine-based eGFR and depressive symptoms (defined as the 15-item Geriatric Depression Scale [GDS-15] score $\geq 5$) [10], and the cross-sectional survey of people over 60 years of age with diabetes in US suggested that only very low eGFR ($< 29$ mL/min/1.73 m$^2$) was associated with an increased risk of depressive symptoms [11]. However, the population-based longitudinal studies of the relationship between measures of kidney function and geriatric depressive symptoms in older adults are still lacking, especially among Chinese elderly people living in rural areas.

Therefore, we hypothesize that increased serum cystatin C or impaired kidney function is associated with an increased risk of geriatric depressive symptoms in older people. We sought to test this hypothesis in this population-based cohort study of older adults who were living in a rural community in China.

# Methods

## Study participants

This is a population-based cohort study. Study participants were derived from the Confucius Hometown Aging Project (CHAP), as fully described elsewhere [12].

Briefly, CHAP was aimed at exploring the role of cardiovascular risk factors and atherosclerotic mechanisms in aging and health. In the current study, we sought to specifically examine the associations of baseline serum cysC levels and impaired kidney function with depressive symptoms both at the baseline (cross-sectional association) and the follow-up (longitudinal association) examinations. At baseline (2010–2011), 1440 (82.6%) of the 1743 eligible participants who were aged $\geq 60$ years and were living in the Xing Long Zhuang community nearby Qufu city (the hometown of Confucius) in Shandong, China were examined for CHAP; of these, 316 persons were defined to have depressive symptoms (GDS-15 score $\geq 5$). In 2014–2016, we carried out the second wave of assessment in the same community for residents who were aged $\geq 60$ years in June 2014, following a procedure similar to that of the baseline survey. In total, 669 (59.5%) of the 1124 persons who were free of depressive symptoms at baseline underwent the follow-up examination. Figure 1 shows the flowchart of the study participants from baseline to the follow-up assessments.

Data collection for all phases of the CHAP study was approved by the Ethics Committee at the Jining No. 1 People's Hospital of Jining Medical University, Shandong, China. Written informed consent was obtained from all participants, or in the case of cognitively impaired persons, from a proxy (usually next-of-kin).

## Data collection and definition

At baseline, data were collected by trained physicians through face-to-face interviews, clinical examination, and laboratory tests, as previously described [12]. We collected data on demographics, lifestyle factors (e.g. smoking and alcohol consumption), health conditions and health history (e.g. hypertension, diabetes, heart disease, stroke, cataract, chronic obstructive pulmonary disease (COPD), arthritis, nephritis, and tumor), and use of medications (e.g., antihypertensive agents and blood glucose-lowering drugs) following a structured questionnaire. Arterial blood pressure was measured twice in the sitting position after resting for at least 5 min, and the mean value of the two measurements was used for analysis. Peripheral blood samples were taken after an overnight fast, and fasting plasma glucose (FPG), serum cystatin C (cysC), high-density lipoprotein (HDL), low-density lipoprotein (LDL), and creatinine were analyzed using the enzymatic methods by an Automatic Biochemistry Analyzer (Olympus AU-400, Japan).

Body mass index (BMI) was calculated as the measured body weight in kilograms divided by the square of height in meters (kg/m$^2$). Smoking status was divided into never and ever (current or former) smoking. Alcohol consumption was assessed based on the frequency

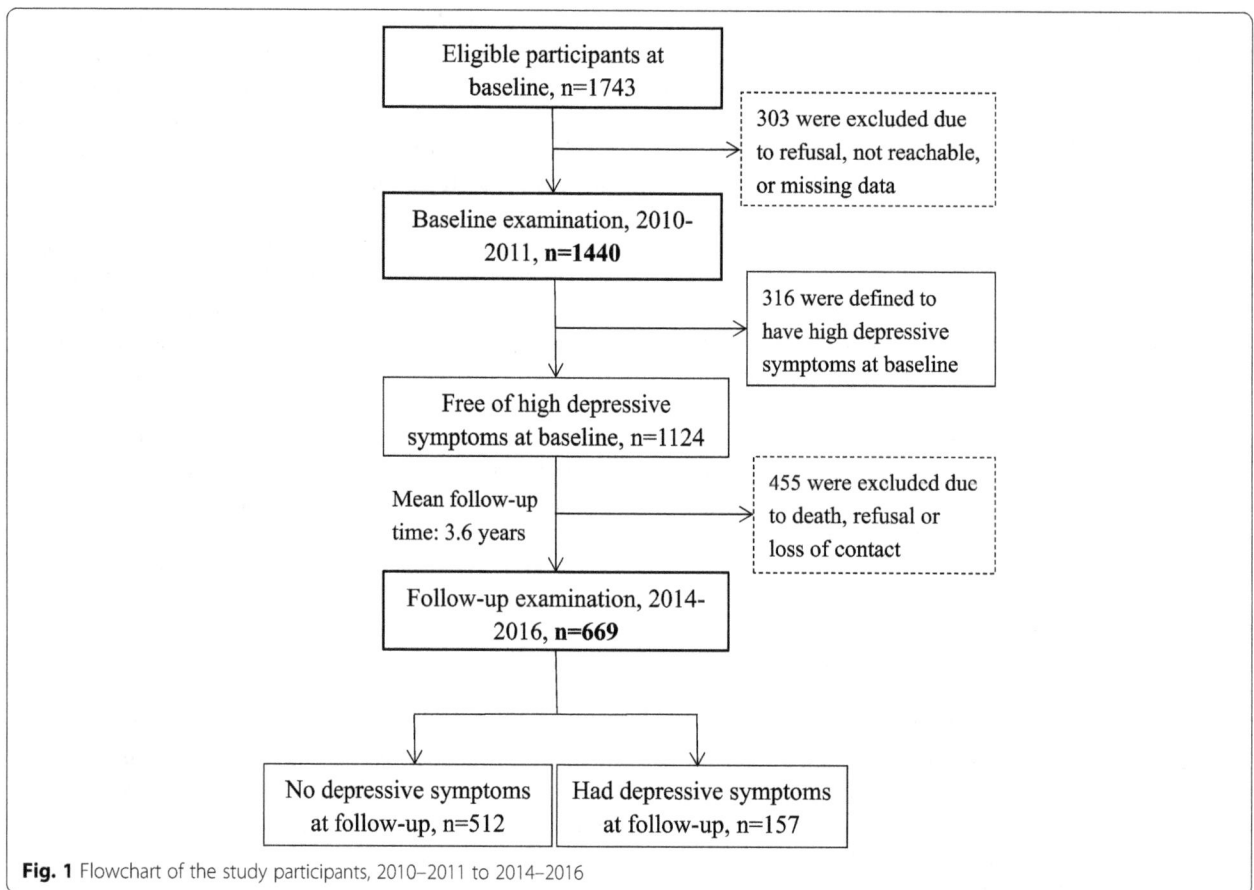

**Fig. 1** Flowchart of the study participants, 2010–2011 to 2014–2016

and amount of alcohol intake in a typical day and was dichotomized into yes vs. no. Hypertension was defined as blood pressure ≥ 140/90 mmHg or currently using antihypertensive drugs [13]. Diabetes was defined as having a self-reported history of physician's diagnosis of diabetes, FPG ≥7.0 mmol/L or current use of hypoglycemic agents or insulin injection [14]. Heart disease, stroke, cataract, COPD, nephritis, and tumor were ascertained through clinical examination, electrocardiogram test, or self-reported physician's diagnosis or currently taking relevant medications.

Global cognitive function was assessed using the validated Chinese version of the Mini-Mental State Examination (MMSE) [15]. Cognitive impairment was defined according to the education-based cutoff scores on MMSE [16], i.e., an MMSE score ≤ 17 for persons without formal schooling, ≤20 for those with 1–6 years of education, and ≤ 24 for those with ≥7 years of education. Physical functioning was assessed using the Katz's basic activities of daily living (ADL) [17], which involves six self-care activities of bathing, dressing, toileting, continence, transferring, and self-feeding. Participants who were not able to carry out at least one of the six tasks were considered to have disability in basic ADL.

## Kidney function

We calculated the eGFR according to the following equations based on serum cysC (eGFR$_{cysC}$) [18]: eGFR$_{cysC}$ = 133× $(cysC/0.8)^{-0.499}$ × $0.996^{age}$ [× 0.932 if female] (if cysC ≤0.8 mg/L); eGFR$_{cysC}$ = 133 × $(cysC/0.8)^{-1.328}$ × $0.996^{age}$ [× 0.932 if female] (if cysC > 0.8 mg/L). Impaired kidney function was defined as eGFR$_{cysC}$ < 60 ml/min/1.73 m$^2$ [19].

## Geriatric depressive symptoms

The GDS-15 tool was used to assess the presence of geriatric depressive symptoms at both baseline and follow-up examinations. We considered depressive symptoms to be present if a GDS-15 score ≥ 5, a cut-off that has been widely used for screening depression in older adults, with fairly high sensitivity and specificity (ranging from ∼ 75% to ∼ 95%) when evaluated against the clinical criteria (e.g., DSM-IV criteria) [10, 20–22].

## Statistical analysis

Baseline characteristics of study participants by having depressive symptoms at baseline were compared using t test for continuous variables and χ$^2$ test for categorical variables. We categorized the serum cysC level into ≤1.0, 1.01–1.25, and > 1.25 mg/L [23]. We examined both cross-sectional and longitudinal associations of serum cysC and impaired kidney function with geriatric depressive symptoms. For the cross-sectional association, we used multiple logistic regression model to estimate the odds ratio (OR) and 95% confidence interval (CI) of having geriatric depressive symptoms associated with baseline serum cysC levels and impaired kidney function. To explore the longitudinal association, Cox proportional-hazards models were constructed in participants who were free of depressive symptoms at baseline to estimate the hazard ratio (HR) and 95% CI of having depressive symptoms at the follow-up associated with serum cysC levels and impaired kidney function at baseline. In the Cox models, the follow-up time from the date of baseline assessment to the date of follow-up examination was used as the time scale. For both cross-sectional and longitudinal associations, we reported results from three models, in which we controlled for different factors that potentially confounded the examined associations: model 1 was controlled for age, gender, and education (in years); model 2 was additionally controlled for alcohol consumption and history of chronic diseases

(e.g. hypertension, heart disease, stroke, cataract, nephritis, arthritis, COPD); and model 3 was further controlled for MMSE score and ADL-disability. We considered $p < 0.05$ ($\alpha$) for a two-tailed test to be statistically significant. IBM SPSS Statistics 19.0 for Windows (Armonk, NY: IBM Corp.) was used for all analyses.

## Results

At baseline, the mean age of the 1440 participants was 68.5 years (SD, 4.9), and 60% were women. Of them, 316 had geriatric depressive symptoms, which resulted in the overall prevalence of 21.9%, with the prevalence being higher in women than in men (24.8% vs. 17.7%, $p = 0.002$). Compared with people without geriatric depressive symptoms, those with depressive symptoms were older and had a higher prevalence of chronic health conditions (e.g., hypertension, heart disease, stroke, COPD, cataract, arthritis, and ADL-disability) (Table 1). Furthermore, people with depressive symptoms had a higher level of LDL, serum cysC, and creatinine, but a lower level of HDL, $eGFR_{cysC}$, and MMSE score than those

**Table 1** Baseline characteristics of study participants according to depressive symptoms at baseline

| Characteristics | Total sample | Depressive symptoms | | |
| --- | --- | --- | --- | --- |
| | (n = 1440) | No (n = 1124) | Yes (n = 316) | p-value |
| Female, n (%) | 864 (60.0) | 650 (75.2) | 214 (24.8) | 0.002 |
| Age (years), mean (SD) | 68.5 (4.9) | 68.3 (4.9) | 69.4 (5.1) | 0.001 |
| Education (years), mean (SD) | 3.9 (3.4) | 4.0 (3.4) | 3.7 (3.3) | 0.180 |
| BMI (kg/m²), mean (SD) | 26.4 (8.1) | 26.5 (8.9) | 26.2 (4.2) | 0.599 |
| Current smoking[a], n (%) | 206 (14.3) | 162 (14.4) | 44 (13.9) | 0.970 |
| Alcohol consumption[a], n (%) | 299 (20.8) | 247 (22.0) | 52 (16.5) | 0.018 |
| Hypertension, n (%) | 768 (53.3) | 573 (51.0) | 195 (61.7) | 0.001 |
| Diabetes, n (%) | 322 (22.4) | 246 (21.9) | 76 (24.1) | 0.415 |
| Heart disease[a], n (%) | 486 (33.8) | 357 (31.8) | 129 (40.8) | 0.009 |
| Stroke[a], n (%) | 124 (8.6) | 86 (7.7) | 38 (12.0) | 0.044 |
| Cataract, n (%) | 200 (13.9) | 145 (12.9) | 55 (17.4) | 0.041 |
| COPD[a], n (%) | 199 (13.8) | 142 (12.6) | 57 (18.0) | 0.029 |
| Arthritis[a], n (%) | 518 (36.0) | 384 (34.2) | 134 (42.4) | 0.015 |
| Nephritis[a], n (%) | 69 (4.8) | 52 (4.6) | 17 (5.4) | 0.763 |
| Tumor, n (%) | 51 (3.5) | 37 (3.3) | 14 (4.4) | 0.333 |
| cysC (mg/L), mean (SD) | 0.99 (0.29) | 0.97 (0.29) | 1.09 (0.26) | < 0.001 |
| HDL (mmol/L), mean (SD) | 1.49 (0.44) | 1.50 (0.42) | 1.44 (0.49) | 0.023 |
| LDL (mmol/L), mean (SD) | 2.69 (0.85) | 2.67 (0.85) | 2.78 (0.87) | 0.045 |
| Creatinine (µmol/L), mean (SD) | 70.5 (21.8) | 69.7 (22.8) | 73.3 (17.7) | 0.010 |
| eGFR (ml/min/1.73 m²), mean (SD) | 81.3 (30.6) | 84.2 (31.7) | 71.2 (23.4) | < 0.001 |
| MMSE score, mean (SD) | 26.2 (4.5) | 26.4 (4.4) | 25.5 (4.8) | 0.002 |
| ADL-disability, n (%) | 32 (2.2) | 12 (1.1) | 20 (6.3) | < 0.001 |

*Abbreviations: BMI* body mass index, *COPD* chronic obstructive pulmonary disease, *cysC* cystatin C, *HDL* high-density lipoprotein, *LDL* low-density lipoprotein, *eGFR* estimated glomerular filtration rate, *MMSE* mini-mental state examination, *ADL* activities of daily living
[a]Numbers of subjects with missing values were 5 for smoking, 11 for alcohol consumption, 1 for stroke, 3 for heart disease, 4 for COPD, 2 for arthritis, and 3 for nephritis. In the subsequent analyses, subjects with missing values were placed in the non-exposure group

without depressive symptoms. The two groups had no significant difference in educational level, BMI, smoking, diabetes, nephritis, and tumor (Table 1).

For the baseline cross-sectional relationship, compared to people with serum cysC level of $\leq 1.00$ mg/l, those with levels of 1.01–1.25 and > 1.25 mg/l had an increased likelihood of having geriatric depressive symptoms, with the multiple-adjusted OR (95% CI) being 1.41 (1.01–1.97) and 3.20 (2.32–4.41), respectively ($p$ for linear trend < 0.001). Impaired kidney function (eGFR$_{cysC}$ < 60 ml/min/1.73 m$^2$) was significantly associated with an increased likelihood of having depressive symptoms (multiple-adjusted OR = 2.95; 95% CI 2.22–3.92) (Table 2).

At an average 3.6 years (SD, 0.62) of follow-up, 157 out of the 669 persons who had no depressive symptoms at baseline were ascertained to have incident geriatric depressive symptoms. People who developed incident depressive symptoms at the follow-up were more likely to be female and to have lower education than those who did not. Cox regression analysis suggested that having an elevated serum cysC level (> 1.25 vs. < 1.00 mg/L) was significantly associated with an increased HR of having incident depressive symptoms, even in model 3 when controlling for multiple potential confounders (HR = 2.16, 95% CI 1.43–3.27) ($p$ for linear trend < 0.001) (Table 3). Impaired kidney function at baseline was significantly associated with a 54% increased risk of incident geriatric depressive symptoms detected at the follow-up assessment (multiple-adjusted HR 1.54; 95% CI 1.03–2.30) (Table 3).

## Discussion

In this community-based cohort study, we found that geriatric depressive symptoms affected more than one-fifth of Chinese older adults who were living in a rural area. In addition, both the cross-sectional and longitudinal data suggested that higher levels of serum cysC were associated with an increased risk of having geriatric depressive symptoms in a dose-response manner, even after adjusting for multiple potential confounders, including sociodemographic factors, lifestyles, cardiovascular disorders, cognitive function, and physical disability. Finally, impaired kidney function, when assessed based on eGFR$_{cysC}$, was associated with both prevalent and incident geriatric depressive symptoms, independent of multiple confounders. This study suggests that high serum cysC levels and impaired kidney function may be risk factors for depressive symptoms in geriatric populations.

The relationship between renal function and depression among older adults has rarely been explored so far in the general population settings. The cross-sectional data from the Maastricht Study of older adults indicated that albuminuria was associated with incidence of depressive symptoms, whereas the reduced eGFR based on creatinine and cystatin C (eGFR$_{Cr-cysC}$) was not associated with minor or major depressive episodes [24]. The follow-up data from the US Health, Aging and Body Composition Study of community-dwelling older adults suggested that an elevated serum cysC level was associated with a 2-fold increased risk of depression, but impaired renal function, assessed based on eGFR$_{Cr-cysC}$ < 60 ml/min/1.73 m$^2$, was not related to depression [25]. Of note, some of the previous studies that do not show an association between reduced eGFR and depressive symptoms in older adults have used either serum creatinine or a combination of serum creatinine and cysC to assess eGFR [10, 24, 25]. Because creatinine excretion

**Table 2** Cross-sectional associations of serum cystatin C and impaired kidney function with prevalent geriatric depressive symptoms ($n = 1440$)

| Serum cystatin C or impaired kidney function | N/n | Odds ratio (95% confidence interval) | | |
|---|---|---|---|---|
| | | Model 1[a] | Model 2[a] | Model 3[a] |
| Cystatin C, mg/L | | | | |
| ≤ 1.00 | 768/119 | 1.00 (reference) | 1.00 (reference) | 1.00 (reference) |
| 1.01–1.25 | 360/79 | 1.43 (1.03–1.98) | 1.40 (1.004–1.95) | 1.41 (1.009–1.97) |
| > 1.25 | 312/118 | 3.25 (2.39–4.42) | 3.30 (2.40–4.50) | 3.20 (2.32–4.41) |
| P for trend | | < 0.001 | < 0.001 | < 0.001 |
| Impaired kidney function | | | | |
| No | 1070/176 | 1.00 (reference) | 1.00 (reference) | 1.00 (reference) |
| Yes | 370/140 | 3.07 (2.34–4.03) | 3.03 (2.30–4.01) | 2.95 (2.22–3.92) |

N/n indicates number of subjects/number of persons with depressive symptoms
*Abbreviations*: *MMSE* mini-mental state examination, *ADL* activities of daily living
[a]Model 1 was adjusted for age, sex, and education; model 2 was additionally adjusted for alcohol consumption, hypertension, stroke, heart disease, cataract, chronic obstructive pulmonary disease, nephritis, and arthritis; and in model 3, MMSE score and ADL-disability were added to model 2

**Table 3** Longitudinal associations of serum cystatin C and impaired kidney function with incident geriatric depressive symptoms ($n = 669$)

| Serum cystatin C or impaired kidney function | N/n | Hazard ratio (95% confidence interval) | | |
|---|---|---|---|---|
| | | Model 1[a] | Model 2[a] | Model 3[a] |
| Cystatin C, mg/L | | | | |
| ≤ 1.00 | 388/78 | 1.00 (reference) | 1.00 (reference) | 1.00 (reference) |
| 1.01–1.25 | 175/40 | 1.11 (0.75–1.65) | 1.22 (0.82–1.81) | 1.21 (0.81–1.80) |
| > 1.25 | 106/39 | 2.20 (1.48–3.27) | 2.23 (1.48–3.34) | 2.16 (1.43–3.27) |
| p for linear trend | | 0.001 | 0.001 | 0.001 |
| Impaired kidney function | | | | |
| No | 544/122 | 1.00 (reference) | 1.00 (reference) | 1.00 (reference) |
| Yes | 125/35 | 1.57 (1.06–2.32) | 1.57 (1.05–2.34) | 1.54 (1.03–2.30) |

N/n indicates number of subjects/number of persons with depressive symptoms
*Abbreviations*: MMSE mini-mental state examination, ADL activities of daily living
[a]Model 1 was adjusted for age, sex, and education; model 2 was additionally adjusted for alcohol consumption, hypertension, stroke, heart disease, cataract, chronic obstructive pulmonary disease, nephritis, and arthritis; and in model 3, MMSE score and ADL-disability were added to model 2

is dependent on age, muscle mass, and nutritional status, especially among older adults, serum cysC has been considered to be more accurate and more sensitive in assessing renal function [26, 27]. Indeed, we did not find any association between serum creatinine and depressive symptoms (data not shown). When estimating the eGFR based on serum cysC, we found that reduced eGFR$_{cysC}$ or impaired kidney function was associated both cross-sectionally and longitudinally with an increased risk of having geriatric depressive symptoms among Chinese older adults. This is consistent with a cross-sectional study among Chinese older people (age 70–84 years), in which impaired kidney function was associated with a 1.71-fold increased likelihood of having depressive symptoms (GDS-15 score ≥ 5) [9].

The biological and pathological mechanisms linking serum cysC and impaired kidney function with geriatric depressive symptoms are not fully understood, but multiple pathways are supposed to be involved. First, impaired kidney function or reduced eGFR$_{cysC}$ due to glomerular small vessel disease has been correlated with subclinical cerebral microvascular disease in older adults [28, 29]. Further, cerebral microvascular dysfunction and diseases in brain regions involved in mood regulation were associated with late-life depression ("vascular depression") [30, 31]. Thus, impaired kidney function or reduced eGFR might be linked with late-life depressive symptoms through cerebral small vessel disease. Second, serum cysC, as a cysteine protease inhibitor, affects the migration of neutrophils and involves the inflammatory process [32, 33], which may impair function of the brain-serotonin system and stimulate the activation of the hypothalamus-pituitary-adrenal axis to cause depressive symptoms through inflammation pathway [34]. In addition, the population-based studies of older adults

have linked inflammatory markers (e.g., C-reactive protein, IL-6, and TNF-α receptor 1) with elevated serum cysC or impaired kidney function defined by eGFR$_{cysC}$ [35, 36]. The meta-analysis of population-based studies also supported an association of several inflammatory markers with depression in older adults [37], suggesting the involvement of inflammation in the development of depression. Thus, inflammatory mechanisms may mediate the relationship between serum cysC and depressive symptoms. Of note, our data showed that the association of high serum cysC and impaired kidney function with depressive symptoms was present independent of the inflammation-related diseases such as atherosclerotic disorders, arthritis, and cognitive and functional impairment, suggesting that additional pathways may be involved in linking high serum cysC with geriatric depressive symptoms.

Our cohort study involved both cross-sectional and longitudinal data of older adults who were living in a rural area in China. Moreover, we collected comprehensive data (e.g., demographics, lifestyles, health history, and cognitive and physical functioning) following a standard approach. Thus, we were able to control for a broad range of potential confounding factors. However, our study also has limitations. First, we used GDS-15 to assess geriatric depressive symptoms instead of a clinical diagnosis of depression, although the GDS-15 cut-off score ≥ 5, as a widely screening instrument for major depressive disorders in older adults, did show high sensitivity and specificity in geriatric populations [10, 21, 22]. Second, we used the cysC-based eGFR as an approximation of glomerular filtration rate instead of a direct measurement, although eGFR has been widely used to define kidney function. Finally, the study population was derived from a single rural community in Eastern China, where people had relatively low education and low socioeconomic position. Thus, caution is needed when generalizing our results to other populations.

## Conclusion

This population-based cohort study showed that depressive symptoms were common among Chinese older adults living in a rural community and that high serum cysC levels and impaired kidney function (assessed using serum cysC-based eGFR) were associated with an increased risk of having geriatric depressive symptoms. While our findings warrant further confirmation in other populations, this study suggests that psychological interventions among older adults with impaired kidney function may help reduce the risk of geriatric depression.

### Abbreviations
ADL: Activities of daily living; BMI: Body mass index; CHAP: The Confucius Hometown Aging Project; CI: Confidence interval; COPD: Chronic obstructive pulmonary disease; CysC: Cystatin C; eGFR$_{cysC}$: Cystatin C-based estimated glomerular filtration rate; FPG: Fasting plasma glucose; GDS-15: The 15-item Geriatric Depression Scale; HDL: High-density lipoprotein; HR: Hazard ratio; LDL: Low-density lipoprotein; MMSE: Mini-Mental State Examination; OR: Odds ratio

### Acknowledgements
The authors would like to thank all the study participants for their contribution to the Confucius Hometown Aging Project.

### Funding
The Confucius Hometown Aging Project (CHAP) was supported in part by grants from the Department of Science and Technology (2008GG30002058), the Department of Health (2009–067), and the Department of Natural Science Foundation (ZR2010HL031) in Shandong, China and by the Young Scholar Grant for Strategic Research in Epidemiology at Karolinska Institutet, Stockholm, Sweden. Dr. C Qiu received grants from the Swedish Research Council (grants no.: 2017–00740 and 2017–05819), the Swedish Research Council for Health, Working Life and Welfare (grant no.: 2014–01382), Stockholm, Sweden, and the Taishan Scholar Program of Shandong Province, China.

### Authors' contributions
LW, ZY, and CQ designed the study. ZY and HJ obtained the data. LW, HX, and HL analyzed the data. LW and CQ drafted the paper. LW, HX, and HL had full access to all the data in this study and take responsibility for the integrity of the data and accuracy of the data analysis. ZY and CQ supervised this study. All authors made critical revisions and approved the submission.

### Competing interests
The authors declare that they have no competing interests.

### Author details
[1]Cheeloo College of Medicine, Shandong University, Jinan, Shandong, China. [2]Department of Neurology, Jining No. 1 People's Hospital, Jiankang Road 6, Jining 272111, Shandong, China. [3]Xing Long Zhuang Hospital, Shandong Yankuang Group, Jining, Shandong, China. [4]Department of Neurology, Shandong Provincial Hospital, Jinan, Shandong, China. [5]Aging Research Center, Department of Neurobiology, Care Sciences and Society, Karolinska Institutet-Stockholm University, Widerströmska Huset, Tomtebodavägen 18A, 171 65 Solna, Sweden.

## References

1. Sivertsen H, Bjørkløf GH, Engedal K, Selbæk G, Helvik AS. Depression and quality of life in older persons: a review. Dement Geriatr Cogn Disord. 2015; 40:311–39.
2. Fiske A, Wetherell JL, Gatz M. Depression in older adults. Annu Rev Clin Psychol. 2009;5:363–89.
3. Ferrari AJ, Charlson FJ, Norman RE, Patten SB, Freedman G, Murray CJ, Vos T, Whiteford HA. Burden of depressive disorders by country, sex, age, and year: findings from the global burden of disease study 2010. PLoS Med. 2013;10: e1001547.
4. Li D, Zhang DJ, Shao JJ, Qi XD, Tian L. A meta-analysis of the prevalence of depressive symptoms in Chinese older adults. Arch Gerontol Geriatr. 2014;58:1–9.
5. Zhang L, Xu Y, Nie H, Zhang Y, Wu Y. The prevalence of depressive symptoms among the older in China: a meta-analysis. Int J Geriatr Psychiatry. 2012;27:900–6.
6. Kok RM, Reynolds CF 3rd. Management of depression in older adults: a review. JAMA. 2017;317:2114–22.
7. Bowling CB, Sharma P, Fox CS, O'Hare AM, Muntner P. Prevalence of reduced estimated glomerular filtration rate among the oldest old from 1988-1994 through 2005-2010. JAMA. 2013;310:1284–6.
8. Coresh J, Selvin E, Stevens LA, Manzi J, Kusek JW, Eggers P, Van Lente F, Levey AS. Prevalence of chronic kidney disease in the United States. JAMA. 2007;298:2038–47.
9. Liu Q, Li YX, Hu ZH, Jiang XY, Li SJ, Wang XF. Reduced estimated glomerular filtration rate is associated with depressive symptoms in elder Chinese: a population-based cross-sectional study. Neurosci Lett. 2017;666:127–32.
10. Feng L, Yap KB, Ng TP. Depressive symptoms in older adults with chronic kidney disease: mortality, quality of life outcomes, and correlates. Am J Geriatr Psychiatry. 2013;21:570–9.
11. Campbell KH, Huang ES, Dale W, Parker MM, John PM, Young BA, Moffet HH, Laiteerapong N, Karter AJ. Association between estimated GFR, health-related quality of life, and depression among older adults with diabetes: the diabetes and aging study. Am J Kidney Dis. 2013;62:541–8.
12. Liang Y, Yan Z, Sun B, Cai C, Jiang H, Song A, Qiu C. Cardiovascular risk factor profiles for peripheral artery disease and carotid atherosclerosis among Chinese older people: a population-based study. PLoS One. 2014;9:e85927.
13. Wang R, Yan Z, Liang Y, Tan EC, Cai C, Jiang H, Song A, Qiu C. Prevalence and patterns of chronic disease pairs and multimorbidity among older Chinese adults living in a rural area. PLoS One. 2015;10:e0138521.
14. Song A, Liang Y, Yan Z, Sun B, Cai C, Jiang H, Qiu C. Highly prevalent and poorly controlled cardiovascular risk factors among Chinese elderly people living in the rural community. Eur J Prev Cardiol. 2014;21:1267–74.
15. Yan Z, Liang Y, Shi J, Cai C, Jiang H, Song A, Qiu C. Carotid stenosis and cognitive impairment amongst older Chinese adults living in a rural area: a population-based study. Eur J Neurol. 2016;23:201–4.
16. Cui GH, Yao YH, Xu RF, Tang HD, Jiang GX, Wang Y, Wang G, Chen SD, Cheng Q. Cognitive impairment using education-based cutoff points for CMMSE scores in elderly Chinese people of agricultural and rural Shanghai China. Acta Neurol Scand. 2011;124:361–7.
17. Welmer AK, Liang Y, Angleman S, Santoni G, Yan Z, Cai C, Qiu C. Vascular risk factor burden, atherosclerosis, and functional dependence in old age: a population-based study. Int J Behav Med. 2014;21:597–604.
18. Inker LA, Schmid CH, Tighiouart H, Eckfeldt JH, Feldman HI, Greene T, Kusek JW, Manzi J, Van Lente F, Zhang YL, et al. Estimating glomerular filtration rate from serum creatinine and cystatin C. N Engl J Med. 2012;367:20–9.
19. Yin Z, Yan Z, Liang Y, Jiang H, Cai C, Song A, Feng L, Qiu C. Interactive effects of diabetes and impaired kidney function on cognitive performance in old age: a population-based study. BMC Geriatr. 2016;16:7.
20. Feng L, Yan Z, Sun B, Cai C, Jiang H, Kua EH, Ng TP, Qiu C. Tea consumption and depressive symptoms in older people in rural China. J Am Geriatr Soc. 2013;61:1943–7.
21. Nyunt MS, Fones C, Niti M, Ng TP. Criterion-based validity and reliability of the geriatric depression screening scale (GDS-15) in a large validation sample of community-living Asian older adults. Aging Ment Health. 2009;13:376–82.
22. Marc LG, Raue PJ, Bruce ML. Screening performance of the 15-item geriatric depression scale in a diverse elderly home care population. Am J Geriatr Psychiatry. 2008;16:914–21.
23. Yaffe K, Lindquist K, Shlipak MG, Simonsick E, Fried L, Rosano C, Satterfield S, Atkinson H, Windham BG, Kurella-Tamura M. Cystatin C as a marker of

cognitive function in elders: findings from the health ABC study. Ann Neurol. 2008;63:798–802.

24. Martens RJH, Kooman JP, Stehouwer CDA, Dagnelie PC, van der Kallen CJH, Kroon AA, Leunissen KML, van der Sande FM, Schaper NC, Sep SJS, et al. Albuminuria is associated with a higher prevalence of depression in a population-based cohort study: the Maastricht study. Nephrol Dial Transplant. 2018;33:128–38.

25. Minev E, Unruh M, Shlipak MG, Simsonick E, Yaffe K, Leak TS, Newman AB, Fried LF, Health ABC Study. Association of cystatin C and depression in healthy elders: the health, aging and body composition study. Nephron Clin Pract. 2010;116:c241–6.

26. Onopiuk A, Tokarzewicz A, Gorodkiewicz E. Cystatin C: a kidney function biomarker. Adv Clin Chem. 2015;68:57–69.

27. Rule AD, Rodeheffer RJ, Larson TS, Burnett JC Jr, Cosio FG, Turner ST, Jacobsen SJ. Limitations of estimating glomerular filtration rate from serum creatinine in the general population. Mayo Clin Proc. 2006;81:1427–34.

28. Akoudad S, Sedaghat S, Hofman A, Koudstaal PJ, van der Lugt A, Ikram MA, Vernooij MW. Kidney function and cerebral small vessel disease in the general population. Int J Stroke. 2015;10:603–8.

29. Wada M, Nagasawa H, Kawanami T, Kurita K, Daimon M, Kubota I, Kayama T, Kato T. Cystatin C as an index of cerebral small vessel disease: results of a cross-sectional study in community-based Japanese elderly. Eur J Neurol. 2010;17:383–90.

30. van Agtmaal MJM, Houben AJHM, Pouwer F, Stehouwer CDA, Schram MT. Association of microvascular dysfunction with late-life depression: a systematic review and meta-analysis. JAMA Psychiatry. 2017;74:729–39.

31. Aizenstein HJ, Baskys A, Boldrini M, Butters MA, Diniz BS, Jaiswal MK, Jellinger KA, Kruglov LS, Meshandin IA, Mijajlovic MD, et al. Vascular depression consensus report - a critical update. BMC Med. 2016;14:161.

32. Arpegård J, Ostergren J, de Faire U, Hansson LO, Svensson P. Cystatin C–a marker of peripheral atherosclerotic disease? Atherosclerosis. 2008;199:397–401.

33. Yalcin S, Ulas T, Eren MA, Aydogan H, Camuzcuoglu A, Kucuk A, Yuce HH, Demir ME, Vural M, Aksoy N. Relationship between oxidative stress parameters and cystatin C levels in patients with severe preeclampsia. Medicina (Kaunas). 2013;49:118–23.

34. van Dooren FE, Schram MT, Schalkwijk CG, Stehouwer CD, Henry RM, Dagnelie PC, Schaper NC, van der Kallen CJ, Koster A, Sep SJ, et al. Associations of low grade inflammation and endothelial dysfunction with depression - the Maastricht study. Brain Behav Immun. 2016;56:390–6.

35. Keller C, Katz R, Cushman M, Fried LF, Shlipak M. Association of kidney function with inflammatory and procoagulant markers in a diverse cohort: a cross-sectional analysis from the multi-ethnic study of atherosclerosis (MESA). BMC Nephrol. 2008;9:9.

36. Carlsson AC, Nordquist L, Larsson TE, Carrero JJ, Larsson A, Lind L, Ärnlöv J. Soluble tumor necrosis factor receptor 1 is associated with glomerular filtration rate progression and incidence of chronic kidney disease in two community-based cohorts of elderly individuals. Cardiorenal Med. 2015;5:278–88.

37. Smith KJ, Au B, Ollis L, Schmitz N. The association between C-reactive protein, Interleukin-6 and depression among older adults in the community: a systematic review and meta-analysis. Exp Gerontol. 2018;102:109–32.

# Permissions

All chapters in this book were first published in GERIATRICS, by BioMed Central; hereby published with permission under the Creative Commons Attribution License or equivalent. Every chapter published in this book has been scrutinized by our experts. Their significance has been extensively debated. The topics covered herein carry significant findings which will fuel the growth of the discipline. They may even be implemented as practical applications or may be referred to as a beginning point for another development.

The contributors of this book come from diverse backgrounds, making this book a truly international effort. This book will bring forth new frontiers with its revolutionizing research information and detailed analysis of the nascent developments around the world.

We would like to thank all the contributing authors for lending their expertise to make the book truly unique. They have played a crucial role in the development of this book. Without their invaluable contributions this book wouldn't have been possible. They have made vital efforts to compile up to date information on the varied aspects of this subject to make this book a valuable addition to the collection of many professionals and students.

This book was conceptualized with the vision of imparting up-to-date information and advanced data in this field. To ensure the same, a matchless editorial board was set up. Every individual on the board went through rigorous rounds of assessment to prove their worth. After which they invested a large part of their time researching and compiling the most relevant data for our readers.

The editorial board has been involved in producing this book since its inception. They have spent rigorous hours researching and exploring the diverse topics which have resulted in the successful publishing of this book. They have passed on their knowledge of decades through this book. To expedite this challenging task, the publisher supported the team at every step. A small team of assistant editors was also appointed to further simplify the editing procedure and attain best results for the readers.

Apart from the editorial board, the designing team has also invested a significant amount of their time in understanding the subject and creating the most relevant covers. They scrutinized every image to scout for the most suitable representation of the subject and create an appropriate cover for the book.

The publishing team has been an ardent support to the editorial, designing and production team. Their endless efforts to recruit the best for this project, has resulted in the accomplishment of this book. They are a veteran in the field of academics and their pool of knowledge is as vast as their experience in printing. Their expertise and guidance has proved useful at every step. Their uncompromising quality standards have made this book an exceptional effort. Their encouragement from time to time has been an inspiration for everyone.

The publisher and the editorial board hope that this book will prove to be a valuable piece of knowledge for researchers, students, practitioners and scholars across the globe.

# List of Contributors

**Emma Säfström**
Sörmland County Council, Nyköping Hospital, Nyköping, Sweden
Department of Medical and Health Sciences, Division of Nursing Science, Linköping University, Linköping, Sweden
Centre for Clinical Research Sörmland, Uppsala University, Eskilstuna, Sweden

**Anna Strömberg**
Department of Medical and Health Sciences, Division of Nursing Science, Linköping University, Linköping, Sweden
Department of Cardiology, Linköping University, Linköping, Sweden

**Tiny Jaarsma**
Department of Social and Welfare Studies, Linköping University, Linköping, Sweden

**Radhika Nair, Mir Siadaty, Nick C. Patel, Leslie Ann Hazel Fernandez and Vishal Saundankar**
Comprehensive Health Insights, Louisville, USA

**Adam S. Fleisher, Michael M. Witte, AnnCatherine M. Downing and Daniel E. Ball**
Eli Lilly and Company, Indianapolis, USA

**Virginia S. Haynes**
Eli Lilly and Company, Indianapolis, USA
Lilly Corporate Center, Drop Code 1730, Indianapolis, IN 46285, USA

**Derek Van Amerongen**
Humana Inc., Louisville, USA

**Elizaveta Fife, Łukasz Kroc, Agnieszka Guligowska, Małgorzata Pigłowska, Bartłomiej Sołtysik and Tomasz Kostka**
Department of Geriatrics, Healthy Ageing Research Centre, Medical University of Lodz, ul. Pieniny 30, 91-647 Łódź, Poland

**Joanna Kostka**
Department of Geriatrics, Healthy Ageing Research Centre, Medical University of Lodz, ul. Pieniny 30, 91-647 Łódź, Poland
Department of Physical Medicine, Medical University of Lodz, Hallera 1, Łódź, Poland

**Agnieszka Kaufman-Szymczyk and Krystyna Fabianowska-Majewska**
Department of Biomedical Chemistry, Medical University of Lodz, Mazowiecka 6/8, Łódź, Poland

**Machelle Wilchesky**
Department of Family Medicine and Division of Geriatric Medicine, McGill University, 5858, Chemin de la Côte-des-Neiges, Montreal, Quebec H3S 1Z1, Canada
Donald Berman Maimonides Centre for Research in Aging, 5795 Caldwell Avenue, Montreal, Quebec H4W 1W3, Canada

**Gerhard Mueller**
Department of Nursing Science and Gerontology, UMIT-The Health and Life Sciences University, Eduard-Wallnoefer-Zentrum 1, A-6060 Hall in Tyrol, Tyrol, Austria

**Martine Marcotte, Michèle Aubin and Pierre-Hugues Carmichael**
Centre d'excellence sur le vieillissement de Québec, Centre integer universitaire de santé et de services sociaux de la Capitale-Nationale, 1050, Chemin Ste-Foy, room L2-30, Quebec City, Quebec G1S 4L8, Canada

**Michèle Morin, Philippe Voyer, Anik Giguère, Pierre Durand, René Verreault and Edeltraut Kröger**
Centre d'excellence sur le vieillissement de Québec, Centre integer universitaire de santé et de services sociaux de la Capitale-Nationale, 1050, Chemin Ste-Foy, room L2-30, Quebec City, Quebec G1S 4L8, Canada
Laval University, 1050, avenue de la Médecine, Quebec City, Quebec G1V 0A6, Canada

**Nathalie Champoux**
Faculté de médecine, Université de Montréal, 2900 Boulevard Edouard-Montpetit, Montreal, Quebec H3T 1J4, Canada

**Johanne Monette**
Division of Geriatric Medicine, McGill University, Jewish General Hospital, 3755 Côte-Ste-Catherine, Montreal, Quebec H3T 1E2, Canada

**Marcel Arcand**
Centre de recherche sur le vieillissement, affilié à l'Université de Sherbrooke, 1036, rue Belvédère Sud, Sherbrooke, Quebec J1H 4C4, Canada

**Colleen J. Maxwell**
Schools of Pharmacy and Public Health and Health Systems, University of Waterloo, 200 University Ave. W, Waterloo, ON N2L 3G1, Canada
Institute for Clinical Evaluative Sciences, 2075 Bayview Ave, Toronto, ON M4N 3M5, Canada

**Michael A. Campitelli, Christina Diong and Susan E. Bronskill**
Institute for Clinical Evaluative Sciences, 2075 Bayview Ave, Toronto, ON M4N 3M5, Canada

**Luke Mondor**
Institute for Clinical Evaluative Sciences, 2075 Bayview Ave, Toronto, ON M4N 3M5, Canada
Health System Performance Research Network, Toronto, ON, Canada

**David B. Hogan**
Division of Geriatric Medicine, Department of Medicine, University of Calgary, HSC-3330 Hospital Drive NW, Calgary, AB T2N 4N1, Canada

**Joseph E. Amuah**
School of Epidemiology, Public Health and Preventive Medicine, University of Ottawa, 451 Smyth Road, Ottawa, ON K1H 8M5, Canada

**Sarah Leslie**
School of Public Health and Health Systems, University of Waterloo, 200 University Ave. W, Waterloo, ON N2L 3G1, Canada

**Dallas Seitz**
Division of Geriatric Psychiatry, Queen's University and Providence Care Hospital, 752 King Street W, Kingston, ON K7L 4X3, Canada

**Sudeep Gill**
Department of Medicine, Queen's University and Providence Care Hospital, 752 King Street W, Kingston, ON K7L 4X3, Canada

**Kednapa Thavorn**
Ottawa Hospital Research Institute, 501 Smyth Road, Ottawa, ON K1H 8L6, Canada

**Walter P. Wodchis**
Institute of Health Policy Management and Evaluation, University of Toronto, 155 College Street, Toronto, ON M5T 3M6, Canada

**Andrea Gruneir**
Department of Family Medicine, University of Alberta, 8440 112 St. NW, Edmonton, AB T6G 2R7, Canada

**Gary Teare**
Department of Community Health and Epidemiology, College of Medicine, University of Saskatchewan, Health Science Building, 107 Wiggins Rd, Saskatoon, SK S7N 5E5, Canada

**Ryota Sakurai, Naoko Sakuma, Hiroyuki Suzuki, Masashi Yasunaga, Susumu Ogawa and Yoshinori Fujiwara**
Research Team for Social Participation and Community Health, Tokyo Metropolitan Institute of Gerontology, 35-2 Sakae-cho, Itabashi-ku, Tokyo 173-0015, Japan

**Kimi Estela Kobayashi-Cuya**
Research Team for Social Participation and Community Health, Tokyo Metropolitan Institute of Gerontology, 35-2 Sakae-cho, Itabashi-ku, Tokyo 173-0015, Japan
Department of Preventive Medicine and Public Health, School of Medicine, Keio University, 35 Shinanomachi, Shinjuku-ku, Tokyo 160-8582, Japan

**Toru Takebayashi**
Department of Preventive Medicine and Public Health, School of Medicine, Keio University, 35 Shinanomachi, Shinjuku-ku, Tokyo 160-8582, Japan

**Su-Hyun Lee and Won Hyuk Chang**
Department of Physical and Rehabilitation Medicine, Center for Prevention and Rehabilitation, Heart Vascular Stroke Institute, Samsung Medical Center, Sungkyunkwan University School of Medicine, Irwon-ro 81, Gangnam-gu, Seoul 06351, Republic of Korea

**Dong-Seok Kim, Hwang-Jae Lee and Yun-Hee Kim**
Department of Physical and Rehabilitation Medicine, Center for Prevention and Rehabilitation, Heart Vascular Stroke Institute, Samsung Medical Center, Sungkyunkwan University School of Medicine, Irwon-ro 81, Gangnam-gu, Seoul 06351, Republic of Korea
Department of Health Sciences and Technology, SAIHST, Sungkyunkwan University, Irwon-ro 81, Gangnam-gu, Seoul 06351, Republic of Korea

**Junwon Jang**
Samsung Advanced Institute of Technology, Samsung Electronics, 130 Samsung-ro, Yeongtong-gu, Suwon-si, Gyeonggi-do 16678, Republic of Korea

**Byung-Ok Choi**
Department of Neurology, Neuroscience Center, Samsung Medical Center, Sungkyunkwan University School of Medicine, Irwon-ro 81, Gangnam-gu, Seoul 06351, Republic of Korea

**Gyu-Ha Ryu**
Office of Biomechanical science, Research Center for Future Medicine, Samsung Medical Center, Sungkyunkwan University, Irwon-ro 81, Gangnam-gu, Seoul 06351, Republic of Korea

**S. Kipfer**
School of Health, University of Applied Sciences and Arts Western Switzerland, Fribourg, Switzerland

**S. Pihet**
School of Health, University of Applied Sciences and Arts Western Switzerland, Fribourg, Switzerland Haute Ecole de Santé Fribourg, Route des Cliniques 15, 1700 Fribourg, Switzerland

**Patrick Roigk, Clemens Becker and Kilian Rapp**
Department of Clinical Gerontology, Robert-Bosch-Hospital, Auerbachstrasse 110, 70376 Stuttgart, Germany

**Claudia Schulz and Hans-Helmut König**
Department of Health Economics and Health Services Research, University Medical Center Hamburg-Eppendorf, Hamburg, Germany

**Kjersti Grønning, Geir A. Espnes, Camilla Nguyen and Beate André**
Department of Public Health and Nursing, Center for Health Promotion Research, Norwegian University of Science and Technology (NTNU), Postbox 8905, 7491 Trondheim, Norway

**Ana Maria Ferreira Rodrigues, Maria Joao Gregorio, Rute Sousa and Helena Canhão**
CEDOC, EpiDoC Unit, NOVA Medical School, Universidade Nova de Lisboa, Lisbon, Portugal EpiSaude Association, Evora, Portugal

**N. Legdeur**
Alzheimer Center Amsterdam, Department of Neurology, Amsterdam Neuroscience, Vrije Universiteit Amsterdam, Amsterdam UMC, PO Box 7057, 1007, MB, Amsterdam, the Netherlands

**P. J. Visser**
Alzheimer Center Amsterdam, Department of Neurology, Amsterdam Neuroscience, Vrije Universiteit Amsterdam, Amsterdam UMC, 1007, MB, Amsterdam, the Netherlands Department of Psychiatry and Neuropsychology, School for Mental Health and Neuroscience, Maastricht University, Maastricht, the Netherlands

**M. W. Heymans**
Department of Epidemiology and Biostatistics, Amsterdam Public Health Research Institute, Vrije Universiteit Amsterdam, Amsterdam, the Netherlands

**M. Huisman**
Department of Epidemiology and Biostatistics, Amsterdam Public Health Research Institute, Vrije Universiteit Amsterdam, Amsterdam, the Netherlands Department of Sociology, Vrije Universiteit Amsterdam, Amsterdam, the Netherlands

**H. C. Comijs**
GGZ inGeest / Department of Psychiatry, Amsterdam Public Health Research Institute, Vrije Universiteit Amsterdam, Amsterdam, the Netherlands

**A. B. Maier**
Department of Medicine and Aged Care, @ AgeMelbourne, Royal Melbourne Hospital, University of Melbourne, Melbourne, Australia Department of Human Movement Sciences, @ AgeAmsterdam, Faculty of Behavioural and Movement Sciences, Vrije Universiteit Amsterdam, Amsterdam, the Netherlands

**Shirin Vellani, Lily Yeung and Martine Puts**
Lawrence S. Bloomberg Faculty of Nursing, University of Toronto, Toronto, ON, Canada

**Katherine S. McGilton**
Lawrence S. Bloomberg Faculty of Nursing, University of Toronto, Toronto, ON, Canada Toronto Rehabilitation Institute, University Health Network, 550 University Avenue, Toronto, ON M6K 2R7 416 597 3422 (2500), Canada

**Jawad Chishtie**
Toronto Rehabilitation Institute, University Health Network, 550 University Avenue, Toronto, ON M6K 2R7 416 597 3422 (2500), Canada

Rehabilitation Sciences Institute, University of Toronto, Toronto, ON, Canada

**Elana Commisso**
Institute of Health Policy, Management and Evaluation, University of Toronto, Toronto, ON, Canada

**Walter P. Wodchis**
Institute of Health Policy, Management and Evaluation, University of Toronto, Toronto, ON, Canada
Institute for Better Health, Trillium Health Partners, Mississauga, ON, Canada

**Jenny Ploeg**
School of Nursing, McMaster University, Hamilton, ON, Canada

**Melissa K. Andrew**
Division of Geriatric Medicine, Dalhousie University, Halifax, NS, Canada

**Ana Patricia Ayala and Mikaela Gray**
Gerstein Information Science Centre, University of Toronto, Toronto, ON, Canada

**Debra Morgan and Amanda Froehlich Chow**
Canadian Centre for Health and Safety in Agriculture, University of Saskatchewan, Saskatoon, SK, Canada

**Edna Parrott, Doug Stephens, Lori Hale and Margaret Keatings**
The Change Foundation, Toronto, ON, Canada

**Jennifer Walker**
Laurentian University, Sudbury, ON, Canada

**Veronique Dubé**
Faculty of Nursing, Université de Montréal, Montreal, Quebec, Canada

**Janet McElhaney**
Health Sciences North Research Institute and Northern Ontario School of Medicine, Sudbury, ON, Canada

**Shaoqing Ge**
Duke University School of Nursing, 307 Trent Drive, Durham, NC, USA

**Eleanor S. McConnell**
Duke University School of Nursing, 307 Trent Drive, Durham, NC, USA
Geriatric Research, Education and Clinical Center (GRECC) of the Department of Veterans Affairs Medical Center, Durham, NC, USA

**Zheng Zhu**
Fudan University School of Nursing, Shanghai, China
Fudan University Center for Evidence-Based Nursing, a Joanna Briggs Institute Center of Excellence, Shanghai, China

**Bei Wu**
New York University Rory Meyers College of Nursing, New York, NY, USA
Hartford Institute for Geriatric Nursing, New York University, New York, NY, USA

**Saruna Ghimire, Dipta Amatya and Prabisha Amatya**
Agrata Health and Education (AHEAD)-Nepal, Kathmandu, Nepal

**Binaya Kumar Baral, Buddhi Raj Pokhrel and Asmita Pokhrel**
Department of Biochemistry, Nepal Medical College and Teaching Hospital, Kathmandu, Nepal

**Anushree Acharya**
Department of Nutrition and Dietetics, College of Applied Food and Dairy Technology, Purbanchal University, Kathmandu, Nepal

**Shiva Raj Mishra**
Nepal Development Society, Bharatpur-10, Nepal

**Hallgeir Viken and Dorthe Stensvold**
K.G. Jebsen Center of Exercise in Medicine at Department of Circulation and Medical Imaging, Faculty of Medicine and Health Sciences, Norwegian University of Science and Technology, Trondheim, Norway

**Line Skarsem Reitlo**
K.G. Jebsen Center of Exercise in Medicine at Department of Circulation and Medical Imaging, Faculty of Medicine and Health Sciences, Norwegian University of Science and Technology, Trondheim, Norway

Department of Cardiology, St Olavs Hospital, Trondheim University Hospital, Trondheim, Norway

**Silvana Bucher Sandbakk**
K.G. Jebsen Center of Exercise in Medicine at Department of Circulation and Medical Imaging, Faculty of Medicine and Health Sciences, Norwegian University of Science and Technology, Trondheim, Norway
Norwegian National Advisory Unit on Exercise Training as Medicine for Cardiopulmonary Conditions, St. Olav's Hospital, Trondheim, Norway

**Ulrik Wisløff**
K.G. Jebsen Center of Exercise in Medicine at Department of Circulation and Medical Imaging, Faculty of Medicine and Health Sciences, Norwegian University of Science and Technology, Trondheim, Norway
School of Human Movement and Nutrition Sciences, University of Queensland, Brisbane, Australia

**Nils Petter Aspvik and Jan Erik Ingebrigtsen**
Department of Sociology and Political Science, Faculty of Social and Educational Sciences, Norwegian University of Science and Technology, Trondheim, Norway

**Xiangchun Tan**
Department of Neuroscience and Movement Science, Faculty of Medicine and Health Sciences, Norwegian University of Science and Technology, Trondheim, Norway

**Nina Karg, Elmar Graessel and Anna Pendergrass**
Department of Psychiatry and Psychotherapy, Center for Health Service Research in Medicine, Friedrich-Alexander-University Erlangen-Nuremberg, Schwabachanlage 6, D-91054 Erlangen, Germany

**Ottilie Randzio**
Medical Service of Compulsory Health Insurance Funds (MDK) of Bavaria, Haidenauplatz 1, D-81667 Munich, Germany

**James L Smith**
Charles R. Drew University of Medicine and Science, 1731 East 120th Street, Los Angeles, CA 90005, USA

**Mohsen Bazargan and Ebony O King**
Charles R. Drew University of Medicine and Science, 1731 East 120th Street, Los Angeles, CA 90005, USA

University of California, Los Angeles, USA

**Carla M. C. Nascimento, Marisa S. Zazzetta, Grace A. O. Gomes, Fabiana S. Orlandi, Karina Gramani-Say, Fernando A. Vasilceac, Aline C. M. Gratão, Sofia C. I. Pavarini and Marcia R. Cominetti**
Department of Gerontology, Federal University of São Carlos, Rod. Washington Luis, Km 235, Monjolinho, São Carlos, SP CEP 13565-905, Brazil

**Yoshiaki Tamura, Hideki Ito, Yuko Chiba and Atsushi Araki**
Department of Diabetes, Metabolism, and Endocrinology, Tokyo Metropolitan Geriatric Hospital, Tokyo, Japan

**Joji Ishikawa, Jun Tanaka, Masamitsu Sugie and Kazumasa Harada**
Department of Cardiology, Tokyo Metropolitan Geriatric Hospital, Tokyo, Japan

**Yoshinori Fujiwara, Ai Iizuka, Sho Kaito, Akihiko Kitamura, Satoshi Seino and Shoji Shinkai**
Research Team for Social Participation and Community Health, Tokyo Metropolitan Institute of Gerontology, Tokyo, Japan

**Masashi Tanaka**
Department of Clinical Laboratory, Tokyo Metropolitan Geriatric Hospital, Tokyo, Japan

**Nobuo Kanazawa**
Department of Surgery, Tokyo Metropolitan Geriatric Hospital, Tokyo, Japan

**Takashi Nishimura and Shunei Kyo**
Department of Cardiac Surgery, Tokyo Metropolitan Geriatric Hospital, Tokyo, Japan

**Akiko Kanemaru**
Department of Rehabilitation, Tokyo Metropolitan Geriatric Hospital, Tokyo, Japan

**Keigo Shimoji**
Department of Diagnostic Radiology, Tokyo Metropolitan Geriatric Hospital, Tokyo, Japan

**Hirohiko Hirano**
Department of Dentistry and Oral Surgery, Tokyo Metropolitan Geriatric Hospital, Tokyo, Japan

**Ko Furuta**
Department of Psychiatry, Tokyo Metropolitan Geriatric Hospital, Tokyo, Japan

**Taishi Tsuji**
Center for Preventive Medical Sciences, Chiba University, 1-8-1 Inohana, Chuo Ward, Chiba City, Chiba 260-8670, Japan

**Merja Rantakokko, Erja Portegijs, Anne Viljanen and Taina Rantanen**
Gerontology Research Center, Faculty of Sport and Health Sciences, University of Jyvaskyla, PO Box 35, FI-40014 Jyväskylä, Finland

**Rosanne Blanchet**
School of Nursing, University of Ottawa, 1 Stewart Street, Room 212, Ottawa, ON K1H 8M5, Canada

**Nancy Edwards**
School of Nursing, University of Ottawa, 1 Stewart Street, Room 205, Ottawa, ON K1H 8M5, Canada

**Gregory J. Norman, Amy J. Wade, Andrea M. Morris and Jill C. Slaboda**
West Health Institute, 10350 North Torrey Pines Road, La Jolla, CA 92037, USA

**Sigurd Evensen, Ingvild Saltvedt and Olav Sletvold**
Department of Geriatrics, St. Olavs hospital, Trondheim University Hospital, Trondheim, Norway
Department of Neuromedicine and Movement Science, Faculty of Medicine and Health Sciences, Norwegian University of Science and Technology (NTNU), N-7491 Trondheim, Norway

**Kristin Taraldsen**
Department of Neuromedicine and Movement Science, Faculty of Medicine and Health Sciences, Norwegian University of Science and Technology (NTNU), N-7491 Trondheim, Norway

**Stian Lydersen**
Regional Centre for Child and Youth Mental Health and Child Welfare, NTNU, Norwegian University of Science and Technology, Trondheim, Norway

**Torgeir Bruun Wyller**
Oslo Delirium Research Group, Department of Geriatric Medicine, Oslo University Hospital, Oslo, Norway
Institute of Clinical Medicine, University of Oslo, Oslo, Norway

**Ling Wu, Huaimei Xing and Haohao Li**
Cheeloo College of Medicine, Shandong University, Jinan, Shandong, China
Department of Neurology, Jining No. 1 People's Hospital, Jiankang Road 6, Jining 272111, Shandong, China

**Zhongrui Yan**
Department of Neurology, Jining No. 1 People's Hospital, Jiankang Road 6, Jining 272111, Shandong, China

**Hui Jiang**
Xing Long Zhuang Hospital, Shandong Yankuang Group, Jining, Shandong, China

**Chengxuan Qiu**
Department of Neurology, Shandong Provincial Hospital, Jinan, Shandong, China
Aging Research Center, Department of Neurobiology, Care Sciences and Society, Karolinska Institutet-Stockholm University, Widerströmska Huset, Tomtebodavägen 18A, 171 65 Solna, Sweden

# Index

www.ingramcontent.com/pod-product-compliance
Lightning Source LLC
Chambersburg PA
CBHW061315190326
41458CB00011B/3811